Medical Management of HIV/AIDS

Medical Management of HIV/AIDS

Edited by Seth Phelps

hayle medical

New York

Hayle Medical,
750 Third Avenue, 9th Floor,
New York, NY 10017, USA

Visit us on the World Wide Web at:
www.haylemedical.com

ISBN: 978-1-63241-887-6

Cataloging-in-Publication Data

Medical management of HIV/AIDS / edited by Seth Phelps.
p. cm.
Includes bibliographical references and index.
ISBN 978-1-63241-887-6
1. HIV infections. 2. AIDS (Disease). 3. HIV infections--Prevention. 4. AIDS (Disease)--Prevention.
5. HIV infections--Treatment. 6. AIDS (Disease)--Treatment. I. Phelps, Seth.
RC606.6 .M43 2020
616.979 2--dc23

Table of Contents

Preface

The human immunodeficiency virus (HIV) causes HIV infection, which later develops into acquired immunodeficiency syndrome (AIDS). This condition leads to a progressive failure of the immune system which allows certain life-threatening, opportunistic infections and cancers to affect the body. HIV infection may be transmitted sexually such as by contact with vaginal fluids, semen or pre-ejaculate. It may also be transferred from an infected mother to child during pregnancy and childbirth, through breast milk, contaminated blood transfer, etc. HIV infects the helper T cells, macrophages and dendritic cells of the human immune system. Such infection results in low levels of $CD4^+$ T cells through various mechanisms. When these cells decline below a critical level, cell-mediated immunity is lost and the body becomes susceptible to opportunistic infections. There is no effective vaccine or cure for HIV/AIDS. Treatment strategies attempt to slow the progression of the disease with highly active antiretroviral therapy and manage the occurrence of opportunistic infections. A healthy diet is generally promoted for the management of AIDS. This book is a valuable compilation of topics, ranging from the basic to the most complex advancements in the understanding of HIV/AIDS. From theories to research to practical applications, case studies related to all contemporary topics of relevance to this infection have been included herein. It is appropriate for students seeking detailed information in this area as well as for experts.

The researches compiled throughout the book are authentic and of high quality, combining several disciplines and from very diverse regions from around the world. Drawing on the contributions of many researchers from diverse countries, the book's objective is to provide the readers with the latest achievements in the area of research. This book will surely be a source of knowledge to all interested and researching the field.

In the end, I would like to express my deep sense of gratitude to all the authors for meeting the set deadlines in completing and submitting their research chapters. I would also like to thank the publisher for the support offered to us throughout the course of the book. Finally, I extend my sincere thanks to my family for being a constant source of inspiration and encouragement.

Editor

Sexual behavior of HIV-positive adults not accessing HIV treatment in Mombasa, Kenya: Defining their prevention needs

Avina Sarna[1*], Stanley Luchters[2], Melissa Pickett[3], Matthew Chersich[2,4], Jerry Okal[5], Scott Geibel[5], Nzioki Kingola[6] and Marleen Temmerman[2]

Abstract

Background: HIV spread continues at high rates from infected persons to their sexual partners. In 2009, an estimated 2.6 million new infections occurred globally. People living with HIV (PLHIV) receiving treatment are in contact with health workers and therefore exposed to prevention messages. By contrast, PLHIV not receiving ART often fall outside the ambit of prevention programs. There is little information on their sexual risk behaviors. This study in Mombasa Kenya therefore explored sexual behaviors of PLHIV not receiving any HIV treatment.

Results: Using modified targeted snowball sampling, 698 PLHIV were recruited through community health workers and HIV-positive peer counsellors. Of the 59.2% sexually-active PLHIV, 24.5% reported multiple sexual partners. Of all sexual partners, 10.2% were HIV negative, while 74.5% were of unknown HIV status. Overall, unprotected sex occurred in 52% of sexual partnerships; notably with 32% of HIV-negative partners and 54% of partners of unknown HIV status in the last 6 months. Multivariate analysis, controlling for intra-client clustering, showed non-disclosure of HIV status (AOR: 2.38, 95%CI: 1.47-3.84, $p < 0.001$); experiencing moderate levels of perceived stigma (AOR: 2.94, 95%CI: 1.50-5.75, $p = 0.002$); and believing condoms reduce sexual pleasure (AOR: 2.81, 95%CI: 1.60-4.91, $p < 0.001$) were independently associated with unsafe sex. Unsafe sex was also higher in those using contraceptive methods other than condoms (AOR: 5.47, 95%CI: 2.57-11.65, $p < 0.001$); or no method (AOR: 3.99, 95%CI: 2.06-7.75, $p < 0.001$), compared to condom users.

Conclusions: High-risk sexual behaviors are common among PLHIV not accessing treatment services, raising the risk of HIV transmission to discordant partners. This population can be identified and reached in the community. Prevention programs need to urgently bring this population into the ambit of prevention and care services. Moreover, beginning HIV treatment earlier might assist in bringing this group into contact with providers and HIV prevention services, and in reducing risk behaviors.

Keywords: PLHIV, Prevention of sexual transmission of HIV, Sexual behavior, Unsafe sex, Africa

Background

HIV transmission remains a significant global concern; in 2009 there were an estimated 2.6 million new infections globally [1]. At the end of 2009, about 36% of the 15 million people in need of antiretroviral treatment (ART) in low- and middle income countries were receiving ART [1].

People living with HIV (PLHIV) who receive ART are in regular contact with health workers and presumably exposed to prevention messages and commodities. Indeed, several studies have documented a reduction in sexual risk behaviors among PLHIV after initiating ART [2-6]. At the same time, studies have shown that PLHIV accessing HIV care services, but not receiving ART, have higher sexual risk behaviors and unprotected sex than those taking ART, even though both groups have contact with health workers and exposure to prevention messages [7-10]. A major gap, however, is evidence

* Correspondence: asarna@popcouncil.org
[1]Population Council, 142 Golf Links, New Delhi 110048, India
Full list of author information is available at the end of the article

about the patterns of sexual behavior among PLHIV in the community who are not receiving ART and are either accessing HIV care services infrequently or not at all. Although newly diagnosed HIV-positive persons are advised to visit treatment centres for routine follow-up, many PLHIV choose not to. HIV related stigma, denial and disclosure concerns constitute important barriers to accessing care [11,12]. The only contact with health services for these people might well be post-test counselling at the time of testing HIV-positive. At the same time, PLHIV are also exposed to HIV prevention messages through mass media and community awareness programs that presumably also influence their knowledge and behaviors.

Studies of the determinants of unprotected sex in HIV-infected people suggest that a range of factors can operate individually or interact to influence sexual behavior [13]. Intention and self-efficacy regarding safe sex; [14,15] myths around condom use; dilemmas around disclosure of HIV status to partner(s) and fears of subsequent rejection; [14,16-20] and motivation to protect partners as well as themselves against re-infection with a new HIV strain or another sexually transmitted infection play an important role in effecting safe sex [13,20]. Partner attitudes and willingness to use condoms, complicated by partner status and willingness to be tested for HIV add further dimensions to safe sex practices [4,18,19,21]. Furthermore, a desire for children may lead to PLHIV ignoring the risks of unprotected sex [19,22,23].

In Kenya, in 2009, an estimated 1.3 to 1.6 million persons were living with HIV and an estimated 40% of PLHIV with advanced disease who are eligible for treatment were not receiving ART [1,24]. At the same time a large number of PLHIV do not yet require ART. Many of these PLHIV are likely to be outside the ambit of regular health care and prevention services. An estimated 100,000 new HIV infections occurred in 2009 in Kenya, highlighting the need for prevention efforts to focus on sexual risk behaviors of PLHIV, including those not accessing HIV care services. In this paper we examine the sexual risk behaviors of PLHIV in the community who were not receiving ART or co-trimoxazole prophylaxis.

Methods

Study participants were recruited for a cross-sectional survey, using modified targeted snowball sampling that uses outreach workers to recruit participants from identified geographic areas and populations of interest [25,26]. In classical snowball sampling a small number of individuals (typically between 4-6 persons initially) from a particular group of interest are identified, who then serve as 'seeds' to identify and recruit peers, that is, individuals who engage in the same type of risk behaviors, to be included into the study sample [27]. These, initial 'seeds' are often selected by program or study staff via convenience sampling. 'Seeds' can recruit an unlimited number of peers from their network till the desired sample size is achieved or sample saturation takes place. A drawback of this method is that the sample obtained is influenced by characteristics of the initial seeds, the size of their personal network and their ability to reach more cooperative subjects, with a possibility of sampling bias [27]. By contrast, modified targeted sampling, aims to overcome some of the limitations of snowball sampling by including an initial ethnographic assessment aimed at identifying the various networks or subgroups that might exist in a given setting [25]. Participants are then recruited through the active efforts of street outreach workers, using snow-ball sampling. CHWs and PTC counsellors are familiar with the community they serve, the socio-demographic profile of the community and clients, and can help reach PLHIV; we used this cadre of health workers to recruit our study sample. Health workers identified PLHIV in their community and asked these PLHIV to bring in others they knew. As our previous study showed us that PLHIV in Mombasa are relatively isolated due to stigma and disclosure concerns [28], health workers were permitted to add new 'seeds' if PLHIV were unable to bring in peers.

Participants were recruited by community health workers (CHWs) and HIV-positive peer counselors (PCs) from post-test clubs. To reduce biases related to the recruiter and the initial sample, especially over representation of more cooperative subjects and respondents with larger networks, the number of clients each health worker could bring into the study was restricted. Four CHWs from each of Mombasa's four districts (n = 16) were each asked to recruit 20 PLHIV; and five PCs from each of eight post-test centers (n = 40) across the four districts were each tasked with recruiting 12 PLHIV. HIV-positive adults who were 18 years or older, not currently taking ART or co-trimoxazole prophylaxis were eligible to participate.

Recruitment followed a detailed protocol on approaching PLHIV, maintaining confidentiality and verifying the participant's HIV-positive status by checking the referral card issued by a VCT center, or HIV clinic registration card or HIV/CD4 cell test results. Each participant received Ksh 200 (1USD = +/-75Ksh) as compensation for their time and transport. CHWs and PCs received Ksh 100 per participant recruited to cover their transport costs. Ethical approval was obtained from the Kenyatta National Hospital's Ethics Committee and Institutional Review Board of the Population Council. Written informed consent was obtained from all participants. After data collection was completed, project staff worked with CHWs and PTC counsellors to counsel each of the clients they had recruited to return to the HIV clinic for further follow up, care and ART.

Data were collected using structured questionnaires administered in Swahili by trained research assistants. Demographic variables were categorized and time since HIV diagnosis was classified as less than 12 months, 12-24 months and > 24 months. Contraception was categorized as: male/female condoms for contraception, other family planning (FP) methods (intra-uterine device, hormonal methods, permanent methods, diaphragm, foam/jelly, or rhythm) and no contraception. Disclosure of HIV status to a sexual partner was recorded as a binary yes/no variable. Perceived stigma was assessed using an adapted Berger's Stigma Scale (Cronbach's alpha of adapted scale: 0.81) and was categorized as minimal or low (16- 40), moderate (41-52) or high stigma (53-64) [29,30]. The recall reference period for sexual behavior was the previous 6 months, with data collected on: having had sexual intercourse, number of sexual partners, type of partners, partner's HIV status and disclosure of own status to partners. A regular partner was defined as a spouse or cohabiting partner, or a long-term friend with whom the respondent has sex frequently. A partner with whom the respondent was not living and had sex once or rarely was classified as a casual partner. Commercial or transactional partners were those where money or gifts were exchanged for sex.

To assess transmission concerns, participants were asked a binary question: "Are you worried about transmitting HIV to this partner?" Attitudes to condom use were assessed with six statements: "I am tired of always having to make sure that I use a condom every time I have sex","using condom reduces physical pleasure from sex","if a cure were discovered I would stop using condom", "using a condom takes away the romance from sex", "condoms are effective in preventing HIV and STDs" and "condom should only be used to prevent pregnancy and not HIV"- responses were scored on a 4-point Likert scale, ranging from strongly agree, agree, disagree, to strongly disagree. Respondents were also given the option of saying don't know. These statements were adapted from other studies [13,31,32] and pretested, validated and used in a previous study with PLHIV in Mombasa [2,19]. STI events were self-reported episodes of genital discharge or genital ulcer in the last 6 months (laboratory confirmation was unavailable). Participants were asked about the number of biological children they had. Fertility intentions were assessed by asking participants about the intention to have children in the future. Unprotected sex (UPS) was defined as inconsistent condom use with any partner in the past 6 months. Unsafe sex (US), a subset of UPS and the primary outcome for multivariate analysis to determine predictors, was defined as inconsistent condom use with HIV-negative or unknown status partners in the last 6 months. UPS at last sex and US at last sex were also reported.

Data management and statistical analysis

Data were entered into handheld computers (Dell Axim × 51) and then uploaded into Microsoft Access 2003 using Perseus 7.0.044 software. The data were analyzed on two levels (respondent-level and partner-level) using Intercooled Stata 8.0 (Stata Corporation, College Station, Texas, USA).

Respondent-level analysis compared demographic and behavioral characteristics of male and female participants. Unpaired Student's *t* test and the Mann-Whitney U test compared continuous variables with normal or non-normal distributions respectively, and a chi-square test identified differences between categorical variables. Unadjusted Mantel Hanzel odds ratios were reported.

Analysis at the level of sexual partner included data for up to 6 partners for each respondent in the last 6 months. Univariate logistic regression analyses were performed to identify associations between variables of interest and US at 6 months and last sex. Variables significant, at alpha level of 0.05, on univariate regression were included in the multivariate model [33]. Although sex of the respondent was not associated with unsafe sex in univariate analysis, it was forced into the model as socio-demographic characteristics varied markedly between women and men (Table 1). Also, a priori, disclosure of HIV status and type of partner were included in initial models, based on previous evidence of association with unprotected sex [7,34-37]. As a participant's sexual behavior with one partner may not be independent from her or his behavior with other partners, we controlled for multiple observations on sexual partners reported by the same study participant (intra-client clustering). Multiple partners of the same participant were also included as separate units of analysis. We adjusted the standard errors for clustering on the participant's ID in both univariate and multivariate logistic regression analyses. A main effects model was used to fit the multivariate model [38]. Separate multivariate models were developed for US at 6 months and at last sex.

Results

Between May and August 2007, 748 PLHIV were identified by CHWs and PCs; 28 persons were found ineligible (receiving treatment) and 720 PLHIV were interviewed. Data from 22 participants were lost due to technical failures with the hand-held computers, leaving data on 698 participants for analysis.

Table 1 Participant characteristics: HIV-positive adults not receiving ART, Mombasa, 2007

Variable	Total (n = 698)	Males (n = 164)	Females (n = 534)	P[a]
Age: median (IQR)	33.5 (28-39)	34.5 (29-42)	33 (28-38)	0.02[b]
Highest education level:% (n)				
No education	7.3 (51)	3.7 (6)	8.4 (45)	0.04
Primary	59.2 (413)	54.9 (90)	60.5 (323)	
Secondary	31.1 (217)	38.4 (63)	28.8 (154)	
University	2.4 (17)	3.1 (5)	2.3 (12)	
Marital status:% (n)				
Married or cohabiting	34.4 (240)	40.9 (67)	32.4 (173)	< 0.001
Never married	21.1 (147)	32.9 (54)	17.4 (93)	
Divorced or separated	20.4 (143)	15.8 (26)	21.9 (117)	
Widowed	24.1 (168)	10.3 (17)	28.2 (151)	
Employment status:% (n)				
Employed	75.9 (530)	82.9 (136)	73.8 (394)	0.02
Type of HIV testing facility used:% (n)				
Government health facility	80.7 (563)	77.4 (127)	81.7 (436)	< 0.001
Private medical centre	15.3 (107)	12.2 (20)	16.3 (87)	
Other	4.0 (28)	10.4 (17)	2.1 (11)	
Time since diagnosis:% (n)[c]				
0-11 months	43.1 (301)	50.0 (82)	41.0 (219)	< 0.001
12-23 months	19.5 (136)	22.6 (37)	18.5 (99)	
24+ months	33.4 (233)	23.2 (38)	36.5 (195)	
Attends HIV clinic:% (n)				
Yes	23.4 (163)	16.5 (27)	25.5 (136)	0.02
No	76.7 (535)	83.5 (137)	74.5 (398)	
Perceived level of stigma:% (n)				
Low	16.2 (113)	18.9 (31)	15.4 (82)	0.5
Moderate	68.8 (480)	67.7 (111)	69.1 (369)	
High	15.0 (105)	13.4 (22)	15.5 (83)	
Drink alcohol weekly:% (n)				
Yes	26.9 (188)	34.2 (56)	24.7 (132)	0.02
Has ever used drugs:% (n)				
Yes	31.5 (220)	68.5 (104)	21.7 (116)	< 0.001
Have biological children:% (n)				
Yes	81.7 (570)	65.9 (108)	86.5 (462)	< 0.001
Want to have children:% (n)				
No	74.8 (522)	61.6 (101)	78.8 (421)	< 0.001
Using family planning method:% (n)[d]				
No	54.8 (280)	45.5 (49)	56.2 (237)	0.072
Reported correct knowledge:%(n)				
HIV cannot spread through mosquitoes	72.8 (508)	72.6 (119)	72.8 (389)	0.93
HIV cannot spread through shared utensils	84.7 (591)	83.5 (137)	85.0 (454)	0.62
HIV can be transmitted from a mother to child	91.5 (639)	90.2 (148)	91.9 (491)	0.70
Treatment can reduce mother-to-child transmission	61.1 (425)	55.5 (91)	62.8 (334)	0.20
HIV+ person can be re-infected with a new virus	68.6 (479)	64.6 (106)	69.9 (373)	0.45

[a] X^2 test unless indicated

[b] Mann-Whitney *U* test

[c] n = 671; 28 respondents did not provide information on the time since diagnosis

[d] of those not wanting children/more children

ART: antiretroviral therapy; IQR: interquartile range

Median age of participants was 33.5 years (IQR = 28-33). Twenty-three percent (163/698) of participants reported visiting HIV clinics (34.4% visited monthly, 16.6% every two to six months, 20.2% when sick and 28.8% off and on). Differences were observed in socio-demographic characteristics between female and male respondents [Table 1]. Women were more likely than men to be widowed (OR 3.40; 95%CI: 1.98-5.88; $p < 0.001$); to attend HIV clinic (OR 1.73; 95%CI: 1.10-2.74; $p = 0.017$) and be unemployed (OR 1.73; 95%CI: 1.10-2.71; $p = 0.018$). Women were also less likely to drink alcohol each week (OR: 0.63; 95%CI: 0.43-0.93; $p = 0.017$) or to report ever using drugs (OR: 0.16; 95%CI: 0.11-0.24; $p < 0.001$). Women knew their HIV-status for longer periods than men. Participants recruited by CHWs and by PCs had a similar age, sex, education and employment status (data not shown).

Participants were asked about their reasons for not taking ART; multiple responses were permitted. About a quarter (27.9%; n = 195) reported high CD4 cell counts that made them ineligible for ART; 16.8% (n = 117) did not want to start ART; 11.2% (n = 78) reported they were afraid of side-effects; 7.7% (n = 54) did not know where to access treatment; 2.9% (n = 20) complained that treatment was expensive; 2.4% (n = 17) were taking herbal remedies and 2.1% (n = 15) had unfavourable beliefs about ART, such as, 'ARVs can make you mad', 'ARVs kill you faster', 'ARV are brought by donors when they stop it will be the end of your life', and ARVs make you sicker'.

Sexual activity

In the 6 months preceding the survey, 59.2% percent of participants were sexually active; similar in females and males [Table 2].

Males were more likely than female participants to report multiple partners (OR: 3.67; 95%CI 2.18-6.18; $p < 0.001$) in the last 6 months. Sexually-active male respondents (90/164) reported a total of 179 sexual partners and female respondents (320/534) reported a total of 437 sexual partners over the reference period [Table 2].

While the majority of male (84.4%) and female participants (98.8%) reported heterosexual partners, 15.5% of males (14/90) and 1.2% of females (n = 4/320) reported same sex partners in the last 6 months [Table 2]. Over a quarter of men's sexual partners were males (26.8%; 48/179).

Twenty percent of male participants reported a mix of sexual partners (regular/casual/transactional) compared to 9.7% of female participants (OR: 2.33; 95%CI: 1.23-4.43; $p < 0.01$). [Table 2] Female participants reported more regular partners than male participants (72.1% vs. 50.8%; OR: 2.50; 95%CI: 1.73-3.61; $p < 0.001$) while male participants had more casual (23.5% vs. 19.7%; OR: 1.25; 95%CI: 0.82-1.90; $p = 0.29$) and transactional partners (25.7% vs. 8.2%; OR: 3.85; 95%CI: 2.35-6.30; p = < 0.001) than women ($p < 0.001$) [Table 2].

Three-quarter of all partners were of unknown HIV status, similar for men and women. Female respondents reported higher disclosure rates to partners than male respondents (39.8% vs. 30.2%.; OR: 1.53; 95%CI: 1.09-2.47; $p = 0.02$) [Table 2].

Prevalence of unprotected sex

UPS-6 months (inconsistent condom use with any partner in the last 6 months) was reported in over half (51.9%) the sexual partnerships, more by women than men (55.2% vs. 44.1%; OR: 1.56; 95%CI: 1.09-2.21; $p = 0.01$) [Table 3]. Males were more likely to report UPS-6 months with their female partners than their male partners (52% vs. 22.9%; OR: 3.63; 95%CI: 1.66-7.95; $p = 0.001$). Both sexes were more likely to have UPS-6 months with regular partners compared to casual or transactional partners ($p < 0.001$). Inconsistent condom use in the last 6 months (US-6 months) was reported with 31% of HIV-negative partners (females 30.4% vs. males 35.3%; OR: 0.80; 95%CI: 0.25-2.63; $p = 0.72$) and with 53.8% of the partners of unknown HIV status (females 57.3% vs. males 45.0%; OR: 1.64; 95%CI: 1.07-2.47; $p = 0.02$). Patterns of UPS at last sex were similar to those of UPS-6 months (data not shown).

Predictors of unsafe sex (inconsistent condom use with HIV negative or unknown status partners)

Risk factors associated with US-6 months were explored (Table 4). In univariate analysis, university level education, more than 12 months since HIV diagnosis, non-disclosure of HIV-status, moderate and high levels of internalized stigma, condom-use fatigue, attending a HIV clinic, knowing that re-infection with a new viral strain is possible, believing that condoms reduce pleasure and using non-condom contraceptive methods were associated with higher risk of US-6 months and were included in the initial model.

In multivariate analysis, after controlling for multiple observations relating to different sexual partners reported by the same study participant, non-disclosure of HIV status to a partner (AOR 2.38, 95%CI: 1.47-3.84; $p < 0.001$), experiencing moderate levels of perceived stigma (AOR 2.94, 95%CI: 1.50-5.75; $p = 0.002$), believing condoms reduce sexual pleasure (AOR 2.81, 95%CI: 1.60-4.91; $p < 0.001$) or being unsure about condoms reducing pleasure (AOR 8.33, 95%CI: 2.38-29.09; $p = 0.001$), using a non-condom contraceptive method (AOR 5.47, 95%CI: 2.57-11.65; $p < 0.001$) or not using any contraception (AOR 3.99, 95%CI: 2.06-7.75; $p < 0.001$) were independently associated with US-6 months. Sex of the respondent, though not significantly

Table 2 Sexual behavior among HIV-positive adults not receiving ART in Mombasa, Kenya 2007

	All Respondents			
	Total (n = 698)	**Males (n = 164)**	**Females (n = 534)**	**P Value[a]**
Lifetime no. of partners: median (IQR)[b]	5 (3,10)	14 (6,25)	4 (3,8)	< 0.001
Sexually active in past 6 months:% (n)	59.2 (413)	55.5 (91)	60.3 (322)	0.27
	Sexually Active Respondents			
	Total (n = 410)[c]	**Male (n = 90)**	**Female n = 320)**	
No. of partners in past 6 months:% (n)[d]				
One partner	75.5 (308)	54.4 (49)	81.5 (259)	
More than one partner	24.5 (100)	45.6 (41)	18.6 (59)	< 0.001
Sex of partner:% (n)				
Only male	79.8 (327)	12.2 (11)	98.8 (316)	
Only female	18.8 (77)	84.4 (76)	0.3 (1)	
Both male & female	1.5 (6)	3.3 (3)	0.9 (3)	< 0.001[e]
Type of partner:% (n)				
Only regular	76.3 (313)	62.2 (56)	80.3 (257)	
Only casual	8.5 (35)	11.1 (10)	7.8 (25)	
Only sex worker	3.2 (13)	6.7 (6)	2.2 (7)	
Multiple types	12.0 (49)	20.0 (18)	9.7 (31)	0.002
	Sexually Active Respondents (partner level analysis: n = 616)			
	Total number of partners reported by 410 sexually active participants	**Number of partners 90 sexually active men reported**	**Number of partners 320 sexually active women reported**	**P Value[a]**
Partners of respondents	n = 616	n = 179	n = 437	
Sex of partner:% (n)				
Male	78.1 (481)	26.8 (48)	99.1 (433)	
Female	21.9 (135)	73.2 (131)	0.9 (4)	< 0.001[e]
Type of partner:%(n)				
Regular	65.9 (406)	50.8 (91)	72.1 (315)	
Casual	20.8 (128)	23.5 (42)	19.7 (86)	
Sex worker	13.3 (82)	25.7 (46)	8.2 (36)	< 0.001
Partner HIV status:% (n)				
Positive	15.3 (94)	17.3 (31)	14.4 (63)	
Negative	10.2 (63)	9.5 (17)	10.5 (46)	
Unknown	74.5 (459)	73.2 (131)	75.1 (328)	0.64
Disclosure:% (n)				
Partner knows	37.0 (228)	30.2 (54)	39.8 (174)	
Partner does not know	63.0 (388)	69.8 (125)	60.2 (263)	0.02

[a] X^2 test unless indicated

[b] n = 684; 14 respondents were excluded if they did not know, did not respond, or reported ≥ 800 partners

[c] n = 410; 3 sexually active respondents did not answer further questions about their sexual partners

[d] n = 408; 2 respondents did not respond

[e] Fisher's exact test

ART, antiretroviral therapy; IQR, interquartile range

Table 3 Prevalence of Unprotected Sex in the past 6 months among sexually-active participants (partner level analysis)

	Total number of partners reported by 410 sexually active respondents n = 616	UPS-6 months Number of partners by 90 sexually active male respondents n = 179	Number of partners reported by 320 sexually active female respondents n = 437
Total Unprotected Sex:% (n)	51.9 (320/616)	44.1 (79/179)	55.2 (241/437)
By sex of partner:% (n)			
Male	52.4 (252/481)	22.9 (11/48)	55.7 (241/433)
Female	50.4 (68/135)	52.0 (68/131)	0 (0/4)
		p = 0.001	p = 0.04[b]
By type of partner:% (n)			
Regular	61.1 (248/406)	59.3 (54/91)	61.6 (194/315)
Casual	34.4 (44/128)	26.2 (11/42)	38.4 (33/86)
Sex worker	34.2 (28/82)	30.4 (14/46)	38.9 (14/36)
	p < 0.001	p < 0.001	p < 0.001
By partner status:% (n)			
Positive	56.4 (53/94)	45.2 (14/31)	61.9 (39/63)
Negative	31.8 (20/63)	35.3 (6/17)	30.4 (14/45)
Unknown	53.8 (247/459)	45.0 (59/131)	57.3 (188/328)
	p = 0.003	p = 0.74	p < 0.001
By disclosure:% (n)			
Partner knows	53.1 (121/228)	38.9 (21/54)	57.5 (100/174)
Partner does not	51.3 (199/388)	46.4 (58/125)	53.6 (141/263)
know	p = 0.67	p = 0.35	p = 0.43

[a] X^2 test unless indicated

[b] Fisher's exact test

ART, antiretroviral therapy

associated with US-6 months in univariate analysis, was associated with US-6 months on multivariate analysis: female respondents were two times more likely to report US-6 months (AOR 2.10; 95%CI: 1.13-3.90; p = 0.018) compared to male respondents. University education and time since HIV diagnosis were not associated with US-6 months. Predictors for US-last sex were similar to those for US-6 months. (Data not shown)

Sexually transmitted infections

Overall, 44% of participants reported ever having a STI other than HIV. Males were twice as likely to ever report a STI compared to females (55.9% vs. 41.0%; OR: 1.82, 95%CI: 1.27-2.61; p < 0.001). Of those who ever had a STI, half (49.5%) had a STI in the last 6 months. A higher proportion of female participants reported genital discharge (42.9% vs. 19.7%, OR: 3.06; 95%CI: 1.68-5.55; p < 0.001) and ulcers (38.2% vs. 25.5%; OR: 1.80; 95%CI: 1.04-3.11; p = 0.046) in the last six months than men. Of note, 46.5% of participants reporting a STI informed their regular partners of their infection, but only 13.9% of those with multiple partners informed other partners.

Other sexual practices

Twenty nine percent of sexually active respondents reported sexual intercourse with a partner during menstruation (24/90 males and 94/318 females). Of those, 78% (18/24 males and 74/94 females) inconsistently or never used condoms for sex during menstrual periods. Eighteen percent of sexually active respondents (23/90 males and 50/318 females) reported ever having anal sex. Of those, 80.8% (14/23 males and 45/50 females) inconsistently or never used condoms during anal sex. (Data not shown)

Discussion

This study, conducted in Mombasa among PLHIV not accessing HIV treatment, shows the population has high levels of unsafe sex. Almost sixty percent of the participants were sexually-active during the last 6 months. This is significantly higher than that reported in our previous study in Mombasa among PLHIV receiving ART (44%) and PLHIV receiving co-trimoxazole prophylaxis without ART (47%) [7], and in other studies among PLHIV accessing care services in Cote d' Ivoire (47%), Uganda (48%) and Cameroon (47%) [8,10,39].

Table 4 Factors associated with Unsafe Sex in the past 6 months among sexually-active participants, adjusted for intra-client clustering

	US-6 months				
Variable	Prevalence % (n)	Crude Odds (95% CI)	P value	Adjusted Odds (95% CI)	P value
Sex of respondent					
Male (n = 179)	36.3 (65)	1.0	—	—	—
Female (n = 437)	46.2 (202)	1.51 (0.88-2.59)	0.14	2.10 (1.13-3.90)	0.018
Age					
18-24 years (n = 106)	42.5 (45)	0.85 (0.44-1.65)	0.64		
25-34 years (n = 291)	46.4 (135)	1.0	—		
35-44 years (184)	39.7 (73)	0.76 (0.46-1.26)	0.29		
45+ (n = 35)	40.0 (14)	0.77 (0.31-1.94)	0.58		
Marital status					
Married or cohabiting (n = 232)	44.8 (104)	1.0	—		
Never married (n = 184)	41.3 (76)	0.87 (0.49-1.51)	0.61		
Divorced, separated, or widowed (n = 200)	43.5 (87)	0.95 (0.59-1.53)	0.83		
Highest education level					
No education (n = 42)	52.4 (22)	1.32 (0.53-3.26)	0.55	0.53 (0.20-1.37)	0.19
Primary (n = 378)	45.5 (172)	1.0	—	—	—
Secondary (n = 179)	39.1 (70)	0.77 (0.47-1.26)	0.30	1.21 (0.63-2.32)	0.56
University (n = 17)	17.7 (3)	0.26 (0.07-0.98)	0.05	0.82 (0.22-3.03)	0.77
Sex of partner					
Male (n = 481)	44.3 (213)	1.0	—		
Female (n = 135)	40.0 (54)	0.84 (0.49-1.42)	0.52		
Type of partner					
Regular (n = 406)	48.3 (196)	1.80 (0.88-3.68)	0.11		
Casual (n = 128)	33.6 (43)	0.98 (0.41-2.32)	0.96		
Sex worker (n = 82)	34.2 (28)	1.0	—		
Attends HIV clinic					
Yes (n = 122)	25.6 (36)	0.47 (0.29-0.78)	0.003	0.60 (0.34-1.06)	0.08
No (n = 494)	46.8 (231)	1.0	—	1.0	—
Time since diagnosis					
< 12 months (n = 265)	52.8 (140)	1.0	—	—	—
12-24 months (n = 131)	37.4 (49)	0.53 (0.30-0.94)	0.03	0.61 (0.33-1.31)	0.12
2 months (n = 197)	35.0 (69)	0.48 (0.28-0.82)	0.01	0.74 (0.42-1.30)	0.31
Knowledge: re-infection with new strain					
Yes (n = 426)	36.8 (157)	1.0		1.0	
No/Does not know (n = 190)	57.9 (110)	2.35 (1.43-3.86)	0.001	1.27 (0.71-2.27)	0.41
Disclosure to partner					
Yes (n = 228)	31.1 (71)	1.0	—	—	—
No (n = 388)	50.5 (196)	2.26 (1.52-3.35)	< 0.001	2.38 (1.47-3.84)	< 0.001
Transmission concerns					
Yes (n = 394)	43.7 (172)	1.0	—		
No (n = 222)	42.8 (95)	0.97 (0.63-1.49)	0.87		
Had STI in past 6 months					
Yes (n = 145)	42.8 (62)	0.97 (0.58-1.63)	0.91		
No (n = 471)	43.5 (205)	1.0	——		
Perceived internalized stigma					
Minimal/Low (n = 98)	17.4 (17)	1.0	—	—	—
Moderate (n = 431)	46.9 (202)	4.20 (2.22-7.95)	< 0.001	2.94 (1.50-5.75)	0.002
High (n = 87)	55.2 (48)	5.86 (2.60-13.21)	< 0.001	1.93 (0.74-5.03)	0.18
Tired of using condoms					
Agree (n = 253)	49.8 (126)	1.99 (1.26-3.14)	0.003	1.35 (0.80-2.25)	0.25

Table 4 Factors associated with Unsafe Sex in the past 6 months among sexually-active participants, adjusted for intra-client clustering *(Continued)*

Disagree (n = 319)	33.2 (106)	1.0	—	—	—
Do not know(n = 44)	79.6 (35)	7.81 (3.31-18.43)	< 0.001	5.01 (1.78-14.07)	0.002
Believe condom reduces pleasure					
Agree (n = 369)	51.0 (188)	2.87 (1.81-4.54)	< 0.001	2.31 (1.60-4.91)	< 0.001
Disagree (n = 222)	26.6 (59)	1.0	—	—	—
Ambivalent (n = 25)	80.0 (20)	11.1 (4.03-30.28)	< 0.001	8.33 (2.38-29.09)	0.001
Family planning					
Using condom (n = 124)	16.1 (20)	1.0	—	—	—
Using other method (n = 117)	53.0 (62)	5.9 (2.87-11.96)	< 0.001	5.47 (2.57-11.66)	< 0.001
No family planning (n = 375	49.3 (185)	5.06 (2.72-9.42)	< 0.001	3.99 (2.06-7.75)	< 0.001
Drink Alcohol Weekly					
Yes (n = 251)	46.6 (117)	1.25 (0.79-1.97)	0.34		
No (n = 365)	41.1 (150)	1.0	—		

ART, antiretroviral therapy; CI, confidence interval; STI, sexually transmitted infection

Further, participants reported unprotected sex with more than half their sexual partners, significantly more with regular partners than non-regular partners. This is much higher than that reported among ART-naïve PLHIV in Uganda and South Africa [4,9,37] as well as among PLHIV on ART and those on co-trimoxazole prophylaxis without ART in Mombasa [2,7]. It is of concern that unprotected sex was reported with a third of HIV-negative partners and half of untested partners (people with unknown HIV status). This presents a serious HIV prevention challenge, particularly as 75 percent of the partners were untested and only 37 percent of the PLHIV had disclosed their HIV status to their partners. In a review article, Kalichman et al. (2000), have also reported high levels of unsafe sex with HIV-negative and unknown status partners [17]. Disclosure of HIV serostatus to partners and perceived stigma emerged as independent determinants of safe sex behaviors. It is important to note the intersection of the two determinants where PLHIV are reluctant to disclose for fear of rejection (perceived stigma) which may or may not happen [18,19]. Loubiere et al. (2009) and King et al. (2008) also link disclosure of HIV status with safe sex behavior in studies from Cameroon and Uganda [21,35]. Our study also highlights the role that the belief that condoms reduce pleasure and condom-use fatigue play in influencing safe sex. Conley and Collins (2005) found condom non-users to be more likely to believe that condom use interferes with pleasure; more commonly among males. Randolph et al. (2007) report similar results on condom use [40,41]. Prevention programs need to develop and implement strategies to change attitudes and beliefs about condoms. Further, more than half of the participants who did not want to have children were not using contraception, indicating high levels of unmet family planning need. Although it has been discussed extensively, effective integration of family planning counseling and services into HIV prevention programs has not been implemented and merits urgent action [42,43].

We documented other risky sexual practices such as unprotected sex during menstruation and unprotected anal sex. Sexual exposure to genital blood during menstruation is believed to facilitate transmission of HIV and other STIs [44,45]. We also report same sex behaviors among male participants: almost a quarter of all sexual partners reported by male participants were male. It is possible that a MSM peer could have recruited MSM participants. Mombasa has a fairly large population of male sex workers and unprotected anal sex is frequently reported in this population [46,47]. Anal intercourse is reported relatively less frequently by women. Fifteen percent of female participants in our study reported ever anal sex and the vast majority did not use condoms. Kalichman et al. (2009) report a 10% prevalence of heterosexual anal sex reported by women interviewed from community and clinic settings in South Africa [48]. The relatively low prevalence of anal intercourse among heterosexual individuals may be offset by its greater efficiency for transmitting HIV [49]. Health workers need to specifically discuss these forms of risky sexual behaviors during prevention counselling.

The study provides evidence that prevention programs can reach PLHIV who are not accessing HIV care services through community health workers or peer counsellors. About three-quarter of the participants were not accessing any HIV care and support services that they could benefit from; and more than half of them had been tested positive more than 12 months previously and were therefore, more likely to have forgotten any prevention messaging at the time of post-test counselling. This occurred despite the increased availability of

HIV care services and ART in recent years. Further research is needed to examine why some PLHIV are not accessing HIV care services.

The study is not without limitations. We recruited participants using non-probability modified targeted snowball sampling. Although our sample is not a randomly recruited representative sample, this technique did allow us to reach PLHIV within the community who are otherwise not accessible. We believe we were able to recruit a sufficiently diverse and representative sample for this study. We did not use Respondent Driven Sampling, a technique used commonly for hidden hard-to-reach populations such as MSM and injecting drug users, as this sampling method relies heavily on the recruitment of peers through their social networks, and we felt this to be unsuitable for our population and setting. In Mombasa, the network of positive people is small and poorly organized and, our previous study showed that PLHIV were reluctant to reveal their status and were poorly networked, with high levels of internalized stigma. This has also been reported by other African studies [11,12,28]. Our study sample consisted of 76% female participants. There could be several reasons for this: women tend to stay at home and therefore may be more easily contacted by health workers, women may access care earlier than men and so are more likely to know their HIV status, and in general, women make up more than 60% of the HIV-positive population in sub-Saharan Africa [1]. Women constituted 64% and 66% of our sample in our two previous studies in Mombasa [2,7].

In our data analysis we did not control for clustering at the recruiter level, which could lead to increased variance in reported behaviors. We did not do so because we did not link data on individual recruiters to participants; we recorded only type of recruiters (CHW or PTC counsellor). However, the fact that we found no significant socio-demographic differences between PLHIV recruited by CHWs and those recruited by PCs, and that each health worker could bring in a limited number of participants into the study and health workers were able to reach different risk groups as there are no geographic areas in Mombasa with a concentration of particular high-risk populations, may have reduced the bias due to clustering at the recruiter level. The study relies on self-reported sexual risk and condom use behaviors which may be subject to social desirability and recall bias. For the partner level analysis, we limited the number of partners each participant could describe to a maximum of six in the reference period; this afforded us the ability to obtain more reliable recall and limit the influence of the outliers in the sample. Reviews of validity and reliability of HIV research have, however, found that sexual behavior data are fairly consistent and self-reported data on sexual acts are reasonably congruent, especially for infrequent acts and short recall periods [50,51]. However, recent studies using biomarkers to validate self-reported condom use suggest over reporting of condom use and recommend interpreting self-reported behaviors with caution [52]. Over reporting would further raise the level of risk found in this study. Finally, the study would have benefited if a control group of PLHIV on treatment had been included for a comparison of sexual behaviors.

In conclusion, a significantly large number of PLHIV in the community are not accessing ART or HIV care services in Mombasa and high risk sexual behaviors are widely prevalent in this population. HIV programs need to bring this population into the ambit of prevention and care services.

Acknowledgements

We acknowledge the contribution of our colleagues from the Population Council: Ms Susan Kaai in Nairobi, in proposal development and training and Dr Waimar Tun, in Washington DC, for her inputs into proposal development and review of the report. We recognize the contribution of our team of research interviewers: Nicodemus Kisengese, Mariam Kassim, Jacqueline Chokwe, Dorothy Mubweka, Caleb Muasya and Nancy Kingola. The study could not have been done without a team of dedicated Community Health Workers and Post Test Club Peers led by Chorongo Salee and Peter Kimani respectively, our thanks to them. Lastly, we thank all study participants for their invaluable contribution. This work was undertaken by the Population Council and was funded by the generous support of the American people through the US Agency for International Development (USAID), Cooperative Agreement Award No: HRN-A-00-97-00012-00. The opinions expressed herein are those of the authors and do not necessarily reflect the views of USAID.

Author details

[1]Population Council, 142 Golf Links, New Delhi 110048, India. [2]International Centre for Reproductive Health, Department of Obstetrics and Gynaecology, Ghent University, Ghent, Belgium. [3]UCLA Center for Health Policy Research, Los Angeles, USA. [4]Centre for Health Policy, School of Public Health, Faculty of Health Sciences, University of the Witwatersrand, Johannesburg, South Africa. [5]Population Council, Nairobi, Kenya. [6]International Centre of Reproductive Health, Mombasa, Kenya.

Authors' contributions

AS was the PI on the study; she contributed to the design of the study, analysis of data and wrote the manuscript. SL participated in the design of the study and contributed to the manuscript. MP conducted the statistical data analysis. MC contributed substantially in reviewing the manuscript and guided data analysis. JO and NK conducted field research and assisted with contextual data and result interpretation. SG set up the data collection using hand held computers and helped with data interpretation. MT provided overall guidance for the research and manuscript preparation. All authors read and approved the final manuscript.

Competing interests

The authors declare that they have no competing interests.

References

1. UNAIDS, Global report: *UNAIDS report on the global AIDS epidemic 2010* 2010 [http://www.unaids.org/globalreport/Global_report.htm].

2. Luchters S, *et al*: **Safer sexual behaviors after 12 months of antiretroviral treatment in Mombasa, Kenya: a prospective cohort.** *AIDS Patient Care STDS* 2008, **22(7)**:587-594.
3. Peltzer K, Ramlagan S: **Safer sexual behaviors after 1 year of antiretroviral treatment in KwaZulu Natal, South Africa: a prospective cohort study.** *Sex Heal* 2010, **7(2)**:135-141.
4. Bunnell R, *et al*: **Changes in sexual behavior and risk of HIV transmission after antiretroviral therapy and prevention interventions in rural Uganda.** *AIDS* 2006, **20(1)**:85-92.
5. Crepaz N, Hart TA, Marks G: **Highly Active Antiretroviral Therapy and Sexual Risk Behavior A Meta-analytic Review.** *JAMA* 2004, **292(2)**:224-236.
6. Wandera B, *et al*: **Sexual behaviors over a 3-year period among individuals with advanced HIV/AIDS receiving antiretroviral therapy in an urban HIV clinic in Kampala, Uganda.** *J Acquir Immune Defic Syndr* 2011.
7. Sarna A, *et al*: **Sexual risk behavior and HAART: a comparative study of HIV-infected persons on HAART and on preventive therapy in Kenya.** *Int J STD AIDS* 2008, **19**:85-89.
8. Moatti J-P, *et al*: **Access to antiretroviral treatment and sexual behaviors of HIV-infected patients aware of their serostatus in Côte d'Ivoire.** *AIDS* 2003, **17(supplementary 3)**:S69-S77.
9. Eisele TP, *et al*: **High levels of risk behavior among people living with HIV initiating and waiting to start antiretroviral therapy in Cape Town, South Africa.** *AIDS Behav* 2008, **12(4)**:570-577.
10. Bateganya M, *et al*: **Antiretroviral therapy and sexual behavior: a comparative study between antiretroviral- naive and -experienced patients at an urban HIV/AIDS care and research center in Kampala, Uganda.** *AIDS Patient Care and STDs* 2005, **19(11)**:760-768.
11. Roura M, *et al*: **Scaling up stigma? The effects of antiretroviral roll-out on stigma and HIV testing. Early evidence from rural Tanzania.** *Sex Transm Infect* 2009, **85(4)**:308-312.
12. Mshana G, *et al*: **Barriers to accessing antiretroviral therapy in Kisesa, Tanzania: a qualitative study of early rural referrals to the national program.** *AIDS Patient Care STDS* 2006, **20(9)**:649-657.
13. Crepaz N, Marks G: **Towards an understanding of sexual risk behavior in people living with HIV: a review of social, psychological, and medical findings.** *AIDS* 2002, **16**:135-149.
14. Shiltz M, Sandfort TGM: **HIV-positive people, risk and sexual behavior.** *Social Sci Med* 2000, **50(11)**:1571-1588.
15. Courtney-Quirk C, *et al*: **Factors associated with sexual risk behavior among persons living with HIV: Gender and sexual identity group differences.** *AIDS Behav* 2008, **12(5)**:685-694.
16. Kiene SM, *et al*: **High rates of unprotected sex occurring among HIV-positive individuals in a daily diary study in South Africa: The role of alcohol use.** *J Acquir Immune Defic Syndr* 2008, **49(2)**:219-226.
17. Kalichman SC: **HIV transmission risk behaviors of men and women living with HIV-AIDS: Prevalence, predictors and emerging clinical interventions.** *Clin Psychological Sci Pract* 2000, **7**:32-47.
18. Kerrigan D, *et al*: **The search for social validation and the sexual behavior of people living with HIV in Rio de Janeiro, Brazil: understanding the role of treatment optimism in context.** *Social Sci Med* 2006, **62(10)**:2386-2396.
19. Sarna A, *et al*: **Changes in sexual risk taking with antiretroviral treatment: influence of context and gender norms in Mombasa, Kenya.** *Cult Heal Sex* 2009, **11(8)**:783-797.
20. King R, *et al*: **The virus stops with me: HIV-infected Ugandans' motivations in preventing HIV transmission.** *Soc Sci Med* 2009, **68(4)**:749-757.
21. King R, *et al*: **Processes and outcomes of HIV serostatus disclosure to sexual partners among people living with HIV in Uganda.** *AIDS Behav* 2008, **12(2)**:232-243.
22. Moore AR, Oppong J: **Sexual risk behavior among people living with HIV/AIDS in Togo.** *Social Sci Med* 2007, **64(5)**:1057-1066.
23. Kanniappan S, Jeyapaul MJ, Kalyanwala S: **Desire for motherhood: exploring HIV-positive women's desires, intentions and decision-making in attaining motherhood.** *AIDS Care* 2008, **20(6)**:625-630.
24. *NACC, UNGASS on HIV and AIDS Country Report: Kenya* National AIDS Control Council: Nairobi; 2010.
25. Watters J, Biernacki P: **Targeted sampling: Options for the study of hidden populations.** *Soc Probl* 1989, **36(4)**:416-430.
26. Rothenberg R: **Commentary: Sampling in Social Networks.** *Connections* 1995, **18(1)**:104-110.
27. Magnani R, *et al*: **Review of sampling hard-to-reach and hidden population for HIV surveillance.** *AIDS* 2005, **19(Supplement 2)**:S67-S72.
28. Kaai S, *et al*: **Perceived stigma among patients receiving antiretroviral treatment: a prospective randomised trial comparing an m-DOT strategy with standard-of-care in Kenya.** *SAHARA J* 2010, **7(2)**:62-70.
29. Sarna A, *et al*: **Short- and long-term efficacy of modified directly observed antiretroviral treatment in Mombasa, Kenya: a randomized trial.** *J Acquir Immune Defic Syndr* 2008, **48(5)**:611-619.
30. Berger BE, Ferrans CE, Lashley FR: **Measuring stigma in people with HIV: psychometric assessment of the HIV stigma scale.** *Res Nurs Health* 2001, **24(6)**:518-529.
31. Kline A, Van Landingham M: **HIV-infected women and sexual risk reduction: the relevance of existing models of behavior change.** *AIDS Educ Prev* 1994, **6(5)**:390-402.
32. VandeVen P, *et al*: **A scale of optimism-scepticism in the context of HIV treatments.** *AIDS Care* 2000, **12(2)**:171-176.
33. Greenland S, Rothman KJ: **Precision and Statistics in Epidemiologic Studies [Chapter 10:].** *Modern Epidemiology.* 3 edition. Lipincott Williams and Wilkins. 758; 2008.
34. Pettifor A, *et al*: **Continued High Risk Sexual Behavior Following Diagnosis with Acute HIV Infection in South Africa and Malawi: Implications for Prevention.** *AIDS Behav* 2010.
35. Loubiere s, *et al*: **HIV disclosure and unsafe sex among HIV-infected women in Cameroon: results from the ANRS-EVAL study.** *Socical Sci Med* 2009, **69(6)**:885-891.
36. Eaton L, *et al*: **HIV transmission risk among HIV seroconcordant and serodiscordant couples: dyadic processes of partner selection.** *AIDS Behav* 2009, **13(2)**:185-195.
37. Wagner G, *et al*: **Factors associated with condom use among HIV clients in stable relationships with partners at varying risk for HIV in Uganda.** *AIDS Behav* 2010, **14(5)**:1055-1065.
38. Bursac Z, *et al*: **A Purposeful Selection of Macro Variables for Logistic Regression.** *SAS Global Forum* 2007.
39. Marcellin F, *et al*: **Higher risk of unsafe sex and impaired quality of life among patients not receiving antiretroviral therapy in Cameroon: results from the EVAL survey (ANRS 12-116).** *AIDS* 2010, **24(suppl 1)**:S17-S25.
40. Randolph ME, *et al*: **Sexual pleasure and condom use.** *Arch Sex Behav* 2007, **36(6)**:844-848.
41. Conley T, Collins B: **Difference between condom users and condom nonusers in their multidimensional condom attitudes.** *J Appl Soc Psychol* 2005, **35**:603-620.
42. Rutenberg N, Baek C: **Field experiences integrating family planning into programs to prevent mother-to-child transmission of HIV.** *Stud Fam Plann* 2005, **36(3)**:235-245.
43. Church K, Mayhew SH: **Integration of STI and HIV prevention, care, and treatment into family planning services: a review of the literature.** *Stud Fam Plan* 2009, **40(3)**:171-186.
44. Kalichman S, Simbayi L: **Sexual exposure to blood and increased risks for heterosexual HIV transmission in Cape Town, South Africa.** *Afr J Reprod Health* 2004, **8(2)**:55-58.
45. Tanfer K, Aral S: **Sexual intercourse during menstruation and self-reported sexually transmitted disease history among women.** *Sex Transm Dis* 1996, **23(5)**:395-401.
46. Geibel S, *et al*: **Factors associated with self-reported unprotected anal sex among male sex workers in Mombasa, Kenya.** *Sex Transm Dis* 2008, **35(8)**:746-752.
47. Geibel S, *et al*: **Are you on the market?: a capture-recapture enumeration of men who sell sex to men in and around Mombasa, Kenya.** *AIDS* 2007, **21(10)**:1361-1362.
48. Kalichman S, *et al*: **Heterosexual anal intercourse among community and clinical settings in Cape Town, South Africa.** *Sex Transm Infect* 2009, **85(6)**:411-415.
49. Kalichman S, Simbayi L, Cain D: **HIV transmission risk behaviors among HIV seropositive sexually transmitted infection clinic patients in Cape Town, South Africa.** *Eur J Public Health* 2010, **20(2)**:202-206.
50. Obermeyer C: **Reframing research on sexual behavior and HIV.** *Stud Fam Plann* 2005, **36(1)**:1-12.

2

HIV-1 virologic failure and acquired drug resistance among first-line antiretroviral experienced adults at a rural HIV clinic in coastal Kenya

Amin S Hassan[1*], Helen M Nabwera[1], Shalton M Mwaringa[1], Clare A Obonyo[2], Eduard J Sanders[1,3], Tobias F Rinke de Wit[4,5], Patricia A Cane[6] and James A Berkley[1,3]

Abstract

Background: An increasing number of people on antiretroviral therapy (ART) in sub-Saharan Africa has led to declines in HIV related morbidity and mortality. However, virologic failure (VF) and acquired drug resistance (ADR) may negatively affect these gains. This study describes the prevalence and correlates of HIV-1 VF and ADR among first-line ART experienced adults at a rural HIV clinic in Coastal Kenya.

Methods: HIV-infected adults on first-line ART for ≥6 months were cross-sectionally recruited between November 2008 and March 2011. The primary outcome was VF, defined as a one-off plasma viral load of ≥400 copies/ml. The secondary outcome was ADR, defined as the presence of resistance associated mutations. Logistic regression and Fishers exact test were used to describe correlates of VF and ADR respectively.

Results: Of the 232 eligible participants on ART over a median duration of 13.9 months, 57 (24.6% [95% CI: 19.2 – 30.6]) had VF. Fifty-five viraemic samples were successfully amplified and sequenced. Of these, 29 (52.7% [95% CI: 38.8 – 66.3]) had at least one ADR, with 25 samples having dual-class resistance mutations. The most prevalent ADR mutations were the M184V (n = 24), K103N/S (n = 14) and Y181C/Y/I/V (n = 8). Twenty-six of the 55 successfully amplified viraemic samples (47.3%) did not have any detectable resistance mutation. Younger age (15–34 vs. ≥35 years: adjusted odd ratios [95% CI], p-value: 0.3 [0.1–0.6], p = 0.002) and unsatisfactory adherence (<95% vs. ≥95%: 3.0 [1.5–6.5], p = 0.003) were strong correlates of VF. Younger age, unsatisfactory adherence and high viral load were also strong correlates of ADR.

Conclusions: High levels of VF and ADR were observed in younger patients and those with unsatisfactory adherence. Youth-friendly ART initiatives and strengthened adherence support should be prioritized in this Coastal Kenyan setting. To prevent unnecessary/premature switches, targeted HIV drug resistance testing for patients with confirmed VF should be considered.

Keywords: HIV, Virologic failure, Acquired drug resistance, Correlates, Rural, Kenya

* Correspondence: ahassan@kemri-wellcome.org
[1]KEMRI/Wellcome Trust Research Programme, Kilifi, Kenya
Full list of author information is available at the end of the article

Background

By the end of 2011, approximately 34 million people were living with HIV globally, with almost all (97%) coming from low and middle income countries (LMIC) [1]. In the same year, more than 8 million HIV-infected individuals in LMIC were receiving antiretroviral therapy (ART), up from just 400,000 in 2003 [2]. In Kenya, approximately 10,000 HIV-infected individuals were on ART in 2003. By the end of 2011, more than 400,000 individuals had initiated ART in the country [3]. The increase in the number of people with access to ART has resulted in substantial declines in HIV related incidence, morbidity and mortality [4-6]. However, emerging HIV-drug resistance and subsequent treatment failure threatens to reverse these gains. This is especially important in sub-Saharan Africa (sSA) where the scale up of ART has not always been done in tandem with the relevant support for virological monitoring and HIVDR testing.

Regular virological monitoring has been shown to be useful both in resource rich and resource limited settings [7,8]. However, due to cost implications, this is not currently recommended for routine use in most developing country settings. Instead, the World Health Organization (WHO) recommend use of clinical and immunological criteria to monitor treatment failure in resource limited settings [9]. These criteria have been demonstrated to be poor indicators of treatment failure, leading to missed opportunities or unnecessary medication switches [10-14], which not only increase treatment costs, but also limit future treatment options.

A systematic review of virological efficacy and drug resistance outcomes of patients on ART programmes in sSA has reported 76% virological suppression after 12 months on ART and 67% after 24 months [15]. Similarly, a recent systematic review from resource limited settings report HIV drug resistance of 11% in patients on ART for 12–23 months, 15% at 24–36 months and 21% at >36 months [16]. The most common resistance profiles identified include the M184V mutation (associated with nucleoside reverse transcriptase inhibitors; NRTIs), followed by the K103N mutation (associated with non-nucleoside reverse transcriptase inhibitors; NNRTIs). Thymidine analogue mutations (TAMs) and the K65R mutation were less common.

Emerging drug resistance and subsequent treatment failure poses a major concern for HIV programs in resource-limited settings where treatment options are limited. This study aimed to describe the prevalence and correlates of HIV-1 virologic failure and acquired drug resistance among first-line ART-experienced adults from a rural HIV clinic in coastal Kenya.

Methods

Study site

The study was carried out at the HIV clinic in Kilifi District Hospital; a rural public health facility located in Coastal Kenya. HIV services in the clinic are provided according to the Kenyan national guidelines [17]. In brief, immunological monitoring is recommended at enrolment into care and six-monthly (or when clinically indicated) thereafter. Individuals meeting the ART eligibility criteria (WHO clinical staging III/IV regardless of CD4 T-cell count or CD4 T-cell count of <350 cells/mm3 regardless of clinical staging) undergo ART preparedness counseling and are initiated on a standard first-line regimen.

At the time of the study, the national recommended first-line therapy comprised two NRTIs (stavudine/zidovudine and lamivudine) and one NNRTI (nevirapine/efavirenz). A gradual phase-out of stavudine as a first-line agent was recommended in mid-2010. Adherence counseling was done by nurse counselors. Individuals failing first-line therapy were switched to an alternative combination of two NRTIs and a boosted protease inhibitor (bPI) as the recommended second line of choice.

At the time of the study, routine HIV-1 virologic monitoring and drug resistance testing were not recommended in the Kenyan national guidelines. Targeted viral load monitoring was introduced in 2011. A switch to the recommended second line regimen was recommended for individuals with virologic failure (persistent viral load ≥1000 copies/ml).

For this study, remnant blood from routine CD4 count samples was centrifuged to obtain plasma, which was archived at −80 degrees centigrade and used for viral load quantification and HIVDR testing.

Study design

An analytical cross-sectional study design was used. We included HIV-infected adults (≥15 years old) who had been on first-line ART for more than six months. Participants with a previous history of ART exposure for prevention of mother to child transmission (PMTCT) or for post-exposure prophylaxis (PEP), and those on second line regimens were excluded from the study.

Eligible participants were recruited in two phases. In the first cross-section, all consenting eligible participants were recruited between November 2008 and January 2009. At the same time, a prospective cohort was established in order to describe long-term outcomes of new clients enrolling for HIV care. All available plasma samples from participants recruited in the prospective cohort and meeting our eligibility criteria as at March 2011 were cross-sectionally retrieved.

Sources of data

These have been previously described elsewhere [18]. In brief, socio-demographic data including date of birth, gender, marital status, level of education, religion and sub-location of residence were routinely collected using standardized questionnaires from all individuals at enrolment into HIV care by trained fieldworkers and counselors. Actual distance to the clinic was estimated from centroid co-ordinates of sub-locations in which participants resided to the clinic using ArcInfo (ArcCatalog version 9.2, ESRI Corp).

Clinical data including anthropometry, opportunistic infections, WHO staging, ART regimen, drug substitutions, drug pick up dates and appointments were routinely collected by trained clinicians on standardized forms at every clinic encounter. Hematology and CD4 T-cell count data were also collected. A trained data entry clerk entered these data into an electronic data system.

Medicine Possession Ratio (MPR), defined as the amount of time a participant is in possession of antiretrovirals divided by the time between ARV drug pick-ups, is increasingly being used as a proxy for assessing adherence in retrospective analyses. We therefore retrospectively retrieved pharmacy drug refill data from 12 months (or from the date of ART initiation if follow up period <12 months) prior to the date of sampling for every individual participant. MPRs were calculated as proportions of the total number of days between drug pick-ups less the equivalent number of days in possession of ART divided by the time between drug pick-ups for all visits. A mean MPR for each individual was computed, subtracted from 100% and stratified to satisfactory (≥95%) and unsatisfactory (<95%) adherence according to previously published conventions [19,20].

Outcome definitions

The primary outcome was HIV-1 virologic failure (VF), defined as a one-off HIV-1 plasma RNA viral load of ≥400 copies/ml. Viral load quantification was done using an in-house assay. In brief, a multiplex real time quantitative probe-based assay with an internal control and a series of quantified HIV-1 standards was used to determine virus concentration. The assay is designed to quantify HIV-1 plasma RNA for thresholds of 100 – 10,000,000 copies/ml.

The secondary outcome was acquired drug resistance (ADR), determined by HIV-1 genotyping. Genotypic resistance testing was done for all samples with VF using an in-house assay which has been described elsewhere [21]. In brief, the assay amplifies and sequences part of the *pol* sub-genomic region containing the protease and part of the reverse transcriptase genes. Sequences were manually edited and assembled against a reference sequence using Sequencher software (GeneCodes, version 4.1). Sequences were submitted to the Stanford HIV drug resistance database to identify and interpret HIV-1 drug resistance mutations [22,23].

Viral subtypes were identified by 'Subtype Classification Using Evolutionary Algorithm tool (SCUEAL)' (http://www.datamonkey.org/dataupload.php) [24].

Sample size

A *post-hoc* sample size calculation was done to describe whether the data would produce results with sufficient statistical precision. This study assessed for HIV-1 VF among 232 patients on first-line antiretroviral therapy. Assuming a HIV-1 VF prevalence of 24% after a median follow-up period of 12 months on ART in our setting (based on 76% virological suppression after 12 months on ART as reported in a systematic review elsewhere [15]), the risk of 232 ART naïve adults started on first-line regimen and developing VF over a median follow up period of twelve months could be estimated with a precision of +/−6% at 95% confidence level.

Data analysis

Continuous data are presented using medians (interquartile ranges, IQR). Because of the relatively small sample size, and except for marital status, all the exposure variables were grouped into two categories. Continuous data were stratified into two categories, using the median as the guide to the stratification threshold. Frequencies and column percentages were used to describe categorical data.

The prevalence of HIV-1 VF was determined as a percentage of plasma samples with detectable viral load ≥400 copies/ml. The prevalence of ADR was determined as a percentage of samples with detectable resistance associated mutations (as identified by the Stanford HIV drug resistance database) over the total number of samples with VF that were successfully amplified and sequenced.

Univariable and multivariable logistic regression was used to determine correlates of VF. Correlates with a likelihood ratio test (LRT) p-value of <0.05 from the univariable analysis were carried to the multivariable models using the forward stepwise approach. Crude and adjusted odd ratios (OR), 95% confidence intervals (CI) and LRT p-values were presented. Because of the low frequency observed, the Fishers exact test was used to assess for correlates of ADR among all the participants included in the study. Frequencies, row percentages and the Fisher's exact p-values were presented.

From a public health perspective, the Kenyan national ART guidelines recommend use of persistent viral loads of ≥1000 copies/ml as indicative of VF [25]. For comparison purposes with the study outcomes, this definition was also considered in the analyses, albeit from a one-off sampling approach.

All analyses were carried out using STATA statistical software (STATA Intercooled version 11, StataCorp, College Station, Texas, USA).

Ethical considerations

The Kenya Medical Research Institute (KEMRI) Scientific Steering Committee and the National ethics review

Table 1 Distribution of characteristics among first-line antiretroviral experienced adults on care at a rural HIV clinic in coastal Kenya (N = 232)

Characteristic	Categories	Frequency [column %]		
		Cross-section 1 (n = 86)	Cross-section 2 (n = 146)	Total (n = 232)
Gender	Male	16 [18.6]	38 [26.0]	54 [23.3]
	Female	70 [81.4]	108 [74.0]	178 [76.7]
***Age (years)**	Median	36.5	39.3	38.5
	[IQR]	[31.4 – 44.4]	[32.7 – 46.1]	[32.2 – 44.8]
Age group (years)	15.0 – 34.9	33 [38.4]	47 [32.2]	80 [34.5]
	≥ 35.0	53 [61.6]	99 [67.8]	152 [65.5]
Marital status	Single	10 [11.6]	9 [6.2]	19 [8.2]
	Married (monogamous/polygamous)	52 [60.5]	80 [54.8]	132 [56.9]
	Separated/divorced/widowed	24 [27.9]	57 [39.0]	81 [34.9]
Religion	Christian	64 [74.4]	88 [60.3]	152 [65.5]
	Muslim	13 [15.1]	28 [19.2]	41 [17.7]
	Others	9 [10.5]	30 [20.6]	39 [16.8]
Education status	Primary schooling/less	68 [79.1]	119 [81.5]	187 [80.6]
	Secondary/higher	18 [20.9]	27 [18.5]	45 [19.4]
***Distance (km)**	Median	7.8	7.8	7.8
	[IQR]	[2.2 – 21.0]	[2.2 – 13.4]	[2.2 – 15.7]
Group distance (km)	< 10.0	50 [58.1]	98 [67.1]	148 [63.8]
	≥ 10.0	36 [41.9]	48 [32.9]	84 [36.2]
Starting 1st line regimen	Zidovudine based	37 [43.0]	81 [55.5]	118 [50.9]
	Stavudine based	49 [57.0]	65 [44.5]	114 [49.1]
***Baseline WHO staging**	I/II	41 [47.7]	90 [61.6]	131 [56.5]
	III/IV	44 [51.2]	56 [38.4]	100 [43.1]
	Missing	1 [0.0]	0 [0.0]	1 [0.4]
***Baseline BMI (Kg/m^2)**	Median	19.3	19.0	19.3
	(IQR)	[17.6 – 20.7]	[17.3 – 21.1]	[17.4 – 21.1]
Baseline BMI groups (Kg/m^2)	< 18.5	32 [37.2]	63 [43.2]	95 [41.0]
	≥ 18.5	53 [61.6]	83 [56.9]	136 [58.6]
	Missing	1 [1.2]	0 [0.0]	1 [0.4]
***Baseline CD4 count (cells/uL)**	Median	124	126	124
	(IQR)	[61 – 197]	[35–193]	[40–196]
Baseline CD4 groups (cells/uL)	< 100	33 [38.4]	63 [43.2]	96 [41.4]
	≥ 100	51 [59.3]	83 [56.9]	134 [57.8]
	Missing	2 [2.3]	0 [0.0]	2 [0.9]
***Duration on ART (months)**	Median	13.3	15.0	13.9
	[IQR]	[9.0 – 16.1]	[10.8 – 20.3]	[10.0 – 18.3]
Group duration on ART (months)	<12.0	32 [37.2]	49 [33.6]	81 [34.9]
	≥ 12.0	54 [62.8]	97 [66.4]	151 [65.1]
Drug substitution	No	68 [79.1]	100 [68.5]	168 [72.4]
	Yes	18 [20.9]	46 [31.5]	64 [27.6]
WHO staging	Stage I/II	54 [62.8]	78 [53.4]	132 [56.9]
	Stage III/IV	32 [37.2]	68 [46.6]	100 [43.1]

Table 1 Distribution of characteristics among first-line antiretroviral experienced adults on care at a rural HIV clinic in coastal Kenya (N = 232) *(Continued)*

***BMI (Kg/m²)**	Median	21.2	21.1	21.1
	(IQR)	[19.2 – 22.2]	[19.4 – 24.5]	[19.4 – 23.6]
BMI groups (Kg/m²)	< 18.5	12 [14.0]	24 [16.4]	36 [15.5]
	≥ 18.5	74 [86.1]	122 [83.6]	196 [84.5]
***CD4 count (cells/uL)**	Median	282	288	286
	(IQR)	[205–419]	[193–387]	[199–388]
CD4 groups (cells/uL)	< 350.0	49 [57.0]	82 [56.2]	131 [56.5]
	≥ 350.1	29 [33.7]	41 [28.1]	70 [30.2]
	Missing	8 [9.3]	23 [15.8]	31 [13.4]
MPR adherence	≥ 95% (Satisfactory)	59 [68.6]	122 [83.6]	181 [78.0]
	< 95% (Unsatisfactory)	24 [27.9]	19 [13.0]	43 [18.5]
	Missing	3 [3.5]	5 [3.4]	8 [3.5]

Baseline refers to indicators at ART initiation; *Follow up* refers to indicators at the time of sampling; *Median [IQR, Inter-quartile ranges] for continuous variables; BMI (Body Mass Index); WHO (World Health Organization); MPR (Medicine Possession Ratio); Zidovudine based (plus lamivudine/Nevirapine [n = 107] or lamivudine/efavirenz [n = 11]); stavudine based (plus lamivudine/Nevirapine [n = 111] or lamivudine/efavirenz [n = 3]).

committee provided scientific and ethics approval respectively (SSC No. 1341). All the participants provided written informed consent.

Results

Study population characteristics

Overall, 232 adults on first-line ART for a median duration of 13.9 (IQR: 10.0 – 18.3) months were recruited. The characteristics of participants recruited in the first cross-section were not substantially different from those recruited in the second cross-section (Table 1).

The majority of the participants were female (n = 178 [77%]), aged more than 35 years (n = 152 [66%]), married (n = 132 [57%]), with a primary education or less (n = 187 [81%]) and living within 10 kilometers of the clinic (n = 148 [64%]) (Table 1). Half of the participants (n = 118) initiated ART on a zidovudine-based regimen (plus lamivudine/nevirapine, n = 107 [46%] or lamivudine/efavirenz, n = 11 [5%]); the other half (n = 114) started on a stavudine-based regimen (plus lamivudine/nevirapine, n = 111 [48%] or lamivudine/efavirenz, n = 3 [1%]). Over the follow up duration on ART, 64 (28%) participants had undergone at least one drug substitution and 43 (19%) had an average unsatisfactory MPR adherence.

HIV-1 virologic failure

Of the 232 samples that underwent HIV-1 RNA viral load quantification, 57 (24.6% [95% CI: 19.2 – 30.6]) demonstrated VF. In univariable analysis, MPR adherence, age group and marital status were significantly correlated with VF. In multivariable analysis, only MPR adherence and age group remained independently associated with VF (Table 2). Participants with an average unsatisfactory MPR adherence had three-fold odds of having VF, compared to those with an average satisfactory MPR adherence (aOR [95% CI], p-value: 3.0 [1.5 – 6.5], p = 0.003). Likewise, participants aged ≥35 years had 70% lower odds of having VF, compared to those aged 15 – 34 years old (0.3 [0.1 – 0.6], $p < 0.001$). Adjusting for age attenuated the effect of marital status on VF towards the null (Separated/divorced/widowed vs. single, 0.4 [0.1 – 1.2], p = 0.137).

HIV-1 acquired drug resistance

Fifty-five of the 57 samples with VF were successfully amplified and sequenced for HIV drug resistance testing. Of the 55 samples that were successfully amplified and sequenced, 29 (52.7% [95% CI: 38.8 – 66.3]) had at least one detectable HIV-1 resistance associated mutation, giving an overall ADR prevalence of 12.5% (95% CI: 8.5 – 17.5) among all participants included in the study. While all 29 samples had mutations conferring resistance to NNRTIs, 25 (86%) of those with resistance had dual-class (both NRTIs and NNRTIs) mutations (Table 3). The most prevalent variant were the M184V mutation (n = 24), the K103N/S mutation (n = 14) and the Y181C/Y/I/V mutation (n = 8) within the reverse transcriptase genome. Thymidine analogue mutations (TAMs) were present in 4 participants. Twenty-six of the 55 successfully amplified viraemic samples (47.3%) did not have any detectable resistance associated mutations.

Viral load, MPR adherence and age group were strongly associated with ADR (Table 4). Participants with higher viral loads (≥ 4.0 log copies/ml) had a higher prevalence of ADR, compared to those with lower viral loads (< 4.0 log copies/ml), (frequency [%]: 20 [62.5] vs 9 [4.6], $p < 0.001$). Likewise, participants with unsatisfactory MPR adherence had a higher prevalence of ADR, compared to those with satisfactory MPR adherence (frequency [%]: 12 [27.9] vs 17 [9.5], p = 0.004). Similarly,

Table 2 Logistic regression analysis describing correlates of HIV-1 virologic failure (viral load ≥400 copies/ml) among first-line antiretroviral experienced adults at a rural HIV clinic in coastal Kenya (N = 232)

			Logistic univariable analysis			Logistic multivariable analysis (n = 201)		
Risk factors	**Categories**	**Viraemia, n = 57 [%]**	**Crude OR**	**95% C.I**	***P-value**	**Adjusted OR**	**95% C. I**	***P-value**
Gender	Male	12/54 [22.2]	1.0					
	Female	45/177 [25.3]	1.2	0.6 – 2.4	0.645	-	-	-
Age group (years)	15.0 – 34.9	31/80 [38.8]	1.0			1.0		
	≥ 35.0	26/152 [17.1]	0.3	0.2 – 0.6	<0.001	0.3	0.2 – 0.7	0.002
Marital status	Single	8/19 [42.1]	1.0					
	Married (monogamous/polygamous)	36/132 [27.3]	0.5	0.2 – 1.4				
	Separated/Divorced/Widowed	13/81 [16.1]	0.3	0.1 – 0.8	0.034	-	-	-
Religion	Christian	38/152 [25.0]	1.0					
	Muslim	7/41 [17.1]	0.6	0.3 – 1.5				
	Others	12/39 [30.8]	1.3	0.6 – 2.9	0.345	-	-	-
Education status	Primary schooling/Less	46/187 [24.6]	1.0					
	Secondary/Higher	11/45 [24.4]	1.0	0.5 – 2.1	0.983	-	-	-
Group distance (km)	<10.0	37/148 [25.0]	1.0					
	≥ 10.0	20/84 [23.8]	0.9	0.5 – 1.8	0.839	-	-	-
Starting 1st line regimen	Zidovudine based	33/118 [28.0]	1.0					
	Stavudine based	24/114 [21.1]	0.7	0.4 – 1.3	0.221	-	-	-
***Baseline* WHO staging**	I/II	28/131 [21.4]	1.0					
	III/IV	28/100 [28.0]	1. 4	0.8 – 2.6	0.246	-	-	-
***Baseline* BMI groups (Kg/m^2)**	< 18.5	26/95 [27.4]	1.0					
	≥ 18.5	30/136 [22.1]	0.8	0.4 – 1.4	0.356	-	-	-
***Baseline* CD4 groups (cells/uL)**	< 100	25/96 [26.0]	1.0					
	≥ 100	30/134 [22.4]	0.8	0.4 – 1.5	0.523	-	-	-
Duration on ART (months)	<12.0	23/81 [28.4]	1.0					
	≥ 12.0	34/151 [22.5]	0.7	0.4 - 1.4	0.325	-	-	-
Drug substitution	No	40/168 [23.8]	1.0					
	Yes	17/64 [26.6]	1.2	0.6 – 2.2	0.665	-	-	-
***Follow up* WHO staging**	Stage I/II	29/132 [22.0]	1.0					
	Stage III/IV	28/100 [28.0]	1.4	0.8 – 2.5	0.292	-	-	-
***Follow up* BMI groups (Kg/m^2)**	< 18.5	10/36 [27.8]	1.0					
	≥ 18.5	47/196 [24.0]	0.8	0.4 – 1.8	0.627	-	-	-

Table 2 Logistic regression analysis describing correlates of HIV-1 virologic failure (viral load ≥400 copies/ml) among first-line antiretroviral experienced adults at a rural HIV clinic in coastal Kenya (N = 232) *(Continued)*

Follow up CD4 groups (cells/uL)	< 350	35/131 [26.7]	1.0					
	≥ 350	12/70 [17.1]	0.6	0.3 – 1.2	0.120	-	-	-
MPR adherence	≥ 95% (Satisfactory)	34/181 [18.8]	1.0			1.0		
	<95% (Unsatisfactory)	18/43 [41.9]	3.1	1.5 – 6.3	0.002	3.0	1.5 – 6.5	0.003

Baseline refers to indicators at ART initiation; *Follow up* refers to indicators at the time of sampling; *Likelihood Ratio Test p-value; BMI (Body Mass Index); WHO (World Health Organization); MPR (Medicine Possession Ratio). Missing data; Baseline WHO staging (n = 1 [0.4%]), Baseline BMI (n = 1 [0.4%]), Baseline CD4 count (n = 2 [0.9%]), CD4 count (n = 31 [13.4%]) and MPR adherence (n = 8 [3.5%]).

Table 3 Distribution and characteristics of first-line antiretroviral experienced adults with HIV-1 acquired drug resistance mutations from a rural HIV clinic in coastal Kenya

No.	Gender	Age (years)	Sample date	ART date	ART duration#	Viral load	Subtype*	NRTI mutations	NNRTI mutations
1.	Male	30.5	28-Nov-08	28-Mar-08	8.0	697796	Complex	D67DG	K103N, G190A
2.	Female	38.5	02-Dec-08	22-May-08	6.4	5006	A1	M184V	K103N, K238T
3.	Male	36.6	06-Jan-09	11-Apr-08	8.9	861730	A1	M184V	Y188L
4.	Female	33.4	17-Nov-08	19-May-08	6.0	64435	A1	M184V, K219EK	V108IV, Y181CY, G190AG
5.	Female	44.5	16-Dec-08	26-Nov-07	12.7	3087	A1	M184V	G190A
6.	Female	26.5	17-Dec-08	01-Nov-07	13.5	1158	D	M184V	K103N, K238T
7.	Female	22.5	05-Dec-08	30-Oct-07	13.2	4051	A1	M184V	K103N
8.	Female	48.4	12-Nov-08	02-Jul-07	16.4	5274	A1	M184V	K103N, M230LM
9.	Female	24.4	12-Nov-08	29-Aug-07	14.5	24529	D	T69NT, M184V	K103N
10.	Female	63.4	21-Nov-08	03-May-07	18.7	576	A1, AE		K103N
11.	Female	25.6	14-Jan-09	22-Oct-07	14.8	219766	A-ancestral, A1	M184V, T215Y	Y181C
12.	Female	31.3	07-Oct-10	22-Aug-08	25.5	315800	A1	M184V	K103N
13.	Female	34.0	22-Jun-10	07-Oct-09	8.5	17248	A1	M184V	Y181C
14.	Female	25.2	13-Sep-10	19-Aug-09	12.8	109090	D	M184V	V106A, F227L
15.	Female	51.2	10-Aug-10	15-Jun-09	13.8	5396	A1	M184V	K103N
16.	Female	23.7	08-Mar-11	22-Sep-09	17.5	12408	A1	M184V	Y181C
17.	Female	32.1	06-Jul-10	15-Dec-08	18.7	199362	A1	M41L, D67N, K70R, M184V, T215Y, K219Q	Y181IV
18.	Female	31.8	23-Mar-11	27-Feb-09	24.8	834656	A-ancestral, A1		K101E, G190A
19.	Female	38.7	16-Feb-10	22-May-09	8.9	34186	A2	M184V	V106A
20.	Female	41.8	20-Apr-10	22-Jun-09	9.9	4729	A1	M184V	Y181C
21.	Female	31.7	04-Mar-11	24-Mar-09	23.3	20392	A1	M184V	V106A
22.	Female	15.1	16-Mar-10	13-Apr-09	11.1	1046760	A1	M184V	K103S, G190A
23.	Female	31.3	29-Sep-10	11-Jan-10	8.6	129493	A1, A2		K103N
24.	Female	41.7	11-Mar-11	18-Aug-09	18.7	1452	A, A1	M184V	Y181C
25.	Female	17.8	07-Mar-11	08-Dec-09	14.9	130222	A1	M184V	K103N, Y318FY
26.	Female	25.7	04-Mar-11	13-Apr-10	10.7	47795	A1	M184V	K101Q, G190A
27.	Female	21.7	11-Mar-11	01-Sep-09	18.3	2029880	A1	L74V, M184V	K103N, Y181C
28.	Female	48.1	02-Aug-10	08-Oct-08	21.8	72430	A1		G190A
29.	Male	29.5	14-Dec-10	06-Jan-10	11.2	74152	A, A1	K65R, M184V	K103N

#Time (in months) since patient started taking antiretroviral therapy, *HIV-1 subtypes identified using the 'Subtype Classification Using Evolutionary ALgorithm (SCUEAL)' tool, available at (www.datamonkey.org/dataupload_scueal.php).

participants aged 15– 34 had a higher prevalence of ADR compared to those aged ≥35 years (frequency [%]: 19 [23.8] vs 10 [6.7], $p < 0.001$).

Age was further stratified to 10-year age bands and its association with VF and ADR explored. The overall prevalence of VF and ADR was highest in participants aged 15–24 years (53.3% and 40.0% respectively) (Figure 1). Strong evidence of a decreasing trend in prevalence of VF and ADR with increasing age groups (non-parametric test for trend, $p = 0.004$ and $p < 0.001$ respectively) was also observed.

For comparison purposes, the above analyses were repeated using viral load threshold of ≥1000 copies/ml to define VF. Of the 232 participants, 48 (20.7% [95% CI: 15.7 – 26.5]) met this criterion of HIV-1 VF. Of these, 28 (58.3% [95% CI: 43.2 – 72.4]) had at least one detectable HIV-1 resistance mutation. Correlates of VF (Additional file 1: Table S1) and ADR (Additional file 1: Table S2) remained the same as those observed when using this study's outcome definition of ≥400 copies/ml for VF.

Discussion

Findings from a HIV clinic in a rural district hospital in coastal Kenya suggest that one in every four adults on first-line antiretroviral regimen for an average of 14 months had VF, with half of those with VF harboring at least one HIV resistance-associated mutation. The most prevalent mutations observed confer high-level resistance to NRTIs (specifically lamivudine, in the case of the M184V mutation) and NNRTIs (specifically nevirapine and efavirenz, in the case of the K103N/S mutation and

Table 4 Distribution and correlates of HIV-1 acquired drug resistance among first-line antiretroviral experienced adults at a rural HIV clinic in coastal Kenya (N = 230)

		Acquired drug resistance [row %]		
Risk factors	**Categories**	**No (n = 201)**	**Yes (n = 29)**	***P-value**
Gender	Male	51 [94.4]	3 [5.6]	
	Female	150 [85.2]	26 [14.8]	0.100
Age group (years)	15.0 – 34.9	61 [76.3]	19 [23.8]	
	≥ 35.0	140 [93.3]	10 [6.7]	<0.001
Marital status	Single	13 [68.4]	6 [31.6	
	Married (monogamous/polygamous)	113 [86.3]	18 [13.7]	
	Separated/divorced/widowed	75 [93.8]	5 [6.3]	0.013
Religion	Christian	132 [87.4]	19 [12.6]	
	Muslim	36 [87.8]	5 [12.2]	
	Others	33 [86.8]	5 [13.2]	1.000
Education status	Primary schooling/less	162 [87.6]	23 [12.4]	
	Secondary/higher	39 [86.7]	6 [13.3]	0.807
Group distance (km)	<10.0	128 [86.5]	20 [13.5]	
	≥10.0	73 [89.0]	9 [11.0]	0.681
Starting 1st line regimen	Zidovudine based	102 [86.4]	16 [13.6]	
	Stavudine based	99 [88.4]	13 [11.6]	0.695
***Baseline* WHO staging**	I/II	117 [90.0]	13 [10.0]	
	III/IV	83 [83.8]	16 [16.2]	0.228
***Baseline* BMI groups (Kg/m^2)**	< 18.5	82 [88.2]	11 [11.8]	
	≥ 18.5	118 [86.8]	18 [13.2]	0.841
***Baseline* CD4 groups (cells/uL)**	<100	82 [86.3]	13 [13.7]	
	> 100	118 [88.7]	15 [11.3]	0.683
Duration on ART (months)	< 12.0	70 [86.4]	11 [13.6]	
	≥ 12.0	131 [87.9]	18 [12.1]	0.836
Drug substitution	No	145 [87.4]	21 [12.7]	
	Yes	56 [87.5]	8 [12.5]	1.000
***Follow up* WHO staging**	Stage I/II	119 [91.5]	11 [8.5]	
	Stage III/IV	82 [82.0]	18 [18.0]	0.044
***Follow up* BMI groups (Kg/m^2)**	< 18.5	30 [83.3]	6 [16.7]	
	≥ 18.5	171 [88.1]	23 [11.9]	0.417
***Follow up* CD4 groups (cells/uL)**	< 350	110 [84.6]	20 [15.4]	
	≥ 350	64 [91.4]	6 [8.6]	0.193
MPR adherence	≥ 95% (Satisfactory)	162 [90.5]	17 [9.5]	
	< 95% (Unsatisfactory)	31 [72.1]	12 [27.9]	0.004
Viral load (log 10, copies/ml)	0.00 – 4.00	189 [95.5]	9 [4.6]	
	> 4.00	12 [37.5]	20 [62.5]	<0.001

Baseline refers to indicators at ART initiation; *Follow up* refers to indicators at the time of sampling; *Fisher's exact p-value; BMI (Body Mass Index); WHO (World Health Organization) MPR (Medicine Possession Ratio). Missing data; Baseline WHO staging (n = 1 [0.4%]), Baseline BMI (n = 1 [0.4%]), Baseline CD4 count (n = 2 [0.9%]), CD4 count (n = 31 [13.4%]) and MPR adherence (n = 8 [3.5%]).

the Y181C/Y/I/V mutation). These results are consistent with findings from systematic reviews of studies on virological efficacy and drug resistance from other resource limited settings [15,26]. The non-complex resistance patterns observed could possibly indicate an advantage of the current recommended first-line regimen in this setting.

The WHO recommends use of drug-refill data as an early warning indicator (EWI) of HIV treatment failure and drug resistance [27]. Recent EWI analyses on prospective HIVDR data from 6 African countries suggest an advantage of MPR over on-time drug pick-up in identifying participants at risk for developing HIV drug resistance [28]. For

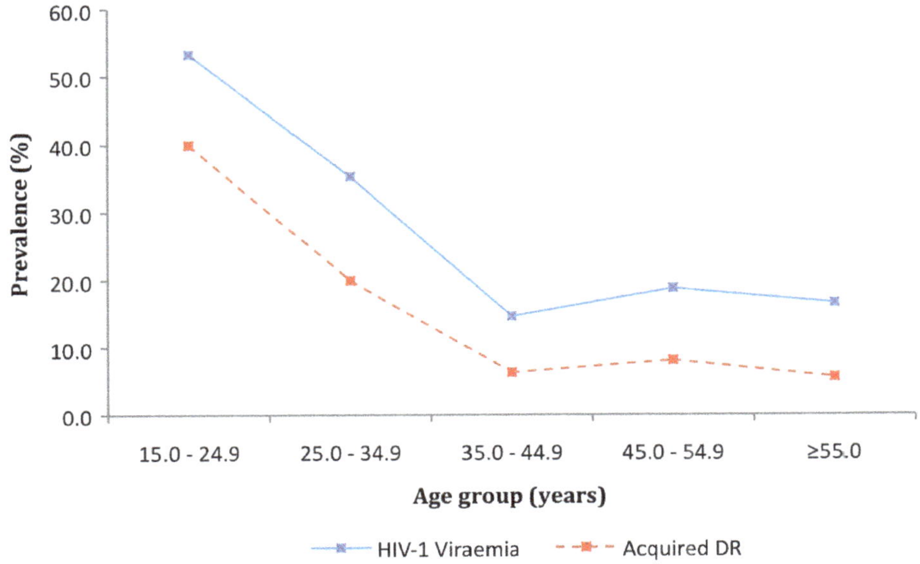

Figure 1 Overall prevalence and distribution of HIV-1 Viraemia (viral load ≥400 copies/ml) and acquired drug resistance by age group, among first-line antiretroviral experienced adults at a rural HIV clinic in coastal Kenya (N=232).

this reason, MPR was used and indeed identified as a practical alternative parameter for assessing adherence, with strong correlation with both VF and ADR in this setting. Similar findings have also been reported elsewhere [19,29-31].

The current study also indicated younger age as a strong risk factor for both HIV-1 VF and ADR. In fact, half of all participants aged 15–24 years had VF, while two in every five had acquired at least one drug resistant strain. Data from a developed setting suggests that the youth face a complex myriad of challenges including peer-related stigma, disclosure, adherence, sexual, reproductive and gender health concerns [32]. If applicable, then these challenges may indirectly contribute to the high burden of virological treatment failure and ADR in our setting.

Higher viral load was strongly associated with ADR, which is consistent with literature [33]. Of interest however, is the finding that only half of participants with VF had detectable ADR. Indeed, if the Kenyan national recommendation of ≥1000 copies/ml was used to suggest VF in this study [25], and assuming sustained viral replication, then a fifth of the participants would have VF. Of these, only 58% had detectable ADR mutations. These data may therefore suggest that up to 42% of participants would have potentially been switched to the more expensive 2nd line regimen prematurely or unnecessarily, thus exhausting and limiting treatment options. This is especially risky in this setting where the only currently recommended second line option is the bPIs, with costs prohibiting the range of other potential alternative regimens.

The findings of this study should be interpreted in light of several limitations. Firstly, the cross-sectional study design and the one-off sampling strategy warrant caution in the interpretation of our findings, as follow up samples were not available to confirm VF. Consequently, blips in viral load cannot be ruled out [34]. It is acknowledged that occasionally, viral blips can occur even during effective treatment [35,36]. This may have resulted to an overestimation of the true burden of VF in this population. In addition, focusing on participants with a median ART follow up duration of more than a year potentially excludes those who may have died or were lost to follow-up within a year of ART due to treatment failure. This may have resulted in an underestimation of the true burden of VF and ADR in this population.

Secondly, it may be argued that the participants may not have achieved virological suppression in the first place, even after being on ART for more than 6 months. This may possibly be attributed to the effect of persisting HIV-1 primary or transmitted resistance mutations, which have been reported to be on the increase in some parts of sSA [37,38]. Transmitted resistant strains have been shown to contribute to VF in clients on ART [39-41]. However, our concurrent data suggest low levels (<5%) of transmitted drug resistance in this rural coastal Kenyan population [42].

Lastly, stigma, disclosure, sexual orientation, reproductive health and gender issues are potential concerns that may contribute to the burden of VF and ADR, especially among the young adults in this setting. Data on these factors were not captured and hence not considered in the analyses.

Conclusions

In conclusion, levels of HIV-1 VF and ADR observed from this rural HIV clinic in coastal Kenya were comparable to those observed in other resource-limited settings. High levels of VF and ADR were observed among younger patients and those with unsatisfactory adherence. Implementation of youth-friendly ART initiatives (e.g. social networks, support clubs) are therefore warranted in this setting. Strengthened adherence support should also be prioritized, more so in cases of suspected virologic treatment failure and before treatment switches. However, if virologic failure is confirmed, targeted HIVDR testing should be considered to prevent unnecessary/premature switches.

Competing interests
The authors declare that they have no competing interest.

Authors' contributions
JAB and PAC conceived the study. ASH coordinated the data/sample collection, analyzed the data and prepared the draft manuscript. SM, HN and CAO assisted with the coordination of the data and sample collection. JAB, PAC, ES and TFRW provided guidance and mentorship during the implementation of the study. All authors reviewed and approved the final manuscript.

Acknowledgments
The authors are grateful to the staff and clients at the Comprehensive Care and Research Clinic for participating in the study. We are also grateful to the members of the Antiviral Unit at Colindale, London for undertaking the HIV drug resistance testing work. We are especially grateful to Dr Simon Carne and his team at the Antiviral Unit at Colindale, London for the HIV-1 RNA viral load quantification. This manuscript was submitted for publication with the permission from the Director of KEMRI.

Sources of funding
This work was supported by the Wellcome Trust foundation (grant number WT089351MA). ASH and JAB were funded by Wellcome Trust fellowships (WT089351MA and WT083579MA respectively). SM and HN were employees of the KEMRI/Wellcome Trust research programme while CAO was an employee of the Kenyan Ministry of Health. EJS was funded by the International AIDS Vaccine Initiative while PAC was financially supported by the Health Protection Agency, UK. TFRW was a member of the PharmAccess African studies to Evaluate Resistance (PASER), which received financial support from the Ministry of Foreign Affairs of the Netherlands. The funding bodies played no part in the design, collection, management, analysis and interpretation of data and manuscript preparation.

Author details
[1]KEMRI/Wellcome Trust Research Programme, Kilifi, Kenya. [2]Kilifi District Hospital, Kilifi, Kenya. [3]Centre for Clinical Vaccinology & Tropical Medicine, University of Oxford, Oxford, UK. [4]PharmAccess Foundation, Amsterdam, Netherlands. [5]Academic Medical Center, University of Amsterdam, Amsterdam, Netherlands. [6]Health Protection Agency, London, UK.

References

1. UNAIDS: *Core slides: Global summary of the AIDS epidemic*; 2012. Available at: [http://www.unaids.org/en/media/unaids/contentassets/documents/epidemiology/2012/201207_epi_core_en.pdf]. Accessed 20 Nov 2012.
2. UNAIDS: *Global AIDS epidemic facts and figures*; 2012. Available at: [http://www.unaids.org/en/media/unaids/contentassets/documents/epidemiology/2012/201207_FactSheet_Global_en.pdf]. Accessed 20 Nov 2012.
3. NACC and NASCOP: *Kenya AIDS Epidemic update*; 2012. Available at: [http://www.unaids.org/en/dataanalysis/knowyourresponse/countryprogressreports/2012countries/ce_KE_Narrative_Report.pdf]. Accessed 04 April 2013.
4. Bendavid E, Bhattacharya J: **The president's emergency plan for AIDS relief in Africa: an evaluation of outcomes.** *Ann Intern Med* 2009, **150**(10):688–695.
5. Jahn A, Floyd S, Crampin AC, *et al*: **Population-level effect of HIV on adult mortality and early evidence of reversal after introduction of antiretroviral therapy in Malawi.** *Lancet* 2008, **371**(9624):1603–1611.
6. UNAIDS: *World AIDS Day Report*; 2011. Available at: [http://www.unaids.org/en/media/unaids/contentassets/documents/unaidspublication/2011/jc2216_worldaidsday_report_2011_en.pdf]. Accessed 20 Nov 2012.
7. Gupta RK, Hill A, Sawyer AW, *et al*: **Virological monitoring and resistance to first-line highly active antiretroviral therapy in adults infected with HIV-1 treated under WHO guidelines: a systematic review and meta-analysis.** *Lancet Infect Dis* 2009, **9**(7):409–417.
8. Keiser O, Tweya H, Boulle A, *et al*: **Switching to second-line antiretroviral therapy in resource-limited settings: comparison of programmes with and without viral load monitoring.** *AIDS* 2009, **23**(14):1867–1874.
9. World Health Organization: *Antiretroviral therapy for HIV infection in adults and adolescents: recommendations for a public health approach - 2010 rev.* Available at: [http://whqlibdoc.who.int/publications/2010/9789241599764_eng.pdf]. Accessed 20 Nov 2012.
10. Badri M, Lawn SD, Wood R: **Utility of CD4 cell counts for early prediction of virological failure during antiretroviral therapy in a resource-limited setting.** *BMC Infect Dis* 2008, **8**:89.
11. Mee P, Fielding KL, Charalambous S, Churchyard GJ, Grant AD: **Evaluation of the WHO criteria for antiretroviral treatment failure among adults in South Africa.** *AIDS* 2008, **22**(15):1971–1977.
12. van Oosterhout JJ, Brown L, Weigel R, *et al*: **Diagnosis of antiretroviral therapy failure in Malawi: poor performance of clinical and immunological WHO criteria.** *Trop Med Int Health* 2009, **14**(8):856–861.
13. Barth RE, Tempelman HA, Moraba R, Hoepelman AI: **Long-term outcome of an HIV-treatment programme in Rural Africa: viral suppression despite early mortality.** *AIDS Res Treat* 2011, **2011**:434375.
14. Kantor R, Diero L, Delong A, *et al*: **Misclassification of first-line antiretroviral treatment failure based on immunological monitoring of HIV infection in resource-limited settings.** *Clin Infect Dis* 2009, **49**(3):454–462.
15. Barth RE, van der Loeff MF, Schuurman R, Hoepelman AI, Wensing AM: **Virological follow-up of adult patients in antiretroviral treatment programmes in sub-Saharan Africa: a systematic review.** *Lancet Infect Dis* 2010, **10**(3):155–166.
16. Stadeli KM, Richman DD: **Rates of emergence of HIV drug resistance in resource-limited settings: a systematic review.** *Antivir Ther* 2013, **18**(1):115–123.
17. National AIDS & STI Control Programme: *Kenya National Clinical Manual For ART Providers.* Available at: [http://nascop.or.ke/library/ART%20guidelines/Kenya%20clinical%20National%20Manual%20for%20ART%20providers.pdf]. Accessed 20 Nov 2012.
18. Hassan AS, Fielding KL, Thuo NM, *et al*: **Early loss to follow-up of recently diagnosed HIV-infected adults from routine pre-ART care in a rural district hospital in Kenya: a cohort study.** *Trop Med Int Health* 2012, **17**(1):82–93.
19. Goldman JD, Cantrell RA, Mulenga LB, *et al*: **Simple adherence assessments to predict virologic failure among HIV-infected adults with discordant immunologic and clinical responses to antiretroviral therapy.** *AIDS Res Hum Retroviruses* 2008, **24**(8):1031–1035.
20. Weidle PJ, Wamai N, Solberg P, *et al*: **Adherence to antiretroviral therapy in a home-based AIDS care programme in rural Uganda.** *Lancet* 2006, **368**(9547):1587–1594.
21. Cane P: **HIV drug resistance testing.** *Methods Mol Biol* 2011, **665**:123–132.
22. Liu TF, Shafer RW: **Web resources for HIV type 1 genotypic-resistance test interpretation.** *Clin Infect Dis* 2006, **42**(11):1608–1618.
23. Rhee SY, Gonzales MJ, Kantor R, *et al*: **Human immunodeficiency virus reverse transcriptase and protease sequence database.** *Nucleic Acids Res* 2003, **31**(1):298–303.
24. Kosakovsky Pond SL, Posada D, Stawiski E, *et al*: **An evolutionary model-based algorithm for accurate phylogenetic breakpoint mapping and subtype prediction in HIV-1.** *PLoS Comput Biol* 2009, **5**(11):e1000581.
25. National aIDS & STI Control Program: *Guidelines for antiretroviral therapy in Kenya.* 4th edition; 2011. [Available at: [http://healthservices.uonbi.ac.ke/sites/default/files/centraladmin/healthservices/Kenya%20Treatment%20Guidelines%202011.pdf]. Accessed 04 May 2013.
26. Stadeli KM, Richman DD: **Rates of emergence of HIV drug resistance in resource-limited settings: a systematic review.** *Antivir Ther* 2013, **18**(1):115–123.

27. World Health Organization: *HIV Drug Resistance Early Warning Indicators. World Health Organization indicators to monitor HIV drug resistance prevention at antiretroviral treatment sites June 2010 Update.* Available at: [http://www2.paho.org/hq/dmdocuments/2010/hivdr-early-warning-indicators—updated-april-2010.pdf]. Accessed 20 Nov 2012.
28. Sigaloff KC, Hamers RL, Menke J, *et al*: **Early warning indicators for population-based monitoring of HIV drug resistance in 6 African countries.** *Clin Infect Dis* 2012, **54**(Suppl 4):S294–S299.
29. El-Khatib Z, Katzenstein D, Marrone G, *et al*: **Adherence to drug-refill is a useful early warning indicator of virologic and immunologic failure among HIV patients on first-line ART in South Africa.** *PLoS One* 2011, **6**(3):e17518.
30. Nachega JB, Hislop M, Dowdy DW, *et al*: **Adherence to highly active antiretroviral therapy assessed by pharmacy claims predicts survival in HIV-infected South African adults.** *J Acquir Immune Defic Syndr* 2006, **43**(1):78–84.
31. Messou E, Chaix ML, Gabillard D, *et al*: **Association between medication possession ratio, virologic failure and drug resistance in HIV-1-infected adults on antiretroviral therapy in Cote d'Ivoire.** *J Acquir Immune Defic Syndr* 2011, **56**(4):356–364.
32. Dowshen N, D'Angelo L: **Health care transition for youth living with HIV/AIDS.** *Pediatrics* 2011, **128**(4):762–771.
33. Assoumou L, Descamps D, Yerly S, *et al*: **Prevalence of HIV-1 drug resistance in treated patients with viral load >50 copies/mL in 2009: a French nationwide study.** *J Antimicrob Chemother* 2013, **68**(6):1400–1405.
34. Nettles RE, Kieffer TL, Kwon P, *et al*: **Intermittent HIV-1 viremia (Blips) and drug resistance in patients receiving HAART.** *JAMA* 2005, **293**(7):817–829.
35. Lee PK, Kieffer TL, Siliciano RF, Nettles RE: **HIV-1 viral load blips are of limited clinical significance.** *J Antimicrob Chemother* 2006, **57**(5):803–805.
36. van Sighem A, Zhang S, Reiss P, *et al*: **Immunologic, virologic, and clinical consequences of episodes of transient viremia during suppressive combination antiretroviral therapy.** *J Acquir Immune Defic Syndr* 2008, **48**(1):104–108.
37. Hamers RL, Wallis CL, Kityo C, *et al*: **HIV-1 drug resistance in antiretroviral-naive individuals in sub-Saharan Africa after rollout of antiretroviral therapy: a multicentre observational study.** *Lancet Infect Dis* 2011, **11**(10):750–759.
38. Gupta RK, Jordan MR, Sultan BJ, *et al*: **Global trends in antiretroviral resistance in treatment-naive individuals with HIV after rollout of antiretroviral treatment in resource-limited settings: a global collaborative study and meta-regression analysis.** *Lancet* 2012, **380**(9849):1250–1258.
39. Hamers RL, Schuurman R, Sigaloff KC, *et al*: **Effect of pretreatment HIV-1 drug resistance on immunological, virological, and drug-resistance outcomes of first-line antiretroviral treatment in sub-Saharan Africa: a multicentre cohort study.** *Lancet Infect Dis* 2012, **12**(4):307–317.
40. Kuritzkes DR, Lalama CM, Ribaudo HJ, *et al*: **Preexisting resistance to nonnucleoside reverse-transcriptase inhibitors predicts virologic failure of an efavirenz-based regimen in treatment-naive HIV-1-infected subjects.** *J Infect Dis* 2008, **197**(6):867–870.
41. Wittkop L, Gunthard HF, de Wolf F, *et al*: **Effect of transmitted drug resistance on virological and immunological response to initial combination antiretroviral therapy for HIV (EuroCoord-CHAIN joint project): a European multicohort study.** *Lancet Infect Dis* 2011, **11**(5):363–371.
42. Hassan AS, Mwaringa SM, Obonyo CA, *et al*: **Low prevalence of transmitted HIV type 1 drug resistance among antiretroviral-naive adults in a Rural HIV clinic in Kenya.** *AIDS Res Hum Retroviruses* 2013, **29**(1):129–135.

3

Boosted protease inhibitor monotherapy in HIV-infected adults: outputs from a pan-European expert panel meeting

José R Arribas[1*], Manuela Doroana[2], Dan Turner[3], Linos Vandekerckhove[4], Adrian Streinu-Cercel[5] and on behalf of the panel members

Abstract

While the introduction of combination highly active antiretroviral therapy (HAART) regimens represents an important advance in the management of human immunodeficiency virus (HIV)-infected patients, tolerability can be an issue and the use of several different agents may produce problems. The switch of combination HAART to ritonavir-boosted protease inhibitor (PI) monotherapy may offer the opportunity to maintain antiviral efficacy while reducing treatment complexity and the risks of toxicity. Current European AIDS Clinical Society (EACS) guidelines recognise ritonavir-boosted PI monotherapy with twice-daily lopinavir/ritonavir or once-daily darunavir/ritonavir as a possible option in patients who have intolerance to nucleoside reverse transcriptase inhibitors, or for treatment simplification. Clinical trials data for PI boosted monotherapy are encouraging, showing substantial efficacy in the majority of patients; however, further data are required before this approach can be recommended as a routine treatment. Available data indicate that the most suitable candidates for the use of boosted PI monotherapy are long-term virologically suppressed patients who have demonstrated good adherence to antiretroviral therapy, who do not have chronic hepatitis B, have no history of treatment failure on PIs and are able to tolerate low-dose ritonavir.

Introduction

While the introduction of highly active antiretroviral therapy (HAART), typically involving three drugs in combination, has been an important advance in the treatment of people infected with human immunodeficiency type-1 virus (HIV-1), many patients do not remain on their original treatment regimen one year after starting HAART (EuroSIDA study; Figure 1) [1]. Common reasons for discontinuing HAART in chronically treated patients include patient/physician choice, treatment failure and tolerability issues such as renal and cardiovascular toxicity with nucleoside reverse transcriptase inhibitors (NRTIs), and, with the non-NRTIs (NNRTIs), dyslipidaemia with efavirenz and rash with nevirapine. Important developments for the future of HAART are to improve its potency and activity against multi-drug resistance viruses, to improve dosing schedules and their convenience, and to improve the tolerability of treatment.

It is relatively common for treatment regimens to be switched in fully suppressed HIV-1-infected patients. These regimen switches can be either proactive (to avoid potential problems) or reactive (in response to poor tolerability or other issues). For example, in pregnant women the regimen may be switched to avoid risk of teratogenicity and to optimise pharmacokinetics, while in other patients regimens may be switched to improve adherence or convenience, to preserve future treatment options, to avoid drug interactions or to reduce costs. Maintenance of virological control is paramount when switching therapies, and treatment switches in virologically suppressed patients was considered by the panel members to be one of the most common therapeutic interventions in HIV therapy in late 2011.

While intermittent therapy, sequential or prolonged treatment interruptions are no longer recommended as switch strategies by HIV treatment guidelines, [2] there remains a

* Correspondence: jrarribas.hulp@salud.madrid.org
[1]Consulta Medicina Interna 2, Hospital La Paz, IdiPAZ, Paseo de la Castellana 261, 28046, Madrid, Spain
Full list of author information is available at the end of the article

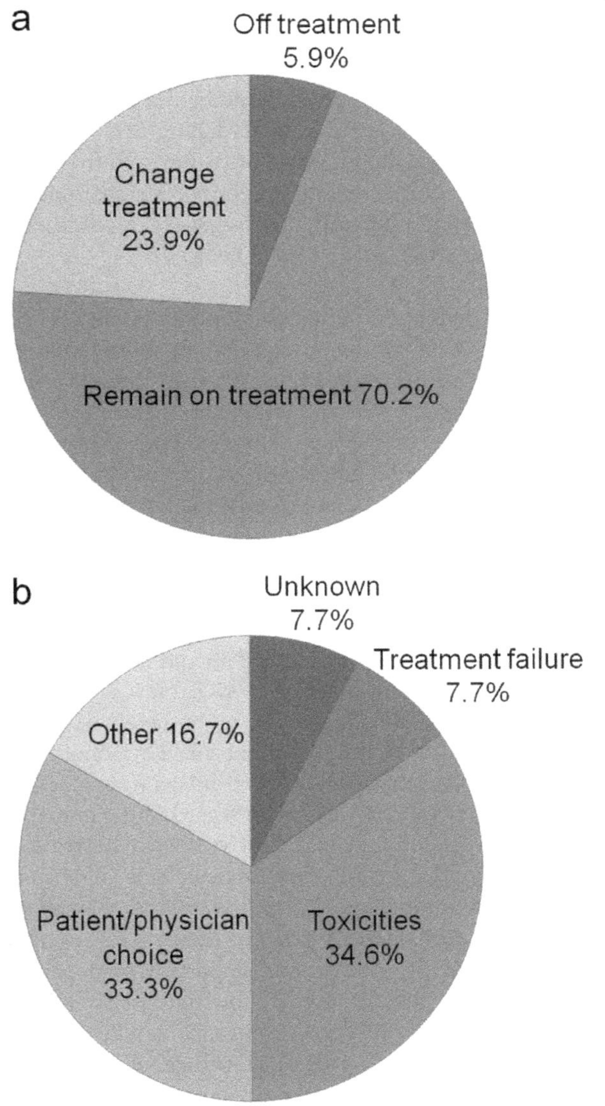

Figure 1 a) Proportion of patients remaining on original treatment regimen 1 year after initiating HAART; b) Reasons for discontinuing HAART between 2002–2004 [1].

variety of switch strategies for use in suppressed patients to deal with toxicity, to simplify treatment regimens and to try to meet patients' wishes for their treatment. These include reducing pill burden, ritonavir-sparing and so-called 'nuc' (NRTI)-sparing regimens. Among the various switching options available, the strategy of switching from a triple-drug regimen to ritonavir-boosted protease inhibitor (PI/r) monotherapy is currently a topic of some interest as it offers a number of potential benefits, including a reduction of NRTI-related toxicity (lipoatrophy, renal disease, bone mineral density [BMD] loss) and reduced cost versus dual or triple therapy while retaining other classes as future treatment options. This review provides an overview of the use of boosted PI monotherapy in Europe and the potential benefits and drawbacks of such therapy.

EACS 2011 guidelines on treatment switch strategies

The current European AIDS Clinical Society (EACS) guidelines for the management of HIV-infected patients list three principal indications for the use of switch strategies in virologically suppressed patients (plasma viral load < 50 HIV-1 RNA copies/mL) [2]:

- switch for toxicity – including documented toxicity, the management of potential drug interactions, side effects, and planned pregnancy
- switch for the prevention of long-term toxicity – including pre-emptive switching; ageing and/or co-morbidity with a possible negative impact of drug(s) in the current regimen (e.g. on cardiovascular risk and metabolic parameters)
- switch for simplification – including the wish to simplify the regimen or because the treatment regimen is no longer recommended.

The EACS 2011 guidelines state that PI/r monotherapy with lopinavir twice daily or darunavir once daily might represent an option in those patients intolerant to NRTIs, or for treatment simplification [2]. The guidelines note that this strategy only applies to patients without a history of failure on prior PI-based therapy and who have had viral load < 50 HIV-1 RNA copies/mL in at least the past 6 months. In considering a switch to boosted PI monotherapy, attention must also be given to the duration of virological suppression prior to the considered switch, to any pharmacokinetic/dynamic considerations, to the expected level of adherence and to the individual patient's needs. Boosted PI monotherapy should not be prescribed to patients co-infected with chronic hepatitis B.

In the USA, PI/r monotherapy is not recommended by the Department of Health and Human Services (DHHS) 2011 guidelines outside of the clinical trial setting, [3] and PI/r monotherapy is only recommended by the International AIDS Society-USA (IAS-USA) 2010 guidelines in exceptional circumstances when other drugs cannot be considered for reasons of toxicity/tolerability. Other treatment guidelines offer differing recommendations with respect to boosted PI monotherapy. At present only the EACS, [2] Italian [4] and Spanish Gesida guidelines [5] recognise PI/r monotherapy as a switch option in the everyday clinical setting. There is currently a lack of consensus in the treatment guidelines with respect to monotherapy. However, this situation may change as the results of ongoing clinical studies of PI/r monotherapy become available.

Current use of boosted PI monotherapy in Europe

At present, there is some variation in clinical practice with regard to the use of boosted PI monotherapy between European countries and regions (e.g. Italy where monotherapy tends to be only used at the larger treatment centres). It is thought there are several reasons for this variation. Some clinicians consider the number of patients included in monotherapy studies to be too few for drawing valid conclusions. It has been suggested that some clinicians could be detracted from initiating boosted PI monotherapy by potential legal implications. Finally, geographic variation may also arise from physicians being influenced by US guidelines and the presence of preexisting PI resistance.

Reasons for variability in the use of boosted PI monotherapy in Europe

Switching from triple-drug HAART regimens to boosted PI monotherapy offers benefits in terms of reduced complexity, the potential for a reduction in some toxicities (though longer-term data are required to more fully assess the tolerability profile of PI/r monotherapy versus HAART), and in terms of cost savings. However, as with any new treatment approach, there are a number of potential issues and concerns about boosted PI monotherapy and such concerns may at least in part account for the observed differences in the adoption of this approach across different European countries. There is evidence that boosted PI monotherapy for maintenance of viral suppression is less effective than triple-drug HAART [6]. However, the observed difference in efficacy between HAART and PI/r monotherapy is small and differences may be PI dependent. Furthermore, although there is an increased risk of low-level viraemia with monotherapy in a subgroup of patients, this has been shown to be reversible after NRTI reintroduction. Clinical trials with darunavir/r [7-9] and lopinavir/r [10] monotherapy have not shown an increased risk of resistance development.

Another potential drawback of PI/r monotherapy is that such regimens are 'less forgiving' of poor adherence than triple-drug regimens, so that a high level of adherence is required for patients switching to PI/r monotherapy. In this regard, clinical trials have shown an association between suboptimal adherence and virological failure in patients treated with lopinavir/r [11,12] or darunavir/r monotherapy [13]. It has been hypothesised that suboptimal adherence may have a greater effect on virological suppression in patients receiving boosted PI monotherapy than it does in those on combination therapy including nucleosides due to the short terminal half-lives of lopinavir and darunavir compared with the long intracellular half-lives of nucleosides [10,14]. It is in any case clear that, in addition to their having had a sufficient period of virological suppression on HAART (at least 6 months), candidates for PI/r monotherapy should demonstrate a history of good adherence to prescribed treatments. In acknowledging the importance of good treatment adherence for the success of boosted PI monotherapy it should be remembered that, as shown in clinical trials, patients failing PI/r monotherapy can be successfully treated with the re-introduction of nucleosides. In this regard, it is important that patients receiving PI/r monotherapy are regularly monitored to allow early detection of 'reversible failures'.

Selection of patients for boosted PI monotherapy

Perhaps the most pertinent question in considering the initiation of PI/r monotherapy is: who are the best candidates and how can we best identify them? The selection of patients and the subsequent demonstration of successful long-term PI/r monotherapy is likely to be critical in the consolidation of monotherapy as an accepted treatment approach. The authors of the MONOI study concluded that good candidates for PI/r monotherapy should have an undetectable viral load (HIV-1 RNA at least < 50 copies/mL) at the time of commencing monotherapy, should be more adherent than for triple therapy and should have been treated with antiretroviral therapy (ART) for a sufficient amount of time before switching to monotherapy [15].

While it is clear that it is important for PI/r monotherapy candidates to have a substantial period with an undetectable viral load, opinions differ with regard to the minimum duration of viral suppression. Most switching studies have used a 6-month period with undetectable viral load, primarily in order to demonstrate that existing therapy was effective prior to the switch and that the patient was adherent. Adherence to treatment is important, and patients who have been stable on HAART for some years and who have shown no signs of poor compliance would appear to be suitable, provided that there are no other factors that would preclude PI/r monotherapy, such as a history of PI failure. With regard to adherence, in MONOI, 48.5% of rebounding PI/r monotherapy patients admitted to having missed at least one treatment dose during follow-up versus 31.6% of other patients [15]. The median duration of prior ART treatment in rebounding PI/r monotherapy patients was 5.1 years versus 8.9 years in other patients.

With regards to pre-HAART HIV DNA, in MONOI the median HIV DNA was 4.2 $\log_{10}$ copies/10^6 cells in patients with virological rebound during 96 weeks of darunavir/r monotherapy (24/112 patients, 21.4%) versus 3.9 $\log_{10}$ copies/10^6 cells in other patients [15]. Furthermore, it was demonstrated (using ultrasensitive plasma RNA assay and quantification of total HIV DNA viraemia) that patients in the MONOI study with the lowest plasma RNA and total HIV DNA viraemia were the most suitable candidates for PI/r monotherapy [13,15].

CD4 cell count status is also an important factor when considering PI/r monotherapy initiation. Analyses to predict PI/r monotherapy failure have shown a significant association between a low baseline CD4 cell count nadir (< 100–200 cells/μL) and subsequent treatment failure [11,16]. Furthermore, in patients co-infected with hepatitis C virus, significantly lower virological response was observed versus non-co-infected patients [17], suggesting that hepatitis C co-infection, likely associated with intravenous drug use, might possibly be a marker of poor adherence.

Maintaining virological efficacy with boosted PI monotherapy

A key consideration for the adoption of boosted PI monotherapy is to achieve a consensus on what constitutes treatment success. It is also important to demonstrate that effective viral suppression can be maintained over the long term. It is worth noting that even with combination therapy, the current 'gold standard' for achieving durable viral suppression, isolated 'blips' (i.e. viral loads that are transiently detectable, but usually no more than 400 HIV-1 RNA copies/mL), are not uncommon in successfully treated patients, so some degree of fluctuation in viral load might also be expected with PI/r monotherapy. In addition to effective viral suppression, the success of treatment must also be defined in terms of its tolerability for the patient and the balance of efficacy/tolerability achieved in relation to other possible treatment approaches. While the success of triple-drug HAART in achieving viral suppression is clear, it is also clear that the long-term success of HAART has, in part, been limited by drug toxicities and drug interactions, as patients are exposed to multiple drugs for prolonged periods of time [18,19].

Although plasma HIV RNA < 50 copies/mL is today consistently considered as undetectable, treatment success has been defined differently across clinical trials e.g. different primary and secondary endpoints providing different power calculations and levels of confidence, as well as different analysis definitions (intent-to-treat [ITT]-time-to-loss of virological response [TLOVR] and TLOVR non-virological failure [VF] censored etc.). It is to be hoped that future studies will adopt similar criteria to assess efficacy and safety parameters for treatments to make it easier to compare their findings. Ideally, treatment decisions would be informed by access to long-term data from controlled clinical trials and cohort studies, but such data are unavailable for most individual treatments and regimens.

Defining treatment failure also remains challenging, with different guidelines offering different perspectives based on different evidence. The EACS guidelines define VF as a confirmed plasma HIV-1 RNA > 50 copies/mL six months after starting therapy (initiation or modification) in patients remaining on ART [2]. In contrast, the US DHHS guidelines define VF as a confirmed viral load > 200 HIV-1 RNA copies/mL, on the basis that it eliminates most cases of apparent viraemia caused by blips or assay variability [3]. However, given the range of viral load assays available, with different sensitivities, it remains possible that different results may be obtained with different assays, such that a patient might be judged to be 'borderline' but still successfully treated using one assay, but a 'failure' requiring consideration of a change in treatment using another assay.

While boosted PI monotherapy offers the potential for reduced toxicity, its adoption depends upon the demonstration of robust efficacy data. Available data show only a small difference in efficacy between triple-drug HAART and boosted PI monotherapy following treatment switch (Figure 2a [lopinavir/r] and 2b [darunavir/r]) and in the MONET study with darunavir/r monotherapy, effective viral suppression was maintained up to three years of treatment [20]. Of note, in the five patients with VF on darunavir/r monotherapy in the MONOI study, re-suppression of viral load (< 50 HIV-1 RNA copies/mL) was successfully achieved with the addition of two NRTIs to the treatment regimen. The emergence of PI resistance on PI/r monotherapy has been rare and re-introduction of HAART remains possible in such cases. It is also important to note that in the PI monotherapy trails reviewed, changes in CD4 cell counts between treatment arms were not considered significant [7,20,21]. In their systematic review of boosted PI monotherapy, Bierman *et al.* reported that mean CD4 cell counts ranged from −40 to +289 cells/μl in patients on monotherapy against +8 to +240 cells/μl in patients on HAART [21]. In summary, the available evidence indicates that, in a large proportion of patients, effective long-term virological control is possible with boosted PI monotherapy and if re-suppression is needed this can be achieved with the re-introduction of NRTIs.

The significance of detectable virus in sanctuary sites

While modern ART can provide effective plasma HIV-1 virus suppression, the importance of viral reservoirs in the genitals and central nervous system (CNS) remains the subject of debate. The principal issues surrounding these reservoirs are whether or not three drugs are still required to control HIV-1 replication in sanctuary sites when plasma HIV-1 RNA is fully suppressed, whether all boosted PIs sufficiently penetrate into the CNS to achieve effective long-term control, and whether boosted PI monotherapy controls HIV-1 RNA in the genital tract. Antiretroviral drug penetration may be important for preventing HIV-1 replication in the CNS, and observational studies have demonstrated a correlation between CNS penetration effectiveness rank (CPE) and HIV-1 levels in the cerebrospinal fluid (CSF) [22]. Further, darunavir/r and lopinavir/r monotherapy have lower CPE scores compared with triple therapy regimens [23]; although it should be noted that CPE score has yet not been validated.

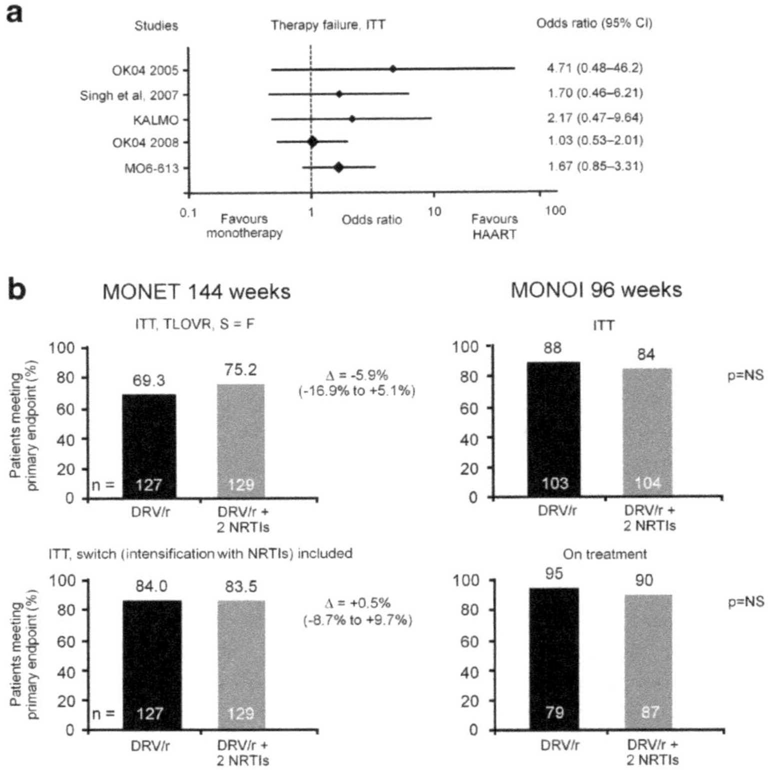

Figure 2 Efficacy of a) Lopinavir/r [21] and b) Darunavir/r monotherapy vs comparator arms [7,20]. Efficacy was assessed in the ITT population and modification of treatment was considered failure in the MONET and MONOI darunavir/r monotherapy trials [7,20]. In the lopinavir/r monotherapy trials [21], there was some variance in what was considered failure. In OK04 2005, treatment modification = failure. In OK04 2008, treatment modification ≠ failure. In KALMO failure was defined as confirmed HIV-1 RNA > 1,000 copies/mL. In MO6-613 non-responders were defined as those who either did not complete 96 weeks of treatment, had HIV-1 RNA at > 50 copies/mL at week 96, or experienced confirmed virological rebound before week 96.

It is thought that the presence of HIV-1 in the CNS results in neurotoxicity [23], with a number of clinical factors associated with its development, including depression, female gender, low CD4 count, advancing age and drug abuse [24,25]. Consequently, an important question is to what degree plasma viral suppression to < 50 HIV-1 RNA copies/mL translates into effective viral suppression in the CNS. It has been suggested that CSF viral load data could be obtained as part of the decision to initiate therapy. In this regard, in the CHARTER study, 96% of patients with undetectable plasma HIV-1 RNA on a triple regimen also had a suppressed CNS viral load [23], indicating that most patients on HAART have effective suppression of HIV-1 in the CNS.

Conversely, since NRTIs potentially have adverse effects on the CNS, monotherapy with boosted PIs have the possible advantage to the CNS of removal of NRTI toxicity. The NRTIs are known to penetrate the CNS and have been associated with improvements in cerebral function. However, administration of the NRTIs can also result in mitochondrial toxicities through CNS penetration. Indeed, several NRTIs have been shown to possess the potential to damage brain tissue and neurones [26,27]. Hence, the use of PI/r monotherapy could decrease some of the CNS toxicities associated with combination therapy.

The current EACS guidelines define potentially CNS-active drugs as antiretrovirals with either demonstrated clear CSF penetration when studied in HIV-infected populations (CSF concentration above the 90% inhibitory concentration [IC_{90}] in > 90% of examined patients), or with proven short-term (3–6 months) efficacy with respect to cognitive function or CSF viral load decay when evaluated as single agents or in controlled studies in peer reviewed papers. According to this definition, agents with demonstrated clear CSF penetration are the NRTIs zidovudine and abacavir, the NNRTIs efavirenz and nevirapine, the boosted PIs darunavir/r, lopinavir/r and indinavir/r, and the entry inhibitor maraviroc, while agents with 'proven efficacy' are the NRTIs zidovudine, stavudine and abacavir, and the boosted PI lopinavir/r [2].

With regard to the genital reservoir for HIV, in a MONOI sub-study investigating the penetration of darunavir into seminal fluid, darunavir seminal plasma concentration was 6-fold higher than the darunavir 50% effective concentration (EC_{50}) against wild-type HIV-1, with the median concentration close to the blood plasma free fraction [28]. In females, in the IMANI-2 study of lopinavir/r first-line monotherapy, lopinavir/r penetration into the cervicovaginal fluid exceeded the reference population median IC_{50} value in all but one sample tested [29].

The available data indicate that both darunavir and lopinavir show moderately good CNS penetration, with both showing high penetration into the genital tract. However, further studies are needed to confirm these findings.

Safety and tolerability benefits with boosted PI monotherapy

One of the main attractions of a switch from multi-drug HAART to boosted PI monotherapy is the potential safety benefit that may result from its use. The tolerability issues of NRTIs in particular are well known, these agents being associated with increased risk of insulin resistance, secondary dyslipidaemia and lipodystrophy/atrophy. Reduced BMD and renal disease may also result with some HAART regimens. Lipodystrophy seems to be associated with particular NRTIs, with regimens containing stavudine or zidovudine appearing to confer highest risk [30]. Data from the M03-613 study in treatment-naïve patients taking lopinavir/r (Figure 3a) and the MONOI trial with darunavir/r (Figure 3b) indicate that boosted PI monotherapy is not associated with the limb fat loss that is observed with some NRTIs [31,32], although longer-term tolerability data are required to confirm the findings.

When considering BMD, while there was a slightly greater decrease in BMD in lopinavir/r monotherapy-treated patients versus triple-therapy patients over 96 weeks in the M03-613 study, in the 48-week MONARCH study in 30 virologically suppressed patients, the switch to darunavir/r monotherapy was associated with a trend for improvement in BMD (and in body fat distribution with stable limb fat and a decrease in visceral adipose tissue) [33]. While long-term data are required, available data indicate that switching to boosted PI monotherapy does not adversely affect BMD. It should be noted, however, that

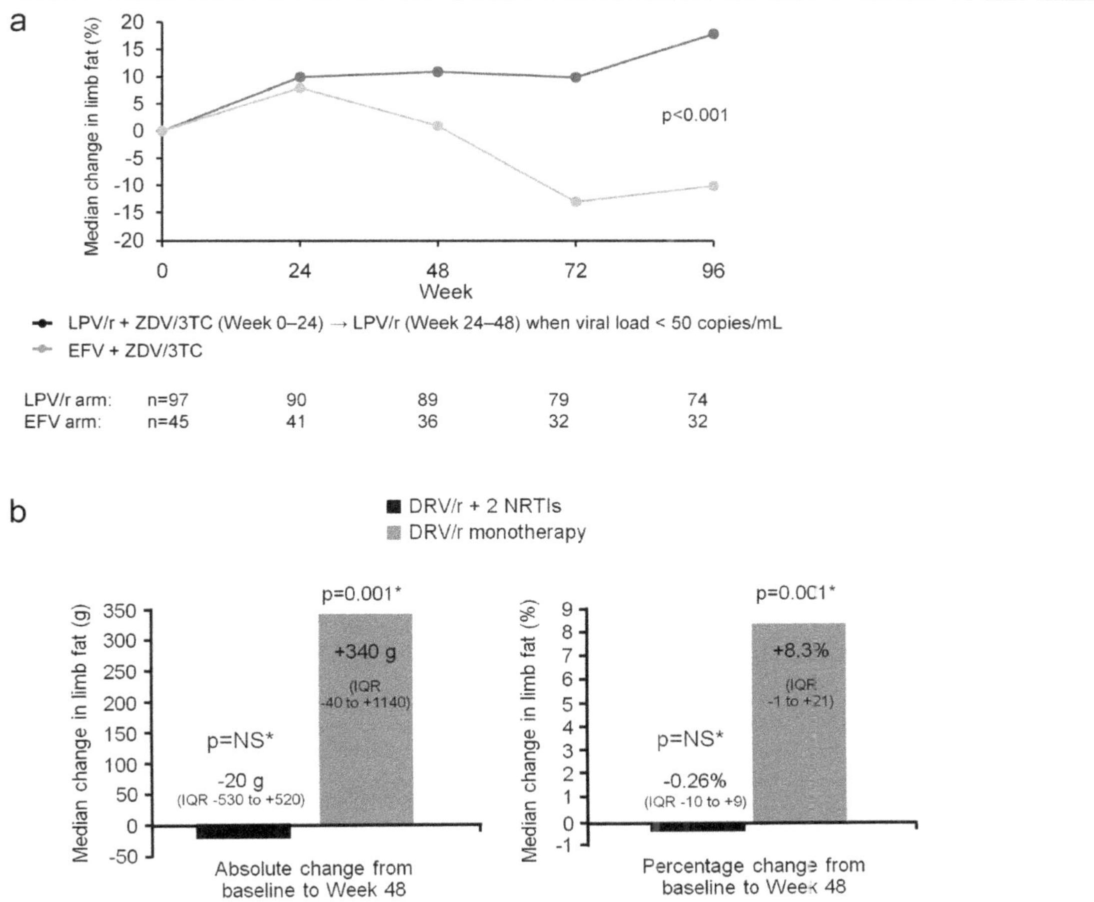

Figure 3 a) Abbott 613 trial: Changes in limb fat over time [30] **b)** MONOI: Median change in limb fat from baseline to week 48 [31].

there were greater increases in total and low density lipoprotein cholesterol with PI/r monotherapy versus triple therapy in MONARCH, though this may reflect the fact that some patients in the triple therapy arm were taking tenofovir, which has a direct lipid-lowering effect [34].

Renal toxicity is a well-recognised risk with tenofovir disoproxil fumarate therapy [35]. From this perspective, boosted PI monotherapy would appear to be a useful treatment option for patients with tenofovir-related renal disease. Finally, while concerns have been expressed about potential CSF viral escape with PI/r monotherapy, after 144 weeks of darunavir/r monotherapy in the MONET study there was no significant difference in the observed change in cognitive functioning between the mono- and triple therapy treatment groups (although the study was not powered to detect differences in neurologic impairment) [36].

Future development of boosted PI monotherapy: ongoing and planned studies

While available data indicate that the switch from multidrug HAART to boosted PI monotherapy in suitable patients represents an attractive treatment option, there remain some questions to be answered, in particular relating to long-term efficacy and tolerability, and efficacy in CNS and genital 'reservoirs' (although in the latter case this is also true for triple therapy).

Two ongoing studies of boosted PI monotherapy are expected to provide a wealth of new efficacy and tolerability data: PIVOT (PI monotherapy Vs Ongoing Triple-therapy in the long-term management of HIV infection) and PROTEA, (PROTEAse inhibitor [darunavir/r] in mono- or triple therapy in suppressed HIV-1-infected patients). The PIVOT trial planned to include 560 patients in the UK and be of 5 years' duration. Patients with a plasma viral load < 50 HIV-1 RNA copies/mL at screening (and for at least 24 weeks prior to screening) and a CD4 cell count > 100 cells/mm^3 are included in the study, which compares boosted PI monotherapy to combination HAART with two NRTIs and either an NNRTI or a PI (boosted or un-boosted). This study, which includes genital secretions and CNS sub-studies, will also measure effects on quality of life, neurocognitive function, cardiovascular risk and costs.

The phase IIIb PROTEA study is investigating the efficacy and tolerability of darunavir/r monotherapy versus darunavir/r-containing triple therapy in approximately 260 virologically suppressed (for at least 48 weeks) HIV-1-infected patients. The primary objective is to demonstrate the non-inferior efficacy of darunavir/r monotherapy (with respect to the percentage of patients with viral load < 50 HIV-1 RNA copies/mL at 48 weeks post-switch to monotherapy) versus triple therapy containing darunavir/r. This study will also assess changes in neurocognitive function over 48 and 96 weeks of treatment and whether there is any correlation between plasma and CSF viral load and neurocognitive function. In addition, PROTEA will study the evolution of the viral genotype and determine whether there is any loss of treatment options at weeks 48 and 96, as defined by the emergence of phenotypic drug resistance.

Summary and conclusions

The switch from triple-drug combination therapy to boosted PI monotherapy appears to be a promising strategy to maintain antiviral efficacy. Available data from PI/r monotherapy trials are encouraging, showing slightly lower efficacy than triple therapy regimens. However, further data – particularly with regard to the long-term efficacy and tolerability of treatment – are required before this approach can be recommended as a routine treatment option. In this regard, further studies are ongoing, which will further elucidate the long-term utility of boosted PI monotherapy. In the meantime, the available data indicate that the most suitable candidates for the use of boosted PI monotherapy are long-term virologically suppressed patients who have demonstrated good adherence to ART, have no history of PI failure, do not have chronic hepatitis B, do not have HIV-associated neurocognitive disorders and who are able to tolerate low dose ritonavir.

Abbreviations

ART: antiretroviral therapy; BMD: bone mineral density; CNS: central nervous system; CPE: CNS penetration effectiveness rank; CSF: cerebrospinal fluid; DHHS: Department of Health and Human Services; EACS: European AIDS Clinical Society; EC: effective concentration; HAART: highly active ART; HIV: human immunodeficiency virus; IAS-USA: International AIDS Society-USA; IC: inhibitory concentration; ITT: intent-to-treat; NNRTI: non-nucleoside reverse transcriptase inhibitor; NRTI: nucleoside reverse transcriptase inhibitor; PI: protease inhibitor; TLOVR: time to loss of virological response; VF: virological failure.

Competing interests

Professor JR Arribas has received advisory fees, speaker fees and grant support from the following sources: Abbott, Bristol-Myers Squibb, Gilead, Janssen, MSD, Tibotec and ViiV Healthcare. Dr M Doroana has received speaker fees from different sources: Gilead, Roche, Janssen and Abbott. Dr D Turner has received honoraria from the following sources: Abbott, Biotis, GlaxoSmithKline, Janssen, MSD, Neopharm, Roche and Schering-Plough. Professor L Vandekerckhove has received advisory fees, speaker fees and grant support from the following sources: Gilead, Janssen, MSD, Bristol-Myers Squibb, Pfizer and ViiV Healthcare. Professor A Streinu Cercel has relationships with all major pharmaceutical companies but without any specific arrangements.

Authors' contributions

All authors substantially contributed to development of all drafts of the manuscript and have read and approved the final draft. The corresponding author had full access to the source literature and takes full responsibility for the content of the paper and for the decision to submit.

Authors' information

Panel members: Professor José Arribas (Spain); Professor Giovanni Di Perri (Italy); Professor Pierre-Marie Girard (France); Dr Alan Winston (UK); Professor Hans-Jürgen Stellbrink (Germany); Professor Adrian Streinu-Cercel (Romania); Professor Linos Vandekerckhove (Belgium); Professor Adriano Lazzarin (Italy); Dr Dan Turner (Israel); Dra Manuela Doroana (Portugal); Dr Esteban Martinez (Spain); Dr Markus Bickel (Germany); Dr Panagiotis Kollaras (Greece); Dr

George Panos (Greece); Dr Giovanni Guaraldi (Italy); Professor Sorin Rugina (Romania); Professor Carmen Dorobat (Romania); Dr Dan Duiculescu (Romania).

Acknowledgements

This clinical review reflects the detailed discussion and opinions of the authors on data and literature reviewed at an expert panel meeting on the use of ritonavir-boosted protease inhibitor monotherapy, held in Bucharest, Romania in November 2011. The meeting was supported by Janssen Pharmaceutica N.V., however the content of this paper does not necessarily reflect the opinions of the meeting sponsor.

Medical writing support was provided by Karen Pilgram, Gardiner-Caldwell Communications (funded by Janssen Pharmaceutica N.V.), who developed the first draft of the manuscript based on the debate and discussions during the meeting.

Author details

[1]Consulta Medicina Interna 2, Hospital La Paz, IdiPAZ, Paseo de la Castellana 261, 28046, Madrid, Spain. [2]Serviço de Doenças Infecciosas, Hospital de Santa Maria, Av Prof Egas Moniz, 1649-035, Lisbon, Portugal. [3]Infectious Diseases Unit, Tel-Aviv Sourasky Medical Center, 6 Weizmann Street, Tel-Aviv 64239, Israel. [4]AIDS Reference Centre, Ghent University Hospital, De Pintelaan 185, 9000, Ghent, Belgium. [5]HIV/AIDS Academy, Str Dr Calistrat Grozovici, Nr 1, 021105, Bucharest, Romania.

References

1. Mocroft A, Phillips AN, Soriano V, *et al*: **Reasons for stopping antiretrovirals used in an initial highly active antiretroviral regimen: increased incidence of stopping due to toxicity or patient/physician choice in patients with hepatitis C coinfection.** *AIDS Res Hum Retroviruses* 2005, **21**:527–536.
2. **European AIDS Clinical Society (EACS) guidelines. Version 6.1. November 2011.** [http://www.europeanaidsclinicalsociety.org/index.php?option=com_content&view=article&id=59&Itemid=41].
3. **DHHS Guidelines for the use of antiretroviral agents in HIV-1-infected adults and adolescents (14 October 2010).** [http://www.aidsinfo.nih.gov/contentfiles/lvguidelines/adultandadolescentgl.pdf].
4. **Aggiornate le linee guida sull'utilizzo degli antiretrovirali nelle persone con infezione HIV-1 (18 luglio 2012).** [http://www.salute.gov.it/hiv/newsHiv.jsp?id=2106&menu=inevidenza&lingua=italiano].
5. **Documento de consenso de Gesida/Plan Nacional sobre el Sida respecto al tratamiento antirretroviral en adultos infectados por el virus de la inmunodeficiencia humana (Actualización enero 2012).** [http://www.gesida-seimc.org/pcientifica/fuentes/DcyRc/gesidadcyrc2012-Documentoconsenso-TAR-adulto-verordenador.pdf].
6. Mathis S, Khanlari B, Pulido F, *et al*: **Effectiveness of protease inhibitor monotherapy versus combination antiretroviral maintenance therapy: a meta-analysis.** *PLoS One* 2011, **6**:e22003.
7. Valantin M, Duvivier C, Lambert C, *et al*: **Long-Term Efficacy of Darunavir/ritonavir Monotherapy in patients with HIV-1 viral suppression in the MONOI-ANRS 136 study: Results at 96 Weeks.** CROI 2011. Abstract P534.
8. Katlama C, Valantin MA, Algarte-Genin M, *et al*: **Efficacy of darunavir/ritonavir maintenance monotherapy in patients with HIV-1 viral suppression: a randomized, open-label, noninferiority trial, MONOI-ANRS 136.** *AIDS* 2010, **24**:2365–2374.
9. Pulido F, Arribas JR, Hill A, Van Delft Y, Moecklinghoff C: **Analysis of drug resistance during HIV RNA viraemia in the MONET trial of darunavir/ritonavir monotherapy.** *Antivir Ther* 2011, **16**:59–65.
10. Arribas JR, Pulido F, Delgado R, *et al*: **Lopinavir/ritonavir as single-drug therapy for maintenance of HIV-1 viral suppression: 48-week results of a randomized, controlled, open-label, proof-of-concept pilot clinical trial (OK Study).** *J Acquir Immune Defic Syndr* 2005, **40**:280–287.
11. Pulido F, Pérez-Valero I, Delgado R, *et al*: **Risk factors for loss of virological suppression in patients receiving lopinavir/ritonavir monotherapy for maintenance of HIV suppression.** *Antivir Ther* 2009, **14**:195–201.
12. Campo RE, Da Silva BA, Cotte L, *et al*: **Predictors of loss of virologic response in subjects who simplified to lopinavir/ritonavir monotherapy from lopinavir/ritonavir plus zidovudine/lamivudine.** *AIDS Res Hum Retroviruses* 2009, **25**:269–275.
13. Lambert-Niclot S, Flandre P, Valantin MA, *et al*: **Factors associated with virological failure in HIV-1-infected patients receiving darunavir/ritonavir monotherapy.** *J Infect Dis* 2011, **204**:1211–1216.
14. Nunes EP, Santini de Oliveira M, Merçon M, *et al*: **Monotherapy with Lopinavir/Ritonavir as maintenance after HIV-1 viral suppression: results of a 96-week randomized, controlled, open-label, pilot trial (KalMo study).** *HIV Clin Trials* 2009, **10**:368–374.
15. Marcelin AG, Lambert-Niclot S, Peytavin G, *et al*: **Baseline HIV RNA ultrasensitive assay and viral DNA predict rise in plasma viral load in patients of MONOI-ANRS 136 trial (DRV/r monotherapy vs 2 NRTI + DRV/r).** CROI 2011. Poster 533.
16. Gutmann C, Cusini A, Günthard HF, *et al*: **Randomized controlled study demonstrating failure of LPV/r monotherapy in HIV: the role of compartment and CD4-nadir.** *AIDS* 2010, **24**:2347–2354.
17. Arribas JR, Montes ML, Prakash M, *et al*: **The MONET trial: correlation between hepatitis C co-infection and HIV RNA responses during darunavir/ritonavir monotherapy, for patients with HIV RNA <50 copies/mL at baseline.** ISHEID 2010. Abstract O-15.
18. Bisson G, Gross R, Miller V, *et al*: **Monitoring of long-term toxicities of HIV treatments: an international perspective.** *AIDS* 2003, **17**:2407–2417.
19. DAD Study Group: **Class of antiretroviral drugs and the risk of myocardial infarction.** *N Engl J Med* 2007, **356**:1723–1735.
20. Arribas JR, Clumeck N, Nelson M, *et al*: **The MONET trial: Week 144 analysis of efficacy of darunavir/ritonavir monotherapy versus DRV/r + 2 NRTIs, for patients with HIV RNA <50 copies/mL at baseline.** 6th IAS Conference on HIV Pathogenesis, Treatment and Prevention 2011. Abstract MOPE216.
21. Bierman WF, van Agtmael MA, Nijhuis M, Danner SA, Boucher CA: **HIV monotherapy with ritonavir-boosted protease inhibitors: a systematic review.** *AIDS* 2009, **23**:279–291.
22. Letendre S, Marquie-Beck J, Capparelli E, *et al*: **Validation of the CNS penetration-effectiveness rank for quantifying antiretroviral penetration into the central nervous system.** *Arch Neurol* 2008, **65**:65–70.
23. Letendre S, FitzSimons C, Ellis R, *et al*: **Correlates of CSF viral loads in 1221 volunteers of the CHARTER cohort.** CROI 2010. Abstract 172.
24. McArthur JC: **HIV dementia: an evolving disease.** *J Neuroimmunol* 2004, **157**:3–10.
25. Arribas J, Hill A: **Neurocognitive disorders during antiretroviral treatment, despite full HIV RNA suppression.** *HIV Ther* 2010, **4**:257–260.
26. Schweinsburg BC, Taylor MJ, Alhassoon OM, *et al*: **Brain mitochondrial injury in human immunodeficiency virus-seropositive (HIV+) individuals taking nucleoside reverse transcriptase inhibitors.** *J Neurovirol* 2005, **11**:356–364.
27. Perez-Valero I, Bayon C, Cambron I, Gonzales A, Arribas JR: **Protease inhibitor monotherapy and the CNS: peace of mind?** *J Antimicrob Chemother* 2011, **66**:1954–1962.
28. Lambert-Niclot S, Peytavin G, Duvivier C, *et al*: **Low frequency of intermittent HIV-1 semen excretion in patients treated with darunavir-ritonavir at 600/100 milligrams twice a day plus two nucleoside reverse transcriptase inhibitors or monotherapy.** *Antimicrob Agents Chemother* 2010, **54**:4910–4913.
29. Yeh RF, Hammill HA, Fiscus SA, *et al*: **Single Agent Therapy (SAT) with lopinavir/ritonavir (LPV/r) controls HIV-1 viral replication in the female genital tract.** EACS 2007. Abstract P7.7/02.
30. Martin A, Smith DE, Carr A, *et al*: **Reversibility of lipoatrophy in HIV-infected patients 2 years after switching from a thymidine analogue to abacavir: the MITOX Extension Study.** *AIDS* 2004, **18**:1029–1036.
31. Cameron DW, da Silva BA, Arribas JR, *et al*: **A 96-week comparison of lopinavir-ritonavir combination therapy followed by lopinavir-ritonavir monotherapy versus efavirenz combination therapy.** *J Infect Dis* 2008, **198**:234–240.
32. Valantin M, Flandre P, Kolta S, *et al*: **Fat tissue distribution changes in HIV-infected patients with viral suppression treated with darunavir/ritonavir (DRV/r) monotherapy versus 2 NRTI + DRV/r in the MONOI-ANRS 136 randomized trial: results at 48 Weeks.** CROI 2010. Abstract 721.
33. Guaraldi G, Zona S, Cossarizza A, *et al*: **Impact of switching to darunavir/ritonavir monotherapy vs. triple-therapy on body fat redistribution and bone mass in virologically suppressed HIV-infected adults. The MONARCH randomized trial.** EACS 2011. Poster PE7.5/4.
34. Rieger A, Banhegyi D, Schmidt W, *et al*: **The MONET trial 96 week analysis: darunavir/ritonavir monotherapy versus DRV/r + 2NRTIs, for patients with HIV RNA < 50 copies/mL at baseline.** IAC 2010. Abstract THLBB209.

4

In vivo effect of statins on the expression of the HIV co-receptors CCR5 and CXCR4

Edwin A Higuita[1*], Fabián A Jaimes[2,3], Maria T Rugeles[1] and Carlos J Montoya[1]

Abstract

Background: During the HIV-1 replication cycle, several molecules including chemokine receptors and cholesterol are crucial, and are therefore potential targets for therapeutic intervention. Indeed statins, compounds that inhibit cellular synthesis of cholesterol and have anti-inflammatory and immunomodulatory properties were shown to inhibit HIV-1 infection by R5 tropic strains but not by X4 strains in vitro, mainly by altering the chemokine receptor/ligands axes. Therefore, the objective of this study was to characterize in vivo, the capacity of statins to modulate in HIV seronegative and chronically HIV-1-infected adults the expression of CCR5 and CXCR4, of their ligands and the tropism of circulating HIV-1 strains.

Methods: Samples from asymptomatic HIV-1-infected adults enrolled in a clinical trial aimed at evaluating the antiretroviral activity of lovastatin were used to evaluate in vivo the modulation by lovastatin of CCR5, CXCR4, their ligands, and the shift in plasma viral tropism over one year of intervention. In addition, ten HIV negative adults received a daily oral dose of 40 mg of lovastatin or 20 mg of atorvastatin; seven other HIV negative individuals who received no treatment were followed as controls. The frequency and phenotype of immune cells were determined by flow-cytometry; mRNA levels of chemokine receptors and their ligands were determined by real-time PCR. Viral tropism was determined by PCR and sequencing, applying the clonal and clinical model of analyses.

Results: Our study shows that long-term administration of lovastatin in HIV-infected individuals does not induce a shift in viral tropism, or induce a significant modulation of CCR5 and CXCR4 on immune cells in HIV-infected patients. Similar results were found in HIV seronegative control subjects, treated with lovastatin or atorvastatin, but a significant increase in CCL3 and CCL4 transcription was observed in these individuals.

Conclusions: These findings suggest that long-term administration of statins at therapeutic doses, does not significantly affect the expression of HIV-1 co-receptors or of their ligands. In addition it is important to point out that based on the results obtained, therapeutic administration of statins in HIV-infected patients with lipid disorders is safe in terms of selecting X4 strains.

Keywords: HIV infection, Statins, CCR5, CXCR4, Viral tropism, Chemokines

Background

Despite the fact that highly active antiretroviral therapy (HAART) is a clinically accepted and cost-effective intervention [1], its efficiency is hampered by limitations in therapy adherence and the emergence of viral resistance, facts closely related to adverse effects and toxicity [2,3]. Thus, it is necessary to develop new medications and therapeutic strategies, with novel mechanisms of action to overcome the limitations of HAART.

HIV infection involves an initial interaction between the viral envelope glycoprotein gp120 and the CD4 molecule on the surface of target cells, followed by a second interaction with a co-receptor; for HIV-1, the classical co-receptor function is provided by one of two different molecules, the C-C chemokine receptor 5 (CCR5) or the C-X-C chemokine receptor 4 (CXCR4), which have a normal physiological function serving as receptors for soluble chemokines [4,5]. The critical role of these molecules in HIV infection encouraged the design of anti-HIV drugs aimed at blocking this molecular interaction [6-8]. Some molecules with ability to exert a

* Correspondence: andreshiguitad@gmail.com
[1]Immunovirology Group, School of Medicine, University of Antioquia, Medellin, Colombia
Full list of author information is available at the end of the article

non-competitive, allosteric, inhibition of the CCR5 receptor have been identified; among them, maraviroc is the first CCR5 antagonist approved for clinical use in HIV-infected patients, and its efficiency has been established in clinical trials [9,10]. However, before receiving maraviroc, it is mandatory to first identify the co-receptor used by the strains infecting each patient, due to the risk on selecting the more pathogenic strains that use the CXCR4 co-receptor.

On the other hand, almost every aspect of the HIV-1 life cycle relies on cholesterol [11-16]; in the absence of this lipid, the attachment of HIV-1 to its host cells is severely impaired because the clustering of HIV-1 receptor/co-receptor in lipid rafts is hindered [17-19], and the conformational status and functions of CCR5 and CXCR4 are critically affected [18]. Indeed, in vitro studies have demonstrated that, in the absence of cholesterol, virus-cell fusion is greatly diminished, viral transcytosis is inhibited, production and budding of viral particles are reduced, and cell signaling is altered [12,20,21]. Cellular synthesis of cholesterol may be effectively inhibited by statins, medications that are competitive analogues of the substrate of the 3-hydroxy-3-methylglutaryl coenzyme A (HMG-CoA) reductase, an enzyme that catalyzes the conversion of hydroxyl-methyl-glutarate into mevalonic acid, a precursor for the biosynthesis of cholesterol and isoprenoids [22-24]. Moreover, a previous in vitro study demonstrated that CD4+ T-cell incubation with statins reduced the level of CCR5 expression in these cells isolated from HIV negative individuals, while it increased the secretion of its natural ligand, RANTES (CCL5), thereby inhibiting HIV-1 infection by R5 tropic strains but no by X4 strains [25]. Consequently, it is important to verify if this effect is reproducible in vivo, mainly because statins are safe medications with other anti-inflammatory and immunomodulatory properties, that could be of potential benefit in the treatment of HIV-1-infected individuals [26-30].

Nevertheless, a therapy with medications that inhibit the surface expression of CCR5 in the absence of complete control of HIV replication, could promote the positive selection of X4 strains of HIV, considered more pathogenic [31-33]. Thus, it is important to determine if the in vivo administration of statins promotes a change in viral tropism with a shift from R5 to X4 strains of HIV-1, as this might alter the natural course of HIV-1 infection and increase the risk of rapid progression to AIDS.

This study was aimed at characterizing the in vivo capacity of statins to modulate, in HIV seronegative and chronically HIV-1 infected adults, the following parameters: i) expression of the HIV-1 co-receptors CCR5 and CXCR4, ii) levels of their ligands RANTES (CCL5), MIP-1α (CCL3), MIP-1β (CCL4) and SDF-1 (CXCL12), and iii) tropism of circulating HIV-1 strains.

Methods

Subjects of study

Samples from chronic asymptomatic HIV-1-infected adults enrolled in a randomized clinical trial aimed at determining the antiretroviral and immunomodulatory activity of lovastatin (LIVE study, NCT00721305) [34], were used to evaluate in vivo the modulation by lovastatin of: i) CCR5 and CXCR4 expression on peripheral blood mononuclear cells (PBMC; lovastatin group n = 41; placebo group n = 43), and ii) the shift in plasma viral tropism throughout one year of intervention (lovastatin n = 44; placebo n = 47). These patients were HAART naïve, had a detectable viral load (>50 and <100.000 RNA copies/ml) and CD4+ T-cell counts higher than 350 cells/μl; the exclusion criteria were previously defined [35].

HIV negative adults, were invited to receive a daily supervised oral dose of lovastatin (40 mg/d, n = 10) or atorvastatin (20 mg/d, n = 9); seven other individuals received no intervention but had the same follow-up as the intervened HIV negative controls for the steady state variation in the expression of the HIV-1 co-receptors.

The study was conducted in accordance with the Declaration of Helsinki, and the protocol was approved by the Institutional Ethical Review Board of the University of Antioquia. All participants provided signed informed consent, prepared according to the Colombian legislation (Resolution 008430 of 1993), before participating in the study.

Statins

Tablets of lovastatin (20 mg), atorvastatin (20 mg) and placebo were kindly provided by Laproff Laboratories (Sabaneta, Colombia). The daily dose of these interventions was administered after the last meal at night, for 45 days in HIV negative controls and 360 days in HIV-infected patients from the LIVE study. The biological activity, safety and tolerance of statins were controlled by clinical evaluation, pharmacotherapeutic follow-up by a pharmacist, and by periodic testing of liver enzymes, creatine phosphokinase (CPK) and creatinine, and by performing a serum lipid profile. The intervention was stopped in the presence of any serious adverse drug event, a three-fold increase in serum hepatic aminotransferases or a five-fold increase in CPK.

Flow cytometry protocols

The frequency and surface phenotype of CD4+ T cells and CD3-/CD4+ monocytes in whole peripheral blood samples were determined by flow cytometry; fluorochrome-labeled mouse monoclonal antibodies (mAbs) against human molecules were from Becton Dickinson (BD, San Jose, CA): CD3 FITC (clone HIT3a), CD4 APC (clone RPA-T4), CD184 PE-Cy5 (clone 12G5), CD195 PE-Cy5 (clone 2D7/CCR5) and the corresponding isotype control antibodies. Briefly, 150 μl of blood were incubated with specific mAbs for 25 min at room temperature in the dark; the erythrocytes were then lysed by incubating for 10 min with 2 ml of 1X Facs lysing solution (Becton Dickinson). The cells were washed twice with 2 ml of cold phosphate-buffered saline (PBS) and fixed with 250 ml of 2% paraformaldehyde. All the preparations were stored at 4°C until acquisition in the cytometer FACS CANTO-II (Becton Dickinson).

Acquisition analyses were performed using the BD FACSDiva, version 6.1.2. Lymphocyte and monocyte gates, identified by side (SSC) versus forward (FSC) light scatter, were used to analyze cell populations identified as $CD3^+/CD4^+$ and $CD3^{-}/CD4^+$ cells, respectively; the surface expression of CCR5 and CXCR4 molecules was analyzed in each cell population; dead cells were excluded from the analysis through SSC vs. FSC.

CD4+ T cell isolation and real time PCR

PBMCs were isolated from heparin anti-coagulated peripheral blood by centrifugation in a Ficoll-Hypaque (Sigma, MO) gradient; CD4+ T lymphocytes were obtained by negative selection using the CD4+ T cell isolation kit II (Miltenyi Biotech, Auburn, CA), according to manufacturer's instructions. From these CD4+ T lymphocytes, total RNA was extracted using the Quiagen RNA tissue extraction kit (Quiagen, CA) following the manufacturer's instructions. The amount and purity of the RNA were determined by spectrometry at 260/280 nm. Total RNA was treated with DNase-I (Fermentas, St. Leon-Rot, Germany), and the DNA copy was synthesized using the RevertAid™ First Strand cDNA Synthesis kit (Fermentas®, Thermo Fisher Scientific, MA), according to manufacturer's instructions.

For real time PCR, each 20 µl of mixture consisted of 0.5 µl of cDNA, 10 µl SYBR® Green PCR Master Mix (Invitrogen, CA) and primers (0.4 µM each). The primer sequences for CCR5, CXCR4, CCL3 (MIP-1alpha), CCL4 (MIP-1beta), CCL5 (RANTES), and CXCL12 (SDF-1) were designed using the PrimerBlast Tool (NCBI web site http://www.ncbi.nlm.nih.gov/). The target for each of this set of primers is directed against exon junctions, to avoid amplifying unspliced mRNA and/or genomic DNA (Table 1); the same cycling profiles were used for all sets of primers according to the SYBR® Green PCR Master Mix instructions (50°C for 2 min, followed by 95°C for 10 min and 40 cycles of 95°C for 15 sec and 60°C for 1 min).

Glyceraldehyde 3-phosphate dehydrogenase (GAPDH) amplification was used to normalize the RNA content of the corresponding transcripts analyzed, and the result was expressed as relative units of transcription ($1.8^{[\Delta Ct \text{ Target gene} - \Delta Ct \text{ GAPDH}]}$). We included a melting curve to confirm the specificity of the PCR product. All real-time RT-PCR amplifications were performed using the CFX96 real-time system and data analysis using the software CFX Manager Version: 1.5.534.0511 (Bio-Rad, Hercules, CA).

Determination of viral tropism

Predictions of co-receptor usage by HIV strains have shown comparable results when performed using either plasma virus or proviral sequences [36]. Genomic DNA was isolated from PBMCs at months 0 and 12 of lovastatin or placebo treatment; briefly, PBMCs were washed twice with PBS and incubated overnight with White Cells Lysis Buffer (Tris–HCl 0.02 M; EDTA 0.02 M; NaCl 0.02 M; SDS 0.2%), and the genomic DNA was isolated using the phenol–chloroform technique. The amount and purity of the DNA samples were determined by spectrometry at 260/280 nm.

For proviral HIV-1 amplification, a nested PCR technique was used as previously described [37]. In the first round, the reaction mixture of 25 µl included 0.5 µg of genomic DNA, 0.4 nM of primer ED3, 0.4 nM of primer

Table 1 Primer pair sequences to detect expression of CCR5, CXCR4, CCL3, CCL4, CCL5 and CXCL12

Primer name	Target mRNA	Primer sequence 5'-3'	Product size (bp)
CCR5F	Exon 2a CCR5	TGATTTGCACAGCTCATCTGGCCA	169
CCR5R	Exon 3 CCR5	CGGGCTGCGATTTGCTTCACATT	
CXCR4F	Exon 1 CXCR4	AGTGACGCCGAGGGCCTGAG	150
CXCR4R	Exon 2b CXCR4	ACGGAAACAGGGTTCCTTCATGGA	
CCL3F	Exon 1 CCL3	CTCTGCAACCAGTTCTCTGCATCA	151
CCL3R	Exon 2/3 junction CCL3	TGGTTAGGAAGATGACACCGGGCT	
CCL4F	Exon 1 CCL4	CTGCCTTCTGCTCTCCAGCG	134
CCL4R	Exon 2 CCL4	GGAGCAGAGGCTGCTGGTCT	
CCL5F	Exon 1 CCL5	CCATGAAGGTCTCCGCGGCA	126
CCL5R	Exon 2 CCL5	GTGGGCGGGCAATGTAGGCAA	
CXCL12F	Exon 2/3b junction CXCL12	CCCTTCAGATTGTAGCCCGGCTG	209
CXCL12R	Exon 3b CXCL12	CTCATGGTTAAGGCCCCCTCCCC	

ED14, and 12.5 μl of 2X PCR Master Mix (Fermentas® Thermo Fisher Scientific, MA). For the second round of PCR, the same proportion of reactants was used for a reaction of 50 μl including the primers ED31 and ED33. In both PCR rounds, the reaction was subjected to a prePCR: 94°C for 3 min, followed by 4 cycles at 94°C for 60 sec, and 55°C for 60 sec. Then, 32 PCR cycles at 94°C for 15 sec, 55°C for 45 sec and 72°C for 60 sec, and a final extension at 72°C for 7 min were performed.

An aliquot of 5 μl of the product of this nested PCR were electrophoresed in 2% agarose, stained with SYBR safe® (Invitrogen, CA), and visualized under UV light for the detection of a band of 550 bp. The remaining product was shipped to Macrogen (Macrogen Inc. Seoul, Korea) to be sequenced using the ED31 and ED33 primers (forward and reverse sequences, respectively).

The contigs were assembled using the Seqman™ II software version 5.01 (DNAStar Inc., Madison, WI) and the sequences obtained, including the V3 loop portion of gp120, served to predict the viral tropism using both the clonal and clinical (CCR5 Δ32 genotype, viral load, CD4+ T cell percentage and count, and CD8+ T cell count) approximations, by means of the geno2pheno (G2P) prediction algorithm (http://coreceptor.bioinf.mpi-inf.mpg.de/index.php). The reported false positive rate (FPR) was used as quantitative output and set to 20% [38].

Data analysis

The overall activity of lovastatin vs. placebo in HIV-infected individuals was established by intention to-treat analysis. The frequency of positive cells and the mean fluorescence intensity of CXCR4 and CCR5 on CD4+ T lymphocytes at 0, 6 and 12 months after the intervention were compared by Generalized Estimating Equations (GEE) for repeated measurements, and informed as estimated average changes (EAC) with 95% Confidence Interval (CI). The frequency of positive cells and the mean fluorescence intensity of CXCR4 and CCR5 on CD4+ T lymphocytes from HIV negative controls at days 0, 7, 30 and 45 were compared by the one way Anova test for paired samples. The mean fluorescence intensity of CXCR4 and CCR5 on CD4+ T lymphocytes from asymptomatic HIV-1 infected patients vs. negative controls was compared by the Student´s t-test. The transcriptional levels of HIV co-receptors and their ligands during 45 days of oral administration of statins were compared by the one way Anova test for paired samples. The Fisher exact test was used to compare the frequency of X4 strains after one year of treatment in placebo- vs. lovastatin-treated groups. In all the comparisons, a value of $p < 0.05$ was considered statistically significant.

Results

Lovastatin administration does not induce a shift in HIV tropism

To determine the in vivo effect of lovastatin on the shift in viral tropism in HIV-1 infected subjects, a total of 91 DNA samples corresponding to month 0, and of 72 DNA samples corresponding to month 12 after daily administration of lovastatin, were amplified and sequenced. However, only 61 samples were paired (from the same patients at months 0 and 12) due to negative Env PCR amplification or low quality of the sequence obtained; 52.5% vs. 47.5% of the samples were from lovastatin and placebo patients, respectively. As shown in Table 2, using the clinical model of analysis, at baseline level, eight patients in the lovastatin treated group (18,1%) and eight (17,0%) in the placebo group were found with X4 X4/R5 circulating virus, and all were predicted to belong to the HIV-1 subtype B. A total shift in viral tropism of 15.6% in lovastatin-treated patients, and 20.7% in placebo patients was observed. The tropism shift from R5 to X4/X4R5 strains was 9.4% and 13.8% in lovastatin and placebo treated patients, respectively ($p = 0.6988$). Similar results were obtained using the clonal model of analysis (Table 2). These results suggest that, in this cohort of patients, the changes in use of the HIV-1 co-receptor were due to the natural course of infection and did not depend on the statin treatment.

Long-term use of statins does not affect the expression of HIV co-receptors on CD4+ T cells

To define in vivo if the long-term administration of lovastatin in HIV-infected patients reproduced a similar regulatory effect on the expression of CCR5 as previously shown in vitro [25], a cohort of chronically HIV-1 infected patients enrolled in the LIVE clinical trial [35] was examined. As shown in Table 3, one year administration of lovastatin had no significant effect on the percentage of CD4+ T cells expressing CXCR4 or CCR5 (EAC = 1.1%, 95% CI = −6.3 to 8.5; and EAC = 2.8%, 95% CI = −4.12 to 9.81, respectively). When the expression level of CXCR4 and CCR5 was measured as the mean fluorescence intensity (MFI) in the same population of CD4 + T cells, the results were similar (EAC = −39.2, 95% CI = −91.1 to 13.5 and EAC = −5.7, 95% CI = −23.9 to 12.4, respectively). The same analysis performed in the population of CD3-/CD4+ monocytes revealed no significant changes in the expression level of CXCR4 and CCR5 (Table 4).

Since the surface expression of CXCR4 and CCR5 could be modulated by the immune activation observed in HIV-1-infected patients, masking the effect of the long-term administration of oral lovastatin on the expression of these molecules, the baseline level of CXCR4 and CCR5 expression was evaluated and compared in

Table 2 Prediction of co-receptor usage shift in proviral sequences from mononuclear cells

	Total sequences obtained	Lovastatin	Placebo	P value (Fisher's exact test)
Baseline	91	44/91	47/9	NA
(Number X4 X4/R5 strains)		(8)	(8)	
12 months post treatment	72	38/72	34/72	NA
Number of paired sequences	61	32/61 (52.5%)	29/61 (47.5%)	NA
Clinical model	Total tropism shift	5/32 (15.6%)	6/29 (20.7%)	0.7426
	R5 shift to X4 or X4R5	3/32 (9.4%)	4/29 (13.8%)	0.6988
Clonal model	Total tropism shift	8/32 (25.0%)	5/29 (17.2%)	0.5411
	R5 shift to X4 or X4R5	4/32 (12.5%)	4/29 (13.8%)	1.0

The geno2pheno (G2P) algorithm was used at the beginning of the study and 12 months post treatment with lovastatin (40 mg/day) or placebo in asymptomatic HIV-1-infected patients. Isolation of peripheral blood mononuclear cells and proviral DNA preparation were as described in Methods. The G2P prediction algorithm is available at http://coreceptor.bioinf.mpi-inf.mpg.de/index.php. NA, No applicable statistical analysis. At the baseline were found 8 individuals with X4 or X4R5 circulating strains in lovastatin treated group, and 8 individuals at placebo treated group.

HIV-1-infected patients and HIV negative controls. Indeed, as shown in Figure 1, the MFI for CXCR4 and CCR5 was significantly higher in CD4+ T cells of HIV-1-infected patients when compared to HIV negative individuals (median MFI CXCR4: 143 +/− 54 vs. 55 +/− 9 relative units, respectively, $p < 0.0001$; MFI CCR5: 76 +/− 36 vs. 37 +/− 26 units, respectively, $p < 0.0001$).

Effect of statins on HIV co-receptor expression in HIV negative control subjects

Due to the differential expression of CXCR4 and CCR5 on resting CD4+ T cells of HIV-infected patients and HIV negative adults, we explored the effect of daily oral statins on the regulation of CXCR4 and CCR5 expression in HIV negative adults. At the different times of observation of statin oral intake, there were not statistically significant differences in the frequency and MFI expression level of CXCR4 by blood CD4+ T cells, when individuals receiving lovastatin or atorvastatin vs. controls were compared (Table 5). Regarding the expression of CCR5, only the administration of atorvastatin at 45 days of intake was associated with a significant increase in the frequency of circulating CD4+ T cells expressing CCR5 (median day 7 = 11.1%; day 45 = 71.4%

Table 3 CXCR4 and CCR5 expression in CD4+ T lymphocytes

Parameter	Time of treatment	Placebo group (n = 43) (95% CI)	Lovastatin group (n = 41) (95% CI)
% CD4+/CXCR4+ T cells	Baseline	68.5 (48.2 - 90.2)	58.5 (32.0 - 87.1)
	6 months post	60.0 (41.0 - 82.0)	66.4 (43.2 - 90.0)
	12 months post	58.5 (33.4 - 87.5)	66.0 (40.1 - 87.0)
	*** EAC by treatment**	**1.1% (−6.3 to 8.5)**	
MFI CXCR4 in CD4+/CXCR4+ T cells	Baseline	157.4 (63.6 - 221.0)	118.7 (76.0 - 176.4)
	6 months post	132.9 (44.4 - 195.6)	117.0 (72.1 - 200.7)
	12 months post	132.1 (35.3 - 231.4)	116.1 (39.3 - 184.6)
	EAC by treatment	**−39.2 (−91.1 to 13.4)**	
% CD4+/CCR5+ T cells	Baseline	17.8 (11.6 - 34.7)	23.6 (12.0 - 64.7)
	6 months post	19.2 (10.5 - 28.3)	26.0 (13.9 - 57.3)
	12 months post	21.5 (9.8 - 60.0)	22.5 (10.5 - 46.0)
	EAC by treatment	**2.84% (−4.1 to 9.9)**	
MFI CCR5 in CD4+/CCR5+ T cells	Baseline	67.9 (50.0 - 94.9)	71.6 (54.1 - 90.6)
	6 months post	63.0 (42.7 - 99.0)	66.2 (44.0 - 98.7)
	12 months post	58.4 (33.5 - 107.3)	83.5 (42.1 - 125.5)
	EAC by treatment	**−5.7 (−23.9 to 12.4)**	

CXCR4 and CCR5 expression levels were measured by flow cytometry at 0 (baseline) 6 and 12 months post treatment with lovastatin (40 mg/day) or placebo in asymptomatic HIV-1-infected patients. * EAC, Estimated average changes with (95% CI) using a GEE model as defined in Data Analysis (see Methods); MFI, Mean fluorescence intensity (in relative units).

Table 4 Expression of CXCR4 and CCR5 in CD3-/CD4+ monocytes

Parameter	Time of treatment	Placebo group (n = 43) (95% CI)	Lovastatin group (n = 41) (95% CI)
% CD3-/CD4+/CXCR4+ monocytes	Baseline	12.0 (3.0 - 23.0)	13.0 (4.0 - 21.0)
	6 months post	14.0 (8.0 - 24.0)	16.5 (5.0 - 29.0)
	12 months post	19.0 (10.5 - 37.5)	24.0 (10.0 - 58.0)
	EAC by treatment	**−2.2% (−7.2 to 2.8)**	
MFI CXCR4 in CD3-/CD4+/CXCR4+ monocytes	Baseline	196.8 (164.1 - 270.6)	192.2 (172.4 - 251.1)
	6 months post	179.7 (28.6 - 236.8)	189.2 (127.1 - 304.9)
	12 months post	149.6 (25.9 - 247.8)	86.2 (26.8 - 184.8)
	EAC by treatment	**8.7 units (−25.3 to 42.6)**	
% CD3-/CD4+/CCR5+ monocytes	Baseline	2.5 (1.0 - 6.0)	2.0 (1.0 - 8.0)
	6 months post	5.9 (1.3 - 16.5)	6.0 (2.3 - 12.2)
	12 months post	6.0 (3.0 - 35.0)	12.0 (6.0 - 33.0)
	EAC by treatment	**−0.99% (−5.1 to 3.1)**	
MFI CCR5 in% CD3-/CD4+/CCR5+ monocytes	Baseline	148.2 (131.7 - 155.9)	146.9 (127.9 - 167.6)
	6 months post	143.9 (38.1 - 168.2)	136.1 (48.9 - 171.0)
	12 months post	104.4 (21.0 - 169.6)	133.9 (33.4 - 164.6)
	EAC by treatment	**11.4 units (−28.0 to 50.9)**	

CXCR4 and CCR5 expression levels were measured by flow cytometry at 0 (baseline) 6 and 12 months post treatment with lovastatin (40 mg/day) or placebo in asymptomatic HIV-1 infected patients. * EAC, Estimated average changes with (95% CI) using a GEE model as defined in Data Analysis (see Methods); MFI, Mean fluorescence intensity (in relative units).

ANOVA $p < 0.05$); there were no differences at other points of evaluation, in the CCR5 MFI level on CD4+ T cells, at different times and with the different treatments (ANOVA $p \geq 0.05$) (Table 5).

In circulating monocytes, the administration of lovastatin for 45 days was not associated with significant modifications in the expression level of CXCR4 or CCR5 at the different times of evaluation (Table 6). In contrast, the daily oral administration of atorvastatin was associated with a significant increase in both molecules on peripheral blood monocytes, at days 30 and 45 of treatment when compared to the values at day 7 (median of cells expressing CXCR4, day 7 = 31.4%; day 30 = 72.3%; day 45 = 69.3%; ANOVA $p < 0.05$; MFI of CXCR4 day 7 = 8.6; day 30 = 25.0; day 45 = 22.4; ANOVA $p < 0.05$). Similar significant differences were observed for the percentage of CCR5+ monocytes and their CCR5 MFI, but only at day 45 of atorvastatin treatment (median of cells expressing CCR5, day 7 = 14.9%; day 45 = 76.1%; ANOVA $p < 0.05$; MFI of CCR5 day 7 = 6.2; day 45 = 26.8; ANOVA $p < 0.05$) (Table 6).

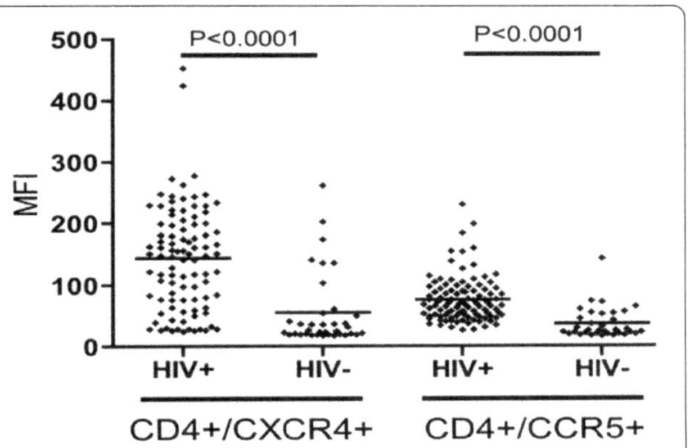

Figure 1 Expression levels of CXCR4 and CCR5 in CD4+ T lymphocytes. A: The mean fluorescence intensity (MFI) of CXCR4 and CCR5 was evaluated in CD4+/CXCR4+ and CD4+/CCR5+ T lymphocytes respectively, by flow cytometry in peripheral blood samples of 84 asymptomatic HIV-1-infected patients (HIV+) and 35 HIV seronegative volunteers (HIV-). Statistical comparison was made using the Student's t-test.

Effect of statins on the transcription level of HIV co-receptors and their ligands in HIV negative controls

Daily administration of lovastatin or atorvastatin was not associated with significant differences at the transcription level of the CXCR4 and CCR5 co-receptors at the different times of sampling (ANOVA $p \geq 0.05$) (Figure 2). Similarly, the transcriptional activity of CCL5 and CXCL12 in CD4+ T cells was not significantly modified by the daily administration of lovastatin or atorvastatin (ANOVA $p \geq 0.05$) (Figure 3, lower panel). In contrast, the administration of lovastatin was associated with a significant increase in the transcription of CCL3 from 0 to day 30 and 45 of treatment (median relative units of transcription = 8.85, 46.71 and 30.78 respectively, ANOVA $p < 0.05$), and in the transcription level of CCL4 at day 30 (median relative units of

Table 5 Follow-up of CXCR4 and CCR5 expression in CD4+ T lymphocytes

CD4+ T lymphocytes	Median (interquartile range)				Comparison by Anova
	Day 0	Day 7	Day 30	Day 45	
% CXCR4+ cells					
Controls without statins (n = 7)	56.2 (22.1 - 66.9)	45.2 (22.9 - 69.5)	68.4 (55.5 - 82.5)	69.2 (61.2 - 97.3)	NS
Lovastatin (n = 10)	54.5 (34.3 - 65.5)	30.9 (6.3 - 43.4)	66.1 (31.0 - 76.2)	63.8 (26.6 - 77.9)	NS
Atorvastatin (n = 9)	45.6 (35.6 - 64.4)	37.1 (24.8 - 44.6)	67.9 (51.0 - 75.6)	18.6 (7.1 - 66.9)	NS
MFI CXCR4 in CXCR4+ cells					
Controls without statins (n = 7)	19.9 (6.6 - 29.1)	15.8 (6.6 - 34.8)	25.1 (19.8 - 43.9)	21.2 (16.7 - 29.3)	NS
Lovastatin (n = 10)	16.5 (10.1 - 23.1)	8.9 (3.7 - 11.2)	16.3 (8.9 - 26.6)	20.4 (7.2 - 39.0)	NS
Atorvastatin (n = 9)	14.1 (10.8 - 27.3)	11.7 (7.8 - 13.2)	23.1 (15.1 - 29.3)	11.8 (4.3 - 33.8)	NS
% CCR5+ cells					
Controls without statins (n = 7)	17.4 (10.9 - 26.9)	28.2 (7.9 - 52.75)	35.0 (26.8 - 56.7)	21.6 (17.6 - 25.9)	NS
Lovastatin (n = 10)	13.3 (6.1 - 19.7)	9.4 (6.5 - 14.1)	14.1 (5.1 - 21.3)	18.1 (9.5 - 54.9)	NS
Atorvastatin (n = 9)	10.4 (7.6 - 18.7)	11.1 (7.1 - 12.0) £	13.5 (9.3 - 18.4)	71.4 (17.1 - 90.1) £	£ $p < 0.05$
MFI CCR5 in CCR5+ cells					
Controls without statins (n = 7)	8.8 (5.8 - 10.6)	13.2 (11.1 - 19.4)	11.1 (9.6 - 17.1)	25.1 (13.1 - 29.1)	NS
Lovastatin (n = 10)	23.0 (18.9 - 29.4)	21.9 (20.1 - 24.6)	29.4 (19.8 - 33.4)	24.1 (18.3 - 33.0)	NS
Atorvastatin (n = 9)	25.9 (20.4 - 50.2)	21.9 (20.0 - 25.4)	36.0 (27.0 - 42.4)	25.1 (23.4 - 39.6)	NS

HIV seronegative volunteers who received or not lovastatin (40 mg/day) or atorvastatin (20 mg/day) during 45 days, were evaluated at 0, 7, 30 and 45 days of treatment by flow cytometry. NS, No statistically significant difference. £: Statistical difference obtained comparing day 7 and day 45 of treatment.

Table 6 Follow-up of CXCR4 and CCR5 expression in CD3-/CD4+ monocytes

CD3-/CD4+ monocytes	Median (Interquartile range)				Comparison by Anova
	Day 0	Day 7	Day 30	Day 45	
% CXCR4+					
Controls without statins (n = 7)	81.1 (61.0 - 83.5)	65.7 (41.9 - 85.4)	89.6 (55.6 - 93.0)	87.2 (60.7 - 91.2)	NS
Lovastatin (n = 10)	48.6 (43.7 - 76.3)	34.8 (16.1 - 50.2)	69.7 (51.5 - 81.6)	57.7 (37.2 - 88.9)	NS
Atorvastatin (n = 9)	40.2 (29.7 - 51.5)	31.4 (25.3 - 41.3) £. †	72.3 (53.6 - 82.4) £	69.3 (36.3 - 89.3) †	£ $p < 0.05$. † $p < 0.05$
MFI CXCR4 in CXCR4+ cells					
Controls without statins (n = 7)	34.6 (17.1 - 37.7)	22.9 (10.6 - 58.4)	40.1 (16.6 - 58.4)	29.9 (13.7 - 33.5)	NS
Lovastatin (n = 10)	16.3 (12.1 - 26.9)	9.2 (5.9 - 12.3)	19.5 (12.8 - 30.3)	13.4 (9.6 - 64.9)	NS
Atorvastatin (n = 9)	10.6 (10.1 - 14.5)	8.6 (7.6 - 10.3) £. †	25.0 (13.5 - 28.2) £	22.4 (9.7 - 57.9) †	£ $p < 0.05$. † $p < 0.05$
% CCR5+					
Controls without statins (n = 7)	56.8 (32.2 - 64.5)	52.9 (15.7 - 70.3)	60.9 (32.1 - 72.3)	79.6 (27.8 - 80.0)	NS
Lovastatin (n = 10)	27.3 (21.6 - 41.5)	22.7 (7.8 - 26.9)	49.2 (24.0 - 61.8)	50.5 (18.9 - 73.7)	NS
Atorvastatin (n = 9)	23.6 (17.0 - 55.7)	14.9 (8.5 - 21.3) †	55.7 (25.8 - 57.2)	76.1 (27.3 - 78.3) †	† $p < 0.05$
MFI CCR5 in CCR5+ cells					
Controls without statins (n = 7)	15.9 (9.0 - 19.4)	16.4 (6.0 - 25.2)	16.1 (10.2 - 29.0)	18.3 (8.0 - 20.7)	NS
Lovastatin (n = 10)	8.6 (7.0 - 13.3)	7.1 (4.7 - 8.3)	12.7 (7.5 - 18.5)	11.8 (6.4 - 27.2)	NS
Atorvastatin (n = 9)	7.1 (6.3 - 19.8)	6.2 (4.7 - 7.5) †	15.3 (8.0 - 16.1)	26.0 (8.0 - 29.5) †	† $p < 0.05$

HIV seronegative volunteers who received or not lovastatin (40 mg/day) or atorvastatin (20 mg/day) during 45 days, were evaluated at 0, 7, 30 and 45 days of treatment by flow cytometry. NS, No statistically significant difference. †: Statistical analysis performed comparing day 7 and day 45 of treatment; £: Statistical difference obtained comparing day 7 and day 30 of treatment.

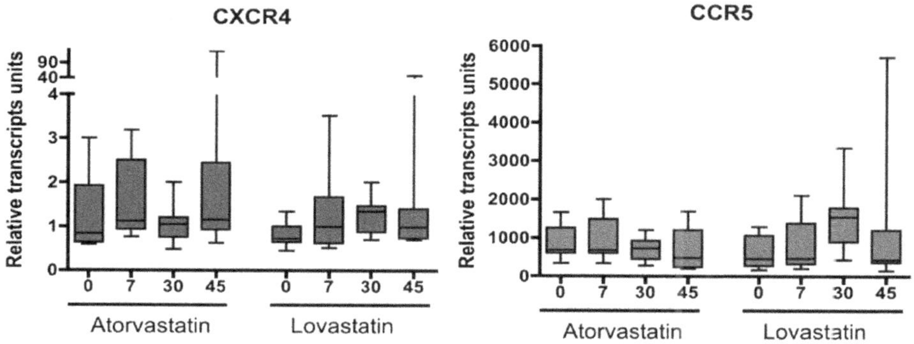

Figure 2 Transcription levels of CXCR4 and CCR5 genes during lovastatin or atorvastatin treatment. Transcription levels of CXCR4 and CCR5 in purified CD4+ T cells of adult HIV negative volunteers, during 45 days of oral administration of atorvastatin (20 mg/day; n = 9) or lovastatin (40 mg/day; n = 10); the measurements were performed by real time PCR at baseline and on days 7, 30 and 45. Statistical comparisons were performed using the One Way Anova test for paired samples.

transcription day 0 = 3.4; day 30 = 10.6, ANOVA $p < 0.05$ (Figure 3, upper panel); however, the administration of atorvastatin was not associated with significant variations in the transcriptional activity of CCL3 and CCL4 (Figure 3, upper panel).

Discussion

In this investigation, evaluating a representative cohort of chronic asymptomatic HIV-1-infected patients without requirements to receive antiretroviral therapy, we demonstrated that a daily oral administration of lovastatin during one year did not result in significant modulation of CCR5 and CXCR4 expression on CD4– T cells or CD4+ monocytes. Also, in HIV negative individuals, the daily administration of two different statins for 45 days did not lead to a significant regulation of these molecules. These findings suggest that long-term administration of statins, at doses commonly used in clinical practice, does not have a significant effect on modulating the expression of HIV-1 co-receptors or their ligands (except for CCL3 and CCL4).

Previous results support the immunomodulatory effects of statins in different inflammatory states [27,39-46].

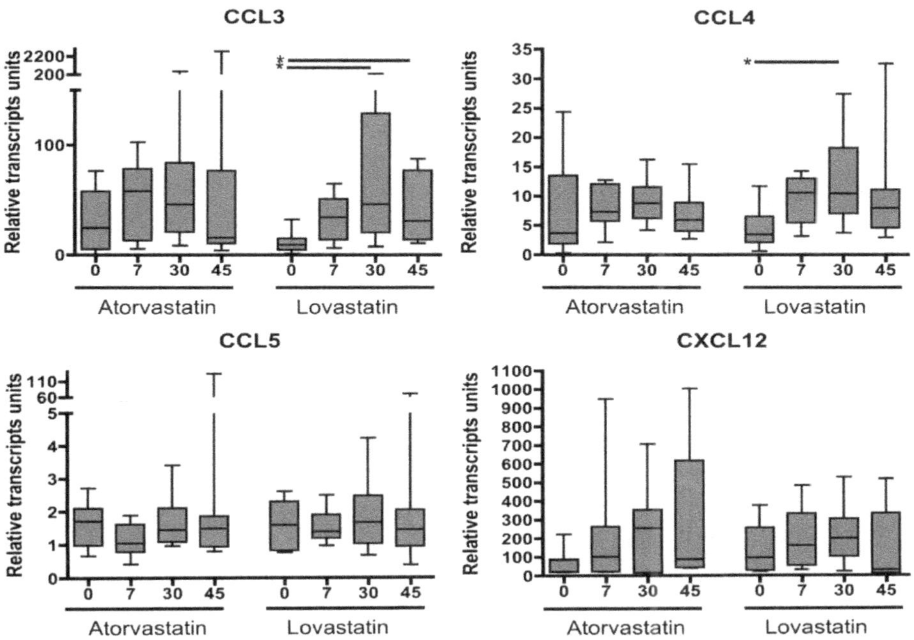

Figure 3 Transcription levels of CCL3, CCL4, CCL5 and CXCL12 genes during lovastatin or atorvastatin treatment. Transcription levels of CCL3, CCL4, CCL5 and CXCL12 in purified CD4+ T cells of adult HIV negative volunteers, during 45 days of oral administration of atorvastatin (20 mg/day; n = 9) or lovastatin (40 mg/day; n = 10); the measurements were performed by real time PCR at baseline and on days 7, 30 and 45. Statistical comparisons were performed using the One Way Anova test for paired samples. (*): p value <0.05, considered significant.

Similarly, the in vitro modulation of the expression of CCR5 and RANTES in CD4+ T lymphocytes by statins, as well as their inhibition of infection by R5 strains of HIV-1, was previously demonstrated [25]. These findings highlighted the importance of verifying whether the administration of statins modulated in vivo the expression of such a receptor and its ligands, and if this treatment could lead to the selection of X4 tropic strains of HIV-1 in infected individuals. Several explanations might account for the apparently contradictory data obtained in the in vitro studies and our in vivo studies regarding the actions of statins. The incubation of CD4+ T cells with statins in well plates allows the direct interaction of these compounds with their cellular targets (HMG-CoA reductase), favouring the molecular effects expected of statins. However, this might not be the case in vivo; considering that HIV replication and immune activation are active on secondary lymphoid organs (lymphoid nodes, mucosal lymphoid tissues), several pharmacokinetic limitations could hamper the effective biological activity of statins. In particular, if the bioavailability of statins in lymphoid tissues is deficient, then the immunomodulatory activities of these compounds will be limited. Thus, statins with better pharmacokinetic profiles would be more suitable to achieve the effects observed in vitro, where direct administration of statins to cells in culture overcomes the potential limitations derived from oral administration. It is also possible that long-term administration of higher doses of statins might be associated with better immunomodulatory effects, but the risks of adverse events and intolerance also increase, questioning the beneficial balance of such doses. Due that several factors could impact the outcome, including drug dose, potency, treatment-time, further investigations are needed in order to carefully demonstrate that statins do not affect the expression of coreceptors and their ligands in HIV infected or uninfected individuals.

The steady state expression of HIV-1 co-receptor molecules has been previously defined in HIV negative individuals, indicating that peripheral blood CD4+ naive T cells (CD45RA+) express high levels of CXCR4, but most of them are negative for CCR5; in contrast, most memory CD4+ T cells express CCR5, becoming the main target cells for efficient HIV-1 replication [47]. Also, in memory T cells, the expression of CCR5 may be modulated by cell activation [17,48-50]. Other observations support the fact that the level of CCR5 expression is associated with the infectious capacity of R5 strains of HIV [51] and give us an important evidence that if we regulate the expression of CCR5 it might act as a target for HIV infection prevention and control of replication. Additionally, HIV gp120 can acts in lymphocytes as "viral chemokines" interacting with CCR5 or CXCR4, and activating downstream signal proteins, induction of ion channel currents and Ca^{2+} flux, quantitatively different to that induced by chemokines. These differences in gp120 and chemokine-elicited Ca^{2+} flux can result in a Long Terminal Repeat (LTR) activation, due to a possible differential transcription factor activation [52]. The importance of the density of CD4 and of HIV CCR5 co-receptor expression for efficient infection has been also investigated in other cells different from human CD4+ T cells. In CD4+ HeLa cells expressing minimal concentrations of CCR5 on their surface, the infection by R5 strains of HIV occurred more efficiently during CCR5 expression concomitantly with a high level of CD4 expression, suggesting that a minimal number of CCR5 molecules are required when cell surface levels of CD4 reach a sufficient density [53]. Along the same line, epidemiological results associated the Δ32 CCR5 homozygous genotype with protection against the acquisition of HIV-1 [54-57], indicating that modulating CCR5 expression or function in HIV-infected individuals could help control progression of HIV infection, as occurs with maraviroc treatment; in despite of this, some Δ32 CCR5 homozygous individuals have become infected with HIV-1, indicating that this genotype may not be fully protective [58,59]. In our study, when compared with HIV negative baseline values a significant increase in the level of CCR5 expression on peripheral blood CD4+ T cells from the HIV-1 infected individuals was observed, which is in agreement with the uncontrolled chronic immune activation characterizing this infection. Furthermore, expression of CXCR4 on these cells was also significantly increased in infected individuals. Taken together, these facts suggest that generation of target cells with higher expression of co-receptors requires niches for persistent viral replication, and could be another pathological event associated with chronic immune activation during HIV infection.

Increased CXCR4 expression in HIV-infected patients is a remarkable finding, since enhanced expression of CXCR4 has been associated with more risk of metastasis in different types of cancers [60-64]; in fact, increased severity of oncogenic processes in chronically HIV-infected individuals has been previously documented [65-71]. These findings highlight the importance of investigating the association between chronic immune activation, enhanced expression of CXCR4 by different cells and cancer progression, and metastasis during HIV infection.

Regarding the expression of the CXCR4 and CCR5 ligands by purified CD4+ T cells of HIV negative adults, we observed an increase in CCL3 and CCL4 transcripts during lovastatin but not during atorvastatin treatment. The increase in both transcripts might correspond to the fact that the CCL3 and CCL4 genes are complexed in a very close genomic region, and their expression is determined by the number of gene copies [72]. It is possible that differences in the chemical structure, potency and molecular activity of lovastatin (natural statin) vs. atorvastatin (synthetic statin) could be associated with the apparently distinct immunomodulatory activities of both statins.

Previous in vitro evidence indicated that statins were not efficient in inhibiting the infection of CD4+ T cells by X4 strains of HIV-1, in contrast to their capacity to hamper the infection by R5 strains [25]; these observations generated the hypothesis that the long-term administration of statins to HIV-1-infected patients could lead to the selection of X4 strains, contributing to accelerate the evolution of HIV infection to AIDS. The frequency of the shift of R5 strains to X4 strains was similar between placebo and patients treated with lovastatin for one year, suggesting that the shifts in co-receptor usage were due to the natural course of infection, rather than to a selective process induced by statins. This finding suggests that the therapeutic administration of statins in HIV-infected patients with lipid disorders could be safe in terms of selecting X4 strains.

Although the role of the CCR5 and CXCR4 co-receptors in HIV-1 infection is well established, little is known regarding the regulation of their expression. Understanding these processes could facilitate the development of new therapeutic interventions with a similar mechanism of action as maraviroc. The investigation of new compounds that block or modulate the expression and function of HIV co-receptors must continue, since they represent conserved host molecules rather than viral proteins susceptible to continued mutations, making them interesting targets for anti-viral therapies.

Competing interests

EAH received a doctoral scholarship from COLCIENCIAS; the other authors declare that they have no competing interest.

Authors' Contributions

EA was the primary researcher, conceived the study, designed, participated in data collection and drafted manuscript, FJ assigned the randomization of patients and conducted statistical analysis, MR and CM assisted in data collection, follow-up the HIV positive patients and reviewed the initial and final drafts of the manuscript. All authors read and approved the final manuscript.

Acknowledgements

The authors acknowledge the excellent assistance of Alba L. León in performing the data analyses and Ana L. Rodríguez for the follow-up of HIV negative volunteers; also, the authors thank the HIV-infected patients and the outpatient program for HIV infection control from EPS SURA - Medellin, for help in detecting potential candidates to be enrolled in this investigation. Laboratorios Laproff (Sabaneta, Colombia) kindly provided lovastatin, atorvastatin and placebo tablets.

Funding

This work was supported by: Instituto Colombiano para el Desarrollo de la Ciencia y la Tecnología "Francisco José de Caldas" (COLCIENCIAS, Bogota, Colombia, grant number: 1115-40-820508) and Universidad de Antioquia "Estrategia de Sostenibilidad 2013-2014 (Medellin, Colombia).

Author details

[1]Immunovirology Group, School of Medicine, University of Antioquia, Medellin, Colombia. [2]Department of Internal Medicine and Academic Group of Clinical Epidemiology (GRAEPIC), School of Medicine, University of Antioquia, Medellín, Colombia. [3]Clinical Research Unit, Hospital Pablo Tobón Uribe, Medellin, Colombia.

References

1. Simpson KN, Roberts G, Hicks CB, Finnern HW: **Cost-effectiveness of tipranavir in treatment-experienced HIV patients in the United States.** *HIV Clin Trials* 2008, **9:**225–237.
2. Calza L: **Renal toxicity associated with antiretroviral therapy.** *HIV Clin Trials* 2012, **13:**189–211.
3. Jones M, Nunez M: **Liver toxicity of antiretroviral drugs.** *Semin Liver Dis* 2012, **32:**167–176.
4. Campbell JD, Stinson MJ, Simons FE, Rector ES, HayGlass KT: **In vivo stability of human chemokine and chemokine receptor expression.** *Hum Immunol* 2001, **62:**668–678.
5. Lee B, Doranz BJ, Ratajczak MZ, Doms RW: **An intricate web: chemokine receptors, HIV-1 and hematopoiesis.** *Stem Cells* 1998, **16:**79–88.
6. Boesecke C, Pett SL: **Clinical studies with chemokine receptor-5 (CCR5)-inhibitors.** *Curr Opin HIV AIDS* 2012, **7:**456–462.
7. Murakami T, Yamamoto N: **Role of CXCR4 in HIV infection and its potential as a therapeutic target.** *Future Microbiol* 2010, **5:**1025–1039.
8. Steen A, Schwartz TW, Rosenkilde MM: **Targeting CXCR4 in HIV cell-entry inhibition.** *Mini Rev Med Chem* 2009, **9:**1605–1621.
9. Gulick RM, Lalezari J, Goodrich J, Clumeck N, DeJesus E, Horban A, Nadler J, Clotet B, Karlsson A, Wohlfeiler M, *et al*: **Maraviroc for previously treated patients with R5 HIV-1 infection.** *N Engl J Med* 2008, **359:**1429–1441.
10. Wasmuth JC, Rockstroh JK, Hardy WD: **Drug safety evaluation of maraviroc for the treatment of HIV infection.** *Expert Opin Drug Saf* 2012, **11:**161–174.
11. Graham DR, Chertova E, Hilburn JM, Arthur LO, Hildreth JE: **Cholesterol depletion of human immunodeficiency virus type 1 and simian immunodeficiency virus with beta-cyclodextrin inactivates and permeabilizes the virions: evidence for virion-associated lipid rafts.** *J Virol* 2003, **77:**8237–8248.
12. Liao Z, Cimakasky LM, Hampton R, Nguyen DH, Hildreth JE: **Lipid rafts and HIV pathogenesis: host membrane cholesterol is required for infection by HIV type 1.** *AIDS Res Hum Retroviruses* 2001, **17:**1009–1019.
13. Liao Z, Graham DR, Hildreth JE: **Lipid rafts and HIV pathogenesis: virion-associated cholesterol is required for fusion and infection of susceptible cells.** *AIDS Res Hum Retroviruses* 2003, **19:**675–687.
14. Manes S, del Real G, Lacalle RA, Lucas P, Gomez-Mouton C, Sanchez-Palomino S, Delgado R, Alcami J, Mira E, Martinez AC: **Membrane raft microdomains mediate lateral assemblies required for HIV-1 infection.** *EMBO Rep* 2000, **1:**190–196.
15. Nguyen DH, Hildreth JE: **Evidence for budding of human immunodeficiency virus type 1 selectively from glycolipid-enriched membrane lipid rafts.** *J Virol* 2000, **74:**3264–3272.
16. Nguyen DH, Taub D: **CXCR4 function requires membrane cholesterol: implications for HIV infection.** *J Immunol* 2002, **168:**4121–4126.
17. Alkhatib G: **The biology of CCR5 and CXCR4.** *Curr Opin HIV AIDS* 2009, **4:**96–103.
18. Kamiyama H, Yoshii H, Tanaka Y, Sato H, Yamamoto N, Kubo Y: **Raft localization of CXCR4 is primarily required for X4-tropic human immunodeficiency virus type 1 infection.** *Virology* 2009, **386:**23–31.
19. Lodowski DT, Palczewski K: **Chemokine receptors and other G protein-coupled receptors.** *Curr Opin HIV AIDS* 2009, **4:**88–95.
20. Saez-Cirion A, Nir S, Lorizate M, Agirre A, Cruz A, Perez-Gil J, Nieva JL: **Sphingomyelin and cholesterol promote HIV-1 gp41 pretransmembrane sequence surface aggregation and membrane restructuring.** *J Biol Chem* 2002, **277:**21776–21785.
21. Vincent N, Genin C, Malvoisin E: **Identification of a conserved domain of the HIV-1 transmembrane protein gp41 which interacts with cholesteryl groups.** *Biochim Biophys Acta* 2002, **1567:**157–164.
22. del Real G, Jimenez-Baranda S, Mira E, Lacalle RA, Lucas P, Gomez-Mouton C, Alegret M, Pena JM, Rodriguez-Zapata M, Alvarez-Mon M, *et al:* **Statins inhibit HIV-1 infection by down-regulating Rho activity.** *J Exp Med* 2004, **200:**541–547.

23. Greenwood J, Steinman L, Zamvil SS: **Statin therapy and autoimmune disease: from protein prenylation to immunomodulation.** *Nat Rev Immunol* 2006, **6**:358–370.
24. Tobert JA: **Lovastatin and beyond: the history of the HMG-CoA reductase inhibitors.** *Nat Rev Drug Discov* 2003, **2**:517–526.
25. Nabatov AA, Pollakis G, Linnemann T, Paxton WA, de Baar MP: **Statins disrupt CCR5 and RANTES expression levels in CD4(+) T lymphocytes in vitro and preferentially decrease infection of R5 versus X4 HIV-1.** *PLoS One* 2007, **2**:e470.
26. Bottaro EG, Caravello O, Scapellato PG, Stambulian M, Vidal GI, Loggia V, Scapellato JL, Thompson F, Cassetti I: **Rosuvastatin for the treatment of dyslipidemia in HIV-infected patients receiving highly active antiretroviral therapy. Preliminary experience.** *Enferm Infecc Microbiol Clin* 2008, **26**:325–329.
27. De Wit S, Delforge M, Necsoi CV, Clumeck N: **Downregulation of CD38 activation markers by atorvastatin in HIV patients with undetectable viral load.** *AIDS* 2011, **25**:1332–1333.
28. Issat T, Nowis D, Jakobisiak M, Golab J: **Lovastatin potentiates antitumor effects of saquinavir against human lymphoma cells.** *Oncol Rep* 2004, **12**:1371–1375.
29. Maganti RM, Reveille JD, Williams FM: **Therapy insight: the changing spectrum of rheumatic disease in HIV infection.** *Nat Clin Pract Rheumatol* 2008, **4**:428–438.
30. Visnegarwala F, Maldonado M, Sajja P, Minihan JL, Rodriguez-Barradas MC, Ong O, Lahart CJ, Hasan MQ, Balasubramanyam A, White AC Jr: **Lipid lowering effects of statins and fibrates in the management of HIV dyslipidemias associated with antiretroviral therapy in HIV clinical practice.** *J Infect* 2004, **49**:283–290.
31. Blaak H, van't Wout AB, Brouwer M, Hooibrink B, Hovenkamp E, Schuitemaker H: **In vivo HIV-1 infection of CD45RA(+)CD4(+) T cells is established primarily by syncytium-inducing variants and correlates with the rate of CD4(+) T cell decline.** *Proc Natl Acad Sci U S A* 2000, **97**:1269–1274.
32. Picchio GR, Gulizia RJ, Wehrly K, Chesebro B, Mosier DE: **The cell tropism of human immunodeficiency virus type 1 determines the kinetics of plasma viremia in SCID mice reconstituted with human peripheral blood leukocytes.** *J Virol* 1998, **72**:2002–2009.
33. Rudensey LM, Kimata JT, Benveniste RE, Overbaugh J: **Progression to AIDS in macaques is associated with changes in the replication, tropism, and cytopathic properties of the simian immunodeficiency virus variant population.** *Virology* 1995, **207**:528–542.
34. Montoya CJ, Higuita EA, Estrada S, Gutierrez FJ, Amariles P, Giraldo NA, Jimenez MM, Velasquez CP, Leon AL, Rugeles MT, Jaimes FA: **Randomized clinical trial of lovastatin in HIV-infected, HAART naive patients (NCT00721305).** *J Infect* 2012, **65**:549–558.
35. Montoya CJ, Jaimes F, Higuita EA, Convers-Paez S, Estrada S, Gutierrez F, Amariles P, Giraldo N, Penaloza C, Rugeles MT: **Antiretroviral effect of lovastatin on HIV-1-infected individuals without highly active antiretroviral therapy (The LIVE study): a phase-II randomized clinical trial.** *Trials* 2009, **10**:41.
36. Verhofstede C, Brudney D, Reynaerts J, Vaira D, Fransen K, De Bel A, Seguin-Devaux C, De Wit S, Vandekerckhove L, Geretti AM: **Concordance between HIV-1 genotypic coreceptor tropism predictions based on plasma RNA and proviral DNA.** *HIV Med* 2011, **12**:544–552.
37. Cardona-Maya W, Velilla P, Montoya CJ, Cadavid A, Rugeles MT: **Presence of HIV-1 DNA in spermatozoa from HIV-positive patients: changes in the semen parameters.** *Curr HIV Res* 2009, **7**:418–424.
38. Lengauer T, Sander O, Sierra S, Thielen A, Kaiser R: **Bioinformatics prediction of HIV coreceptor usage.** *Nat Biotechnol* 2007, **25**:1407–1410.
39. Brinkkoetter PT, Gottmann U, Schulte J, van der Woude FJ, Braun C, Yard BA: **Atorvastatin interferes with activation of human CD4(+) T cells via inhibition of small guanosine triphosphatase (GTPase) activity and caspase-independent apoptosis.** *Clin Exp Immunol* 2006, **146**:524–532.
40. Dunn SE, Youssef S, Goldstein MJ, Prod'homme T, Weber MS, Zamvil SS, Steinman L: **Isoprenoids determine Th1/Th2 fate in pathogenic T cells, providing a mechanism of modulation of autoimmunity by atorvastatin.** *J Exp Med* 2006, **203**:401–412.
41. Kwak B, Mulhaupt F, Veillard N, Pelli G, Mach F: **The HMG-CoA reductase inhibitor simvastatin inhibits IFN-gamma induced MHC class II expression in human vascular endothelial cells.** *Swiss Med Wkly* 2001, **131**:41–46.
42. Oka M, Fagan KA, Jones PL, McMurtry IF: **Therapeutic potential of RhoA/Rho kinase inhibitors in pulmonary hypertension.** *Br J Pharmacol* 2008, **155**:444–454.
43. Overmeyer JH, Maltese WA: **Isoprenoid requirement for intracellular transport and processing of murine leukemia virus envelope protein.** *J Biol Chem* 1992, **267**:22686–22692.
44. Serhan CN, Chiang N, Van Dyke TE: **Resolving inflammation: dual anti-inflammatory and pro-resolution lipid mediators.** *Nat Rev Immunol* 2008, **8**:349–361.
45. Waiczies S, Prozorovski T, Infante-Duarte C, Hahner A, Aktas O, Ullrich O, Zipp F: **Atorvastatin induces T cell energy via phosphorylation of ERK1.** *J Immunol* 2005, **174**:5630–5635.
46. Weber C, Erl W, Weber KS, Weber PC: **HMG-CoA reductase inhibitors decrease CD11b expression and CD11b-dependent adhesion of monocytes to endothelium and reduce increased adhesiveness of monocytes isolated from patients with hypercholesterolemia.** *J Am Coll Cardiol* 1997, **30**:1212–1217.
47. Berkowitz RD, Beckerman KP, Schall TJ, McCune JM: **CXCR4 and CCR5 expression delineates targets for HIV-1 disruption of T cell differentiation.** *J Immunol* 1998, **161**:3702–3710.
48. Camargo JF, Quinones MP, Mummidi S, Srinivas S, Gaitan AA, Begum K, Jimenez F, VanCompernolle S, Unutmaz D, Ahuja SS, Ahuja SK: **CCR5 expression levels influence NFAT translocation, IL-2 production, and subsequent signaling events during T lymphocyte activation.** *J Immunol* 2009, **182**:171–182.
49. Soares R, Foxall R, Albuquerque A, Cortesao C, Garcia M, Victorino RM, Sousa AE: **Increased frequency of circulating CCR5+ CD4+ T cells in human immunodeficiency virus type 2 infection.** *J Virol* 2006, **80**:12425–12429.
50. Stoddart CA, Keir ME, McCune JM: **IFN-alpha-induced upregulation of CCR5 leads to expanded HIV tropism in vivo.** *PLoS Pathog* 2010, **6**:e1000766.
51. Paxton WA, Liu R, Kang S, Wu L, Gingeras TR, Landau NR, Mackay CR, Koup RA: **Reduced HIV-1 infectability of CD4+ lymphocytes from exposed-uninfected individuals: association with low expression of CCR5 and high production of beta-chemokines.** *Virology* 1998, **244**:66–73.
52. Juno JA, Fowke KR: **Clarifying the role of G protein signaling in HIV infection: new approaches to an old question.** *AIDS Rev* 2010, **12**:164–176.
53. Ketas TJ, Kuhmann SE, Palmer A, Zurita J, He W, Ahuja SK, Klasse PJ, Moore JP: **Cell surface expression of CCR5 and other host factors influence the inhibition of HIV-1 infection of human lymphocytes by CCR5 ligands.** *Virology* 2007, **364**:281–290.
54. Dean M, Carrington M, Winkler C, Huttley GA, Smith MW, Allikmets R, Goedert JJ, Buchbinder SP, Vittinghoff E, Gomperts E, *et al*: **Genetic restriction of HIV-1 infection and progression to AIDS by a deletion allele of the CKR5 structural gene. Hemophilia growth and development study, multicenter AIDS cohort study, multicenter hemophilia cohort study, San Francisco city cohort, ALIVE study.** *Science* 1996, **273**:1856–1862.
55. Huang Y, Paxton WA, Wolinsky SM, Neumann AU, Zhang L, He T, Kang S, Ceradini D, Jin Z, Yazdanbakhsh K, *et al*: **The role of a mutant CCR5 allele in HIV-1 transmission and disease progression.** *Nat Med* 1996, **2**:1240–1243.
56. Samson M, Libert F, Doranz BJ, Rucker J, Liesnard C, Farber CM, Saragosti S, Lapoumeroulie C, Cognaux J, Forceille C, *et al*: **Resistance to HIV-1 infection in caucasian individuals bearing mutant alleles of the CCR-5 chemokine receptor gene.** *Nature* 1996, **382**:722–725.
57. Zimmerman PA, Buckler-White A, Alkhatib G, Spalding T, Kubofcik J, Combadiere C, Weissman D, Cohen O, Rubbert A, Lam G, *et al*: **Inherited resistance to HIV-1 conferred by an inactivating mutation in CC chemokine receptor 5: studies in populations with contrasting clinical phenotypes, defined racial background, and quantified risk.** *Mol Med* 1997, **3**:23–36.
58. Biti R, Ffrench R, Young J, Bennetts B, Stewart G, Liang T: **HIV-1 infection in an individual homozygous for the CCR5 deletion allele.** *Nat Med* 1997, **3**:252–253.
59. Theodorou I, Meyer L, Magierowska M, Katlama C, Rouzioux C: **HIV-1 infection in an individual homozygous for CCR5 delta 32. Seroco study group.** *Lancet* 1997, **349**:1219–1220.
60. Dubrovska A, Elliott J, Salamone RJ, Telegeev GD, Stakhovsky AE, Schepotin IB, Yan F, Wang Y, Bouchez LC, Kularatne SA, *et al*: **CXCR4 expression in prostate cancer progenitor cells.** *PLoS One* 2012, **7**:e31226.
61. Dubrovska A, Hartung A, Bouchez LC, Walker JR, Reddy VA, Cho CY, Schultz PG: **CXCR4 activation maintains a stem cell population in tamoxifen-**

resistant breast cancer cells through AhR signalling. *Br J Cancer* 2012, **107**:43–52.
62. Hiller D, Chu QD: **CXCR4 and axillary lymph nodes: review of a potential biomarker for breast cancer metastasis.** *Int J Breast Cancer* 2011, **2011**:420981.
63. Kahan BD, Rutzky L, Berlin B, Tomita J, Wiseman F, LeGrue S, Noll H, Tom BH: **Cell surface alterations on colon adenocarcinoma cells.** *Cancer Res* 1976, **36**:3526–3534.
64. Sun X, Cheng G, Hao M, Zheng J, Zhou X, Zhang J, Taichman RS, Pienta KJ, Wang J: **CXCL12/CXCR4/CXCR7 chemokine axis and cancer progression.** *Cancer Metastasis Rev* 2010, **29**:709–722.
65. Mani D, Haigentz M Jr, Aboulafia DM: **Lung cancer in HIV Infection.** *Clin Lung Cancer* 2012, **13**:6–13.
66. Newsom-Davis T, Bower M: **HIV-associated anal cancer.** *F1000 Med Rep* 2010, **2**:85.
67. Shiels MS, Pfeiffer RM, Gail MH, Hall HI, Li J, Chaturvedi AK, Bhatia K, Uldrick TS, Yarchoan R, Goedert JJ, Engels EA: **Cancer burden in the HIV-infected population in the United States.** *J Natl Cancer Inst* 2011, **103**:753–762.
68. Strehl JD, Mehlhorn G, Koch MC, Harrer EG, Harrer T, Beckmann MW, Agaimy A: **HIV-associated hypertrophic herpes simplex genitalis with concomitant early invasive squamous cell carcinoma mimicking advanced genital cancer: case report and literature review.** *Int J Gynecol Pathol* 2012, **31**:286–293.
69. White HL, Mulambia C, Sinkala M, Mwanahamuntu MH, Parham GP, Moneyham L, Grimley DM, Chamot E: **'Worse than HIV' or 'not as serious as other diseases'? Conceptualization of cervical cancer among newly screened women in Zambia.** *Soc Sci Med* 2012, **74**:1486–1493.
70. Yannam GR, Gutti T, Poluektova LY: **IL-23 in infections, inflammation, autoimmunity and cancer: possible role in HIV-1 and AIDS.** *J Neuroimmune Pharmacol* 2012, **7**:95–112.
71. Zanet E, Berretta M, Di Benedetto F, Talamini R, Ballarin R, Nunnari G, Berretta S, Ridolfo A, Lleshi A, Zanghi A, *et al*: **Pancreatic cancer in HIV-positive patients: a clinical case–control study.** *Pancreas* 2012, **41**:1331–1335.
72. Colobran R, Pedrosa E, Carretero-Iglesia L, Juan M: **Copy number variation in chemokine superfamily: the complex scene of CCL3L-CCL4L genes in health and disease.** *Clin Exp Immunol* 2010, **162**:41–52.

Mutations in variable domains of the HIV-1 envelope gene can have a significant impact on maraviroc and vicriviroc resistance

Odalis Asin-Milan[1,2], Annie Chamberland[1,2], Yi Wei[1], Alpha Haidara[1,2], Mohamed Sylla[1,2] and Cécile L Tremblay[1,2,3,4*]

Abstract

Background: Resistance to CCR5 inhibitors, such as maraviroc and vicriviroc is characterized by reduction of maximal percent inhibition which indicates the use of an inhibitor-bound conformation of CCR5 for human immunodeficiency virus-1(HIV-1) entry. It is accompanied by substitutions in gp120 and gp41. Variable domain 3 (V3) plays the most important role, but substitutions outside V3 could also be involved in phenotype resistance. In this work, we investigated how mutations in variable regions of the viral envelope protein gp120 can contribute to CCR5 inhibitor resistance.

Methods: Resistant isolates were selected by passaging CC1/85 and BaL viruses with sub-inhibitory MVC and VCV concentrations. Mutations in gp160 were identified and mutants containing V2 (V169M), V3 (L317W) and V4 (I408T) were constructed.

Results: MVC and VCV susceptibility and viral tropism were assessed by single cycle assay. Mutant I408T showed 4-fold change (FC) increase in the half maximal inhibitory concentration (IC_{50}) to MVC, followed by L317W (1.52-FC), V169M (1.23-FC), V169M/I408T (4-FC) L317W/I408T (3-FC), V169M/L317W (1.30-FC), and V169M/L317W/I408T (3.31-FC). MPI reduction was observed for mutants I408T (85%), L317W (95%), V169M/I408T (84%), L317W/I408T (85%) and V169M/L317W/I408T (83%). For VCV, I408T increased the IC_{50} by 2-FC and few mutants showed MPI reduction less than 95%: I408T (94%), L317W/I408T (94%) and V169M/L317W/I408T (94%). All mutants remained R5-tropic and presented decreased infectivity.

Conclusions: These results suggest that mutations in the V4 loop of HIV-1 may contribute to MVC and VCV resistance alone or combined with mutations in V2 and V3 loops.

Keywords: Maraviroc, Vicriviroc, Resistance, CCR5 Inhibitors

Background

HIV-1 entry into target cells is initiated by interactions between the viral envelope (Env) protein gp120 and the host cell receptor CD4. It triggers conformational changes in gp120, forming the co-receptor binding site [1-3]. gp120 interaction with C-C chemokine receptor 5 (CCR5) or C-X-C chemokine receptor 4 (CXCR4) induces other conformational changes in gp120, which evoke structural re-arrangement of gp41 and enables the viral and cellular membrane fusion, permitting viral entry [4]. CCR5 inhibitors, including maraviroc (MVC), vicriviroc (VCV), aplaviroc, TAK-779 and TAK-220, antagonize this process and have strong anti-viral activity against HIV-1 *in vitro* [5,6]. Although they bind the hydrophobic pocket within transmembrane domains of CCR5 with high affinity, they occupy different sub-cavities by interacting with different amino acids [6]. MVC is the first CCR5 inhibitor approved for the treatment of R5-tropic HIV-1 infection in both naïve and treatment-experienced adult patients. VCV development was stopped because of suboptimal efficacy [5]. Since

* Correspondence: c.tremblay@umontreal.ca
[1]Centre de recherche, Centre hospitalier de l'Université de Montréal (CRCHUM), Montréal, QC, Canada
[2]Department of Microbiology and Immunology, Faculty of Medicine, Université de Montréal, Montréal, QC, Canada
Full list of author information is available at the end of the article

MCV and VCV are allosteric inhibitors of virus entry, resistance to these drugs is evidenced by reduction in the plateau of virus inhibition curves rather than by increases in 50 percent inhibitory concentration (IC_{50}) [7,8]. The magnitude of this decrease can be expressed as maximum plateau inhibition (MPI) [9]. Plateau height depends on the relative affinity of HIV-1 for inhibitor-bound versus free CCR5, the greater the affinity for inhibitor-bound CCR5, the lower the height of the plateau [7]. MOTIVATE clinical trials of MVC revealed that the MPI of most MVC-resistant viruses in subjects failing therapy ranged from 80 to 95% [9]. In VICTOR-E1 clinical trials of VCV, phenotypic resistance was manifested by reductions in relative MPI. The cut-off value was 0.94 [8]. Changes in susceptibility to CCR5 inhibitors are usually accompanied by substitutions in gp120, with V3 domain appearing to play a critical role. However, substitutions outside this region also contribute to the resistance phenotype [10]. The aim of this study is to investigate how mutations in other variable loops of the HIV-1 Env can contribute to MVC and VCV resistance.

Results

Selection of resistance mutations by *in vitro* passage

After 4 passages of CC1/85 virus in the presence of sub-inhibitory MVC concentrations, some mutations, such as V169M and N192K in V2, L317W in V3, I408A in V4, D462N, N463T, S464T and N465aD in V5, and L820I, I829V and Y837C in gp41,were associated with increased p24 levels (Table 1). After 16 passages, 2 new mutations materialized: I408T in V4 and P849Q in gp41 (Table 1). It is noteworthy that the mutation I408A in V4 appeared after 4 passages and disappeared at passage 16, when a new mutation, I408T, surfaced at the same position.. For VCV, 2 mutations emerged after 4 passages: V169M in V2 and L317W in V3. After 16 passages, the mutation I840Y arose in gp41. No amino acid change was observed with either drug in the Env region of laboratory-adapted BaL virus after 16 passages (Additional file 1).

Susceptibility of mutant clones to MVC and VCV

Significant (85%) reduction in MVC's MPI was apparent for I408T, 84% for the double mutant V169M/I408T, 85% for L317W/I408T, and 83% for the triple mutant V169M/L317W/I408T. L317W and V169M/L317W mutants presented intermediate resistance of 95% and 94%, respectively. No significant MPI diminution occurred for the single mutant V169M (96%). A similar pattern was observed when measuring fold-change (FC) increase in the IC_{50}, with I408T showing 4-FC, L317W 1.52-FC, and V169M, 1.23-FC increase. The double mutants V169M/L317W exhibited 1.30-FC, V169M/I408T 4-FC and L317W/I408T 3-FC, and 3.31-FC was evident for the triple mutant V169M/L317W/I408T (Table 2 and Figure 1A). The single mutants V169M and L317W and the double mutants V169M/L317W and V169M/I408T retained their susceptibility to VCV, reaching 100% inhibition in some cases. For VCV, I408T increased the IC_{50} by 2-FC, and the mutants I408T, L317W/I408T and V169M/L317W/I408T showed MPI of 94%, 93% and 94%, respectively (Table 3 and Figure 1B).

Mutations affect virus infectivity differentially

The CC1/85 parental clone and mutants exhibited different levels of infectivity. All mutants manifested decreased infectivity that ranged from 20 to 38%. Infectivity percentage was 75% for V169M, 76% for L317W, 80% for I408T, 76% for the double mutants V169M/L317W, 63% for V169M/I408T, 67% for L317W/I408T, and 67% for the triple mutant V169M/L317W/I408T (Figure 2).

Tropism and V3 net charge

All CC1/85-derived mutants remained R5-tropic. None of them was able to replicate in U87CD4CXCR4+ cells, but did so well in U87CD4CCR5+ cells (Tables 2 and 3). R5-tropism was also confirmed by 2 different genotypic predictors, $PSSM_{X4R5}$ [11,12] and geno2pheno co-receptor [13]. No change in V3 net charge was observed.

Discussion

Our findings indicate that viruses resistant to MVC can retain the use of CCR5 coreceptor as reported previously [14-16]. CCR5 inhibitors are associated with mutations in the Env V3 region of R5 isolates [14,17]. Our passage experiments revealed only 1 polymorphism in the V3 loop crown, L317W, which was associated with reduced infectivity, but not with resistance to CCR5 inhibitors or changes in V3 net charge (Tables 1 and 2). The selection of HIV-1 resistance to CCR5 inhibitors is relatively difficult [14,18], the V3 loop being the least variable of the HIV-1 Env variable regions [19]. Marozsan et al. found no amino acid changes in the V3 loop of CC1/85 resistant to VCV generated *in vitro* [15]. Wesby et al. reported a MVC-resistant CC1/85 virus generated in passage experiments with only 2 changes in amino acid positions 316 and 323 in the V3 loop [14]. Anastassopoulou et al. described D1/86.16, a VCV escape mutant that has no mutations in V3 [20].

Interestingly, when V3 substitution L317W is associated with V4 substitution I408T or triple substitution V169M/L317W/I408T, it confers further reduction of infectivity to 70% of the parental clone (Figure 2). This decreased infectivity could be due to lower fusion activity or binding affinity to the CCR5 co-receptor molecule of the mutant L317W.

The same polymorphism was found by Yu et al. in V3 region of the gp120 isolates CRF07_BC and CRF01_AE,

Table 1 Summary of sequence changes in env gene associated with decreased susceptibility to MVC and VCV in passages experiments

Virus, drug	Passage no.	gp 120 V2 loop amino acid sequence
CC1/85	start	158 198 SFNITTSIRNKVQKQYALFYKLDVVPIDNDSNNTNYRLISC
CC1/85 control	4	--
CC1/85, maraviroc	4	--------------------**M**---**K**-------
CC1/85, vicriviroc	4	--------------------**M**--
CC1/85 control	16	--
CC1/85, maraviroc	16	--------------------**M**---**K**-------
CC1/85, vicriviroc	16	--------------------**M**--
		gp 120 V3 loop amino acid sequence
CC1/85	start	296 331 CTRPNNYTRKSIHIGPGRALYATGDIIGDIRQAHC
CC1/85 control	4	---
CC1/85, maraviroc	4	-----------------------------------**W**--------------------------
CC1/85, vicriviroc	4	-----------------------------------**W**--------------------------
CC1/85 control	16	---
CC1/85, maraviroc	16	-----------------------------------**W**--------------------------
CC1/85, vicriviroc	16	-----------------------------------**W**--------------------------
		gp 120 V4 loop amino acid sequence
CC1/85	start	385 418 CNSTKLFNSTWTWNNSTWNNTKRANDIEEIITLPC
CC1/85 control	4	--
CC1/85, maraviroc	4	---**A**-------------
CC1/85, vicriviroc	4	---
CC1/85 control	16	---**A**-------------
CC1/85, maraviroc	16	---**T**--------------
CC1/85, vicriviroc	16	--
		gp 120 V5 loop amino acid sequence
CC1/85	start	461 469 KDNSTNEIFR
CC1/85 control	4	-----------------
CC1/85, maraviroc	4	**TN--T----N---**
CC1/85, vicriviroc	4	-------------------
CC1/85 control	16	---------------
CC1/85, maraviroc	16	**TNTT-D----**
CC1/85, vicriviroc	16	-------------
		gp 41 amino acid sequence
CC1/85	start	642 681 IYNLLEESQNQQEKNEQELLELDKWANLWNWFDISNWLWY
CC1/85 control	4	---
CC1/85, maraviroc	4	---
CC1/85, vicriviroc	4	---
CC1/85 control	16	--------------------------------------**A**--------------------------------------
CC1/85, maraviroc	16	--------------------------------------**A**--------------------------------------
CC1/85, vicriviroc	16	---

Table 1 Summary of sequence changes in env gene associated with decreased susceptibility to MVC and VCV in passages experiments *(Continued)*

		gp 41 amino acid sequence
CC1/85	start	812 850
		IKIFINATALAVAEGTDRILEVLCRAYRAILHIPRRIRP
CC1/85 control	4	----------------I--
CC1/85, maraviroc	4	----------------I----------------V----------C-------------------
CC1/85, vicriviroc	4	---
CC1/85 control	16	----------------I----------------V---A-----C-------------------
CC1/85, maraviroc	16	----------------I----------------V----------C-----------------Q
CC1/85, vicriviroc	16	---------------------------------------A---------Y--------------

Residues are numbered according to the HXB2 gp120 sequence.

the predominant HIV-1 subtypes in China in patients naïve to CCR5 inhibitors. In their study, R5 isolates harboring 2 dominant polymorphisms, R315Q and F317W in V3, were less susceptible than B isolates to MVC and TAK779. They postulated that baseline resistance to entry inhibitors may be associated with naturally-occurring polymorphisms [21]. Yuan et al. [22] studied a combination of polymorphisms in the gp120 V3 loop of HIV-1JR-FL virus that can confer non-competitive resistance to MVC with a V3 loop library containing a set of random combinations of 0-10 polymorphic mutations *in vitro*. After 17 passages, they found pseudoviruses containing the polymorphism F317W (F312W from the V3 library) with typical non-competitive resistance to MVC. The polymorphism F317W was also found by Muñoz-Nieto et al. in 2008 in the env region from primary isolates during follow-up of dual natural infection with subtypes B and G [23].

In our study, I408T in V4 was the mutation that conferred the highest level of resistance. This mutation

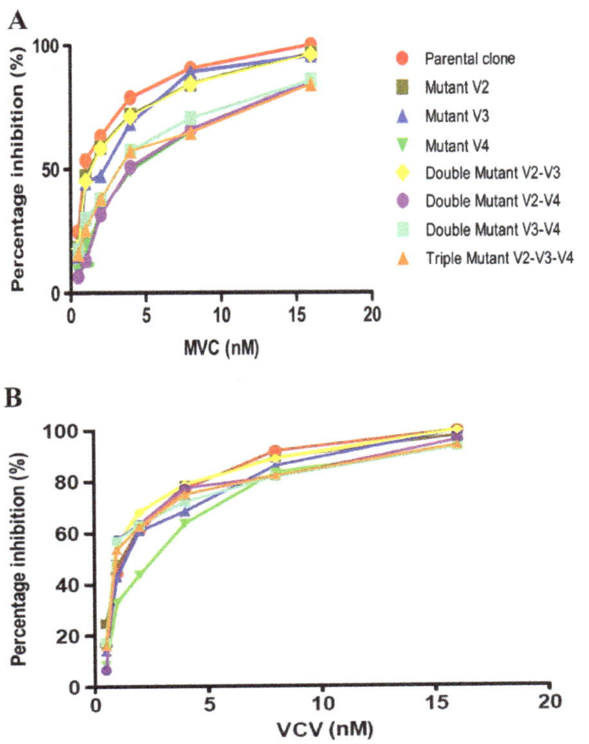

Figure 1 Sensitivity of parental and mutant clones to MVC (A) and VCV (B). HIV-1 Env pseudoviruses bearing the parental clone or Env-selected mutations V2 (V169M), V3 (L317W) and V4 (I408T) in single, double and triple combinations served to infect U87-CD4-CCR5 cells in the presence of increasing MVC and VCV concentrations. Infectivity was assessed by measuring luciferase activity 3 days after infection. The GraphPad Prism program generated inhibition curves. In each graph, the percentages of inhibition of parental clones are shown in red, and all results are the means of 3 experiments, each performed in triplicate.

Table 2 Susceptibility and phenotypic properties of V2, V3 and V4 single, double and triple mutants against maraviroc

Loop	Mutant	Tropism	IC_{50}	IC_{50} FC increase	MPI
Parental clone	Wild type	R5	1.47 nM	-	-
V2	V169M	R5	1.82 nM	1.23	96%
V3	L317W	R5	2.24 nM	1.52	95%
V4	I408T	R5	5.46 nM	4.00	85%
V2-V3	V169M L317W	R5	1.92 nM	1.30	94.3%
V2-V4	V169M I408T	R5	5.76 nM	4.00	84%
V3-V4	L317W I408T	R5	4.29 nM	3.00	85%
V2-V3-V4	V169M L317W I408T	R5	4.88 nM	3.31	83%

IC_{50}, 50% effective concentration or concentration needed to inhibit 50% of HIV. IC_{50} FC was calculated as the ratio IC_{50} for resistant virus/IC_{50} for wild type virus. MPI (maximum percent inhibition) was calculated as described in Methods.

Table 3 Summary of susceptibility and phenotypic properties of V2, V3 and V4 single, double and triple mutants against vicriviroc

Loop	Mutant	Tropism	IC_{50}	IC_{50} FC increase	MPI
Parental clone	Wild type	R5	1.56 nM	-	-
V2	V169M	R5	1.61 nM	1.03	100%
V3	L317W	R5	1.90 nM	1.21	100%
V4	I408T	R5	3.16 nM	2.02	94%
V2-V3	V169M L317W	R5	1.56 nM	1.57	100%
V2-V4	V169M I408T	R5	1.62 nM	1.03	96%
V3-V4	L317W I408T	R5	1.68 nM	1.07	93%
V2-V3-V4	V169M L317W I408T	R5	1.59 nM	1.01	94%

IC_{50}, 50% effective concentration or concentration needed to inhibit 50% of HIV. IC_{50} FC was calculated as the ratio IC_{50} for resistant virus/IC_{50} for wild type virus. MPI (maximum percent inhibition) was calculated as described in Methods.

occurred only in viruses resistant to MVC in passage experiments. It was a change from medium size and hydrophobic I to medium size and polar T. The mutation conferred resistance to MVC and was linked with cross-resistance to VCV, as indicated by MPI values. Although cross-resistance was observed for VCV, the virus was more resistant to MVC. Cross-resistance is commonly seen among CCR5 inhibitors [5]. Even if VCV had a favorable resistance profile, its virological activity was sub-optimal in phase II and III studies, possibly because of its pharmacokinetic profile and the dose chosen [5,24]. Tilton et al. [25] analyzed viruses from 11 treatment-experienced patients in whom virologic failure occurred on regimens containing MVC and noted that resistance was dependent upon mutations within the V3 loop which was only modulated by additional mutations in the V4 loop. The V4 mutations consisted of D407G and loss of a glycosylation site at residue 386.

Platt et al. [26] described HIV-1 CCR5 (ΔNt)-adapted mutants of the JR-CSF strain that had mutations in regions V3, V2 and C3 with 4 mutations in the V4 loop: N403S, N403K, T405A, and T405N. They concluded that loss of N-glycan at position 403 helps to convert the HIV-1 env into a hairpin-trigger form that no longer requires strong interactions with both the CCR5 amino terminus and ECL2 but efficiently targets either site alone [27-32]. Based on these models, we could postulate that the presence of T in position 408 of the V4 loop could alter the quaternary structure of the gp120-gp41 trimeric complex, eliciting conformational transition from a high-energy to a low-energy state (fusogenic conformation), enhancing membrane fusion, and promoting the next step in the virus entry pathway. Since positions 403 and 408 of the V4 loop are close proximity, we imagine that the resistance conferred by I408T mutation in our study could alter the quaternary structure of the HIV-1

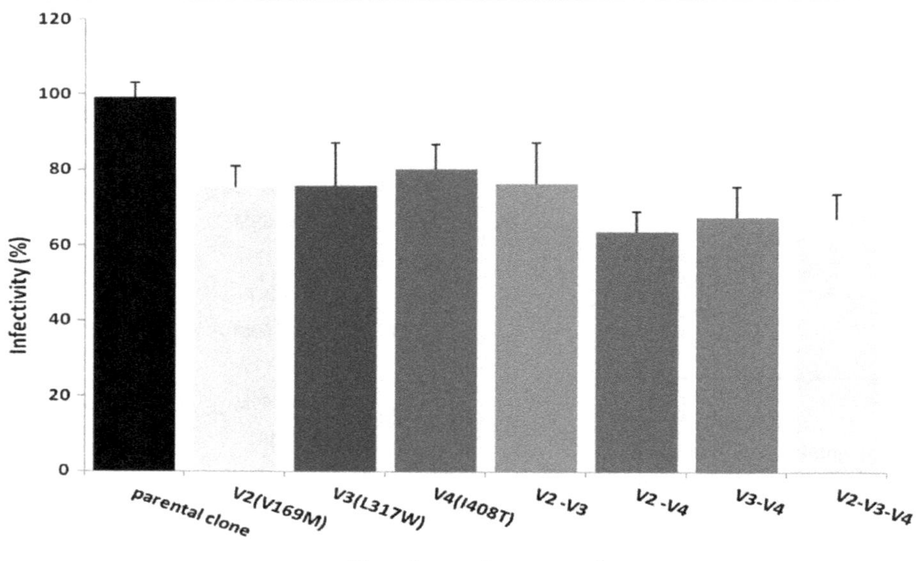

Figure 2 Effect of Env glycoprotein mutations on infectivity of the HIV-1 strain CC1/85. U87-CD4-CCR5 cells were infected with HIV-1 Env pseudoviruses bearing parental clone (wild type) or Env single mutants V169M, L317W, I408T, double mutants V169M/L317W, V169M/I408T, L317W/I408T and the triple mutant V169M/L317W/I408T. Means from 3 independent experiments performed in triplicate are reported. Pseudovirus infectivity was calculated as RLU of the mutant/RLU of the wild type × 100%.

Env, thus sterically masking the glycosylation site in position 403.

Mutations in V2, C3 and gp41 have also been observed in CC1/85-derived, MVC-resistant viruses [14]. The mutation V169M, identified in our study, was also found by Marozsan et al. in VCV escape mutant, which was resistant to VCV, but they did not investigate the contribution of each individual mutation to the resistant phenotype [15]. Recently, Thielen et al. [33] demonstrated that mutations at position 169 of the V2 loop can serve in HIV-1 co-receptor prediction. In their study, the mutation V169T showed strong association with CXCR4 usage while V169K was coupled with CCR5 usage. In another study, the mutation V169K in V2 was predictive of the R5 phenotype [34]. Our results disclosed that mutant V169M exploits R5 exclusively as a co-receptor. V169M mutation was coupled with reduced infectivity but not with a resistant phenotype. Unexpectedly, our triple mutant was less infective than single and double mutants as the emergence of mutations throughout gp120 and gp41 indicated general envelope gene (env) re-arrangement to compensate for decreased replicative capacity [35,36].

Conclusions

Several mutations outside the V3 loop were shown to contribute to CCR5 inhibitor resistance. Our results showed that I408T, L317W/I408T and V169M/L317W/I408T mutants had the highest impact on MVC susceptibility, mostly due to I408T in V4. This mutation could lower the activation energy needed to enable gp41 to undergo the next conformational changes and acquire a more stable low-energy state. All mutants retained the CCR5 co-receptor, supporting the concept that resistant viruses maintained the ability to use inhibitor-bound CCR5, depending on co-receptor density on the cellular surface and the degree of CCR5 co-receptor occupancy by drugs.

Methods

Compounds, cells and viruses

MVC and VCV were obtained from ViroChem Inc. Canada, now Vertex Canada Inc., reconstituted in DMSO 100% (Sigma, St. Louis, MO, USA) and diluted in RPMI 1640 culture medium (Sigma). Peripheral blood mononuclear cells (PBMCs) from 3 HIV-negative donors were isolated by Ficoll-Paque gradient separation (Sigma), stimulated for 3 days with phytohemagglutinin (Sigma) at 1 mg/ml and re-suspended at 2×10^6 cells/ml in RPMI 1640 supplemented with 20% heat-inactivated fetal calf serum (FCS, Invitrogen, Carlsbad, CA, USA), 50 U/ml penicillin (Invitrogen), 50 μg/ml streptomycin (Invitrogen)., 2 mM L-glutamine, 10 mM hydroxyethylpiperazine N-2 ethanesulfonic acid (HEPES) and 1 μg/ml interleukin-2 (Hoffmann-La Roche, Nutley, NJ, USA) in 6-well plates (Becton Dickinson, Lincoln Park, N.J USA.). 293T cells were cultured in Dulbecco's modified Eagle medium (DMEM) and supplemented with 10% FCS, 100 U/ml penicillin and 0.1 mg of streptomycin/ml U87CD4CXCR4 and U87CD4CCR5 cells were cultured in DMEM and supplemented with 10% FCS, 100 U/ml of penicillin, 0.1 mg of streptomycin/ml, 1 μg/mL of puromycin (Sigma) and 300 μg of G418 (Invitrogen). All cells were maintained at 37°C and 5% CO_2. Cells and the viruses BaL and CC1/85 (R5 tropic), III B (X4-tropic) and 85.6 (dual-tropic) were obtained from the National Institutes of Health.

Generation of HIV-1 mutants resistant to MVC and VCV by *in vitro* passage in PBMCs

2×10^6 PBMCs/ml were infected with 3,000 tissue culture infective doses 50% of BaL and CC1/85 viruses, in a final volume of 2 ml containing sub-inhibitory concentrations of 0.04 nM MVC and 0.02 nM VCV. Every 7 days, the culture supernatant was passaged onto fresh cells with MVC- and VVC-containing medium, and virus growth was monitored by enzyme-linked immunosorbent assay (ELISA) to measure supernatant p24 levels (Perkin-Elmer, Norwalk, CT, USA). MVC and VCV were added every 4 days at concentrations depending on p24 levels. MVC and VCV control passages were set up in parallel. Full length sequences of gp120 and gp41 were obtained for different time points, and mutations from resistant viruses were identified. Resistance was defined as MPI <95% or ≥3-FC in IC_{50}. Viral tropism was predicted according to 11/25 and net charge rules [37] as well as $PSSM_{X4R5}$ [11,12] and geno2pheno co-receptor algorithms [13].

Amplification and sequence analysis of the HIV env gene from selected time-points

HIV-1 RNA was extracted from culture supernatants with QIAmp Viral RNA mini-kit (Qiagen, Mississauga, ON, Canada). Full-length gp160 was amplified with reverse transcription -polymerase chain reaction (RT-PCR) primers (5' NewFHindIII GGCCAAGCTTATGAGAGT GACGGAGATCAG and 5' YW15XhoI GGCCCTCGA GTTATCCAGTCCCCCCTTTTC), followed by nested polymerase chain reaction (PCR) with primers (5' NewFHindIII GGCCAAGCTTATGAGAGTGACGGAG ATCAG and 5' YW16XhoI GGCCCTCGAGTTATTTT GACCACTTGCCAC). PCR products were separated on 1% agarose gel and purified with QIAprep Spin Miniprep Kit (Qiagen). Sequencing was undertaken at the Génome-Québec sequencing facilities in a 3730 × l DNA analyser from Applied Biosystems (McGill University and the Genome Quebec Innovation Centre, Montreal, QC, Canada) with Sequencer 4.7 (Gene Code Software

Corporation, Ann Arbor, MI, USA) and aligned by ClustalW version 1.83 [10]. Nucleotide sequences of CC1/85 have been deposited in GenBank under accession numbers JQ924495 (start), JQ924496 (controlP4), JQ924497 (MVCP4), JQ924498 (VCVP4), JQ924499 (controlP16), JQ92450 (MVCP16), and JQ924501 (VCVP16).

Site-directed mutagenesis

Primers were designed with the Stratagene's web-based QuikChange® Primer Design Program [38]. Mutagenesis procedures were carried out according to an overlapping-extension PCR-based procedure [39,40].

Cloning and pseudovirus construction

The expression plasmid pcDNA3.1day/V5HisTOPO (Invitrogen) and Env PCR products of CC1/85, BaL, III B, 85.6 viruses and selected mutants (V169M in V2, L317W in V3 and I408T in V4) in single, double and triple combinations were digested with HindIII and Xhol restriction enzymes (Invitrogen), purified and ligated with T4 DNA Ligase (Invitrogen). The ligation product was transformed into *E. coli* TOP10 competent cells. Pseudoviruses were produced by co-transfection of Env expression plasmid and backbone pNL4-3. Luc.E-R-, as described previously [41,42]. Pseudovirus stocks were normalized with p24 ELISA prior to testing infectivity. Assays were performed with 25 ng of p24 per well.

Luciferase assays to determine infectivity and tropism

A luminescence assay using U87CD4CXCR5 and U87CD4CXCR4 cells was used to measure infectivity and tropism. On the day prior to infection, $1{\times}10^6$ cells per well were seeded in 96-well plates. On the day of infection, MVC and AMD 3100 were added to wells designated for treatment with an inhibitor and incubated for 1 h at 37°C prior to infection. 50 μl of normalized pseudovirus stocks were added in each well. The plates were incubated for 2 days at 37°C with 5% CO_2. The medium was removed, and 100 μl of lysis buffer (Promega Inc., Madison, WI, USA) was added to each well for 30 min. Then, 100 μl of luciferase assay reagent (Promega) was added immediately prior to reading the plates in a luminometer (Tecan, Morrisville, NC, USA). Luciferase activity was recorded as relative light units (RLU). Viral entry was determined as percent reduction of viral infectivity compared to the controls. All experiments were performed in duplicate. IC_{50}-FC was calculated as the ratio of IC_{50} for resistant virus/IC_{50} for wild type virus. MPI was calculated as [1- (RLU in the presence of drug/RLU in the absence of drug)] × 100, and infectivity as RLU of the mutant/RLU of the wild type × 100%. Inhibition curves were generated by GraphPad Prism software (San Diego, CA, USA).

Abbreviations

(HIV-1): Human immunodeficiency virus-1 entry; (V3): Variable domain 3; (IC_{50}): Half maximal inhibitory concentration; (Env): Envelope protein; (CCR5): C-C chemokine receptor 5; (CXCR4): C-X-C chemokine receptor 4; (MVC): Maraviroc; (VCV): Vicriviroc; (MPI): As maximum percent inhibition; (FC): Measuring fold-change; (env): Envelope gene.

Competing interests

CT is the Pfizer/University of Montreal Chair in HIV Translational Research and a scholar from Fonds de la recherche en santé du Québec. The other authors declare no conflicts of interest.

Authors' contributions

OA-M participated in study conception and design, data collection, analysis and interpretation as well as manuscript drafting; AC supervised the study, analyzed and interpreted the data, and reviewed the manuscript; YW participated in study conception and design; AH participated in data collection; MS participated in data collection, analysis and interpretations; CT participated in study conception and design, data analysis and interpretation, study supervision, and manuscript review. All authors read and approved the final manuscript.

Acknowledgments

We thank Dr. Andrés Finzi for reading our manuscript and offering valuable suggestions, Dr. Amal Nadiri for discussions on and assistance with mutagenesis, and the NIH AIDS Research and Reference Reagent Program for the viruses, the backbone pNL4-3. Luc.E-R- and U87CD4CXCR4, U87CD4CCR5 and 293T cells.

Funding

This work was supported by the Réseau Fonds de la recherche en santé du Québec (FRSQ)-SIDA.

Author details

[1]Centre de recherche, Centre hospitalier de l'Université de Montréal (CRCHUM), Montréal, QC, Canada. [2]Department of Microbiology and Immunology, Faculty of Medicine, Université de Montréal, Montréal, QC, Canada. [3]Laboratoire de santé publique du Québec/Institut national de santé publique du Québec (INSPQ), Québec, Canada. [4]CRCHUM – Hôtel-Dieu, Pavillon Jeanne-Mance, bureau 7-355, 3840 rue St-Urbain, Montréal, QC H2W 1T8, Canada.

References

1. Chen B, Vogan EM, Gong H, Skehel JJ, Wiley DC, Harrison SC: **Structure of an unliganded simian immunodeficiency virus gp120 core.** *Nature* 2005, **433:**834–841.
2. Kwong PD, Wyatt R, Robinson J, Sweet RW, Sodroski J, Hendrickson WA: **Structure of an HIV gp120 envelope glycoprotein in complex with the CD4 receptor and a neutralizing human antibody.** *Nature* 1998, **393:**648–659.
3. Pfaff JM, Wilen CB, Harrison JE, Demarest JF, Lee B, Doms RW, Tilton JC: **HIV-1 resistance to CCR5 antagonists associated with highly efficient use of CCR5 and altered tropism on primary CD4+ T cells.** *J Virol* 2010, **84:**6505–6514.
4. Tilton JC, Doms RW: **Entry inhibitors in the treatment of HIV-1 infection.** *Antiviral Res* 2010, **85:**91–100.
5. Berro R, Klasse PJ, Moore JP, Sanders RW: **V3 determinants of HIV-1 escape from the CCR5 inhibitors Maraviroc and Vicriviroc.** *Virology* 2012, **427:**158–165.

6. Kondru R, Zhang J, Ji C, Mirzadegan T, Rotstein D, Sankuratri S, Dioszegi M: **Molecular interactions of CCR5 with major classes of small-molecule anti-HIV CCR5 antagonists.** *Mol Pharmacol* 2008, **73:**789–800.
7. Strizki JM, Tremblay C, Xu S, Wojcik L, Wagner N, Gonsiorek W, Hipkin RW, Chou CC, Pugliese-Sivo C, Xiao Y, *et al*: **Discovery and characterization of vicriviroc (SCH 417690), a CCR5 antagonist with potent activity against human immunodeficiency virus type 1.** *Antimicrob Agents Chemother* 2005, **49:**4911–4919.
8. McNicholas PM, Mann PA, Wojcik L, Phd PQ, Lee E, McCarthy M, Shen J, Black TA, Strizki JM: **Mapping and characterization of vicriviroc resistance mutations from HIV-1 isolated from treatment-experienced subjects enrolled in a phase II study (VICTOR-E1).** *J Acquir Immune Defic Syndr* 2011, **56:**222–229.
9. Roche M, Jakobsen MR, Sterjovski J, Ellett A, Posta F, Lee B, Jubb B, Westby M, Lewin SR, Ramsland PA, *et al*: **HIV-1 escape from the CCR5 antagonist maraviroc associated with an altered and less-efficient mechanism of gp120-CCR5 engagement that attenuates macrophage tropism.** *J Virol* 2011, **85:**4330–4342.
10. McNicholas P, Wei Y, Whitcomb J, Greaves W, Black TA, Tremblay CL, Strizki JM: **Characterization of emergent HIV resistance in treatment-naive subjects enrolled in a vicriviroc phase 2 trial.** *J Infect Dis* 2010, **201:**1470–1480.
11. Jensen MA, Li FS, van't Wout AB, Nickle DC, Shriner D, He HX, McLaughlin S, Shankarappa R, Margolick JB, Mullins JI: **Improved coreceptor usage prediction and genotypic monitoring of R5-to-X4 transition by motif analysis of human immunodeficiency virus type 1 env V3 loop sequences.** *J Virol* 2003, **77:**13376–13388.
12. Jensen MA, Coetzer M, van't Wout AB, Morris L, Mullins JI: **A reliable phenotype predictor for human immunodeficiency virus type 1 subtype C based on envelope V3 sequences.** *J Virol* 2006, **80:**4698–4704.
13. Lengauer T, Sander O, Sierra S, Thielen A, Kaiser R: **Bioinformatics prediction of HIV coreceptor usage.** *Nat Biotechnol* 2007, **25:**1407–1410.
14. Westby M, Smith-Burchnell C, Mori J, Lewis M, Mosley M, Stockdale M, Dorr P, Ciaramella G, Perros M: **Reduced maximal inhibition in phenotypic susceptibility assays indicates that viral strains resistant to the CCR5 antagonist maraviroc utilize inhibitor-bound receptor for entry.** *J Virol* 2007, **81:**2359–2371.
15. Marozsan AJ, Kuhmann SE, Morgan T, Herrera C, Rivera-Troche E, Xu S, Baroudy BM, Strizki J, Moore JP: **Generation and properties of a human immunodeficiency virus type 1 isolate resistant to the small molecule CCR5 inhibitor, SCH-417690 (SCH-D).** *Virology* 2005, **338:**182–199.
16. Trkola A, Kuhmann SE, Strizki JM, Maxwell E, Ketas T, Morgan T, Pugach P, Xu S, Wojcik L, Tagat J, *et al*: **HIV-1 escape from a small molecule, CCR5-specific entry inhibitor does not involve CXCR4 use.** *Proc Natl Acad Sci USA* 2002, **99:**395–400.
17. Kuhmann SE, Pugach P, Kunstman KJ, Taylor J, Stanfield RL, Snyder A, Strizki JM, Riley J, Baroudy BM, Wilson IA, *et al*: **Genetic and phenotypic analyses of human immunodeficiency virus type 1 escape from a small-molecule CCR5 inhibitor.** *J Virol* 2004, **78:**2790–2807.
18. Roche M, Jakobsen MR, Ellett A, Salimiseyedabad H, Jubb B, Westby M, Lee B, Lewin SR, Churchill MJ, Gorry PR: **HIV-1 predisposed to acquiring resistance to maraviroc (MVC) and other CCR5 antagonists in vitro has an inherent, low-level ability to utilize MVC-bound CCR5 for entry.** *Retrovirology* 2011, **8:**89.
19. Zolla-Pazner S, Cardozo T: **Structure-function relationships of HIV-1 envelope sequence-variable regions refocus vaccine design.** *Nat Rev Immunol* 2010, **10:**527–535.
20. Anastassopoulou CG, Ketas TJ, Klasse PJ, Moore JP: **Resistance to CCR5 inhibitors caused by sequence changes in the fusion peptide of HIV-1 gp41.** *Proc Natl Acad Sci USA* 2009, **106:**5318–5323.
21. Yu X, Yuan L, Huang Y, Xu W, Fang Z, Liu S, Shao Y, Jiang S, Ma L: **Susceptibility of HIV-1 Subtypes B', CRF07_BC and CRF01_AE that Are Predominantly Circulating in China to HIV-1 Entry Inhibitors.** *PLoS One* 2011, **6:**e17605.
22. Yuan Y, Maeda Y, Terasawa H, Monde K, Harada S, Yusa K: **A combination of polymorphic mutations in V3 loop of HIV-1 gp120 can confer noncompetitive resistance to maraviroc.** *Virology* 2011, **413:**293–299.
23. Munoz-Nieto M, Perez-Alvarez L, Thomson M, Garcia V, Ocampo A, Casado G, Delgado E, Miralles C, de Parga EV, Sierra M, *et al*: **HIV type 1 intersubtype recombinants during the evolution of a dual infection with subtypes B and G.** *AIDS Res Hum Retroviruses* 2008, **24:**337–343.
24. Wilkin TJ, Gulick RM: **CCR5 antagonism in HIV infection: current concepts and future opportunities.** *Annu Rev Med* 2012, **63:**81–93.
25. Tilton JC, Wilen CB, Didigu CA, Sinha R, Harrison JE, Agrawal-Gamse C, Henning EA, Bushman FD, Martin JN, Deeks SG, Doms RW: **A maraviroc-resistant HIV-1 with narrow cross-resistance to other CCR5 antagonists depends on both N-terminal and extracellular loop domains of drug-bound CCR5.** *J Virol* 2010, **84:**10863–10876.
26. Platt EJ, Shea DM, Rose PP, Kabat D: **Variants of human immunodeficiency virus type 1 that efficiently use CCR5 lacking the tyrosine-sulfated amino terminus have adaptive mutations in gp120, including loss of a functional N-glycan.** *J Virol* 2005, **79:**4357–4368.
27. Wyatt R, Kwong PD, Desjardins E, Sweet RW, Robinson J, Hendrickson WA, Sodroski JG: **The antigenic structure of the HIV gp120 envelope glycoprotein.** *Nature* 1998, **393:**705–711.
28. Wyatt R, Sodroski J: **The HIV-1 envelope glycoproteins: fusogens, antigens, and immunogens.** *Science* 1998, **280:**1884–1888.
29. Xiang SH, Finzi A, Pacheco B, Alexander K, Yuan W, Rizzuto C, Huang CC, Kwong PD, Sodroski J: **A V3 loop-dependent gp120 element disrupted by CD4 binding stabilizes the human immunodeficiency virus envelope glycoprotein trimer.** *J Virol* 2010, **84:**3147–3161.
30. Cormier EG, Dragic T: **The crown and stem of the V3 loop play distinct roles in human immunodeficiency virus type 1 envelope glycoprotein interactions with the CCR5 coreceptor.** *J Virol* 2002, **76:**8953–8957.
31. Cormier EG, Tran DN, Yukhayeva L, Olson WC, Dragic T: **Mapping the determinants of the CCR5 amino-terminal sulfopeptide interaction with soluble human immunodeficiency virus type 1 gp120-CD4 complexes.** *J Virol* 2001, **75:**5541–5549.
32. Huang CC, Lam SN, Acharya P, Tang M, Xiang SH, Hussan SS, Stanfield RL, Robinson J, Sodroski J, Wilson IA, *et al*: **Structures of the CCR5 N terminus and of a tyrosine-sulfated antibody with HIV-1 gp120 and CD4.** *Science* 2007, **317:**1930–1934.
33. Thielen A, Sichtig N, Kaiser R, Lam J, Harrigan PR, Lengauer T: **Improved prediction of HIV-1 coreceptor usage with sequence information from the second hypervariable loop of gp120.** *J Infect Dis* 2010, **202:**1435–1443.
34. Monno L, Saracino A, Scudeller L, Punzi G, Brindicci G, Altamura M, Lagioia A, Ladisa N, Angarano G: **Impact of mutations outside the V3 region on coreceptor tropism phenotypically assessed in patients infected with HIV-1 subtype B.** *Antimicrob Agents Chemother* 2011, **55:**5078–5084.
35. Gonzalez-Ortega E, Ballana E, Badia R, Clotet B, Este JA: **Compensatory mutations rescue the virus replicative capacity of VIRIP-resistant HIV-1.** *Antiviral Res* 2011, **92:**479–483.
36. Lucas GM: **Antiretroviral adherence, drug resistance, viral fitness and HIV disease progression: a tangled web is woven.** *J Antimicrob Chemother* 2005, **55:**413–416.
37. Poveda E, Alcami J, Paredes R, Cordoba J, Gutierrez F, Llibre JM, Delgado R, Pulido F, Iribarren JA, Garcia Deltoro M, *et al*: **Genotypic determination of HIV tropism - clinical and methodological recommendations to guide the therapeutic use of CCR5 antagonists.** *AIDS Rev* 2010, **12:**135–148.
38. **The stratagene's web-based Primer Design Program QuikChange® available at website at** [http://www.genomics.agilent.com/primerDesignProgram.jsp]
39. Kanoksilapatham, GJM W, Robb FT: **Directed-Mutagenesis and Deletion Generated through an Improved Overlapping-Extension PCR Based Procedure.** *Silpakorn U Sci Tech J Vol* 2007, **1:**7–12.
40. Aiyar A, Xiang Y, Leis J: **Site-directed mutagenesis using overlap extension PCR.** *Methods Mol Biol* 1996, **57:**177–191.
41. Connor RI, Sheridan KE, Lai C, Zhang L, Ho DD: **Characterization of the functional properties of env genes from long-term survivors of human immunodeficiency virus type 1 infection.** *J Virol* 1996, **70:**5306–5311.
42. Singh A, Page T, Moore PL, Allgaier RL, Hiramen K, Coovadia HM, Walker BD, Morris L, Ndung'u T: **Functional and genetic analysis of coreceptor usage by dualtropic HIV-1 subtype C isolates.** *Virology* 2009, **393:**56–67.

6

Predictors of mortality among HIV infected patients taking antiretroviral treatment in Ethiopia

Sibhatu Biadgilign[1], Ayalu A Reda[2*] and Tesfaye Digaffe[3]

Abstract

Background: Studies indicate that there is high early mortality among patients starting antiretroviral treatment in sub-Saharan Africa. However, there is paucity of evidence on long term survival of patients on anti-retroviral treatment in the region. The objective of this study is to examine mortality and its predictors among a cohort of HIV infected patients on anti-retroviral treatment retrospectively followed for five years.

Methods: A retrospective cohort study was conducted among HIV infected patients on ART in eastern Ethiopia. Cox regression and Kaplan-Meier analyses were performed to investigate factors that influence time to death and survival over time.

Result: A total of 1540 study participants were included in the study. From the registered patients in the cohort, the outcome of patients as active, deceased, lost to follow up and transfer out was 1005 (67.2%), 86 (5.9%), 210 (14.0%) and 192 (12.8%) respectively. The overall mortality rate provides an incidence density of 2.03 deaths per 100 person years (95% CI 1.64 - 2.50). Out of a total of 86 deaths over 60 month period; 63 (73.3%) died during the first 12 months, 10 (11.6%) during the second year, and 10 (11.6%) in the third year of follow up. In multivariate analysis, the independent predictors for mortality were loss of more 10% weight loss, bedridden functional status at baseline, ≤ 200 CD4 cell count/ml, and advanced WHO stage patients.

Conclusion: A lower level of mortality was detected among the cohort of patients on antiretroviral treatment in eastern Ethiopia. Previous history of weight loss, bedridden functional status at baseline, low CD4 cell count and advanced WHO status patients had a higher risk of death. Early initiation of ART, provision of nutritional support and strengthening of the food by prescription initiative, and counseling of patients for early presentation to treatment is recommended.

Introduction

Development of highly active antiretroviral treatment (ART) in the mid-1990s revolutionized the care of HIV-infected patients and led to marked reductions in HIV-associated morbidity and mortality in many industrialized countries [1,2]. ART has clearly shown to be effective in reducing mortality among those who remain in treatment and adhere to therapy [2-4]. In recent years in developing countries with a high burden of AIDS, ART has become more widely available. According to estimation by the World Health Organization (WHO), about 6 650 000 patients were receiving ART in low- and middle-income countries by the end of 2010 [5], this is a huge improvement from the levels in 2003 [6,7]. Two sub-Saharan African countries, Botswana and Rwanda, have achieved universal access target (treatment coverage of 80% or more of patients in need) at the end of 2009 [7], while countries such as Ethiopia, Zambia, Namibia and Senegal are moving closer to the same target having covered 50-80% of patients in need of treatment [7]. Due to this morbidity and mortality among HIV-infected persons have dramatically decreased [8,9].

The primary goals of antiretroviral therapy are preventing HIV-related morbidity and mortality, and improving quality of life by restoring immunologic function through suppression of viral load [10]. Many studies

* Correspondence: ayaluaklilu@yahoo.com; a.reda@haramaya.edu.et
[2]Department of Public Health, College of Health Sciences, Haramaya University, P. O. Box 235, Harar, Ethiopia
Full list of author information is available at the end of the article

have reported high early mortality among patients starting antiretroviral treatment in sub-Saharan Africa [4]. One of the reasons cited for this is that despite better availability of ART, people are still diagnosed late and thus start ART at later stages of the HIV disease [11].

In Ethiopia, there were more than 222,000 patients on antiretroviral treatment at the end of 2010 [6]. ART has improved survival of patients with HIV/AIDS and improved the quality of life of patients in the country [12]. In Ethiopia, there are no studies reporting the long term survival of patients on antiretroviral treatment. Such studies could provide valuable information to evaluate the ART program in the country. The objective of this study is to examine mortality and its predictors among a cohort of HIV infected patients on antiretroviral treatment retrospectively followed for five years.

Methods

Study area and period

The study was conducted in Hiwot Fana, Jugal and Dil Chora hospitals located in eastern Ethiopia. Data was collected from September to November 2010.

Study design

A retrospective cohort study was conducted among HIV patients on ART. A random sample of 1537 patients that started treatment between September 11, 2005 and September 10, 2008 were included in the study and retrospectively followed up for an additional two years until September 10, 2010. The patients' identification numbers were used to generate the necessary sample from the records of the hospitals for extracting data.

Socio-demographic characteristics, baseline and follow up clinical and laboratory measurement information, and treatment outcomes were abstracted from patients' cards. The primary outcome measure was patient survival, while secondary outcome measures included CD4 count and body weight.

Data collection and quality control

A standard questionnaire was used for recording information extracted from patients' cards. This form is developed using the standardized ART entry and follow up form employed by the ART clinic. The CD4 count laboratory results recorded before starting ART were used as a base line values. If there is no pre-treatment laboratory test, however, results obtained within one month of ART initiation were considered as baseline values. Four experienced ART nurses who were trained on comprehensive HIV care and involved in patient follow ups collected the data. Data collection was supervised by the researchers. All completed data collection forms were examined for clarity and consistency. The data were entered and cleaned by trained data clerks and the investigators before analysis.

Death was ascertained by reviewing cards and death certificates. Patients who died from unrelated diseases or accident were considered as censored, as well as those alive at the end of the follow up period.

Table 1 Baseline characteristics of HIV infected patients initiating antiretroviral therapy

	All patients, ¥N (%)	Patients with CD4 count≤200 (n = 1149)	Patients with CD4 count>200 (n = 361)
Sex			
Male	574 (37.3)	431 (37.6)	131 (36.3)
Female	963 (62.5)	715 (62.4)	230 (63.7)
Age (Median, IQR)	32 (28–40)	32 (28.0–40.0)	35 (28.0–40.0)
Religion			
Muslim	305 (19.8)	220 (19.1)	76 (21.1)
Orthodox	1074 (69.9)	812 (70.7)	241 (66.8)
Protestant	144 (9.4)	103 (9.0)	41 (11.4)
Others	14 (0.9)	14 (1.2)	3 (0.8)
Education			
No education	261 (17.0)	185 (16.1)	67 (18.6)
Primary	681 (44.3)	490 (42.7)	178 (49.3)
Secondary	500 (32.5)	391 (34.1)	102 (28.3)
Tertiary	96 (6.2)	81 (7.1)	14 (3.9)
Marital status			
Never Married	287 (18.6)	217 (18.9)	65 (18.0)
Married	606 (39.4)	475 (41.4)	124 (34.3)
Separated	288 (18.7)	206 (17.9)	74 (20.5)
Divorced	116 (7.5)	89 (7.8)	22 (6.1)
Widowed	242 (15.7)	161 (14.0)	76 (21.1)
Occupation			
Merchant	75 (7.4)	60 (7.7)	15 (6.7)
Gov. Employee	157 (15.5)	122 (15.6)	33 (14.8)
Non-Gov. Employee	41 (4.1)	34 (4.4)	7 (3.1)
Day Laborer	174 (17.2)	130 (16.7)	44 (19.7)
Job-less	402 (39.7)	303 (38.8)	94 (42.2)
Other	163 (16.2)	131 (16.8)	30 (13.5)
Past co-trimoxazole treatment			
Yes	758 (49.2)	576 (50.1)	171 (47.4)
No	782 (50.8)	573 (49.9)	190 (52.6)
WHO stage at baseline			
Stage I	92 (6.0)	76 (6.7)	15 (4.2)
Stage II	348 (22.7)	282 (24.7)	63 (17.5)
Stage III	890 (58.2)	633 (55.5)	239 (66.6)
Stage IV	200 (13.1)	150 (13.1)	42 (11.7)
Baseline CD4 count, median (IQR)	135 (76.0–198.3)	107 (64.0–154.0)	253 (223.3–304.0)
Weight at baseline in kgs, median (IQR)	50.0 (44.0–56.0)	50 (44.0–56.0)	50 (45.0–57.0)

¥Number and percentages unless indicated otherwise. IQR, inter-quartile rage.

Data analysis

Descriptive statistics such as median, mean, SDs and tables were be used to investigate the characteristics of the cohort. Person years of follow up were calculated by assessing the date of enrollment for ART and death or censoring. Survival analysis and the Kaplan-Meier test were used to investigate factors that influence time to death. Hazard ratios (HR), as well as 95% confidence intervals were used as effect measures. A p-value of 0.05 was used. Descriptive statistics and Cox regression were conducted using SPSS® version 16. Proportionality of hazards test on Schoenfeld residuals and graph were conducted using STATA® version 10.

Ethical consideration

Ethical clearance was obtained from the Institutional Research Ethics Review Committee (IRERC) of Haramaya University. All information collected from patients cards were kept strictly confidential and names were not included in the abstracted data.

Results

Characteristics of patients

A total of 1540 study participants were included in the study. The sample comprised 963 (62.5%) females and 574 (37.3%) males respectively. The median and inter-quartile range (IQR) age was 32 and 28–40. The majority of participants 1074 (69.9%) were Orthodox Christians and 305 (19.8) were Muslim. Clinically, 890 (58.2%) and 348 (22.7%) patients were on the stage III and II. The median (IQR) baseline CD4 count was 135 (76.0–198.3) per milliliter (Table 1).

Follow up and survival patterns of the cohort

From the registered patients in this cohort analysis, the outcome of patients as active, deceased, lost to follow up and transfer out were 1005 (67.2%), 86 (5.9%), 210 (14.0%) and 192 (12.8%) respectively. There were 86 deaths in 4234.8 person years of retrospective follow up Figure 1 displays the survival patterns of the cohort based on WHO clinical stage categories. The overall mortality rate provides an incidence density of 2.03 deaths per 100 person years (95% CI 1.64–2.50). Out of a total of 86 deaths over 60 month period; 63 (73.3%) died during the first 12 months, 10 (11.6%) during the second year, and 10 (11.6%) in the third year of follow up. When the follow-up period was divided into 1-year time bands (from ART initiation through 1 year, from 1 year through 2 years, and from 2 years though 3 years), the mortality rates per 100 person years at risk were 55.67 (95% CI 43.48–71.26), 4.03 (95% CI 2.17–7.51), and 0.31 (95% CI 0.18–0.54) respectively.

Predictors of mortality

In univarite analysis, factors associated with the predictor of mortality were previous weight loss of more than 10%, bedridden functional status at baseline, less than 200 CD4 cells/ml and WHO stage IV patients. Those patients who reported to have lost a weight of more than 10% at baseline were 5 times more likely to die compared to those who did not (hazard ratio, HR 4.41; 95% CI 1.08–17.92). Those patients who were bedridden or non-ambulatory at the initiation of treatment were five times more likely to die compared with those that were working (HR 5.33; 95% CI 3.05–9.30). Those patients whose CD4 cell count lied between 201–300

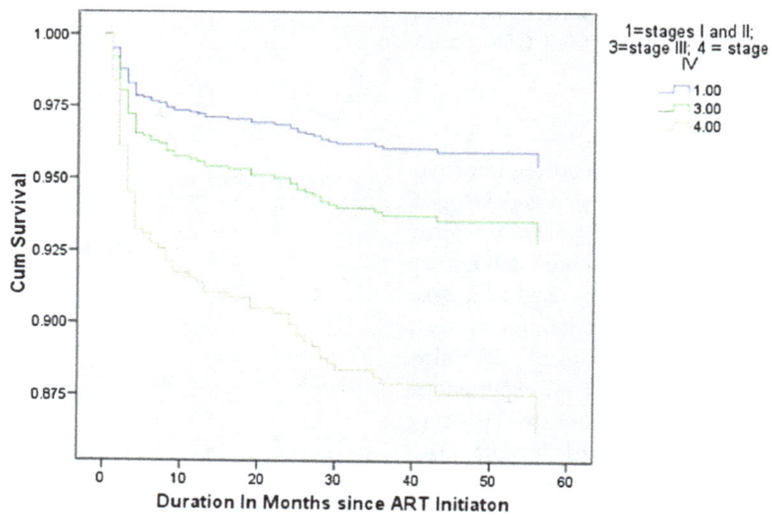

Figure 1 Survival functions stratified according to WHO clinical staging in HIV infected patients in a cohort of patients on antiretroviral treatment in eastern Ethiopia (y-axis truncated to improve visibility).

were 58% less likely to die as compared to those patients whose CD4 count was less than 200 cells per milliliter (HR 0.42; 95% CI 0.19–0.92).

In the multivariate analysis, five baseline factors were independent predictors of mortality. WHO stage IV patients were 3 times more likely to die compared to stage I and II patients (HR 3.19; 95% CI 1.51–6.76). Bedridden patients were four times more likely to die compared with those patients who are working (HR 4.09; 95% CI 2.12–7.90). Patients who reported to have lost more than 10% of their weight at baseline were 5 times more likely to die compared to those patients who did not (HR 4.93; 95% CI 1.20–20.41). Patients whose CD4 cell counts between 201–300 were 60% less likely to die compared to those whose CD4 counts less than 200 (HR 0.40; 95% CI 0.17–0.93). Those patients with primary education were almost 3 times more likely to die than illiterate counterpart (HR 2.79; 95% CI 1.26–6.16) (Table 2).

Discussions

The findings indicate that from the registered cohort, there were 86 deaths in 4234.8 years of retrospective follow up, providing an incidence density of 2.03 deaths per 100 person years (95% CI 1.64–2.51). About 210 (14.0%) patients were lost to follow up. Factors that were

Table 2 Predictors of mortality among a sample of HIV infected cohorts on anti-retroviral treatment in eastern Ethiopia

Independent variables	Unadjusted HR (95% CI)	P-value	¥Adjusted HR (95% CI)	P-value
Age	1.02 (0.99–1.04)	0.131	1.02 (0.99–1.05)	0.156
Sex				
Male	1.00		1.00	
Female	1.05 (0.68–1.64)	0.819	1.16 (0.68–2.00)	0.584
Religion				
Muslim	1.00		1.00	
Christian	0.85 (0.51–1.42)	0.539	0.98 (0.55–1.75)	0.939
Employment				
Employed	1.00		1.00	
Not employed	1.05 (0.66–1.67)	0.827	0.94 (0.58–1.52)	0.788
Marital status				
Not married	1.00		1.00	
Married	0.92 (0.60–1.41)	0.694	0.97 (0.60–1.56)	0.884
Education				
No education	1.00		1.00	
Primary	1.58 (0.79–3.16)	0.193	2.79 (1.26–6.16)	0.011
Secondary or above	1.42 (0.70–2.87)	0.331	1.40 (0.61–3.22)	0.435
Baseline functional status				
Working	1.00		1.00	
Ambulatory	1.28 (0.77–2.13)	0.337	1.14 (0.64–2.04)	0.651
Bedridden	5.33 (3.05–9.30)	0.000	4.09 (2.12–7.90)	0.000
10% weight loss				
No	1.00		1.00	
Yes	4.41 (1.08–17.92)	0.038	4.93 (1.20–20.41)	0.027
CD4 category				
≤ 200	1.00		1.00	
201–300	0.42 (0.19–0.92)	0.029	0.40 (0.17–0.93)	0.034
>300	0.67 (0.24–1.82)	0.428	0.86 (0.30–2.41)	0.77
WHO category				
Stage I and II	1.00		1.00	
Stage III	1.35 (0.77–2.36)	0.294	1.60 (0.85–3.04)	0.15
Stage IV	3.35 (1.80–6.24)	0.000	3.19 (1.51–6.76)	0.002

¥Global test of proportionality of hazards derived from Schoenfeld residuals not significant (df = 13, ch2 = 13, p = 0.108).

associated with mortality were 10% weight loss, bedridden functional status at baseline, ≤200 CD4 cells/ml and advanced stage patients.

Long-term retention of patients in antiretroviral treatment is a prerequisite for achieving any adherence at all. Various studies have shown that mortality during the first 6 months after initiating ART is much higher than in developed countries and retention of patients in programs is poor [4,13]. However, most longitudinal studies conducted in Africa have been either short-term or have involved small numbers of participants.

In our study, the overall mortality rate of 2.03 deaths per 100 person years is lower or comparable to that reported elsewhere; however the mortality rate at the first year (55.67; 95% CI 43.5–71.3; or 4.3%) is high. In the ART-LINC Collaboration, which analyzed data from 18 cohorts across the developing world, mortality averaged 4.2% across all 18 cohorts in the first year after initiation [11]. In Yaounde, Cameroon, from 312 patients, the incidence rate of mortality rate was 21.2 per 100 person years (95% CI 15–31) [14]. In southern Ethiopia, the mortality rate was 15.4 per 100 person-years of observation [12]. The majority or 74.1% of the deaths occurred in the first year after treatment. The study highlights the high early mortality in ART cohorts in resource-limited settings that has been observed by other groups in similar settings [4,15,16].

The primary causes of death in AIDS patients could be the causes such immune reconstitution syndrome and opportunistic infections as a result of very weak immunity levels. In our study one of the factors associated with early mortality is late presentation for ART. This may also account for the high rate of death in the first year. According to reports, patients that start ART at WHO Stage III and IV are at an increased risk of dying [17,18]. Furthermore, early mortality risk is higher among those with low CD4 cell count [4,19]. The CD4 count is a proxy indicator of severity of disease which corresponds to the functional status and reflects the immune state of patients [20]. In our study, the functional status of patients at the entry level had a positive correlation with their disease stage and negative correlation with CD4 count. In a report from Hong Kong, there was a 79% reduction in mortality among ART taking patients with CD4 counts of less than 200/ml [21]. The majority of morbidity and mortality seen among individuals starting ART with low baseline CD4 cell count occurs during the first 3–6 months on treatment [2,3,15,16,22]. In one study patients initiating ART with a base-line CD4 cell count of less than 50 cells/mm3 had a 3.2-fold higher mortality rate (p 0.004) compared with patients with a CD4 cell count between 51 and 200 cells/mm3 at the time of ART initiation [23]. Patients starting treatment with CD4 cell count below 100 cells/mm3 were at significantly greater risk of death during the follow-up period (OR 2.69; 95% CI 1.12–6.44) [12].

Nutritional and physical status can predict early mortality. In our study, 10% weight loss determines mortality during the course of treatment. In a district hospital in Ethiopia, weight loss was seen in about a third of patients who survived up to the fourth week, and it was associated with increased death [18]. Higher body weight at baseline was found to be associated with lower risk of mortality with a HR of 0.58 for weight groups of 40–50 kilograms compared with the reference of less than 40 kilograms, and HR of 0.25 for groups ≥60 kilograms compared with the reference groups ($p < 0.013$). The two year patient survival was significantly related with co-trimoxazole initiation at or before treatment, clinical stage IV disease, working functional status and weight greater than 60 kilograms [24]. In another study, baseline body mass index (BMI) of less than 18.5 was independently associated with early mortality risk [19].

About 61% of patients in this study had education below secondary school. According to reports, low educational level among patients is a contributing factor to late presentation for ART [25]. This is understandable since the more educated a patient is the better their understanding of the disease state and comprehension of instructions given on drug usage. These could enhance treatment outcomes [26]. A report from British Columbia reported a protective effect of educational level on mortality from all causes among intravenous drug users receiving anti-retroviral treatment [27,28]. Most reports suggest that low educational level has consistently been associated with higher mortality, both overall and cause-specific [29,30]. In our study lower educational level was associated with a higher risk of mortality. However, patients with primary education seem to be at higher risk of death compared to those with no education. This is an interesting finding for which we could not find explanation due to the nature of our data, however it needs further investigation in future research.

This study has limitations. CD4 cell counts and HIV RNA measurements were not available for all patients because of cost issues. Diagnostic tests that would confirm the presence of certain opportunistic infections were limited; as a result we were not able to include these in our analysis. The retrospective cohort study design limited our ability to gather data about factors that may influence the risk of mortality, for instance factors such as lack of social supports networks, disclosure of infection status and depression. Data was collected from those who were attending ART centers mostly through self-reporting and hence may have reporting and recall bias. In ART programs of developing countries like Ethiopia, poor ascertainment of deaths and recording of information on losses to follow up may lead to underestimation of mortality rates.

In conclusion, we detected a relatively lower level of mortality among the cohort of patients on antiretroviral treatment in eastern Ethiopia. Previous history of weight loss, bedridden functional status at baseline, low CD4 cell count and advanced WHO patients had a higher risk of death among the retrospective cohort. So early initiation of ART while CD4 counts are higher and opportunistic infections limited, provision of nutritional support and strengthening the food by prescription initiative, and counseling of patients for early presentation during testing for HIV is recommended.

Competing interests

All authors declare that they have no competing interest associated with the publication of this manuscript.

Acknowledgements

We would like to thank Haramaya University for funding this project. We also acknowledge the cooperation of the Research and Publication Office of Harar Campus, and the office of the Dean of Harar College of Health Sciences. We thank Yordanos Asalif for her secretarial assistance and for helping in the download and printing of scientific articles. We also thank all the health facilities staff for their cooperation and the patients involved in this study.

Author details

[1]Department of Epidemiology and Biostatistics, College of Medical and Health Science, Jimma University, Jimma, Ethiopia. [2]Department of Public Health, College of Health Sciences, Haramaya University, P. O. Box 235, Harar, Ethiopia. [3]Department of Medical Laboratory Science, College of Health Sciences, Harar, Ethiopia.

Authors' contributions

AAR and SB contributed significantly in the design, manuscript writing and review. AAR conceived and designed the study, collected data in the field, performed the data analysis, interpreted the data, and drafted the manuscript and critically reviewed it. TD was significantly involved in data collection and has reviewed the manuscript. All authors approved and read the final manuscript.

References

1. Palella FJ, Deloria-Knoll M, Chmiel JS, Moorman AS, Wood KC, Greenberg AE, Holmberg SD, HIV Outpatient Study (HOPS) Investigators: **Survival benefit of initiating antiretroviral therapy in HIV-infected persons in different CD4+ cell Strata.** *Ann Intern Med* 2003, 138:620–626.
2. Egger M, May M, Chêne G, Phillips AN, Ledergerber B, Dabis F, Costagliola D, D'Arminio Monforte A, de Wolf F, Reiss P, *et al*: **Prognosis of HIV-1-infected patients starting highly active antiretroviral therapy: a collaborative analysis of prospective studies.** *Lancet* 2002, **360:**119–129.
3. Coetzee D, Hildebrand K, Boulle A, Maartens G, Louis F, Labatala V, Reuter H, Ntwana N, Goemaere E: **Outcomes after two years of providing antiretroviral treatment in Khayelitsha, South Africa.** *AIDS* 2004, **18:**887–895.
4. Lawn SD, Harries AD, Anglaret X, Myer L, Wood R: **Early mortality among adults accessing antiretroviral treatment programmes in sub-Saharan Africa.** *AIDS* 2008, **22:**1897–1908.
5. UNAIDS: *Global report: UNAIDS report on the global AIDS epidemic 2010. vol. 10.11E | JC1958E.* Geneva: Joint United Nations Programme on HIV/AIDS (UNAIDS); 2010.
6. UNAIDS, WHO, UNICEF: *Global HIV/AIDS response - Epidemic update and health sector progress toward univeral access - Progress report 2011.* Geneva: UNAIDS; 2011.
7. WHO: *Towards universal access - Scaling up priority HIV/AIDS interventions in the health sector - Progress report 2010.* Geneva: World Health Organization; 2010.
8. Centers for Disease Control and Prevention (CDC): *HIV/AIDS Surveillance Report.* Atlanta: (US Department of Health and Human Services ed; 2001.
9. Mocroft A, Vella S, Benfield TL, Chiesi A, Miller V, Gargalianos P, D'Arminio Monforte A, Yust I, Bruun JN, Phillips AN, Lundgren JD: **Changing patterns of mortality across Europe in patients infected with HIV-1. EuroSIDA Study Group.** *Lancet* 1998, **352:**1725–1730
10. Hoffmann C, JK R, Kamps S, Eds.): *HIV Medicine 2007.* Paris: Flying Publishers; 2007.
11. Braitstein P, Brinkhof MW, Dabis F, Schechter M, Boulle A, Miotti P, Wood R, Laurent C, Sprinz E, Seyler C, *et al*: **Mortality of HIV-1-infected patients in the first year of antiretroviral therapy: comparison between low-income and high-income countries.** *Lancet* 2006, **367:**817–824.
12. Jerene D, Naess A, Lindtjørn B: **Antiretroviral therapy at a district hospital in Ethiopia prevents death and tuberculosis in a cohort of HIV patients.** *AIDS Res Ther* 2006, **3:**10.
13. Jaffar S, Munderi P, Grosskurth H: **Adherence to antiretroviral therapy in Africa: how high is it really?** *Tropical Medicine and International* 2008, **13:**1096–1097.
14. Rougemont M, Stoll BE, Elia N, Ngang P: **Antiretroviral treatment adherence and its determinants in Sub-Saharan Africa: a prospective study at Yaounde Central Hospital.** *Cameroon. AIDS Research and Therapy* 2009, **6:**21.
15. Stringer JS, Zulu I, Levy J, Stringer EM, Mwango A, Chi BH, Mtonga V, Reid S, Cantrell RA, Bulterys M, *et al*: **Rapid scale-up of antiretroviral therapy at primary care sites in Zambia: feasibility and early outcomes.** *JAMA* 2006, **296:**782–793.
16. Weidle PJ, Malamba S, Mwebaze R, Sozi C, Rukundo G, Downing R, Hanson D, Ochola D, Mugyenyi P, Mermin J, *et al*: **Assessment of a pilot antiretroviral drug therapy programme in Uganda: patients' response, survival, and drug resistance.** *Lancet* 2002, **360:**34–40.
17. Amuron B, Levin J, Birunghi J, Namara G, Coutinho A, Grosskurth H, Jaffar S: **Mortality in an antiretroviral therapy programme in Jinja, south-east Uganda: a prospective cohort study.** *AIDS Res Ther* 2011, **8:**39.
18. Jerene D, Endale A, Hailu Y, Lindtjørn B: **Predictors of early death in a cohort of Ethiopian patients treated with HAART.** *BMC Infect Dis* 2006, **6:**136.
19. Lawn SD, Little F, Bekker LG, Kaplan R, Campbel E, Orrell C, Wood R: **Changing mortality risk associated with CD4 cell response to antiretroviral therapy in South Africa.** *AIDS* 2009, **23:**335–342.
20. May M, Sterne JA, Sabin C, Costagliola D, Justice AC, Thiébaut R, Gill J, Phillips A, Reiss P, Hogg R, *et al*: **Prognosis of HIV-1-infected patients up to 5 years after initiation of HAART: collaborative analysis of prospective studies.** *Lancet* 2007, **21:**1185–1197.
21. Chan CW, Cheng LS, Chan WK, Wong KH: **Highly active antiretroviral therapy per se decreased mortality and morbidity of advanced human immunodeficiency virus disease in Hong Kong.** *Chin Med J* 2005, **118:**1338–1345.
22. Duncombe C, Kerr SJ, Ruxrungtham K, Dore GJ, Law MG, Emery S, Lange JM, Phanuphak P, Cooper DA: **HIV disease progression in a patient cohort treated via a clinical research network in a resource limited setting.** *AIDS* 2005, **19:**169–178.
23. Wester CW, Kim S, Bussmann H, Avalos A, Ndwapi N, Peter TF, Gaolathe T, Mujugira A, Busang L, Vanderwarker C, *et al*: **Initial response to highly active antiretroviral therapy in HIV-1 C-infected adults in a public sector treatment program in Botswana.** *J Acquir Immune Defic Syndr* 2005, **40:**336–343.
24. Worku A: *Pattern and determinants of survival in adult HIV patients on antiretroviral therapy, Ethiopia. Umeå university, Umeå International School of Public Health, Department of Epidemiology and Public Health sciences*; 2009.
25. Bello SI: **Management Outcomes of HIV/aids Patients on Haart in a Secondary Health Institution in North Central, Nigeria.** *Pharmacologia* 2012, **3:**336–343.
26. Bello SI, Itiola OA: **Drug adherence amongst tuberculosis patients in the University of Ilorin Teaching Hospital, Ilorin, Nigeria.** *African Journal of Pharmacy and Pharmacology* 2010, **4:**109–114.
27. Jarrin ILB, Ferreros I, *et al*: **Effect of education on overall and causespecific mortality in injecting drug users, according to HIV and introduction of HAART.** *Int J Epidemiol* 2007, **36:**e187–e194.

28. Wood EMJ, Chan K, *et al*: **Socioeconomic status, access to triple therapy, and survival from HIV-disease since 1996.** *AIDS* 2002, **16:**e2065–e2072.
29. Jarrin I, Lumbreras B, Ferreros I, Pérez-Hoyos S, Hurtado I, Hernández-Aguado I: **Effect of education on overall and cause-specific mortality in injecting drug users, according to HIV and introduction of HAART.** *Int J Epidemiol* 2007, **36:**187–194.
30. Wood E, Montaner JS, Chan K, Tyndall MW, Schechter MT, Bangsberg D, O'Shaughnessy MV, Hogg RS: **Socioeconomic status, access to triple therapy, and survival from HIV-disease since 1996.** *AIDS* 2002, **16:**2065–2072.

7

Race/ethnicity and HAART initiation in a military HIV infected cohort

Erica N Johnson[1,2], Mollie P Roediger[1,3], Michael L Landrum[1,2], Nancy F Crum-Cianflone[1,4], Amy C Weintrob[1,5], Anuradha Ganesan[1,5], Jason F Okulicz[1,2], Grace E Macalino[1], Brian K Agan[1*] and the Infectious Disease Clinical Research Program HIV Working Group

Abstract

Background: Prior studies have suggested that HAART initiation may vary by race/ethnicity. Utilizing the U.S. military healthcare system, which minimizes confounding from healthcare access, we analyzed whether timing of HAART initiation and the appropriate initiation of primary prophylaxis among those at high risk for pneumocystis pneumonia (PCP) varies by race/ethnicity.

Methods: Participants in the U.S. Military HIV Natural History Study from 1998-2009 who had not initiated HAART before 1998 and who, based on DHHS guidelines, had a definite indication for HAART (CD4 <200, AIDS event or severe symptoms; Group A), an indication to consider HAART (including CD4 <350; Group B) or electively started HAART (CD4 >350; Group C) were analyzed for factors associated with HAART initiation. In a secondary analysis, participants were also evaluated for factors associated with starting primary PCP prophylaxis within four months of a CD4 count <200 cells/mm^3. Multiple logistic regression was used to compare those who started vs. delayed therapy; comparisons were expressed as odds ratios (OR).

Results: 1262 participants were evaluated in the analysis of HAART initiation (A = 208, B = 637, C = 479 [62 participants were evaluated in both Groups A and B]; 94% male, 46% African American, 40% Caucasian). Race/ethnicity was not associated with HAART initiation in Groups A or B. In Group C, African American race/ethnicity was associated with lower odds of initiating HAART (OR 0.49, p = 0.04). Race and ethnicity were also not associated with the initiation of primary PCP prophylaxis among the 408 participants who were at risk.

Conclusions: No disparities in the initiation of HAART or primary PCP prophylaxis according to race/ethnicity were seen among those with an indication for therapy. Among those electively initiating HAART at the highest CD4 cell counts, African American race/ethnicity was associated with decreased odds of starting. This suggests that free healthcare can potentially overcome some of the observed disparities in HIV care, but that unmeasured factors may contribute to differences in elective care decisions.

Keywords: HIV, HAART, Race, Ethnicity, Indications for HIV treatment, Disparities in care, African Americans

Introduction

HIV has become a treatable illness in the era of highly active antiretroviral therapy (HAART), and HAART is associated with a reduction in morbidity and mortality among those with severe immunosuppression [1]. There is increasing evidence that HAART is associated with reduced mortality among those initiating HAART at higher CD4 cell counts as well [2-7]. Thus the optimal timing of HAART initiation may result in a more robust immunologic and virologic response, which may improve outcomes. However there are factors other than the degree of immune suppression involved in the decision to start HAART.

Despite the known benefits of HAART, certain groups appear to be more vulnerable to treatment disparities, and these disparities have persisted over time. In a U.S. study of HIV-infected persons, delays of three or more months

* Correspondence: bagan@idcrp.org
[1]Department of Preventive Medicine and Biometrics, Infectious Disease Clinical Research Program, Uniformed Services University of the Health Sciences, Bethesda, MD, USA
Full list of author information is available at the end of the article

between diagnosis and an initial specialty encounter occurred more frequently among patients who lacked access to care at diagnosis and among those of African American or Latino race/ethnicity [8]. Delays in the initiation of HAART and failure to receive PCP prophylaxis occurred more frequently among blacks or Latinos, women, and the underinsured compared with other HIV patients [9]. Among a national sample of patients eligible to receive HAART by published guidelines, African American race/ethnicity, female gender and injection drug use were all associated with decreased likelihood of receipt of HAART [10]. Finally, in patients with HIV treated at multiple clinical sites in the United Kingdom, black race was associated with starting antiretroviral therapy at a lower CD4 count [11].

The etiology of these disparities is complex and likely multifactorial. Factors that have been hypothesized from previous studies include lack of health insurance or other barriers impeding healthcare access, variations in patient education or health literacy, and aspects of the physician-provider relationship [12,13]. Understanding the role these factors play in creating barriers to optimal care is needed and may offer an explanation for some of these observed differences in HIV care and outcomes [14-17].

In this study, we evaluated factors associated with HAART initiation within a defined time window in a United States military cohort of persons with HIV. As a secondary analysis, we also analyzed factors associated with the initiation of primary pneumocystis pneumonia (PCP) prophylaxis among persons at highest risk for PCP. Our population consists of an ethnically diverse group of early-diagnosed HIV patients with free healthcare and medications [18]. Furthermore, since military service for those on active duty provides a stable source of income and members have a minimum high school education, this cohort may offer somewhat less confounding due to socioeconomic status. Time windows to evaluate HAART initiation were established based on military policy requiring that HIV infected active duty members with stable disease undergo medical evaluation every six months and standard practice to evaluate those with advanced HIV disease more frequently, at least every three to four months. HAART initiation was assessed in accordance with the U.S. Department of Health and Human Services (DHHS) guidelines for the use of antiretroviral agents [19], which, since 1998, have been adopted into the practice of many U.S. physicians who specialize in HIV care, including those practicing within the U.S. military system.

Methods

Study population

The U.S. Military HIV Natural History Study (NHS), a cohort study of military beneficiaries with HIV infection including active duty personnel, retirees and dependents, enrolled 5261 participants from 1986 to 2009. Active duty personnel must be HIV negative prior to entry into U.S. military service, and subsequently undergo HIV screening every one to five years. Service members and beneficiaries identified with HIV are referred to military treatment facilities (MTFs) across the U.S. for evaluation and treatment. Those participating in the study provide written informed consent prior to assuming a schedule of evaluations by an HIV specialist at least every six months at one of five participating MTFs. Data including demographic characteristics, medical history, and laboratory measurements are collected at each study visit as previously described [18]. In compliance with the Helsinki Declaration, the NHS protocol has been reviewed and approved by the institutional review boards (IRBs) centrally and at the study sites. All subjects provided informed consent for participation. This analysis was reviewed and approved by the central IRB.

Participants who were enrolled in the NHS from 1998-2009 and who had not initiated HAART before 1998 were included in this substudy. Participants were excluded from these analyses if they had died (N = 1195), were lost-to-follow-up (N = 969), or had initiated HAART prior to January 1, 1998 (N = 1514). The analysis also excluded those participants who, prior to the three-month window preceding the first study date, i.e. September 1, 1997, had a CD4 cell count below 200 cells/mm^3, an AIDS-defining condition, or any severe symptoms (category B symptoms according to the 1993 Revised Classification System for HIV Infection, including refractory mucosal candidiasis, wasting syndrome, pre-invasive cervical cancer, bacillary angiomatosis, oral hairy leukoplakia, and chronic diarrhea) [20] (N = 233).

Study design

Participants were followed from the later of January 1, 1998 or their date of initial diagnosis with HIV until meeting criteria for assignment in one of three groups based on concurrent DHHS criteria. The details of this classification as well as changes in DHHS criteria during the study period of 1998-2009 are summarized in Table 1. The three groups included:

- Group A – those participants with a definite indication for HAART. Participants were classified as "initiators" if they started HAART within four months of classification or "delayers" if they did not. Those with less than four months of follow-up between the date of classification and last study visit were excluded from analysis (N = 18).
- Group B – those participants with an indication to consider HAART. Initiators started HAART within six months of classification and delayers did not start HAART within this timeframe. Those with less

Table 1 Study group classifications according to changes in the DHHS guidelines for initiation of antiretroviral therapy in chronically-infected HIV patients[1]

Group	1998-2000	2001	2002-2004	2005-2007	2008-2009
A	• AIDS-defining condition	• AIDS-defining condition	• AIDS-defining condition	• AIDS-defining condition	• AIDS-defining condition
	• Severe symptoms	• Severe symptoms	• Severe symptoms	• Severe symptoms	• Severe symptoms
		• $CD4^+$ <200	• $CD4^+$ <200	• $CD4^+$ <200	• $CD4^+$ <200
B	• $CD4^+$ <500	• $CD4^+$ >200 but ≤350	• $CD4^+$ >200 but ≤350	• $CD4^+$ >200 but ≤350	• $CD4^+$ >200 but ≤350
	• VL >10,000 (bDNA) or >20,000 (RT-PCR)				
C	• Elective decision	• VL >30,000 (bDNA) or >55,000 (RT-PCR)	• VL >55,000 (bDNA or RT-PCR)	• VL >100,000 (RT-PCR)	• $CD4^+$ >350
		• $CD4^+$ >350	• $CD4^+$ >350	• $CD4^+$ >350	• Other elective decision
		• Other elective decision	• Other elective decision	• Other elective decision	

[1]Guideline statements of "some would treat" were interpreted as indicating the elective nature of this decision. Therefore viral load was not included as a Group B criterion after 2000.

than six months of follow-up between the date of classification and last study visit were excluded from analysis (N = 77).

- Group C – those participants who may have electively started HAART; initiators started HAART prior to being categorized into either Groups A or B; delayers were HAART-naive as of their last study visit and had not yet been categorized into Groups A or B.

The different initiator/delayer classification timeframes for Groups A and B were selected based on practice patterns unique to the military, specifically that some participants do not live near an MTF offering specialty HIV care and receive care on an approximately four to six month cycle. Participants could be evaluated in more than one group if they later met criteria for inclusion in another group, up until the time when they initiated HAART, at which point they could no longer be analyzed in any other group.

To further assess for evidence of disparity, the analysis was repeated evaluating the association between study factors and starting primary pneumocystis pneumonia (PCP) prophylaxis within four months of the first verified CD4 count <200 cells/mm^3 (i.e. at least one subsequent CD4 count within three months that was also <200 cells/mm^3). This analysis included those without a history of PCP who met CD4 criteria for primary PCP prophylaxis and had not yet started this treatment. Initiators started PCP prophylaxis within four months and delayers did not.

Data analysis

Factors studied included demographic characteristics (age, gender, self-reported race/ethnicity, duty status, and rank), HIV-specific factors (time since HIV infection, CD4 cell counts, HIV RNA levels, history of prior AIDS-defining condition and history of HIV symptoms), comorbid medical conditions (cerebrovascular disease, chronic kidney disease, chronic obstructive pulmonary disease, chronic viral hepatitis, cirrhosis, coronary artery disease, diabetes, and malignancy other than basal cell carcinoma) and history of a mental health disorder (anxiety disorder, bipolar disorder, major depression, obsessive-compulsive disorder, post-traumatic stress disorder, schizophrenia, substance abuse, and prior suicide attempt).

Descriptive statistics are presented as means with standard deviations (SD) or medians with interquartile ranges (IQR). For Groups A and B, factors were compared as of the date the participant was categorized into the group. For Group C, comparisons used the date of HAART initiation for initiators and date of last visit for delayers. Within each group, study variables among participants who initiated vs. delayed HAART were compared using logistic regression. Analyses were repeated among participants who initiated vs. delayed primary PCP prophylaxis when indicated. All multivariate models adjusted for gender, age, race/ethnicity, marital status, rank, duty status, military site, branch of service, duration of HIV disease, prior ART use, prior comorbid illnesses, and history of mental health diagnosis. The Group A analyses additionally adjusted for HIV RNA and reason for classification (CD4 cell count <200 cells/mm^3, AIDS-defining condition, or severe symptoms). The Group C analyses additionally adjusted for HIV RNA and CD4 cell count. To account for changes in recommendations, models for the analyses were stratified by HIV treatment guideline era. Odds ratios are given with 95% confidence intervals (CI). All p-values are two-sided. Analyses were conducted using SAS (version 9.1, Cary, NC).

Results

We evaluated 1262 participants who were predominantly male (94%) with a mean age of 33.8 years (SD 8.7). Forty percent of participants were Caucasian, 46% African

American, 10% Hispanic and 5% other ethnic groups. Sixty-two participants were evaluated in both Group A and Group B.

Of the 1262 participants, 208 were categorized as having a definite indication to start HAART (Group A), including 99 (48%) due to a CD4 count below 200 cells/mm^3, 99 (48%) due to severe symptoms, and 10 (5%) for an AIDS-defining condition. Of these, 121 (58%) initiated HAART within 4 months of indication, with a median of 11 days (IQR 3-36) from indication to HAART initiation. The remaining 87 (42%) were defined as delayers; reasons for delay were not captured in the study database. The median CD4 cell count was 176 (IQR 131 – 207) among initiators and 417 (IQR 267-554) among delayers.

In both the univariate (UV) and multivariate (MV) models, race/ethnicity and other demographic variables were not significantly associated with the timing of HAART in Group A. Participants with higher HIV RNA levels were more likely to initiate HAART (OR 2.19, 95% CI 1.32-3.64 per 1-log_{10} increase). Participants classified into Group A due to severe symptoms were less likely to initiate HAART when compared to those classified because their CD4 cell count fell below 200 cells/mm^3 (OR = 0.07, 95% CI 0.03-0.17). There was no significant difference between participants classified into Group A for an AIDS-defining condition when compared with those classified for a CD4 cell count <200 cells/mm^3 (OR = 0.36, 95% CI 0.07 – 1.93) (Table 2).

Group B included 637 participants, with 248 (39%) initiators and 389 (61%) delayers. Of these, 476 (75%) were classified into this group because of CD4 count, 82 (13%) due to HIV RNA level, and 79 (12%) because of meeting a combination of these factors. As in Group A, race/ethnicity was not significantly associated with the timing of HAART in Group B in either model. Factors associated with initiating HAART in both the UV and MV models were duration of HIV infection (OR 0.87, 95% CI 0.0.80-0.94 per 1-year increase) and prior non-HAART antiretroviral therapy (ART) use (OR 0.51, 95% CI 0.27-0.97). Additional factors that were significant only in univariate analyses were age, military status, and comorbid illnesses (Table 3).

Among the 479 participants in Group C, 144 (30%) participants initiated HAART. In UV models, African Americans were half as likely to initiate HAART in this group when compared to Caucasians (OR 0.50, 95% CI 0.32-0.78). In the MV model, African American race remained significantly associated with delayed HAART initiation (OR 0.49, 95% CI 0.25-0.97) (Table 4).

There were 408 participants with a CD4 count <200 cells/mm^3 included in the analysis of factors associated with the initiation of primary PCP prophylaxis. Race/ethnicity, age, and gender were not associated with the timing of primary PCP prophylaxis. HAART-experienced participants were less likely to start PCP prophylaxis (OR 0.48, 95% CI 0.25-0.91, compared to ART-naive participants) as were those with CD4 cell counts closer to 200 cells/mm^3 (OR 0.55, 95% CI 0.42 – 0.70 per 50 cells/mm^3) (Table 5).

Discussion

The interplay of factors surrounding the timing of HAART initiation is complex, and involves not only biologic factors such as immune function and disease progression, but also psychosocial and systems-based factors. A better understanding of these factors may help eliminate treatment barriers and enable healthcare providers to offer optimal care to all patients with HIV. This study's findings show that in an environment providing no-fee open access care, certain factors previously demonstrated to affect the timing of HAART, namely race/ethnicity, age, gender and depression did not have the same impact in most patients in this cohort. This remained true with respect to timely initiation of primary PCP prophylaxis when indicated. However in the subset of patients in Group C who electively started HAART at higher CD4 cell counts without an indication, African American race/ethnicity was associated with lower odds of initiation.

The Department of Defense provides a healthcare system ensuring access to visits and medications for its beneficiaries. In addition, keeping appointments is reinforced for active duty members by their chain of command. This practice and the military's culture of health provide a potential explanation for the absence of a statistically significant difference in the timing of HAART initiation when indicated across demographic groups in this cohort. However the potential impact of command-directed follow-up among active duty personnel may be suggested by the observation of a non-significant trend towards lower odds of HAART initiation among retired participants. Previous studies have underscored the importance of regular clinic follow-up on appropriate HAART use. In one study which showed a longer time to HAART initiation among black patients, the most common reasons for delays in referral to case conferences (where decisions were made about HAART) were lack of regular follow-up, active substance use, and the patient's desire to not use HAART [21]. There are fewer issues with access and follow-up in the U.S. military healthcare system. Also, the DoD Drug Demand Reduction Program with random urine drug screening has been very successful in decreasing substance abuse among active duty, especially with regard to intravenous drug use [22]. Cultural differences in medication uptake and adherence have yet to be fully explored in the military setting, but preliminary evaluation suggests HAART adherence levels are equally high among a subset of African Americans and Caucasians [18].

Table 2 Factors associated with the initiation of HAART from 1998-2009 among those with a definite indication to start (Group A)

	Initiators (N = 121) N (%) or median (IQR)	Delayers (N = 87) N (%) or median (IQR)	Univariate models OR (95% CI)	P	Multivariate model* OR (95% CI)	P
Demographics						
Gender (% Male)	107 (88%)	77 (89%)	0.99 (0.42 - 2.35)	0.99	0.55 (0.11 - 2.61)	0.45
Age	35.1 ± 9.4	33.9 ± 9.7	1.01 (0.98 - 1.04)	0.35	1.03 (0.98 - 1.08)	0.26
Race/ethnicity						
Caucasian	41 (33.9%)	35 (40.2%)	Referent		Referent	
American	53 (43.8%)	41 (47.1%)	1.10 (0.60 - 2.03)	0.75	0.69 (0.28 - 1.71)	0.43
Hispanic/Latino/other	27 (22.3%)	11 (12.6%)	2.09 (0.91 - 4.82)	0.08	1.71 (0.53 - 5.50)	0.37
Marital status (% married)	45 (38.5%)	27 (32.5%)	1.30 (0.72 - 2.34)	0.39	1.08 (0.46 - 2.56)	0.86
Military characteristics						
Rank						
Officer/warrant	8 (6.6%)	8 (9.2%)	0.70 (0.25 - 1.95)	0.50	0.34 (0.08 - 1.49)	0.15
Enlisted	100 (82.6%)	70 (80.5%)	Referent		Referent	
N/A	13 (10.7%)	9 (10.3%)	1.01 (0.41 - 2.49)	0.98	0.73 (0.08 - 6.73)	0.78
Duty status						
Active	83 (68.6%)	66 (75.9%)	Referent		Referent	
Retired	22 (18.2%)	14 (16.1%)	1.23 (0.59 - 2.60)	0.58	1.34 (0.35 - 5.19)	0.67
Dependent	15 (12.4%)	7 (8.0%)	1.68 (0.65 - 4.37)	0.28	2.56 (0.29 - 22.80)	0.40
HIV characteristics						
Duration of HIV infection (years)	1.3 (0.1 - 4.8)	1.9 (0.2 - 7.1)	0.95 (0.90 - 1.02)	0.14	0.92 (0.83 - 1.03)	0.15
Log_{10} HIV RNA	4.7 (4.3 - 5.2)	4.3 (3.7 - 4.8)	2.10 (1.46 - 3.04)	**<0.001**	2.19 (1.32 - 3.64)	**0.002**
CD4 count in cells/mm^3	176.0 (131.0 - 207.0)	417.0 (267.0 - 554.0)				
Prior ART (non-HAART) use	18 (15%)	13 (15%)	0.99 (0.46 - 2.16)	0.99	0.97 (0.26 - 3.55)	0.96
Prior comorbid illness(es)	10 (8%)	10 (11%)	0.69 (0.28 - 1.75)	0.44	0.30 (0.08 - 1.14)	0.08
History of mental health diagnosis						
Depression	11 (9%)	9 (10%)	0.87 (0.34 - 2.21)	0.77	0.65 (0.18 - 2.42)	0.52
Other mental health diagnosis	9 (7%)	6 (7%)	1.07 (0.36 - 3.14)	0.90	1.13 (0.27 - 4.83)	0.86
None	101 (83%)	72 (83%)	Referent		Referent	
Reason for classification						
Severe symptoms	34 (28%)	65 (75%)	0.12 (0.06 - 0.22)	**<0.001**	0.07 (0.03 - 0.17)	**<0.001**
AIDS defining condition	6 (5%)	4 (5%)	0.33 (0.09 - 1.30)	0.11	0.36 (0.07 - 1.93)	0.23
CD4 count <200 cells/mm^3	81 (67%)	18 (21%)	Referent		Referent	

*Multivariate model additionally adjusts for branch and site of service.
P-values < 0.05 are presented in bold text.

African Americans in this study were less likely than Caucasians to electively start HAART at higher CD4 counts. And while there were no statistically significant ethnic differences among those with an indication for HAART, there remained a trend towards lower odds of HAART initiation at lower CD4 count thresholds among African American participants when compared with Caucasian participants. A number of previous studies observed disparities in HAART use among certain race/ethnic groups and women although these did not specifically evaluate the elective initiation of HAART at high CD4 counts [8-10,14,21,23-26]. While the etiology of these disparities is largely attributed to differences in healthcare access, other factors have also been shown to contribute and perhaps offer an explanation for the findings in this study. For example, racial discordance of the physician-patient relationship may be associated with cultural miscommunication that could explain delays in

Table 3 Factors associated with the initiation of HAART from 1998-2009 among those classified into the consider offering treatment group (Group B)

	Initiators (N = 248) N (%) or median (IQR)	Delayers (N = 389) N (%) or median (IQR)	Univariate models		Multivariate model*,**	
			OR (95% CI)	p	OR (95% CI)	p
Demographics						
Gender (% Male)	236 (95%)	368 (95%)	1.04 (0.50 - 2.16)	0.92	1.19 (0.44 - 3.22)	0.74
Age	31.7 ± 7.3	33.1 ± 8.4	0.98 (0.96 - 1.00)	**0.04**	1.00 (0.97 - 1.03)	0.93
Race/ethnicity						
Caucasian	102 (41.1%)	141 (36.2%)	Referent		Referent	
African American	109 (44.0%)	195 (50.1%)	0.80 (0.56 - 1.13)	0.20	0.83 (0.56 - 1.24)	0.37
Hispanic/Latino/other	37 (14.9%)	53 (13.6%)	0.91 (0.55 - 1.49)	0.71	1.05 (0.60 - 1.82)	0.88
Marital status (% married)	83 (34.6%)	120 (33.9%)	1.05 (0.74 - 1.49)	0.78	1.10 (0.75 - 1.62)	0.62
Military characteristics						
Rank						
Officer/warrant	19 (7.7%)	28 (7.2%)	1.01 (0.55 - 1.86)	0.97	1.14 (0.56 - 2.32)	0.72
Enlisted	214 (86.3%)	334 (85.9%)	Referent		Referent	
N/A	15 (6.0%)	27 (6.9%)	0.95 (0.49 - 1.84)	0.88	0.97 (0.20 - 4.77)	0.97
Duty status						
Active	219 (88.3%)	297 (76.3%)	Referent		Referent	
Retired	17 (6.9%)	77 (19.8%)	0.34 (0.19 - 0.59)	**<0.001**	0.61 (0.28 - 1.32)	0.21
Dependent	12 (4.8%)	15 (3.9%)	1.15 (0.53 - 2.52)	0.72	2.20 (0.36 - 13.35)	0.39
HIV characteristics						
Duration of HIV infection (years)	0.3 (0.1 - 1.9)	1.8 (0.2 - 5.2)	0.84 (0.78 - 0.89)	**<0.001**	0.87 (0.80 - 0.94)	**<0.001**
Log_{10} HIV RNA	4.5 (4.1 - 4.9)	4.1 (3.4 - 4.5)				
CD4 cell count	323.0 (287.0 - 422.5)	352.0 (316.0 - 461.0)				
Prior ART (non-HAART) use	22 (9%)	100 (26%)	0.30 (0.18 - 0.51)	**<0.001**	0.51 (0.27 - 0.97)	**0.04**
Prior comorbid Illness (es)	12 (5%)	40 (10%)	0.45 (0.23 - 0.89)	**0.02**	0.76 (0.35 - 1.66)	0.49
History of mental health diagnosis						
Depression	18 (7%)	37 (10%)	0.73 (0.40 - 1.32)	0.30	1.02 (0.53 - 1.98)	0.95
Other mental health diagnosis	13 (5%)	20 (5%)	0.96 (0.47 - 1.99)	0.92	1.16 (0.53 - 2.55)	0.71
None	217 (88%)	332 (85%)	Referent		Referent	
Reason for classification						
CD4 <500 (1998-2000) CD4 <350 (2001-2008)	168 (68%)	308 (79%)				
HIV RNA >20,000 copies/ml (1998-2000 only)	32 (13%)	50 (13%)				
CD4 <500 and HIV >20,000 copies/ml (1998-2000 only)	48 (19%)	31 (8%)				

*All models are stratified by guideline era (1998-2000, 2001-2009).
**Multivariate model additionally adjusts for branch and site of service.
P-values < 0.05 are presented in bold text.

receipt of HAART [12,27]. Additionally, patients who reported that their provider "knows me as a person" were more likely to receive HAART than those who did not report this belief [13]. Other factors may also impact decisions about HAART including health literacy and attitudes toward health [28,29]. It is important to note that not all studies have shown racial/ethnic differences in the receipt of HAART. In a study performed among HIV-positive patients in Denmark, where healthcare is free, both white and nonwhite patients had similar rates of receiving HAART, and race/ethnicity did not have an apparent effect on the outcomes associated with HAART [30].

Table 4 Factors associated with the elective initiation of HAART from 1998-2009, Group C

	Initiators (N = 144) N (%) or median (IQR)	Delayers (N = 335) N (%) or median (IQR)	Univariate models		Multivariate model*,**	
			OR (95% CI)	p	OR (95% CI)	P
Demographics						
Gender (% Male)	140 (97%)	310 (93%)	3.19 (1.08 - 9.47)	**0.04**	1.50 (0.34 - 6.63)	0.59
Age	33.6 ± 9.4	32.2 ± 8.5	1.01 (0.99 - 1.04)	0.20	1.04 (0.99 - 1.09)	0.08
Race/ethnicity						
Caucasian	70 (48.6%)	117 (34.9%)	Referent		Referent	
African American	47 (32.6%)	162 (48.4%)	0.50 (0.32 - 0.78)	**0.002**	0.49 (0.25 - 0.97)	**0.04**
Hispanic/Latino/other	27 (18.8%)	56 (16.7%)	0.88 (0.51 - 1.53)	0.66	0.85 (0.40 - 1.82)	0.68
Marital status (% married)	38 (27.7%)	95 (31.8%)	0.67 (0.41 - 1.08)	0.10	0.67 (0.34 - 1.33)	0.25
Military characteristics						
Rank						
Officer/warrant	23 (16.0%)	30 (9.0%)	1.79 (0.99 - 3.24)	**0.05**	1.30 (0.56 - 3.04)	0.54
Enlisted	116 (80.6%)	275 (82.1%)	Referent		Referent	
N/A	5 (3.5%)	30 (9.0%)	0.27 (0.10 - 0.74)	**0.01**	1.53 (0.19 - 12.62)	0.69
Duty status						
Active	121 (84.0%)	284 (84.8%)	Referent		Referent	
Retired	18 (12.5%)	32 (9.6%)	1.09 (0.58 - 2.06)	0.78	0.52 (0.13 - 2.13)	0.36
Dependent	5 (3.5%)	19 (5.7%)	0.50 (0.18 - 1.39)	0.18	0.38 (0.04 - 3.52)	0.40
HIV characteristics						
Duration of HIV Infection (years)	1.2 (0.3 - 4.0)	2.1 (0.7 - 4.8)	0.92 (0.86 - 0.98)	**0.009**	0.91 (0.80 - 1.04)	0.18
Log_{10} HIV RNA^{+}	4.5 (3.7 - 5.0)	3.7 (3.0 - 4.4)	3.11 (2.30 - 4.21)	**<0.001**	3.25 (2.15 - 4.93)	**<0.001**
CD4 cell count***	496.5 (398.5 - 627.5)	606.0 (496.0 - 775.0)	0.83 (0.78 - 0.89)	**<0.001**	0.82 (0.75 - 0.90)	**<0.001**
Prior ART (non-HAART) use	29 (20%)	19 (6%)	3.49 (1.82 - 6.71)	**<0.001**	50.56 (9.94 - 257.1)	**<0.001**
Prior comorbid illness (es)	12 (8%)	21 (6%)	1.32 (0.62 - 2.77)	0.47	0.51 (0.16 - 1.62)	0.25
History of mental health diagnosis						
Depression	14 (10%)	43 (13%)	0.74 (0.39 - 1.41)	0.36	0.44 (0.17 - 1.10)	0.08
Other mental health diagnosis	8 (6%)	35 (10%)	0.52 (0.23 - 1.15)	0.11	0.37 (0.13 - 1.04)	0.06
None	122 (85%)	257 (77%)	Referent		Referent	

*All models are stratified by guideline era (1998-2000, 2001-2009).
**Multivariate model additionally adjusts for branch and site of service.
$^{+}$Per 1.0 log_{10} increase.
***Univariate and Multivariate models are per 50 cells/mm^3.
P-values < 0.05 are presented in bold text.

The implication of the ethnic difference in elective HAART initiation in this study is important because some studies have demonstrated a differential response to HAART between Caucasian and non-Caucasian groups [16,17,21,31,32]. In an analysis of antiretroviral-naïve patients with HIV who started HAART between 1997 and 2003, African American race/ethnicity was associated with failure to reach virologic suppression at 12 months [16] and at 6 months and 12 months after initiating HAART [17]. And despite continuous use of HAART, black women experienced increased rates of AIDS-defining illness and death from AIDS when compared with white women [32]. Interestingly, two studies suggest that in spite of decreased rates of virologic suppression, African Americans and Caucasians treated with HAART in the DoD have equivalent long-term outcomes [15,18]. Pharmacogenomic and adherence differences are being explored as possible explanations for the lower virologic suppression rates.

Depression was not associated with the timing of HAART in this study among those with an indication to start, although it has been shown to impact the decision to start HAART in some previous studies [33,34] but not all [35]. There was a delay in HAART initiation in Group A due to the presence of severe symptoms, which may reflect the high median CD4 cell count among delayers in this group, a prioritization of disease management, or possibly a concern about immune reconstitution inflammatory

Table 5 Factors associated with early initiation of primary PCP prophylaxis from 1998-2009

	Initiators (N = 156) N (%) or median (IQR)	Delayers (N = 252) N (%) or median (IQR)	Univariate models OR (95% CI)	p	Multivariate model* OR (95% CI)	P
Demographics						
Gender (% Male)	144 (92%)	227 (90%)	1.32 (0.64 - 2.71)	0.45	1.00 (0.33 - 3.03)	>0.99
Age	36.9 (29.2 - 43.0)	37.4 (32.2 - 42.5)	0.99 (0.97 - 1.01)	0.36	0.98 (0.95 - 1.01)	0.27
Race/ethnicity						
Caucasian	61 (39%)	100 (40%)	Referent		Referent	
African American	72 (46%)	122 (48%)	0.97 (0.63 - 1.49)	0.88	1.21 (0.71 - 2.09)	0.48
Hispanic/Latino/other	23 (15%)	30 (12%)	1.26 (0.67 - 2.36)	0.48	1.35 (0.61 - 3.00)	0.46
Marital status (% married)	63 (41%)	71 (31%)	1.50 (0.98 - 2.30)	0.06	1.52 (0.89 - 2.59)	0.12
Military characteristics						
Rank						
Officer/warrant	19 (12%)	24 (10%)	1.33 (0.70 - 2.54)	0.38	1.76 (0.74 - 4.15)	0.20
Enlisted	121 (78%)	199 (79%)	Referent		Referent	
N/A	16 (10%)	24 (10%)	1.12 (0.57 - 2.20)	0.73	1.72 (0.54 - 5.47)	0.36
Duty status						
Active	82 (53%)	109 (43%)	Referent		Referent	
Retired	63 (40%)	118 (47%)	0.71 (0.47 - 1.08)	0.11	1.16 (0.59 - 2.25)	0.67
Dependent	11 (7%)	25 (10%)	0.58 (0.27 - 1.26)	0.17	0.36 (0.09 - 1.53)	0.17
HIV characteristics						
Duration of HIV infection (years)	2.5 (0.1 - 8.8)	6.6 (1.8 - 10.9)	0.93 (0.89 - 0.97)	**<0.001**	0.99 (0.93 - 1.05)	0.70
Log_{10} HIV RNA	4.8 (4.3 - 5.2)	4.5 (3.6 - 5.0)	1.49 (1.21 - 1.83)	**<0.001**	1.25 (0.98 - 1.60)	0.07
CD4 count*	130.0 (68.5 - 167.0)	169.0 (131.5 - 187.0)	0.59 (0.49 – 0.72)	**<0.001**	0.55 (0.42 – 0.70)	**<0.001**
Prior ART use						
None	92 (59%)	81 (32%)	Referent		Referent	
ART	14 (9%)	24 (10%)	0.51 (0.25 - 1.06)	0.07	0.81 (0.30 - 2.15)	0.67
HAART	50 (32%)	147 (58%)	0.30 (0.19 - 0.46)	**<0.001**	0.48 (0.25 - 0.91)	**0.03**
Prior AIDS	24 (15%)	36 (14%)	1.09 (0.62 - 1.91)	0.76	1.00 (0.45 - 2.19)	>0.99
History of mental health diagnosis						
Depression	19 (12%)	46 (18%)	0.63 (0.35 - 1.13)	0.12	0.82 (0.41 - 1.65)	0.58
Other mental health diagnosis	13 (8%)	16 (6%)	1.24 (0.58 - 2.68)	0.58	1.52 (0.61 - 3.79)	0.36
None	124 (79%)	190 (75%)	Referent		Referent	

*Univariate and Multivariate models are per 50 cells/mm^3.

syndrome (IRIS) among those with lower nadir CD4 cell counts. Prior mono- and dual-NRTI use was associated with decreased odds of starting HAART in Group B, but increased odds in Group C. This effect was highly associated with calendar year and may reflect delays in changing to HAART in the early HAART era in participants stable on non-HAART ART in Group B versus a preference for newer therapies in those electing to start HAART in Group C. A similar phenomenon in the early HAART era is suggested in a study examining the reasons why 28 of 60 patients treated for HIV in a U.S. health clinic were not treated with HAART in 1997-1998 in accordance with DHHS guidelines at the time [36]. Another study also suggested delays in transitioning to the use of protease inhibitors in a U.S. practice in 1996 among 190 patients; higher CD4 cell count (200-500 cells/mm^3) was a prominent factor in multivariate models [37].

There are some study limitations. It is a retrospective analysis covering a broad timeframe and involves five DoD research sites among which practice patterns may vary. Statistical models were adjusted to account for site of visit and service affiliation. While the cohort has a balance of male African American and Caucasian participants, other ethnic groups and women are represented in much smaller proportions, making it difficult to draw conclusions about the timing of HAART among these groups. Overall, the cohort is relatively small, and while we observed many trends that did not reach statistical significance, it is possible that these trends would represent clinically important differences in a larger cohort. Further, it is likely that there are additional confounding factors that we were not able to fully account for in the analysis. The criteria for determining eligibility for HAART initiation in this study are limited to the DHHS guidelines, even though other societies in the U.S. and worldwide have published guidelines that may have influenced practice patterns. And importantly, there are limited data on substance use in this cohort, although it is estimated to be quite low, with no IVDU reported at last survey [22].

Conclusion

In a cohort with free access to HIV care and medications, race/ethnicity, age, and gender did not impact HAART timing among those with an indication for therapy, but African American race/ethnicity was associated with lower odds of electively initiating antiretrovirals. This study reinforces that free healthcare can potentially overcome some of the observed disparities in HIV care, particularly those related to access. However additional unmeasured factors may result in persistent differences in elective care decisions.

Competing interests

The authors declare that they have no competing interests.

Authors' contributions

ENJ, MPR, and BKA designed and conducted the study, interpreted the data, and prepared and edited the manuscript. MLL, NFC, ACW, AG, JFO, and GEM assisted with study design, data interpretation, and editing the manuscript. All authors read and approved the final manuscript.

Acknowledgements

Support for this work (IDCRP-000-13) was provided by the Infectious Disease Clinical Research Program (IDCRP), a Department of Defense (DoD) program executed through the Uniformed Services University of the Health Sciences. This project has been funded in whole, or in part, with federal funds from the National Institute of Allergy and Infectious Diseases, National Institutes of Health (NIH), under Inter-Agency Agreement Y1-AI-5072. We would like to express our gratitude to the current members of the IDCRP HIV Working Group and the long line of military HIV researchers who have supported the HIV NHS and for the research coordinators and support staff for their countless hours of work. Most importantly, we would like to thank the volunteers for their participation, without which this research would not have been possible. Members of the IDCRP HIV Working Group in addition to the Authors: Uniformed Services University of the Health Sciences, Bethesda, MD- M. Kortepeter; Walter Reed National Military Medical Center Bethesda, Bethesda, MD - C. Decker, S. Fraser, J. Hartzell, R. Ressner, P. Waterman, T. Warkentien, T. Whitman, G. Wortmann, M. Zapor; Naval Medical Center, Portsmouth, VA- T. Lalani; San Antonio Military Medical Center, San Antonio, TX- S. Merritt; Naval Medical Center, San Diego, CA- M. Bavaro, H. Chun; Tripler Army Medical Center, Honolulu, HI- G. Hsue, A. Johnson; Walter Reed Army Institute of Research, Silver Spring, MD- C. Eggleston, R. O'Connell, S. Peel; National Institute of Allergy and Infectious Diseases, Bethesda, MD- M. Polis, J. Powers, E. Tramont.

Disclaimer

The content of this publication is the sole responsibility of the authors and does not necessarily reflect the views or policies of the NIH or the Department of Health and Human Services, the DoD or the Departments of the Army, Navy or Air Force. Mention of trade names, commercial products, or organizations does not imply endorsement by the U.S. Government.

Author details

[1]Department of Preventive Medicine and Biometrics, Infectious Disease Clinical Research Program, Uniformed Services University of the Health Sciences, Bethesda, MD, USA. [2]Infectious Disease Service, San Antonio Military Medical Center, San Antonio, TX, USA. [3]Biostatistics Division, University of Minnesota, Minnesota, MN, USA. [4]Naval Health Research Center, San Diego, CA, USA. [5]Infectious Disease Clinic, Walter Reed National Military Medical Center, Bethesda, MD, USA.

References

1. Palella FJ Jr, Delaney KM, Moorman AC, *et al*: **Declining morbidity and mortality among patients with advanced human immunodeficiency virus infection.** *N Engl J Med* 1998, **338**:853–860.
2. Palella FJ Jr, Deloria-Knoll M, Chmiel JS, *et al*: **Survival benefit of initiating antiretroviral therapy in HIV-infected persons in different CD4+ cell strata.** *Ann Intern Med* 2003, **138**:620–626
3. Gras L, Kesselring AM, Griffith JT, *et al*: **CD4 cell counts of 800 cells/mm^3 or greater after 7 years of highly active antiretroviral therapy are feasible in most patients starting with 350 cells/mm^3 or greater.** *J Acquir Immune Defic Syndr* 2007, **45**:183–192.
4. Moore RD, Keruly JC: **CD4+ cell count 6 years after commencement of highly active antiretroviral therapy in persons with sustained virologic suppression.** *Clin Infect Dis* 2007, **44**:441–446.
5. Emery S, Neuhaus JA, Phillips AN, *et al*: **Major clinical outcomes in antiretroviral therapy in (ART)-naive participants and in those not receiving ART at baseline in the SMART study.** *J Infect Dis* 2008, **197**:1133–1144.
6. Kitahata MM, Gange SJ, Abraham AG, *et al*: **Effect of early versus deferred antiretroviral therapy for HIV on survival.** *N Engl J Med* 2009, **360**:1815–1826.
7. Sterne JA, May M, Costagliola D, *et al*: **Timing of initiation of antiretroviral therapy in AIDS-free HIV-1-infected patients: a collaborative analysis of 18 HIV cohort studies.** *Lancet* 2009, **373**:1352–1363.
8. Turner BJ, Cunningham WE, Duan N, *et al*: **Delayed medical care after diagnosis in a US national probability sample of persons infected with human immunodeficiency virus.** *Arch Intern Med* 2000, **160**:2614–2622.
9. Shapiro MF, Morton SC, McCaffrey DF, *et al*: **Variations in the care of HIV-infected adults in the United States: results from the HIV Cost and Services Utilization Study.** *J Am Med Assoc* 1999, **281**:2305–2315.
10. Gebo KA, Fleishman JA, Conviser R, *et al*: **Racial and gender disparities in receipt of highly active antiretroviral therapy persist in a multistate sample of HIV patients in 2001.** *J Acquir Immune Defic Syndr* 2005, **38**:96–103.
11. Easterbrook PJ, Phillips AN, Hill T, *et al*: **Patterns and predictors of the use of different antiretroviral drug regimens at treatment initiation in the UK.** *HIV Med* 2008, **9**:47–56.
12. Cargill VA, Stone VE: **HIV/AIDS: a minority health issue.** *Med Clin North Am* 2005, **89**:895–912.
13. Beach MC, Keruly J, Moore RD: **Is the quality of the patient-provider relationship associated with better adherence and health outcomes for patients with HIV?** *J Gen Intern Med* 2006, **21**:661–665.
14. Anastos K, Schneider MF, Gange SJ, *et al*: **The association of race, sociodemographic, and behavioral characteristics with response to highly active antiretroviral therapy in women.** *J Acquir Immune Defic Syndr* 2005, **39**:537–544.
15. Silverberg MJ, Wegner SA, Milazzo MJ, *et al*: **Effectiveness of highly-active antiretroviral therapy by race/ethnicity.** *AIDS* 2006, **20**:1531–1538.
16. Hartzell JD, Spooner K, Howard R, *et al*: **Race and mental health diagnosis are risk factors for highly active antiretroviral therapy failure in a military cohort despite equal access to care.** *J Acquir Immune Defic Syndr* 2007, **44**:411–416.
17. Weintrob AC, Grandits GA, Agan BK, *et al*: **Virologic response differences between African Americans and European Americans initiating highly active antiretroviral therapy with equal access to care.** *J Acquir Immune Defic Syndr* 2009, **52**:574–580.
18. Marconi VC, Grandits GA, Weintrob AC, *et al*: **Outcomes of highly active antiretroviral therapy in the context of universal access to healthcare: the U.S. Military Natural History Study** *AIDS Res Ther* 2010, **7**:14.

19. Panel on Antiretroviral Guidelines for Adults and Adolescents: **Guidelines for the use of antiretroviral agents in HIV-1-infected adults and adolescents.** *Dep Health Hum Serv* 2008, **1**:139. Available at http://www.aidsinfo.nih.gov/ContentFiles/AdultandAdolescentGL.pdf. Accessed 19 November 2009.
20. Centers for Disease Control and Prevention: **1993 revised classification system for HIV infection and expanded surveillance case definition for AIDS among adolescents and adults.** *MMWR Recomm Rep* 1992, **41**:1–19.
21. Lemly DC, Shepherd BE, Hulgan T, *et al*: **Race and sex differences in antiretroviral therapy use and mortality among HIV-infected persons in care.** *J Infect Dis* 2009, **199**:991–998.
22. Brodine SK, Starkey MJ, Shaffer RA, *et al*: **Diverse HIV-1 subtypes and clinical, laboratory and behavioral factors in a recently infected US military cohort.** *AIDS* 2003, **17**:2521–2527.
23. Palacio H, Kahn JG, Richards TA, Morin SF: **Effect of race and/or ethnicity in use of antiretrovirals and prophylaxis for opportunistic infection: a review of the literature.** *Public Health Rep* 2002, **117**:233–251.
24. Cohen MH, Cook JA, Grey D, *et al*: **Medically eligible women who do not use HAART: the importance of abuse, drug use, and race.** *Am J Public Health* 2004, **94**:1147–1151.
25. McNaghten AD, Hanson DL, Dworkin MS, Jones JL: **Differences in prescription of antiretroviral therapy in a large cohort of HIV-infected patients.** *J Acquir Immune Defic Syndr* 2003, **32**:499–505.
26. Oramasionwu CU, Brown CM, Lawson KA, *et al*: **Differences in national antiretroviral prescribing patterns between black and white patients with HIV/AIDS, 1996-2006.** *South Med J* 2011, **104**:794–800.
27. King WD, Wong MD, Shapiro MF, *et al*: **Does racial concordance between HIV-positive patients and their physicians affect the time to receipt of protease inhibitors?** *J Gen Intern Med* 2004, **19**:1146–1153.
28. Osborn CY, Paasche-Orlow MK, Davis TC, Wolf MS: **Health literacy: an overlooked factor in understanding HIV health disparities.** *Am J Prev Med* 2007, **33**:374–378.
29. Reynolds NR, Testa MA, Marc LG, *et al*: **Factors influencing medication adherence beliefs and self-efficacy in persons naive to antiretroviral therapy: a multicenter, cross-sectional study.** *AIDS Behav* 2004, **8**:141–150.
30. Jensen-Fangel S, Pedersen L, Pedersen C, *et al*: **The effect of race/ethnicity on the outcome of highly active antiretroviral therapy for human immunodeficiency virus type 1-infected patients.** *Clin Infect Dis* 2002, **35**:1541–1548.
31. Losina E, Schackman BR, Sadownik SN, *et al*: **Racial and sex differences in life expectancy losses among HIV-infected persons in the United States: impact of risk behavior, late initiation, and early discontinuation of antiretroviral therapy.** *Clin Infect Dis* 2009, **49**:1570–1578.
32. Murphy K, Hoover DR, Shi Q, *et al*: **Association of self-reported race with AIDS death in continuous HAART users in a cohort of HIV-infected women in the United States.** *AIDS* 2013, **27**:2413–2423.
33. Lazo M, Gange SJ, Wilson TE, *et al*: **Patterns and predictors of changes in adherence to highly active antiretroviral therapy: longitudinal study of men and women.** *Clin Infect Dis* 2007, **45**:1377–1385.
34. Bogart LM, Kelly JA, Catz SL, Sosman JM: **Impact of medical and nonmedical factors on physician decision making for HIV/AIDS antiretroviral treatment.** *J Acquir Immune Defic Syndr* 2000, **23**:396–404.
35. Himelhoch S, Brown CH, Walkup J, *et al*: **HIV patients with psychiatric disorders are less likely to discontinue HAART.** *AIDS* 2009, **23**:1735–1742.
36. Maisels L, Steinberg J, Tobias C: **An investigation of why eligible patients do not receive HAART.** *AIDS Patient Care STDs* 2001, **15**:185–191.
37. Fairfield KM, Libman H, Davis RB, Eisenberg DM: **Delays in protease inhibitor use in clinical practice.** *J Gen Intern Med* 1999, **14**:395–401.

8

Self-care practices and experiences of people living with HIV not receiving antiretroviral therapy in an urban community of Lusaka, Zambia: implications for HIV treatment programmes

Maurice Musheke[1,2,3*], Virginia Bond[1,4] and Sonja Merten[2,3]

Abstract

Background: Despite the increasingly wider availability of antiretroviral therapy (ART), some people living with HIV (PLHIV) and eligible for treatment have opted to adopt self-care practices thereby risking early AIDS-related mortality.

Methods: A qualitative study was conducted in urban Zambia to gain insights into PLHIV self-care practices and experiences and explore the implications for successful delivery of ART care. Between March 2010 and September 2011, in-depth interviews were conducted with PLHIV who had dropped out of treatment (n=25) and those that had opted not to initiate medication (n=37). Data was entered into and managed using Atlas ti, and analysed inductively using latent content analysis.

Results: PHIV used therapeutic and physical health maintenance, psychological well-being and healthy lifestyle self-care practices to maintain physical health and mitigate HIV-related symptoms. Herbal remedies, faith healing and self-prescription of antibiotics and other conventional medicines to treat HIV-related ailments were used for therapeutic and physical health maintenance purposes. Psychological well-being self-care practices used were religiosity/spirituality and positive attitudes towards HIV infection. These practices were modulated by close social network relationships with other PLHIV, family members and peers, who acted as sources of emotional, material and financial support. Cessations of sexual relationships, adoption of safe sex to avoid re-infections and uptake of nutritional supplements were the commonly used risk reduction and healthy lifestyle practices respectively.

Conclusions: While these self-care practices may promote physical and psychosocial well-being and mitigate AIDS-related symptoms, at least in the short term, they however undermine PLHIV access to ART care thereby putting PLHIV at risk of early AIDS-related mortality. The use of scientifically unproven herbal remedies raises health and safety concerns; faith healing may create fatalism and resignation with death while the reported self-prescription of antibiotics to treat HIV-related infections raises concerns about future development of microbial drug resistance amongst PLHIV. Collectively, these self-care practices undermine efforts to effectively abate the spread and burden of HIV and reduce AIDS-related mortality. Therefore, there is need for sensitization campaigns on the benefits of ART and the risks associated with widespread self-prescription of antibiotics and use of scientifically unproven herbal remedies.

Keywords: HIV, Self-care, Faith healing, Herbal remedies, Zambia

* Correspondence: maurice.musheke@unibas.ch
[1]Zambia AIDS-related TB Research Project, University of Zambia, P.O Box 50697, Lusaka, Zambia
[2]Swiss Tropical and Public Health Institute, Socinstrasse 57, Basel CH-4002, Switzerland
Full list of author information is available at the end of the article

Background

While an estimated 5.9 million people in low and middle-income countries were on antiretroviral therapy (ART) by end of 2009, saving 14.4 million life-years since 1996 [1], this only represented half the estimated people eligible for treatment [2]. Previous studies indicate that patient retention in ART care is problematic. For instance, in sub-Saharan Africa (SSA), only an estimated 60% of patients were retained in ART programmes after 2 years of starting treatment [3,4]. This is despite the proven efficacy of ART in reducing AIDS-related deaths [5-8]. The reasons for patient attrition from ART care and failure to initiate treatment are varied and include financial costs associated with accessing treatment [9,10], fear of side effects [9,11-15], fear of drug toxicity and long-term harm to the body [14,15] and feeling healthy [11,14-17]. Other barriers are stigma [9,11], belief in faith healing [11,18-21], use of traditional medicine [17,18,20,22] and perceived burden of being on life-long treatment [12,14,23].

Zambia is one of the countries in SSA worst hit by the HIV pandemic, with an estimated HIV prevalence of 14.3% in the Zambian population aged 15–49 years [24]. The national HIV prevalence peaked at around 16% in the 1990s before levelling off and marginally declining to current rates [25]. Since 2005 when Zambia started providing free ART services in public sector health facilities, there has been a steady increase in the number of PLHIV accessing treatment, from 57,164 in 2005 to an estimated 344, 407 (adults and children) at the end of 2010, representing 68.4% of those in need of treatment [25]. Similar to studies elsewhere, barriers to accessing ART in Zambia include financial and logistical costs [26,27], concerns about side effects [15,27,28], negative perceptions of medication [15,26,28] and overcrowded health facilities [15,27]. Other barriers are stigma and fear of straining interpersonal relationships [27,28], fear of being on life-long treatment and inadequate/lack of food and nutritional support [28].

While the reasons for non-uptake of ART are known, there is paucity of evidence on how PLHIV eligible for but not on treatment manage their health condition; how PLHIV perceive and experience their health on account of any self-care practices; and the implications of self-care practices for successful delivery of ART care. Therefore, within a wider ethnographic study, this study explored the self-care practices and health experiences of PLHIV not receiving ART care in an urban community of Lusaka, Zambia. Self-care in this paper is defined as "the individual's ability to manage the symptoms, treatment, physical and psychosocial consequences and lifestyle changes inherent in living with a chronic condition [in this case HIV] ability to monitor one's condition and to effect the cognitive, behavioural and emotional responses necessary to maintain satisfactory quality of life" [29].

Methods

Research setting

The study was conducted in a predominantly low-income, high-density urban residential area of Lusaka, Zambia. Observations and interviews with study participants indicate that the area comprises multilingual ethnic groups with *Bemba* and *Nyanja* the most widely spoken local languages. Most residents are embedded in strong kin and non-kin social network relationships. Most of the families are large, in part due to the affect of HIV with some individuals growing up as orphans under the care of extended family members. Although not all family members lived together, they still maintained reciprocal social and economic support ties. Other social network relationships are a product of similar religious affiliations and occupational and social lifestyle activities. Due to lack of public social amenities, social lifestyle activities mostly revolve around patronising the ubiquitous bars and drinking places, often a prime source of sexual network relationships.

Most of the residents are poor. A few people are employed in low-paid jobs in the public and private sectors of the formal economy. The majority earned their living in the informal economic sector: as cross-border traders and local market traders mainly selling fruits, vegetables, meat products, charcoal and second-hand clothes either in the city centre markets or in the open-air local markets. Small makeshift shops, locally called *'tuntemba'* are ubiquitous in the area - along the dusty and seasonally muddy roads and in the local open-air markets or next to homes. Unemployment is also endemic in the area especially among the lowly educated youth. The unemployment situation is further exacerbated by rural–urban migration as people move into the city in search of job opportunities and better life.

Health services are mainly provided by a public sector clinic which provides both in-patient and out-patient health services. The clinic also provides ART services. By mid-2010, the health centre had an estimated catchment population of over 150,000 with over 5,000 people on ART and over 5,000 registered for pre-ART care. Alongside the formal health system are traditional healers and herbalist who also provide 'health' care services, including for HIV. There is also a plethora of drug stores, some unlicensed, which provide over-the-counter medication.

Christianity is the dominant religion with a myriad of charismatic evangelical Pentecostal churches, some of which provide healing sessions for people with different ailments, including HIV.

Research design and study participants

The paper draws on data from two exploratory qualitative lines of enquiry nested within a wider 18-month ethnographic study: namely patient attrition from ART care and barriers to patient initiation of ART. For the former, participants were PLHIV who had not reported for pharmacy pick up for at least 6 months hence being classified by the local ART clinic as lost-to-follow up (LTFU). The revised Zambian ART treatment guidelines have reduced the LTFU threshold to at least 60 days from the previous 180 days [30]. In the latter, participants comprised PLHIV recommended to start treatment by ART providers but declined. Only participants aged ≥18 years old constituted our study participants.

Sampling strategy and recruitment of study participants

Purposive sampling using maximum variation sampling procedure was used to select study participants. The sampling technique allows for selection of participants with unique and diverse characteristics in order to generate in-depth unique insights and shared patterns that cut across cases. In this study, the diverse characteristics used to select study participants were demographic characteristics and length of time on and off HIV treatment. The sampling strategy facilitated collection of wide ranging, in-depth insights into self-care behavioural practices and experiences of PLHIV associated with not being on ART.

Due to the difficulties of identifying PLHIV who had dropped out of ART and those who had refused to initiate treatment, some PLHIV not on ART were first contacted and recruited through ART staff. They were contacted by mobile phone and/or physically followed up using locator information (physical address and mobile phone details) they had provided to ART providers at the time of enrolment for treatment. Other research participants were identified and recruited through community-based lay home-based care providers. Given that PLHIV had formed or belonged to social networks, a few study participants were recruited through snowball sampling in which PLHIV interviewed nominated and contacted on behalf of the researchers, friends and family members that they knew had discontinued HIV treatment or had opted not to start treatment despite it being recommended to them by ART providers. For both categories of PLHIV, only those that agreed to be interviewed were later contacted and followed up for interviews by the researchers.

Data collection and analysis

Face-to-face, one-on-one, open ended in-depth interviews were conducted between March 2010 and September 2011. The main research question asked was: "how do you manage your HIV condition in the absence of ART?' Follow-up interviews were conducted during the study period. The initial interviews usually lasted between 30–45 minutes and for those re-interviewed, follow-up interviews lasted between 15–20 minutes. All the interviews were recorded using a digital audio recorder. The majority of the interviews were conducted in the local language, *Nyanja,* and a few in English.

All interviews were transcribed verbatim. Data collection and preliminary data analysis was cyclical with some participants being re-interviewed and analysis continuously informing ensuing interviews. At the completion of data collection and transcription, all interview transcripts were entered into and organised and managed using Atlas ti version 6. Latent content analysis as described by Graneheim and Lundman [31] was undertaken. The transcripts were read several times to develop a sense of the whole data followed by open coding of the transcripts. The codes were compared for similarities and differences and then grouped into categories on a manifest level. Themes were generated by interpreting the categories for their underlying meaning (Figure 1). For instance, codes such prayer, anointing oil, anointing water were categorized as faith healing. Similarly, codes such as antibiotics, anti-diarrheal medication and pain killers were categorized as conventional non-HIV medication while garlic (*allium sativum*), ginger (*zingiber officinale*) aloe vera and *moringa* were categorized as herbal remedies. As a theme, the categories were collectively interpreted as therapeutic and physical health maintenance practices.

Protection of research participants

Ethical approval was granted by the Ethics Committee of the State of Basel (Ethik-Kommission beider Basel) and the University of Zambia Humanities and Social Sciences Research Ethics Committee as part of a bigger research study, 'Improving equity of access to HIV care and treatment in Zambia.' The Ministry of health at national and district levels provided administrative clearance.

To ensure confidentiality and prevent involuntary disclosure of research participants' HIV status, locations for interviews were based on the preferences of the respondents. Some interviews were conducted at the local public sector clinic and private spaces within the homes of respondents' friends. A few PLHIV preferred being interviewed at home. This was done in the absence of family members to ensure privacy. Written informed consent was obtained from all research participants, including for quotes to be used anonymously in published reports.

Results

A total of thirty-seven (37) PLHIV who declined to be enrolled into ART care and twenty-five (25) PLHIV who had abandoned ART care were interviewed. The majority of the respondents (n=41) were women and almost half (n=29) were aged between 25–34 years old. More than two-thirds

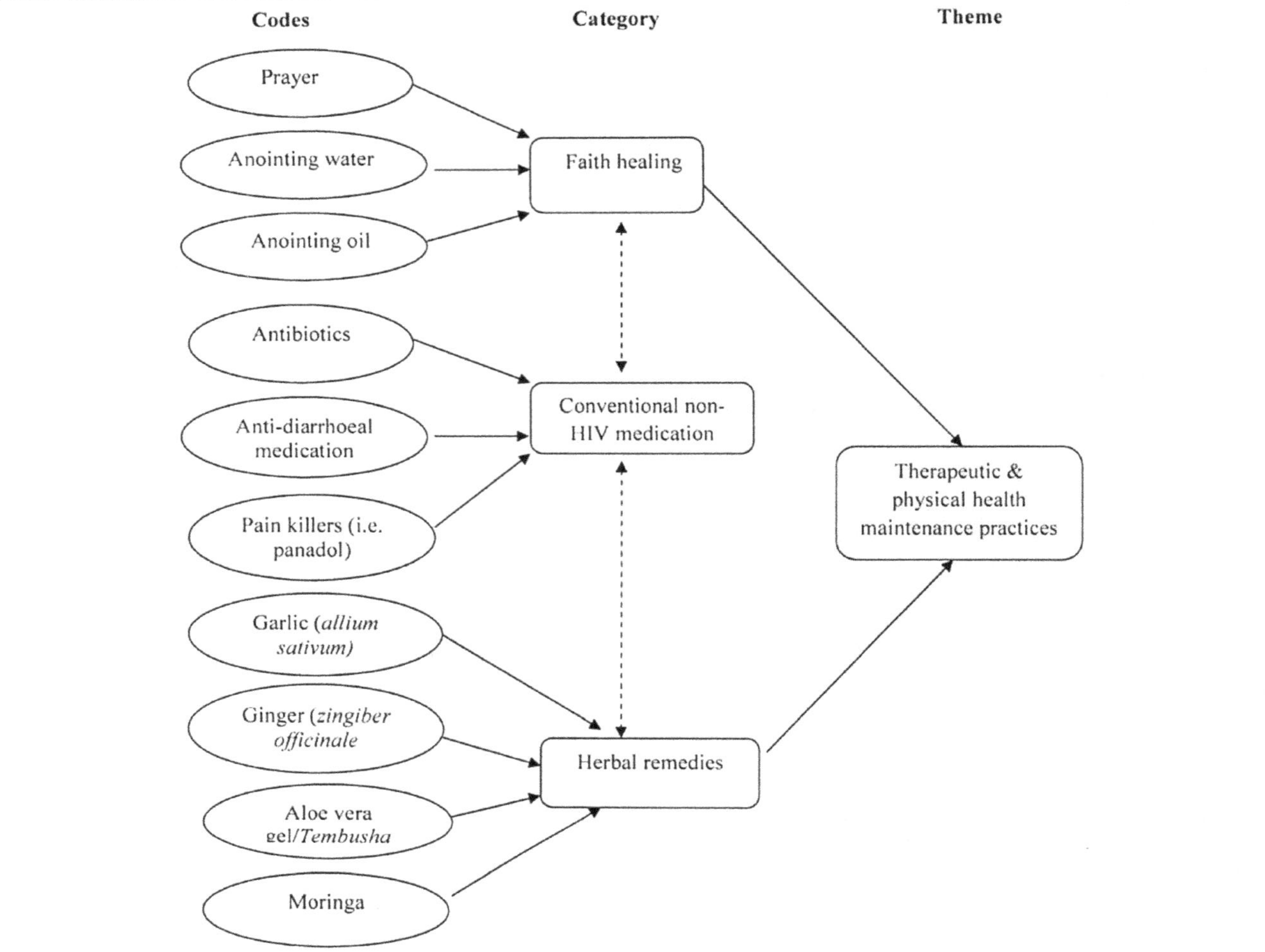

Figure 1 Example of coding framework of PLHIV self-care practices.

(n=42) of the PLHIV were in informal employment. For the PLHIV who had stopped ART, eight (8) of the 25 PLHIV had been on treatment for less than a year; and less than half (n=10) abandoned medication in less than a year of being initiated on treatment. For PLHIV who had never been on ART, almost half (17 out of 37) were recommended ART within the year preceding the interviews (Table 1).

Self-care practices of PLHIV not on ART

Seven (7) self-care practices were identified subsumed under four (4) main themes: Therapeutic and physical health maintenance; psychological well-being; healthy lifestyle and risk reduction practices.

Therapeutic and physical health maintenance practices

Taking herbal therapies

Sustaining physical health involved taking herbal remedies to treat opportunistic infections and mitigate HIV symptoms, 'wash toxins' from the body, replace nutrients and improve appetite levels. Garlic (*allium sativum*), ginger (*zingiber officinale*), aloe vera gel (also locally available in herbal plant form called *tembusha*), *moringa oleifera*, *Ngetwa* from Tanzania, crocodile fats, Chinese herbal remedies, *stametta* (aloe mixed with vitamins and herbs) and some herbs simply labeled *'Back to Eden'* were the most commonly used herbal remedies. Two PLHIV elucidated their experiences of herbal remedies:

> *"I take some moringa. It is a tree with small leaves; we have it in the backyard of our house.... I just put it in tea or even in vegetables; we cook and mix it with other vegetables. Sometimes we "sashila" (add pounded groundnuts] to moringa and cook it as relish. Or you can even add the moringa to porridge."* (50-year old woman; never been on ART)

> *"You know with herbs, if you are coughing, you get guava leaves, lemon leaves, boil and drink them and*

Table 1 Characteristics of PLHIV not on ART

Characteristic	No. of PLHIV who dropped out of ART	No. of PLHIV never on ART
Age (Years)		
18-24	5	4
25-34	11	18
35-44	3	14
>44	6	1
Sex		
Male	8	13
Female	17	24
Marital status		
Single	4	5
Married	12	22
Divorced/separated	7	6
Widowed		4
Source of livelihood		
Formal employment	4	5
Informal employment	15	27
Not working/dependant	6	5
Time on treatment		
<12 months	8	-
1-<2 years	6	-
2-<3 years	6	-
3-<4 years	2	-
≥4 years	3	-
Duration not on treatment (up to time of interview)		
6-<12 months	10	17
1-<2 years	8	10
2-<3 years	5	6
3-<4 years	2	4
4-<5 years	-	-
≥5 years	-	-

then you are done. Even now, when my daughter is coughing, I would just take garlic, I mix with lemons, honey and make cough syrup and it is done." (42-year old woman; never been on ART)

For many PLHIV, herbal remedies were taken as a routine part of life regardless of whether they were experiencing illness-related symptoms or not. Some herbal remedies were cheap while others like aloe vera gel were expensive, fetching as high as US$30 per one litre container. Those with financial means were able to buy these herbal remedies from drug stores, pharmacies, herbal medicine traders and herbal medicine shops. Some PLHIV periodically relied on financial support of relatives to procure these herbal remedies. Some herbal remedies like *moringa* and *ginger*, comparatively cheap, were routinely added to food or tea or juice to treat or prevent illnesses such as cold and flu, diarrhoea or generally to allegedly 'boost' the immune system and reinvigorate the body.

Some PLHIV reported planting these 'health-enhancing' herbs, particularly *moringa* and *tembusha* at home to ensure easy and unfettered access. While ART required high levels of adherence, this was reportedly not the case with herbal remedies. PLHIV reported taking them if and when they wanted. The flexibility of herbal treatment requirements was in part the reason why some PLHIV found herbal remedies attractive compared to conventional HIV medication which required strict adherence. One woman proudly expressed her affection for these herbal remedies:

> *"For me, I take tembusha and my CD4 cell count is high; that explains that the herbal remedy is working. So, why should I start ART?"* (32-year old woman; never been on ART)

One of the recurring themes was that while the study participants acknowledged the efficacy of ART, the burden of taking treatment for life, stringent adherence requirements and concerns about treatment side effects attracted them to use herbal remedies. One woman said:

> *"Even if the ARVs work, people say they are for life and that they have side effect. So when people hear that, they decide to go for herbs because no one wants to experience the side effects or to take the medication for life. They say that herbs have no side effects."* (23-year old woman; never been on ART)

Faith healing as HIV cure

Faith healing was also sought for curative purposes. Some PLHIV reported travelling outside Zambia in search of healing while others relied on their faith in God to secure healing:

> *"When I went [to Nigeria] for healing, I was never the same person again...No one can deceive me that the power of God cannot work or does not work. I saw blind people gaining back their sight; I saw people in wheelchair walk; I saw people who could not hear start hearing. What more evidence does one need to believe that God performs miracles?* (48-year old man; stopped ART)

> *"The thing is that when I pray, God tells me what to do. So God told me in a vision that you are healed*

and from the time that I prayed and stopped treatment, I have never been sick and have never taken any form of medication. The only secret which is there is to pray, and to believe in God, to have faith in Him." (45-year old man; stopped ART)

Ironically, some health workers with HIV, including those working in the ART clinic and eligible for ART also opted for faith healing and/or herbal remedies:

"I have also taken anointing water from [....]. They say it cures if you have faith because it is prayed for by the man of God." (27-year old woman; Pharmacy Technologist)

Using conventional medicine, but only to treat HIV-related infections

Acutely aware of their fledgling health and limitations of other self care strategies, some PLHIV did not completely cut-off ties with the formal health system. In the absence of herbal medication or whenever symptoms did not abate, some PLHIV sought formal health care, but only to use conventional medicine to treat opportunistic infections. Skin infections, respiratory infections and gastrointestinal tract infections were the most commonly reported HIV-related ailments. In other instances, PLHIV got over-the -counter medication, from a plethora of drug outlets in the area and the city centre. Antibiotics such as septrin (co-trimoxazole prophylaxis), flagyl, amoxicillin, anti-diarrhoeal medication were the most reported conventional drugs used. Some PLHIV reportedly used antibiotics used by their spouses on ART. Two PLHIV narrated:

"I just go to the clinic, they give me amoxil, and at times I go to the drug store and buy panadol or septrin or drugs for diarrhoea.... At the clinic, I just pretend as if I was never on ARVs because if I tell them, they [nurses] will just tell me to go to the ART clinic and get ARVs." (43 years old woman; stopped ART)

"I take two tablets of septrin in the morning every day. When the drugs get finished, I go and buy.... Like today, I took my last drugs and I am planning to go and get some drugs from my friend on credit. She runs a drug store. She gives me on credit each time I do not have money to buy." (31-year old woman; stopped ART)

Periodic monitoring of CD4 cell count

Coupled with uptake of herbal remedies, faith healing and conventional non-HIV medication, some PLHIV also monitored their immune system through periodically seeking CD4 cell count testing. Those with the financial means went to private clinics while others made private arrangements with public sector clinic staff to access CD4 cell count testing. At private clinics, charges for CD4 count testing ranged between ZMK50, 000 (US$10) and ZMK 150,000 (US$30) per test. Financial support from family members enabled some PLHIV to meet the costs. One PLHIV explained this strategy:

"I do my tests at a private clinic, there at Dr [.....]'s clinic. He tests for CD4 count. The last time I tested my CD4 count, it was in 2009 but time has elapsed since I last did my CD4 count." (43-year old woman; never been on ART)

Healthy lifestyle practices

Dietary improvements

Good nutrition was a recurring theme as a self-care practice. While many PLHIV found this hard to sustain due to fragile livelihoods characterised by lack of job opportunities and steady and 'adequate' income, this problem was attenuated by improvising local food menus, for instance adding pounded groundnuts to vegetables like rape, cabbage, pumpkin leaves, locally called *"kusashila"* to nourish their bodies and improve their health condition. Other PLHIV heavily relied on nutritional supplements, sometimes supplied by relatives outside the country – in Europe, South Africa and United States of America:

"I usually depend on a food supplement called 'Shake herbal life'. It comes from America. It is in powder form. When you want, you can add it to milk or you can add even fruit juice. It is like powdered milk. What I do is, in the morning, I just take a glass of water and put two full tea spoons of the same 'Shake' and then I mix it and then I drink. If I have money, instead of water, I put milk, I mix it with milk and then I drink. If I have money and I have bananas, I blend and add it to my water and milk and then I drink. Those are my ARVs." (38-year old woman; never been on ART)

Risk reduction practices

Safe sex and cessation of sexual relationships

To avoid re-infections particularly through unprotected sex, some PLHIV, especially those not married - either widowed or divorced/separated - reported either practicing safe sex or ceasing sexual relationships altogether. Some PLHIV drew lessons from the experiences of other PLHIV who had reportedly continued to live 'healthy' and 'normal' lives without ART partly because they had reportedly avoided re-infections. Two PLHIV explained:

"From the time my husband died, I have vowed to abstain from sex. This has helped me because I learnt it from my HIV positive sister who has not been on

any form of treatment since 1995 but is still alive and healthy today. Her secret is good diet and no sex." (42-year old woman; never been on ART)

"Then we developed a culture in the house to say that let us start using condoms. In the house, it is condomising now. Then I think sometimes God comes in, you know. I have been praying to ensure that he would be agreeing to it, you know and for sure, he was not like, no what, what, and so we have been on condoms like that. He has been comfortable with it and we have been living like that." (38-year old woman; never been on ART)

Psychological well-being self-care practices

"I rely on Jesus Christ"- religiosity and spirituality

Religiosity, particularly Christianity, was found to be woven into the day-to-day lives of some PLHIV, thus becoming a powerful self-care practice. Despite anticipation of stigma in religious circles due to the perceived association of HIV infection with improper sexual behaviour and a sinful lifestyle, through self-identification as Christians, some PLHIV, mostly women, drew on the biblical assurances of healing as a source of comfort and hope. Through organized religion, some PLHIV belonged to Christian denominations that were more accepting to PLHIV, particularly churches whose leaders or pastors professed to offer healing for people with HIV. While hoping for healing, some PLHIV reportedly put 'everything in the hands of God'. They reported conducting private individual prayers with their pastors, going for collective intercessory prayers in which they opened up to one another and religious leaders about their HIV condition. One PLHIV who disclosed her status to her pastor described her unflinching belief in God:

"As for me, I rely on Jesus Christ.... I just told myself that it is better I face Jesus Christ, God himself since He is the one that gave me life, not a human being. In John 14:1 [Bible], Jesus says 'I am the way, the truth, and the Life.' You know if God wants to take my life now, He can do it, whether I am on ARVs or not. I have a lot of friends who were on ARVs but have since died. Why? It is because man cannot preserve life; only God can." (48 year old HIV positive woman; stopped ART)

Another PLHIV explained her prayer life:

"Even if you take the medicine, if you do not look to God for healing, you cannot get cured. So everything only works if you also involve God. So I also pray to God for me to be cured. I go for prayers every morning. There are inter-denominational prayer meetings here in Chawama, there at Pentecostal holiness in Kuku compound. Prayers are held every morning, everyday, Monday to Saturday. The prayers start at 06 hours up to 7 hours." (21-year old young woman; stopped ART)

To complement their prayer lives, some PLHIV reported using 'anointing water' - water believed to have healing properties after being prayed for by a Pastor believed to have spiritual healing powers - in order to ward off illnesses. They bought it from their churches that sold it or ordered it from Nigeria where a renowned Pentecostal tele-evangelist was reported to have spiritual healing powers. It cost at least US$100 for a 100 mls bottle. At a time when ART was free in public sector clinics, some PLHIV still opted for faith healing despite the associated financial costs. One PLHIV who went to Nigeria for prayers and bought the 'anointing water' explained:

"It is called anointing water. I have got it right with me in the car. What happens is that he [Pastor] does not heal you, you heal yourself. The belief that you have got yourself that God can heal you is what heals you. The belief that tomorrow I will walk, that tomorrow my immunity will rise, it will. It is you and God, and I believe it. Belief is not medicine, but it also heals. You do not just need medicine to get healed. You also need belief." (48-year old man; stopped ART)

'I avoid thinking about it too much': positive attitudes towards HIV infection

Some PLHIV acknowledged the relationship between psychological well-being and their immune system. Therefore, developing and maintaining positive attitude towards their HIV condition was viewed as another precondition for improved physical well-being. This meant reconstructing their lives to attain a sense of normalcy. PLHIV avoided 'thinking too much' about HIV and treated HIV as any other infection: *"I just try by all means to ignore it; I just pretend as if it does not exist. I tend to live a normal life"*, said a 23-year old man, who had never been on ART. *"I do exercises; and I keep my mind very free. I avoid thinking about it too much,"* said another 24-year old man who has never been on ART. This enabled them to treat HIV not as a fatal condition; rather as something that they could live with and manage while acknowledging episodic periods of good and poor health.

The role of social network relationships

The self-care practices were modulated by kin and non-kin social network relationships. PLHIV treatment seeking behaviour was influenced by relationships with friends/family members and some formal health care providers. For instance, limited disclosure of HIV status to close and trusted friends and family members as well as formation of or belonging to informal networks of PLHIV facilitated coping and self-management of HIV. The social support received could be delineated into two: illness-specific support such as provision of financial resources to access herbal remedies and over-the-counter conventional medication to mitigate the HIV-related symptoms and obtain nutritional supplements. This type of support was mainly provided by family members:

> *"So me, I just use herbal remedy called 'palibe kantu' (there is no problem) which my mother organises for me from the farm in Mumbwa (another district). This herb grows and spreads on the ground like sweet potatoes. So you peel it and boil it and start drinking the water. So she brings that for me from time to time."* (32-year old woman; never been on ART)

The second form of social support mainly provided through religious groupings and networks with other people living with HIV involved psychosocial support. In addition, PLHIV also provided informational support to each other on illness management including which herbal remedies to use for what symptoms or ailments. They also shared information about sources of herbal remedies. As one PLHIV explained:

> *"You know, you come to know each other when you start treatment because in a day, they enroll may be 10 people which means these ten people will be coming to the clinic on the say day plus those that have already started treatment. So, even when you stop taking ARVs, you reach a stage where you know each other, support each other, and even encourage one another."* (39-year old woman; stopped ART)

In some cases, driven in part by their own treatment and health beliefs, it appeared that some health workers encouraged PLHIV to use faith healing and herbal remedies either in combination with or to the exclusion of ART care. Asked how she reconciled her non-uptake of treatment and counselling PLHIV to start and adhere to ART, one lay ART support worker explained:

> *"You know, me even when I am at the ART clinic, I also encourage those people to say that it is not only ARVs, even herbs, because sometimes you find that somebody is taking ARVs, but still more the CD4 count keeps on dropping. You see, I would also advise them that can you also try this, try herbs."* (42-year old ART support worker; never been on ART)

For better and for worse: PLHIV perceptions and experiences of self-care practices

Some PLHIV reported a rebound in their CD4 cell count or improved physical health due to the use of herbal remedies or after going through prayer sessions and therefore believed that it was possible to live a normal and healthy life if one used herbal medication and/or 'surrendered' his life to God for care. One lay health worker who has never been on ART explained her experience:

> *"When they told me that 'your CD4 count is low,' I just started using herbs like moringa, and after that, my CD4 count improved a bit up to 460 something."* (32-year old Treatment support worker; never been on ART)

Another PLHIV - an ART support worker - who went to South Africa for prayers instead of seeking ART care also reported a rebound in her CD4 cell count. She recounted:

> *"We were taught how to receive healing. We were learning about how to have faith, and how to receive healing. And when we [with the husband] came back from there, I was just ok. When I came back, I went to the clinic to check my CD4 count and it had been boosted from 165 to 365. So that is it."* (37-year old woman; never been on ART)

For some PLHIV, a rebound in physical health was not associated with previous use of ART. Instead, they attributed 'good' health to the effectiveness of their non-ART related self-care practices. One PLHIV who had gone to Nigeria for healing prayers explained his experience:

> *"When I went there, I was not walking. Other people were assisting me to walk. But when I came from there, I was walking. He never gave me any herbs; he never gave me any medicine. He just gave me water and prayer."* (48-year old man; stopped ART)

Notwithstanding the perceived effectiveness of these self-care strategies, some PLHIV reported noticeable decline in their health and all PLHIV contemplated starting ART if all other efforts failed. For others, a decline in health status was attributed to either lifestyle behaviour deemed incompatible with their condition or due to psychosocial distress. These included beer drinking, smoking, challenges of maintaining a nutritious diet, pregnancy and psychological distress due to strained family relationships. As two PLHIV explained:

> *"The only problem why I develop these health problems, I look sick, is that I started drinking again. After two years of stopping treatment, I was ok. But that habit of drinking came back....The only mistake I made was that*

I started excessive drinking. Again I realized that this beer will kill me. So I stopped. I do not drink beer anymore." (48-year old man; stopped ART)

"I used to monitor my CD4 count, and it was high... until 2008 when I was pregnant that is when my CD4 count came down.... But I think my CD4 count is also low because most of the time, we are quarrelling with my husband, so I think my mind is often disturbed." (32-year old woman; never been on ART)

Despite reporting a decline in health status, some PLHIV still remained upbeat, viewing their poor health as temporal - a period which every individual, regardless of their HIV status went through - and not an indication that they needed to start treatment. HIV treatment was viewed as not a guarantor of good health and their lives. To them, the death of PLHIV despite being on ART was emblematic of the shortcomings of ART:

"It happens in life. Sometimes you can have good days and sometimes you can have bad days. So, if my health is not good today, it does not mean that it will be like that forever. Things change; starting treatment does not guarantee that you will become healthy forever. What about those people who have died despite taking ARVs?" (24-year old man; stopped ART)

Discussion

Our study explored the different self-care practices that PLHIV used as alternatives to ART care. We found that PLHIV used - often concurrently - herbal remedies, over-the-counter conventional medicine and faith healing, augmented by adoption of healthy lifestyle practices to promote physical and psychosocial well-being. If PLHIV opting for self care alternatives subsequently accessed health services, they never mentioned to non-ART prescribing health workers that they had opted to discontinue accessing ART or that they had opted not to start treatment. Neither did health workers inquire about the health and treatment history of these PLHIV. Thus, health workers missed the opportunity to bring these PLHIV back into ART care and treat them for the underlying cause of their ill-health. These self-care practices were modulated by availability of social support (Figure 2). These findings have implications for successful delivery of ART care.

Herbal remedies may mitigation HIV symptoms but undermine access to treatment

Our findings show that herbal remedies were widely used as a self-care practice. The herbs were reportedly used to 'cleanse' the body of toxins, to treatment opportunistic infections, 'boost' the immune system and enhance physical functioning. The pressure associated with adhering to ART compared with herbal remedies that were taken on "if and when they want" basis motivated PLHIV to opt for herbal remedies. These herbs were perceived to be as effective as ART, albeit with perceived fewer side effects and no strict dosage and adherence requirements. Our findings are consistent with previous studies that have reported wide use of herbal medication as a self-care strategy [32-37].

Worryingly, the growth of the market for herbal remedies, their popularity and perceived effectiveness without scientific proof, risks undermining the success of ART care and consequently increasing the burden of HIV care in the long term. This could happen in three ways: first, by inhibiting patient (re-) entry into ART care and second, by 'pulling' out of ART care PLHIV already receiving medication due to the perception that herbal remedies were effective. Consequently, delayed initiation of ART may create

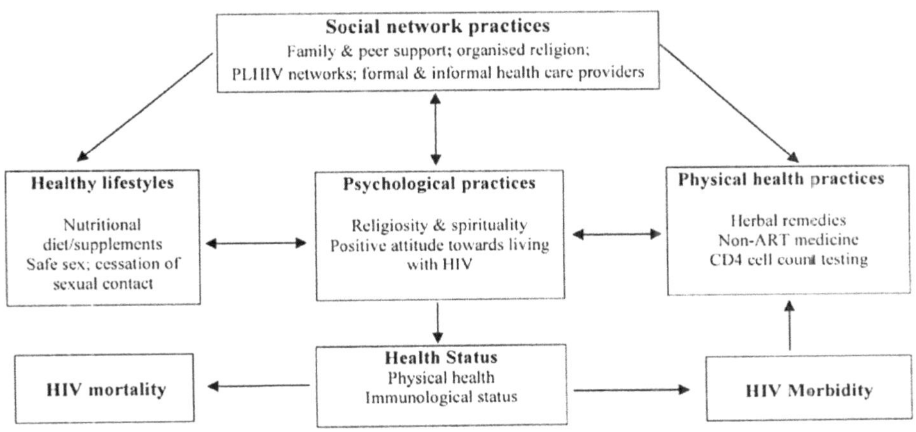

Figure 2 Nested relationships of self-care practices of PLHIV not on ART.

additional therapeutic costs when PLHIV eventually return for ART care, albeit in poor health. The reported decline in health by some PLHIV clearly suggests that it is just a matter of time before PLHIV seek ART care. Third, the perceived effectiveness of herbal remedies could also attract even those already in ART care to use them. For these PLHIV, combining herbal remedies and antiretrovirals could affect the pharmacokinetics of antiretrovirals. This could either lead to higher antiretroviral plasma levels thus putting PLHIV at greater risk of developing serious side effects or lower the optimal therapeutic level of antiretrovirals thereby leading to treatment failure and an enhanced risk of developing drug resistance [38]. For instance, garlic, which is widely used as herbal therapy or nutritional supplement, has been reported to affect the pharmacokinetic concentration of HIV medication [39,40]. Bepe and colleagues [41] found that concomitantly using herbal remedies with antiretrovirals elevates some adverse events. Other studies have also reported reduced adherence to ART by those using herbal remedies and other alternative forms of care [42,43].

Importantly too, with growing demand for these herbal remedies and drawing on the desperation and naiveté of PLHIV, scientifically unproven herbal remedies could pose a health-risk to PLHIV. There have been reports about bogus HIV 'cures' or 'immune boosters' in Zambia and the dangers they presented to the lives and health of PLHIV. For instance in 2007, one of the purported AIDS 'cure' or 'immune booster' was found to be a pesticide, tetrasil, used for cleaning swimming pools [44]. Therefore, to ensure successful delivery of ART care, there is need for HIV care providers to step up sensitisation campaigns during ART counselling sessions and more widely about the health risks associated with use of unproven herbal remedies. This is critical not only to improve uptake of and adherence to treatment, avert possible negative interaction effects with antiretroviral treatment, but also to protect the health and lives of PLHIV and ensure patient retention in ART care.

Religiosity and spirituality may simulate counselling but undermine uptake of ART care

Our study also found that some PLHIV sought recourse to religiosity and spirituality as a self-care practice. This is consistent with previous studies that have reported use of religiosity and spirituality as coping strategies by those with chronic health conditions, including HIV [45,46]. Religiosity has been associated with less psychological distress [47] and less depression [48], suggesting that it provides beneficial psychological outcomes. This is despite the reported stigmatizing influence of religious beliefs due to the association of HIV infection with improper sexual relationships [49,50].

In our study, religion and Christianity in particular was not only used to secure complete healing, but also to provide hope, comfort and assurances in the face of an incurable disease. While PLHIV were exposed to stigmatizing attitudes within religious settings, they often navigated their spiritual lives by moving to churches that preached healing and deliverance and whose leadership was perceived as open and receptive to PLHIV. Some PLHIV that were not publicly open about their HIV status only confided in and sought healing from their religious leaders. Two lessons can be drawn which have implications for successful delivery of ART care: On a positive note, these findings suggest that prayer simulates aspects of counselling [45] and can therefore be a useful coping mechanism for living with HIV. However, there is a thin line between faith healing as a psychosocial coping strategy and faith healing as a cure, with the latter posing a threat to patient access to and retention in ART care. More so, religious beliefs can trigger a fatalistic attitude and passive resignation with death, thus hindering uptake of treatment. Therefore, during group sensitisation and individual counselling sessions at ART clinics, health workers should tap into PLHIV belief systems to identify and harness those beliefs that promote psychosocial well-being without hindering PLHIV uptake of treatment. At community level, sensitisation efforts are required to encourage PLHIV claiming to have experienced healing through prayers to undergo formal medical tests to substantiate these claims. This is critical to ensure that PLHIV get (back) into ART care.

PLHIV self-prescription of antibiotics raises concerns about development of microbial resistant strains

Due to the experiential limitations of faith healing and herbal remedies in addressing HIV-related ailments, we found that the use of conventional medicine, particularly antibiotics as a self-care strategy was common amongst PLHIV. Since the onset of ART roll-out, western medicines like co-trimoxazole prophylaxis have become widely available in low-income countries to treat microbial infections in PLHIV. The World Health Organisation (WHO) guidelines recommend provision of co-trimoxazole prophylaxis to all HIV symptomatic adults with CD4 count lower than 350 cells per μL in resource-limited settings [51]. Co-trimoxazole prophylaxis has been found to reduce mortality and morbidity amongst PLHIV through prevention and control of opportunistic infections [52,53]. Based on their knowledge of these conventional medicines and experiences with the formal health system and social network ties, PLHIV opted to obtain antibiotics in order to manage AIDS-related ailments. Our findings suggest that there was widespread use of antibiotics obtained either privately from the public sector clinics or purchased from a plethora of drug stores and pharmacies. The self-prescription of antibiotics raises great concern about future development of microbial resistance to antibiotics amongst PLHIV which could undermine future efforts to deal with HIV-related opportunistic infections. In the past, WHO has raised concerns about bacterial resistance to antibiotics due to their inappropriate use [54]. The reported widespread self-prescription and use of antibiotics by PLHIV therefore calls for sensitization measures about the dangers of self-prescription of antibiotics, especially amongst PLHIV. There is also need for enforcement of pharmaceutical regulations to control self-prescription and use of antibiotics, including clamping down on unregistered drug stores. This is even more critical for effective care of patients in ART care.

Social support may also undermine uptake of ART care

As a corollary, self-care practices were found to be socially delineated and modulated by social support mechanisms. Social support "entails the structure of an individual's social life (i.e. group memberships, existence of familial ties) and the explicit functions they serve such as emotional support" [55]. Previous studies have reported that social support was a strong predictor of utilization of formal HIV care services [56] and improved the odds of entry into and use of ART care [57]. Our findings suggest that while social support may serve as a stress-buffer and enables individuals through their social support networks to easily come to terms with their condition and develop a more positive outlook to life in the face of an incurable condition, social support is also a key self-care input factor that undermines access to ART care (Figure 2). For instance, social pressure and influence existed at family and interpersonal level to shun ART. Conversely, social support in the form of material, financial and moral support was provided to access herbal remedies, over-the-counter conventional medication to treat AIDS-related symptoms, and faith healing as cure for HIV. This places PLHIV at risk of AIDS-related morbidity and early mortality (Figure 2).

While the physical and psychological self-care practices complemented by adoption of healthy lifestyles and risk reduction such as practicing safe sex/cessation of sexual relationships to avoid re-infections are vital in the overall management of HIV, these behavioural practices in the absence of ART care are not sufficient to effectively prevent disease progression. The long-term benefits, therefore, reside in encouraging PLHIV to access ART care.

Study limitations

Caution has to be taken when generalising the study findings. Some PLHIV were recruited in the community through their caregivers or snowball sampling and their eligibility for the study was based on self-reports of being eligible for treatment. Snowball sampling may have led to clustering of shared ideas and views. However, over two thirds of the study participants were identified, contacted and recruited through the ART clinic staff who were aware of which individuals had dropped out of ART or declined ART despite being eligible, suggesting that our sample largely comprised of treatment-eligible PLHIV who were independent from each other. Also, this study was descriptive and exploratory, aimed at providing wide ranging insights into how PLHIV managed their health in the absence of ART and how these self-care practices impacted uptake of ART. Thus, the purpose of the study was neither to establish causal relationships (i.e. effect of herbal remedies on immune system) nor to assess the effectiveness of these self-care strategies.

The paucity of data on PLHIV self-care practices meant that the study had to focus on identifying a wide range of themes rather than securing a representative sample of non-uptakers of treatment. To mitigate the potential for bias in the selection of study participants, we endeavoured to ensure that our study sample was diverse in terms of demographic, length of time since diagnosis and treatment-related characteristics. Therefore, similar studies are needed in other settings for comparability of findings. Despite these possible limitations, our findings could be generalised to similar settings in urban areas in the country and provide useful insight to inform policy and practice to improve ART uptake.

Conclusions

This study explored the self-care practices of PLHIV not receiving ART. These PLHIV comprised those to whom ART was recommended by ART providers but for other reasons opted not to initiate treatment and PLHIV who had completely discontinued their medication. Our findings show that the use of herbal remedies and faith healing were dominant self-care practices. In addition, PLHIV used conventional medicines, but only to deal with AIDS-related ailments. It was also common for PLHIV to concomitantly use these different self-care practices. While these self-care practices were perceived by PLHIV to be effective, some PLHIV still reported slow and intermittent decline in health status, an indication that these self-care strategies were not as effective as reported and experienced. For PLHIV that had dropped out of ART, the perceived effectiveness of self-care practices could be attributed to previous use of antiretrovirals. These self-care practices undermine patient uptake of treatment and risk compromising future effectiveness of medical therapies and increase likelihood of microbial resistance and HIV resistant strains amongst PLHIV. In turn, this could increase the costs of ART care and family and community resources. Therefore, to ensure effective delivery of ART care, there is need to compile and include evidence of complementary HIV care practices into counselling guidelines and encourage those self-care practices that do not affect the effectiveness of antiretrovirals and do not put the health of PLHIV at risk. On the other hand, some of the self-care practices like self-prescription and indiscriminate use of antibiotics and use of scientifically unproven herbal remedies may cause long-term harm to PLHIV hence the need for sensitization campaigns and enforcement of pharmaceutical regulations to address them.

Competing interests
The authors declare that they have no competing interests.

Authors' contributions
MM conceptualized the study, conducted data collection and analysis and wrote the draft manuscript. VB and SM contributed towards the conceptualization of the study, provided input in the analysis, interpretation of the findings and drafting of the manuscript. All authors have given final approval of the version to be published.

Acknowledgements
The study was funded by the Swiss National Science Foundation (SNSF) through the research study 'Improving equity of access to HIV care and treatment in Zambia.' The authors are grateful to the home-based care providers and VCT/ART workers of the local public health centre who helped identify and recruit research participants; the research participants for agreeing to share their time and experiences.
The funder played no role in the design and conduct of the study; the interpretation of the data; and the write up of this paper.

Author details
[1]Zambia AIDS-related TB Research Project, University of Zambia, P.O Box 50697, Lusaka, Zambia. [2]Swiss Tropical and Public Health Institute, Socinstrasse 57, Basel CH-4002, Switzerland. [3]University of Basel, Faculty of Science, Basel CH-4003, Switzerland. [4]Department of Global Health and Development, London School of Hygiene and Tropical Medicine, Keppel Street, London WC1E 7HT, UK.

References
1. UNAIDS: *Global Report: UNAIDS Report on the Global AIDS Epidemic*. Geneva: UNAIDS; 2010.
2. WHO/UNAIDS/UNICEF: *Global AIDS Response - Progress Report 2011*. Geneva: WHO; 2011.
3. Harries AD, Zachariah R, Lawn SD, Rosen S: **Strategies to retain patients on antiretroviral therapy in sub-Saharan Africa.** *Trop Med Int Health* 2010, **15**(Suppl 1):70–75.
4. Rosen S, Fox MP, Gill CJ: **Patient retention in antiretroviral therapy programs in sub-Saharan Africa: a systematic review.** *PLoS Med* 2007, **4:**e298.
5. Hammond R, Harry TC: **Efficacy of antiretroviral therapy in Africa: effect on immunological and virological outcome measures: a meta-analysis.** *Int J STD AIDS* 2008, **19:**291–296.
6. Coetzee D, Hildebrand K, Boulle A, Maartens G, Louis F, Labatala V, Reuter H, Ntwana N, Goemaere E: **Outcomes after two years of providing antiretroviral treatment in Khayelitsha, South Africa.** *AIDS* 2004, **18:**887–895.
7. Ivers LC, Kendrick D, Doucette K: **Efficacy of antiretroviral therapy programs in resource-poor settings: a meta-analysis of the published literature.** *Clin Infect Dis* 2005, **41:**217–224.
8. Egger M, May M, Chene G, Phillip AN, Ledergerber B, Dabis F, Costagliola D, D'Arminio Monforte A, de Wolf F, Reiss P, Lundgren JD, Justice AC, Staszewski S, Leport C, Hogg RS, Sabin CA, Gill MJ, Salzberger B, Sterne JA: **Prognosis of HIV-1-infected patients starting highly active antiretroviral therapy: a collaborative analysis of prospective studies.** *Lancet* 2002, **360:**119–129.
9. Miller CM, Ketlhapile M, Rybasack-Smith H: **Why are antiretroviral treatment patients lost to follow-up? A qualitative study from South Africa.** *Trop Med Int Health* 2010, **15**(Suppl. 1):48–54.
10. Zachariah R, Harries AD, Manzi M, Gomani P, Teck R, Phillips M, Firmenich P: **Acceptance of antiretroviral therapy among patients infected with HIV and Tuberculosis in rural Malawi is low and associated with cost of transport.** *PLoS One* 2010, **1**(1):e121.
11. Beer L, Fagan JL, Valverde E, Bertolli J: **Health-related beliefs and decisions about accessing HIV medical care among HIV-infected persons who are not receiving care.** *AIDS Patient Care STDS* 2009, **23:**785–792.
12. Alfonso V, Bermbach N, Geller J, Montaner JSG: **Individual variability in barriers affecting people's decision to take HAART: A qualitative study identifying barriers to being on HAART.** *AIDS Patient Care STDS* 2006, **20:**848–857.
13. Gellaitry G, Cooper V, Davies C, Fisher M, Leake M: **Patients' Perception of information about HAART: impact on treatment decisions.** *AIDS Care* 2005, **17:**367–376.
14. Gold RS, Ridge DT: **"I will start treatment when I think time is right": HIV positive gay men talk about their decision not to access antiretroviral therapy.** *AIDS Care* 2001, **13:**693–708.
15. Musheke M, Bond V, Merten S: **Individual and contextual factors influencing patient attrition from antiretroviral therapy in an urban community of Lusaka Zambia.** *J Int AIDS Soc* 2012, **15**(Suppl 1):17366.
16. Katz IT, Essien T, Marinda ET, Gray GE, Bangsberg DR, Martinson NA, De Bruyn G: **Antiretroviral therapy refusal among newly diagnosed HIV-infected adults.** *AIDS* 2011, **25:**2177–2181.
17. Murphy RA, Sunpath H, Taha B, Kappagoda S, Maphasa KTM, Kuritzkes DR, Smeaton L: **Low uptake of antiretroviral therapy and high mortality after tuberculosis and opportunistic infection in Kwazulu-Natal, South Africa.** *Int J Tuberc Lung Dis* 2010, **14**(7):903–908.
18. Unge C, Ragnarsson A, Ekström AM, Indalo D, Belita A, Carter J, Ilako F, Sodërgard B: **The influence of traditional medicine and religion on discontinuation of ART in an urban informal settlement in Nairobi.** *Kenya. AIDS Care* 2011, **23**(7):851–858.
19. Roura M, Nsigaye R, Nhandi B, Wamoyi J, Busza J, Urassa M, Todd J, Zaba B: **"Driving the devil away": qualitative insights into miraculous cures for AIDS in a rural Tanzanian ward.** *BMC Publ Health* 2010, **10:**427.
20. Wringe A, Roura M, Urassa M, Busza J, Athanas V, Zaba B: **Doubts, denial and divine intervention: understanding delayed attendance and poor retention rates at a HIV treatment programme in rural Tanzania.** *AIDS Care* 2009, **21:**632–637.
21. Wanyama J, Castelnuovo B, Wandera B, Mwebaze P, Kambungu A, Bangsberg DR, Kamya MR: **Belief in divine healing can be a barrier to antiretroviral therapy adherence in Uganda.** *AIDS* 2007, **21**(11):1486–1487.
22. Babb DA, Pemba L, Seatlanyane P: **Use of traditional medicine by HIV-infected individuals in South Africa in the era of antiretroviral therapy.** *Psychol Health Med* 2007, **12**(3):314–320.
23. Stevens PE, Hilderbrandt E: **Pill taking from the perspective of HIV-infected women who are vulnerable to antiretroviral treatment failure.** *Qual Health Res* 2009, **19**(5):593–604.
24. Central Statistics Office (CSO), Ministry of Health (MoH), Tropical Disease Research Centre (TDRC), University of Zambia, Macro International Inc: *Zambia Demographic and Health Survey 2007*. Calverton, Maryland, USA: CSO and Macro International Inc; 2009.
25. National AIDS Council: *Zambia Country Report. Monitoring the Declaration of Commitment on HIV and AIDS and the Universal Access - Biennial report for January 2010 – December 2011. Submitted to the United Nations General Assembly Special Session on AIDS*. Lusaka: NAC; 2012.
26. Fox MP, Mazimba A, Seidenberg P, Crooks D, Sikateyo B, Rosen S: **Barriers to initiation of antiretroviral treatment in rural and urban Zambia: A cross-sectional study of cost, stigma and perception of treatment.** *J Int AIDS Soc* 2010, **13:**8.
27. Grant E, Logie D, Masura M, Gorman D, Murray SA: **Factors facilitating and challenging access and adherence to antiretroviral therapy in a township in the Zambian Copperbelt: A qualitative study.** *AIDS Care* 2008, **20**(10):1155–1160.
28. Murray LK, Semrau K, McCauley E, Thea DM, Scott N, Mwiya M, Kankasa C, Bass J, Bolton P: **Barriers to acceptance and adherence of antiretroviral therapy in urban Zambian women: A qualitative study.** *AIDS Care* 2009, **21**(1):78–86.

29. Barlow J, Wright C, Sheasby J, Turner A, Hainsworth J: **Self-management approaches for people with chronic conditions: a review.** *Patient Educ Couns* 2002, **48**:177–187.
30. Ministry of Health: *Adult and adolescent antiretroviral therapy protocols (2nd edition).* Lusaka: MoH; 2010.
31. Graneheim UH, Lundman B: **Qualitative content analysis in nursing research: concepts, procedures and measures to achieve trustworthiness.** *Nurse Educ Today* 2004, **24**:105–112.
32. Marie Modeste RR, Majeke SJ: **Self-care symptom management strategies among women living with HIV in urban Kwazulu-Natal.** *Health* 2010, **15**:1.
33. Monera TG, Maponga CC: **Moringa oleifera supplementation by patients on antiretroviral therapy.** *J Int AIDS Soc* 2010, **13**(Suppl 4):P188.
34. Hsiao AF, Wong MD, Kanouse DE, Collins RL, Liu H, Andersen RM, Gifford AL, McCutchan A, Bozzette SA, Shapiro MF, Wenger NS: **Complementary and alternative medicine use and substitution for conventional therapy by HIV-infected patients.** *J Acquir Immune Defic Syndr* 2003, **33**:157–165.
35. Thorne S, Paterson B, Russell C, Schultz A: **Complementary/alternative medicine in chronic illness as informed self-care decision making.** *Int J Nurs Stud* 2002, **39**:671–683.
36. Duggan J, Peterson WS, Schutz M, Khudar S, Charkraborty J: **Use of complementary and alternative therapies in HIV infected individuals.** *AIDS Patient Care STDS* 2001, **15**(3):159–167.
37. Ernst E: **Prevalence of use of complementary/alternative medicine: a systematic review.** *Bull World Health Organ* 2000, **78**(2):252–257.
38. Van den Bout-van den Beukel CJ, Koopmans PP, van der Ven AJ, De Smet PA, Burger DM: **Possible drug metabolism interactions of medicinal herbs with antiretroviral agents.** *Drug Metab Rev* 2006, **38**:477–514.
39. Borrelli F, Capasso R, Izzo AA: **Garlic (allium sativum L): Adverse effects and drug interactions in humans.** *Mol Nutr Food Res* 2007, **51**:1386–1397.
40. Piscitelli SC, Burstein AH, Welden N, Gallicano KD, Falloon J: **The effect of garlic supplements on the pharmacokinetics of Saquinavir.** *Clin Inf Dis* 2002, **34**:234–238.
41. Bepe N, Madanhi N, Mudzviti T, Gavi S, Maponga CC, Morse GD: **The impact of herbal remedies on adverse effects and quality of life in HIV-infected individuals on antiretroviral therapy.** *J Infect Dev Ctries* 2011, **5**(1):048–053.
42. Peltzer K, Friend-du Preez N, Ramlagan S, Fomundam H, Anderson H, Chanetsa L: **Antiretrovirals and the use of traditional, complementary and alternative medicine by HIV patients in Kwa-Zulu Natal, South Africa. A longitudinal study.** *Afr J Tradit Complement Altern Med* 2011, **8**(4):337–345.
43. Owen-Smith A, Diclemente R, Wingood G: **Complementary and alternative medicine use decreases adherence to HAART in HIV-positive women.** *AIDS Care* 2007, **19**(5):589–593.
44. Amon JJ: **Dangerous medicines: Unproven AIDS cures and counterfeit antiretroviral drugs.** *Global health* 2008, **4**:5.
45. Ridge D, Williams I, Anderson J, Elford J: **Like a prayer: the role of spirituality and religion for people living with HIV in the UK.** *Sociol Health Illn* 2007, **30**(3):413–428.
46. Woods TE, Ironson GH: **Religion and spirituality in the face of illness: how cancer, cardiac and HIV patients describe their religiosity/spirituality.** *J Health Psychol* 1999, **4**(3):393–412.
47. Simoni JM, Martone MG, Kerwin JF: **Spirituality and psychological adaptation among women with HIV/AIDS: implications for counselling.** *J Counsel Psychol* 2002, **49**:139–147.
48. Simoni JM, Ortiz MZ: **Mediational models of spirituality and depressive symptomatology among HIV-positive Puerto Rican women.** *Cultur Divers Ethnic Minor Psychol* 2003, **9**:3–15.
49. Zou J, Yamanaka Y, Muze J, Watt M, Ostermann J, Thielman N: **Religion and HIV in Tanzania: influence of religious beliefs on HIV stigma, disclosure, and treatment attitudes.** *BMC Publ Health* 2009, **9**:75.
50. Genrich GL, Brathwaite BA: **Response of religious groups to HIV/AIDS as a sexually transmitted infection in Trinidad.** *BMC Publ Health* 2005, **5**:121.
51. WHO: *Guidelines on co-trimoxazole prophylaxis for HIV-related infections among children, adolescents and adults: recommendations for a public health approach.* Geneva: WHO; 2006.
52. Walker AS, Ford D, Gilks CF, Munderi P, Ssali F, Reid A, Katabira E, Grosskurth H, Mugyenyi P, Hakim J, Darbyshire JH, Gibb DM, Babiker AG: **Daily co-trimoxazole prophylaxis in severely immune-suppressed HIV-infected adults in Africa started on combination antiretroviral therapy: an observational analysis of the DART cohort.** *Lancet* 2010, **375**:1278–1286.
53. Walker AS, Mulenga V, Ford D, Kabamba D, Sinyinza F, Kankasa C, Chintu C, Gibb DM, CHAP Team: **The impact of daily Cotrimoxazole prophylaxis and antiretroviral therapy on mortality and hospital admissions in HIV-infected Zambian children.** *Clin Infect Dis* 2007, **44**:1361–1367.
54. WHO: *Antimicrobial resistance: the facts. Essential drugs monitor Issue Number 28 & 29.* Geneva: WHO; 2000.
55. Uchino NN: **Social support and health: a review of physiological processes potentially underlying links to disease outcomes.** *Int J Behav Med* 2006, **29**(4):377–387.
56. Uphold CR, Mkanta WN: **Use of health care services among persons living with HIV infection: state of the science and future directions.** *AIDS Patient Care STDS* 2005, **19**(8):473–485.
57. Waddell EN, Messeri PA: **Social support, disclosure and use of antiretroviral therapy.** *AIDS Behav* 2006, **10**:263–272.

9

Levels of circulating myeloid subpopulations and of heme oxygenase-1 do not predict CD4+ T cell recovery after the initiation of antiretroviral therapy for HIV disease

Lillian Seu[1,2], Gabriel M Ortiz[1,3], Trevor D Burt[4,5], Steven G Deeks[6], Jeffrey N Martin[6,7] and Joseph M McCune[1*]

Abstract

The level (or frequency) of circulating monocyte subpopulations such as classical ($CD14^{hi}CD16^{-}$) and non-classical ($CD14^{dim}CD16^{+}$) monocytes varies during the course of HIV disease progression and antiretroviral therapy (ART). We hypothesized that such variation and/or differences in the degree to which these cells expressed the immunoregulatory enzyme, heme oxygenase-1 (HO-1), would be associated with $CD4^{+}$ T cell recovery after the initiation of ART. This hypothesis was tested in a cross-sectional study of four groups of HIV-infected subjects, including those who were seronegative, untreated virologic controllers [detectable viral load (VL) of <1000 copies/mL], untreated virologic non-controllers [VL > 10,000 copies/mL], and ART-mediated virologic controllers [VL < 75 copies/mL]. A longitudinal analysis of ART-treated subjects was also performed along with regression analysis to determine which biomarkers were associated with and/or predictive of $CD4^{+}$ T cell recovery. Suppressive ART was associated with increased levels of classical monocyte subpopulations ($CD14^{hi}CD16^{-}$) and decreased levels of non-classical monocyte populations ($CD14^{dim}CD16^{+}$). Among peripheral blood mononuclear cells (PBMCs), HO-1 was found to be most highly up-regulated in $CD14^{+}$ monocytes after *ex vivo* stimulation. Neither the levels of monocyte subpopulations nor of HO-1 expression in $CD14^{+}$ monocytes were significantly associated with the degree of $CD4^{+}$ T cell recovery. Monocyte subpopulations and HO-1 gene expression were, however, restored to normal levels by suppressive ART. These results suggest that the level of circulating monocyte subpopulations and their expression of HO-1 have no evident relationship to $CD4^{+}$ T cell recovery after the initiation of ART.

Keywords: HIV, HO-1, Immune activation, Monocytes, $CD4^{+}$ T cell recovery

Background

Circulating myeloid cells are a heterogeneous population of monocytes and dendritic cells with diverse immunoregulatory capacities [1]. $CD14^{dim}CD16^{+}$ "non-classical" monocytes have gene expression profiles that are generally considered to be pro-inflammatory in nature and are found at higher frequencies in the blood of subjects with chronic inflammatory diseases such as HIV infection [2]. $CD14^{hi}CD16^{-}$ "classical" monocytes comprise the bulk of the circulating myeloid pool and are anti-inflammatory in function, as demonstrated by their low potential to migrate to inflammatory sites [3], their production of IL-10 after stimulation with lipopolysaccharide (LPS) [4], and their propensity to mature into tolerogenic antigen presenting cells (APCs) in the context of appropriate cytokine stimulation [5]. Consistent with their pro-inflammatory properties, non-classical $CD14^{dim}CD16^{+}$ monocytes are found at 2- to 8-fold higher levels in HIV-infected subjects compared to uninfected controls [6]. Additionally, untreated HIV-infected subjects with elevated frequencies of circulating $CD14^{hi}CD16^{+}$ "intermediate" monocytes have increased viral loads and decreased $CD4^{+}$ T cell counts which decline after virologically suppressive ART [7]. How these changes in monocyte subpopulations might impact SIV/HIV disease progression remains unclear.

* Correspondence: mike.mccune@ucsf.edu
[1]Division of Experimental Medicine, Department of Medicine, University of California, San Francisco, CA 94110, USA
Full list of author information is available at the end of the article

Heme oxygenase-1 (HO-1), the rate-limiting enzyme in the catabolism of heme, has potent immunoregulatory activity. HO-1 activity within myeloid cells is generally thought to be anti-inflammatory- resulting in decreased TNFα expression, increased IL-10 expression, and is associated with differentiation into tolerogenic APCs [8]. We have previously demonstrated that monocytes represent one of the most prevalent sources of HO-1, and HO-1 inhibitors cause monocyte-dependent T cell proliferation *in vitro* [9]. HO-1 levels are elevated in the peripheral blood cells of HIV-infected individuals [10], and functional HO-1 promoter polymorphisms correlate with circulating markers of inflammation in ART-treated subjects [11]. Given these data, we wondered whether increased levels of certain monocyte subpopulations and/or of their expression of HO-1 might be generally anti-inflammatory in nature and thereby facilitate the $CD4^+$ T cell response to suppressive ART. Altering the balance of the immune system towards a less activated state (e.g., by increasing the frequency of the anti-inflammatory classical monocytes) may prevent immunopathology associated with chronic HIV disease and, ultimately, improve HAART-mediated $CD4^+$ T cell recovery. In this study, we sought to determine if $CD4^+$ T cell recovery after the initiation of ART was predicted by the frequency of monocyte subpopulations and/or of HO-1 expression in $CD14^+$ monocytes.

Results

Antiretroviral therapy is associated with an increased frequency of classical monocytes

As shown in Figure 1A, three blood myeloid subpopulations were defined by expression of HLA-DR, CD14, CD16, and CD11c: $CD14^{hi}CD16^-$ classical monocytes, $CD14^{dim}CD16^+$ non-classical monocytes, and $CD11c^+$ myeloid dendritic cells (mDCs) (Figure 1A, and Additional file 1: Figure S1A) [12].

To determine the relative frequency of various myeloid subpopulations in the context of HIV disease, PBMCs from untreated viral controllers, untreated viremics, ART-suppressed subjects, and HIV-seronegative subjects (Table 1) were studied by flow cytometry. The highest circulating frequencies of classical monocytes were observed in HIV-seronegative subjects, a group known to have low levels of T cell activation, while the highest frequencies of pro-inflammatory non-classical monocytes were observed in untreated viremic subjects, a group known to have high levels of T cell activation (Figure 1B and Additional file 2: Figure S2) [13]. These results confirm and extend existing reports of altered monocyte populations during HIV disease progression [7,14].

To understand the cellular characteristics of circulating monocyte populations in more detail, we performed a comprehensive analysis of the geometric mean fluorescence intensities (gMFI) of various myeloid markers in these defined monocyte populations within patients on early ART n = 24 (Early ART suppressed, Table 2). The following markers were assessed: HLA-DR (a Class II major histocompatibility receptor [15]), CD11c (a type 1 transmembrane integrin), CD11b (a Mac-1 integrin forming the complement receptor 3), and CD33 (a myeloid-restricted transmembrane protein of the sialic acid binding Ig-like lectin family). (Additional file 3: Figure S3) The $CD14^{hi}$ classical monocytes had the highest levels of CD11b and CD33 expression ($P < 0.0001$) whereas the $CD14^{dim}CD16^+$ non-classical monocytes had the highest levels of CD11c expression ($P < 0.0001$). $CD11c^+$ mDCs that were $CD14^-CD16^-$ did not display high levels of CD11b, CD11c, or CD33 (Additional file 3: Figure S3). These findings indicate that classical and non-classical monocytes can be further characterized by cell surface expression levels of CD11c, CD11b, and CD33, molecules that have implications on trafficking through the circulation and in tissue sites of infection [16]. A recent study showed that other monocyte markers such as CD62L, CD115, neopterin, and soluble CD163 and CXCL10 are dynamically altered in HIV patients [17].

ART is known to result in both decreases in plasma virus as well as in T cell activation levels [13]. Based on our cross-sectional analysis (Figure 1B), classical monocytes were hypothesized to increase over time on ART. To directly test this hypothesis, myeloid cell subpopulations were analyzed longitudinally over time in the "pre-ART" subjects (described in Table 2). Pre-ART subjects (n = 12) were not on ART and had a median viral load of 33,123 copies/mL (IQR 19,383 - 100,092) and a median CD4 count of 173.5 cells/mm3 (149.3 - 251.8). After 2.5 years on suppressive therapy (IQR 1.7 – 3), viral loads were at levels below 75 copies/mL, the limit of viremia detection. During this time, classical monocyte frequencies increased from 54.1% (IQR 44.5-60.2%) to 69.2% (IQR 64.3 – 71.1%) ($P < 0.001$) whereas non-classical monocyte frequencies decreased from 16.0% (IQR 11.1- 20.3%) to 10.7% (IQR 8.1 – 12.9%) ($P = 0.01$) (Figure 1C). These results corroborate previous findings where non-classical monocyte populations appear to diminish after suppressive ART [7,18].

HO-1 is induced in $CD14^+$ monocytes by cobalt protoporphyrin IX (CoPP)

To determine which of the various myeloid subpopulations circulating in HIV-seropositive subjects might be the main producers of HO-1, stimulation experiments were carried out to detect intracellular HO-1 before and after *ex vivo* induction with Cobalt protoporphyrin IX (CoPP) [9]. At baseline prior to CoPP stimulation,

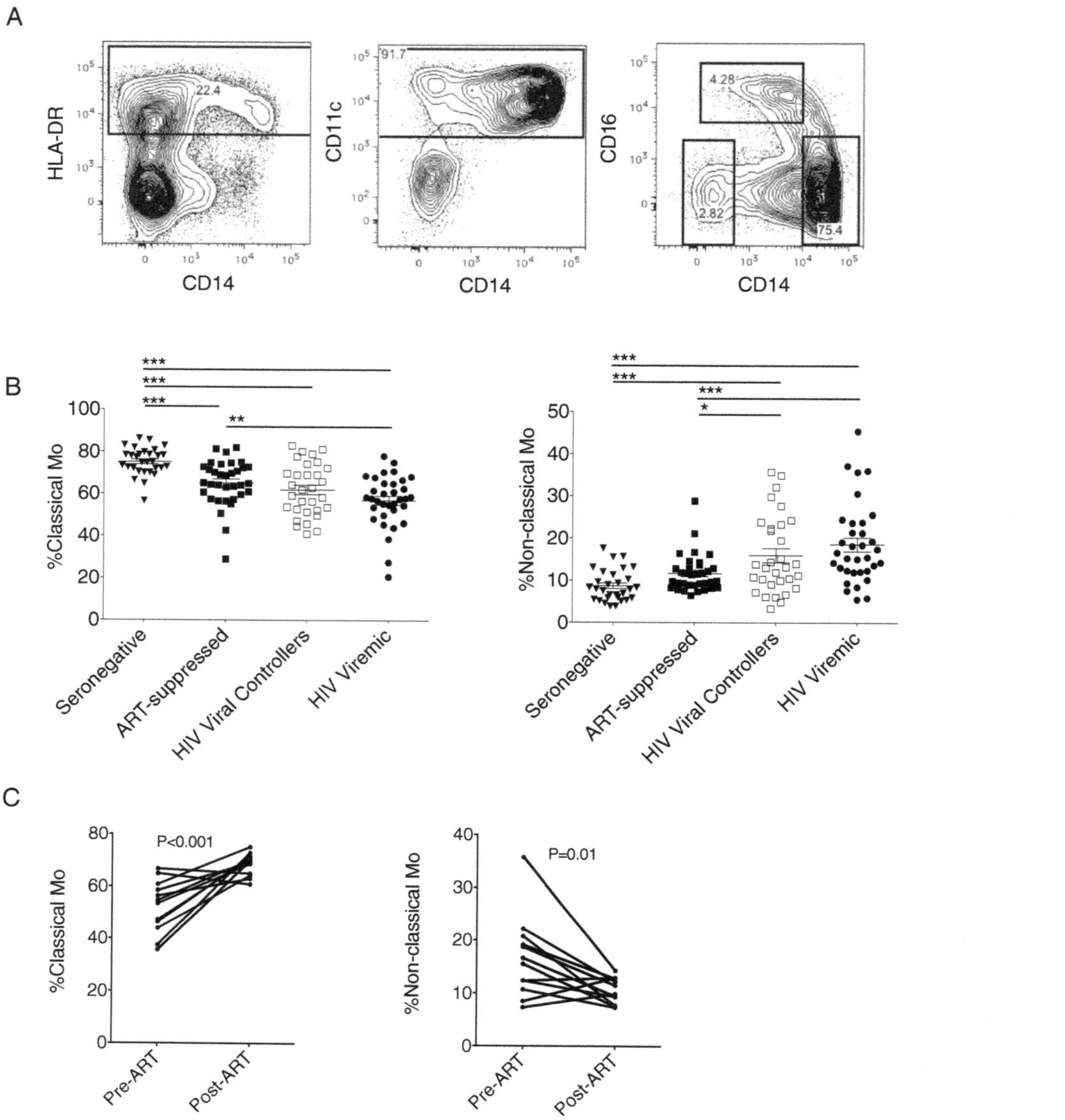

Figure 1 Prolonged ART results in an increased frequency of classical monocytes. (A) Thawed PBMCs from HIV patients were stained with antibodies recognizing cell-surface and intracellular myeloid markers. Analysis was performed by sequentially gating on live cells, singlets (FSC-A/ FSC-H), non-lymphocyte (SSC-A high/FSC-A high), lineage negative ($CD3^-$ $CD19^-$ $CD56^-$), and HLA-DR and CD11c positive populations. Myeloid cells were further defined by expression of CD14 and CD16 into three subsets ($CD14^{hi}CD16^-$, $CD14^{dim}CD16^+$, and $CD14^-CD16^-$ cells). Frequencies of $CD14^{hi}CD16^-$ classical monocytes (lower right gate), $CD14^{dim}CD16^+$ non-classical monocytes (upper left gate), and $CD11c^+$ $CD14^-CD16^-$ mDCs (lower left gate) and in relation to the parent myeloid gate were calculated. **(B)** Column statistics were performed by 1-way ANOVA on patients described in Table 1. Statistical significance is denoted as *$p < 0.05$, **$p < 0.01$, and ***$p < 0.001$. **(C)** Myeloid subpopulations were measured during pre-ART to post-ART time points from thawed PBMCs of ART-treated subjects (see "pre- ART-suppressed" subjects described in Table 2). Student's paired t-test was performed and corresponding p values are described.

HO-1 expression was higher in the $CD14^+$ monocyte subpopulation than in the $CD11c^+$ mDC population (Figure 2B).

Cell culture and stimulation resulted in classical and non-classical monocyte populations to combine into one subpopulation of $CD14^+$ monocytes with intermediate expression of CD14 and CD16 compared to baseline expression patterns (Figure 2A). Upon CoPP stimulation, the $CD14^+$ monocytes expressed higher HO-1 levels compared to their PBS (Figure 2C; $p < 0.0001$, 2-way ANOVA post-test). Consistent with prior findings [9,11], our observations suggest that $CD14^+$ monocytes are the most

Table 1 Clinical descriptions for cross-sectional HIV patients

Patients	N	VL (copies/mL)[#]	CD4 (cells/ul)[#]	Mean age[#]	Male%
HIV Viral Controllers[a]	31	75 (75–184.3)	710 (514–945.5)	45.5 (43–52.7)	64.5%
HIV Viremic[b]	34	89246 (45295.5–174381)	304 (202.2–451)	43 (39.2–47.7)	79.4%
ART-suppressed[c]	34	75 (50–75)	388.5 (313.5–500.2)	47 (41.7–50)	79.4%
Seronegative	30	NA	NA	42 (37.2–45.7)	100.0%

[a]HIV viral controllers were defined as untreated subjects with at least three plasma HIV VL < 1,000 copies/mL during a 12 month period.
[b]HIV viremics were defined as untreated individuals with VL > 10,000 copies/ml.
[c]ART-suppressed subjects had VL < 75 copies/mL for a period between 2–4 years after treatment initiation, with only one viral blip >1000 copies/mL permissible during the analysis time.
[#]Values are expressed as median ± interquartile range.

biologically relevant producers of HO-1 in the peripheral blood.

Antiretroviral therapy is associated with decreased PBMC levels of HO-1

Relative transcript levels of HO-1 were assessed from thawed PBMCs from untreated viral controllers, untreated viremic subjects, ART-treated subjects, and HIV-seronegative subjects (Table 1). There were no statistically significant differences in the levels of HO-1 transcript across all patient groups (Figure 3A).

We tested whether *HMOX1* transcript changed after the initiation of suppressive ART in patients that were followed longitudinally (Table 2). *HMOX1* relative gene expression levels decreased from 142.5 (98.0 - 182) to 78.8 (56.5 - 104.5) (P = 0.05) (Figure 3B).

Circulating monocyte frequencies and levels of HO-1 expression are not predictive of better $CD4^+$ T cell recovery in ART-treated subjects

$CD4^+$ T cell recovery was longitudinally assessed in early ART-suppressed cohort (n = 24, Table 2). All subjects achieved durable ART-mediated viral suppression by seven months of treatment. We hypothesized that subjects with higher pro-inflammatory non-classical $CD14^{dim}CD16^+$ monocyte frequencies may experience lower $CD4^+$ T cell gains during suppressive ART (Table 3). We performed regression analysis to determine if classical monocytes or non-classical monocytes measured at a time point early after ART initiation may be predictive of the subsequent rate of $CD4^+$ T cell count gain (cells/mm3/month). There was no strong evidence of a significant association between either the level of classical monocytes (Spearman's rho $\rho = -0.24$, P < ns) (Figure 4A) or of non-classical monocytes (Spearman's rho $\rho = -0.069$, P < ns) and $CD4^+$ T cell counts (cells/mm3) measured during early or late ART, nor with the subsequent rate of gain in $CD4^+$ T cell count (cells/mm3/month) (Figure 4B).

To perform more in-depth analysis of monocyte populations and their role in $CD4^+$ T cell recovery, we further analyzed HO-1 [9] and tested the possibility that its expression within $CD14^+$ monocytes might be high in HIV subjects with improved $CD4^+$ T cell recovery after ART in an analysis similar to a prior cohort study [19]. HO-1 expression in $CD14^+$ monocytes measured at the first

Table 2 Biomarkers in pre-ART suppressed subjects prior to and during suppressive ART[a]

	n = 12	Pre-ART timepoint [Median (IQR)]	Post-ART timepoint [Median (IQR)]	P value[a]
Gender		83.30%		/
Age	Years	46.5 (41.5–47)	49 (43.2–50)	/
Viral Load	copies/mL	33,123 (19,383–100,092)	75 (75–75)	0.03
$CD4^+$ T cells	Total (cells/uL)	173.5 (149.3–251.8)	435 (343.8–594.3)	0.0006
$CD8^+$ T cells	Total (cells/uL)	1320 (792–1630)	1561 (1105–2313)	ns
Activation (+%)	$CD4^+CD38^+HLADR^+$	13.0 (9.6–26.6)	3.6 (2.6–4.7)	0.0007
	$CD8^+CD38^+HLADR^+$	22.5 (13.9–24.1)	6.8 (5.2–10.2)	0.0007
$SSC^{++}Lin^-$ (+%)	Classical Monocytes ($HLADR^+CD11c^+CD14^{hi}CD16^-$)	54.1 (44.5–60.2)	69.2 (64.3–71.1)	0.0009
	Non-Classical Monocytes ($HLADR^+CD11c^+CD14^{dim}CD16^+$)	16.0 (11.1–20.3)	10.7 (8.1–12.9)	0.01
PBMC gene transcript expression	HO-1/HPRT	142.5 (98.0–182)	78.8 (56.5–104.5)	0.05

[a]Pre-ART suppressed subjects were un-treated subjects with un-suppressed viral load.

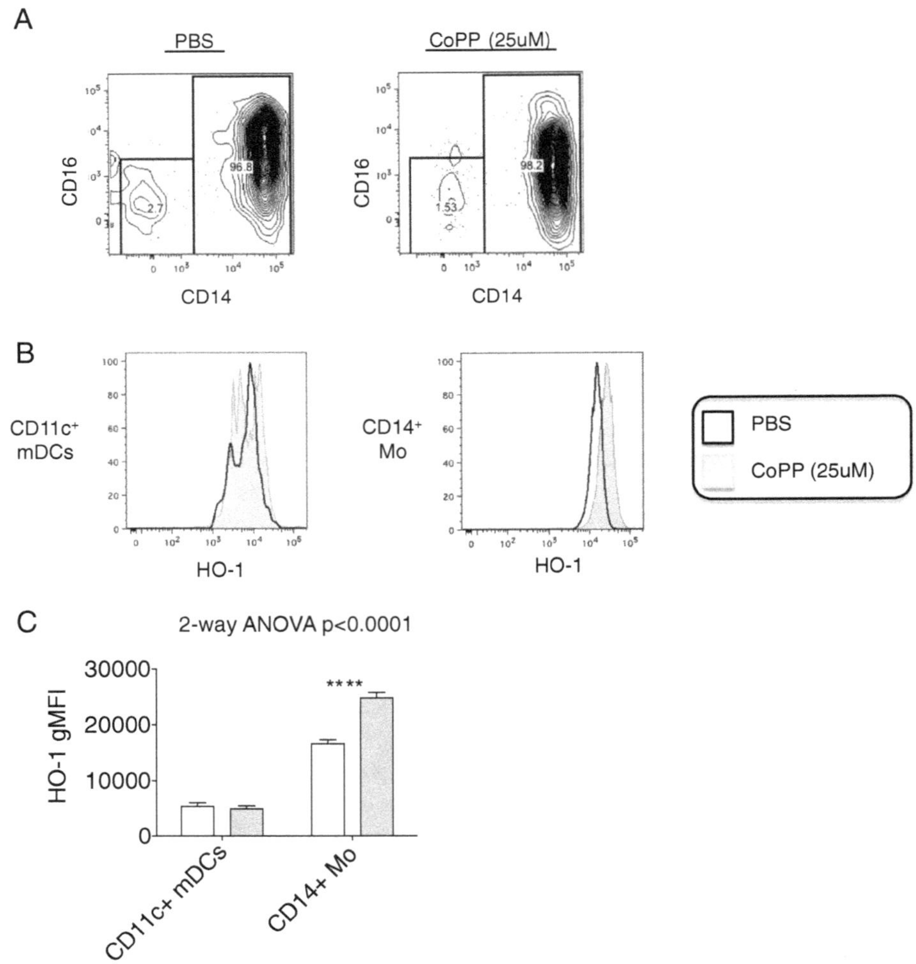

Figure 2 CD14⁺ monocytes are the main site of HO-1 induction after *ex vivo* CoPP stimulation. Thawed PBMC samples from Early ART Patients (Table 3) (n = 24) were analyzed for cell surface expression of monocyte markers. **(A)** Scatter plots showing the expression of CD14 and CD16 after monocyte cell culture in PBS (left) and stimulation with CoPP (right) on UpCell™ plates are depicted **(B)** Histograms representing the fluorescence intensities of HO-1, CD14, CD16, and CD11c in $CD14^+$ monocytes and in $CD11c^+$ mDCs after treatment with saline or CoPP are shown. Thawed PBMCs were cultured with saline or 25 μM CoPP for 48 hours on UpCell™ plates, harvested, and then stained with antibodies recognizing cell-surface and intracellular myeloid markers. Data from a representative subject are shown. **(C)** CoPP-induced changes in HO-1 among $CD14^+$ monocytes or $CD11c^+$ DCs. The ****symbol represents a $p < 0.0001$ for differences in culture conditions (saline vs. CoPP).

time point available after complete viral suppression (ART time point 1) was not significantly associated with more robust $CD4^+$ T cell recovery over the course of ART (Figure 4C).

In summary, these results demonstrate that neither circulating levels of monocyte populations nor high HO-1 expression in classical monocytes measured at a time point early after ART initiation predict greater $CD4^+$ T cell gains at later ART time points, despite being differentially altered during the course of untreated HIV disease.

Discussion

Immune activation is a cardinal feature of HIV disease and contributes to pathologic outcomes before and after the initiation of ART [20]. In each instance, it is not clear if immune activation is due directly to viral replication and/or to the host response to such replication. It is clear, however, that the higher the level of activation, the faster the course of disease progression in untreated subjects [13,20] and the lower the level of $CD4^+$ T cell recovery in those provided ART.

We demonstrate that suppressive ART restores homeostatic levels of monocyte population frequencies (Figure 1B, C). There may be multiple explanations for these findings. For example, diminished levels of $CD14^+$ myeloid cells could arise if CD14 cell surface receptors are actively shed after activation. The CD14 molecule serves as the bacterial lipopolysaccharide (LPS) receptor

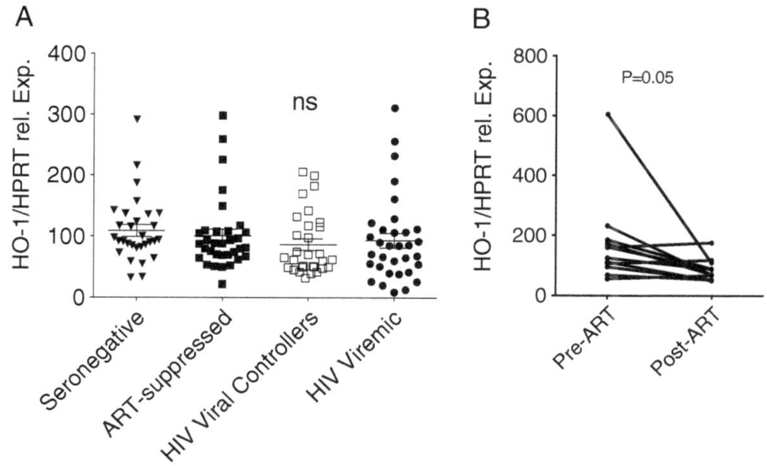

Figure 3 Antiretroviral therapy is associated with decreased PBMC mRNA levels of *HMOX1*. (A) Cross-sectional analysis of the relative transcript expression levels of *HMOX1/HPRT* in patients described in Table 1. Column statistics were performed by 1-way ANOVA. Statistical significance is denoted as *$p < 0.05$, **$p < 0.01$, and ***$p < 0.001$. **(B)** Longitudinal changes in relative transcript expression levels of HO-1/HPRT were measured during pre-ART to post-ART time points from thawed PBMCs of ART-treated subjects (see "pre-ART suppressed subjects" described in Table 2). Student's paired t-test was performed with p value = 0.05.

Table 3 Cellular expression levels (+ %) of immunological biomarkers in early- ART suppressed HIV-infected subjects[a]

	n = 24	ART time point 1	ART time point 2	P value[a]
Gender		58.30%		/
Age	Years	46 (42–48.7)	48 (44–50)	/
Length of time on ART	Months	6.4 (4.8–13.9)	29.3 (27.3–38.9)	/
Viral Load	copies/mL	75 (56.2–75)	75 (56.2 - 75)	ns
$CD4^+$ T cells	Total (cells/uL)	300.0 (222.5–360.7)	425 (328.25–513.5)	<0.0001
$CD8^+$ T cells	Total (cells/uL)	1085 (710–1396)	1114 (750.3–1593)	ns
$SSC^{++}Lin^-$ (+%)	$CD11c^+$ mDCs ($HLADR^+CD11c^+$)	3.9 (2.7–5.4)	2.8 (2.3–4.4)	ns
	Classical Monocytes ($HLADR^+CD11c^+CD14^{hi}CD16^-$)	70.3 (67.8–75.1)	78.8 (74.35–83.1)	0.004
	Non-Classical Monocytes ($HLADR^+CD11c^+CD14^{dim}CD16^+$)	3.0 (1.6–6.2)	3.8 (2.3–5.7)	ns
Classical Monocytes ($HLADR^+CD11c^+CD14^{hi}CD16^-$)	HLA-DR gMFI	14375(10569–16546)	12516 (10343–15220)	ns
	CD11b gMFI	31139 (26954–34508)	31096 (27432–34876)	ns
	CD11c gMFI	13514 (10406–14970)	12069 (10430–13956)	0.008
	CD33 gMFI	29624 (20462–36580)	29938 (19164–37687)	ns
Non-Classical Monocytes ($HLADR^+CD11c^+CD14^{dim}CD16^+$)	HLA-DR gMFI	12311 (10047–14272)	12993 (11328–14673)	ns
	CD11b gMFI	2123 (1726–3767)	2421 (1756–2957)	ns
	CD11c gMFI	21517 (17876–24957)	22780 (20620–24761)	ns
	CD33 gMFI	8678 (6510–11084)	8956 (6472–11433)	ns
$CD14^+$ monocytes	HO-1 gMFI	16290 (14784–18027)	15785 (13875–18535)	ns

[a]Early HAART-suppressed subjects had VL <100 copies/mL after initial viral suppression, with only one blip of >1000 copies/mL permissible during the time frame of analysis on HAART. Early HAART time point refers to a period between 2–10 months of treatment initiation, at a time when VL had achieved an undetectable level.

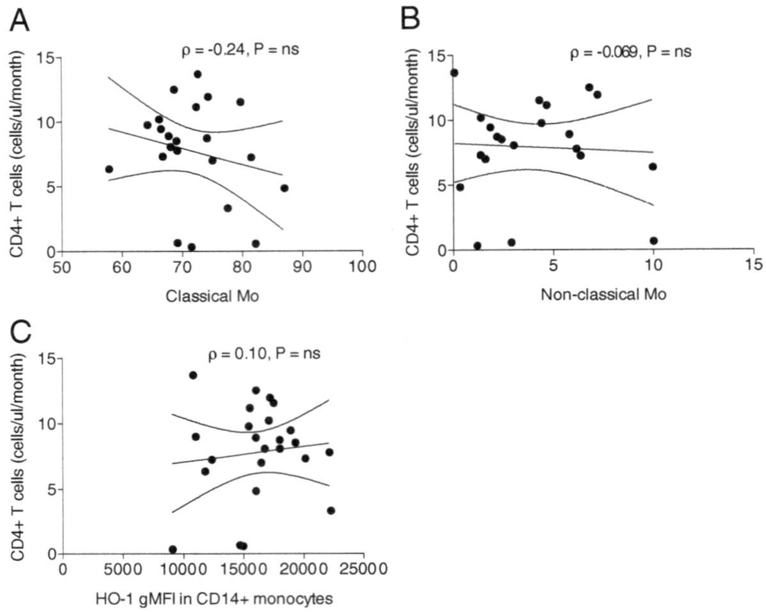

Figure 4 Circulating monocyte frequencies measured at time points early after ART initiation are not predictive of better subsequent CD4$^+$ T cell recovery in ART-treated subjects. Thawed PBMC samples from Early ART Patients (Table 2) were analyzed for cell surface expression of monocyte markers. Regression analysis of CD4$^+$ T cell recovery between time point 1 and time point 2 was performed using the Spearman rank correlation. Rho coefficient (ρ) reveals lack of association between CD4$^+$ T cell recovery and the following parameters measured at ART time point 1: **(A)** percentage of classical monocytes, **(B)** percentage of non-classical monocytes, and **(C)** HO-1 gMFI levels in CD14$^+$ monocytes.

that is cleaved when engaged by LPS, resulting in circulating soluble CD14. The increase in the frequency of classical monocytes observed after suppressive ART may reflect decreased plasma LPS, allowing persistent expression of CD14 on these cells [21]. Moreover, and as suggested by the current studies, expression of immunomodulatory enzymes such as HO-1 by classical monocytes may contribute to control of immune activation after ART-mediated viral suppression. Cellular phenotyping of monocytes was performed on cryopreserved samples, and previous studies have comparable results upon the freeze-thawing process of peripheral blood mononuclear cells [22,23].

We hypothesized that frequencies of circulating monocyte subpopulations may not only be differentially altered during the course of HIV disease [7] but may also predict the rate of CD4$^+$ T cell recovery in patients that are suppressed on ART. Our study was designed such that the first time point of analysis occurred after the early months of ART (when there is substantial patient-to-patient variation in the kinetics of suppression of viremia [24] and of T cell redistribution [25]) as well as after the virus load has been effectively suppressed (thereby avoiding the confounding effects of unsuppressed and variable viral loads that would have otherwise been a major driver of most if not all of the measured parameters [13]). In the cohort studied, however, circulating classical or non-classical monocyte percentages were not predictive of CD4$^+$ T cell recovery in early ART-suppressed patients (Figure 4A, B). However, the possibility of missing an association due to low statistical power could be related to the relatively small sample size and/or small effect size of CD4$^+$ T cells (cells/uL) gain per patient.

A similar study looking at a panel of candidate T cell biomarkers within the same patient cohort described in Table 2 (Early ART suppressed) [19] demonstrated that poor levels of CD4$^+$ T cell recovery are predicted by high levels of CD8$^+$ T cells with a senescent phenotype, i.e., increased cell surface expression of CD57 and/or decreased cell surface expression of CD27 and of CD28.

The altered monocyte populations observed during the context of HIV disease have further implications as they may constitute a viral reservoir. It appears that CD16-positive monocytes (5% of monocyte population [2]) are both more susceptible to infection and preferentially harbor the virus long-term [26] *in vitro.* We have also reported that immunoregulatory enzymes like HO-1 and indoleamine 2, 3-dioxygenase (IDO), may have beneficial effects in HIV-seropositive subjects [27]. While HO-1 expression in CD14$^+$ monocytes was not predictive of CD4$^+$ T cell recovery when measured at time points early after ART-mediated viral suppression, (Figure 4C) suppressive ART did restore homeostatic levels of *HMOX1* gene expression (Figure 3B). HO-1 is an important immune modulator, with effects that are anti-proliferative, anti-oxidant, anti-apoptotic, and cytoprotective. (Reviewed in [28]) HO-1 deficiency results in macrophages that produce greater amounts of TNFα, IFNα, IL-6, and IL-2 after LPS stimulation in mouse models [29]. Reciprocally, increased levels of HO-1 are associated with decreased levels of HIV replication in monocytes *in vitro* [8]. Therefore, PBMC HO-1 levels may be reflective of the overall immune activation state, resulting in parallel decreases in both parameters over time on ART.

Conclusions

We performed a comprehensive assessment of the relationship between circulating monocyte populations and HIV disease outcome among ART patients (as defined by CD4 reconstitution) in a cohort of well-characterized HIV- infected and -uninfected adults. We show that suppressive ART restores homeostatic levels of monocyte population frequencies as well as HO-1 gene expression levels. These results suggest that monocyte populations may be dysregulated during chronic untreated HIV disease, that suppressive ART restores their frequencies to normal levels, and that, at least at this level of discrimination, neither the levels of circulating monocyte populations, nor the levels of the immunoregulatory enzyme, HO-1, do not predict $CD4^+$ T cell recovery after the initiation of ART but rather parallel the overall immune activation levels. This homeostatic recovery of different monocyte populations upon successful ART may contribute to the extent of immunological restoration and overall disease management in chronic HIV patients.

Methods

Human subjects

Healthy, HIV-seronegative adults (n = 30) and HIV-seropositive subjects (n = 135) were recruited from the San Francisco-based UCSF SCOPE (Study of the Consequences of the Protease Inhibitor Era) cohort. All subjects provided written informed consent for all biologic specimens and clinical data used in this study, and research records were kept confidential meeting specifications for this project approved by the UCSF Committee on Human Research (IRB #10-01330, reference #046371). For cross-sectional studies, HIV-infected subjects were categorized into four groups: virologic controllers (VL < 1000 copies/mL) (n = 31), virologic non-controllers (VL > 10,000 copies/mL) (n = 34), and ART-mediated virologically suppressed subjects (n = 34) (Table 1). Pre-ART subjects (n = 12) were followed longitudinally at time points from a time prior to ART initiation as well as 2.5 years post-suppressive therapy (Table 2). "Early ART" subjects (n = 24), were followed at a time point from early ART (median 6.4 months, interquartile range [IQR] 4.8 – 13.9 months) as well as 1 – 2 years of follow-up (median 19.8 months, IQR 18.3 – 24.6 months) were used for analysis as described in Table 3.

Isolation of plasma and primary peripheral bloods cells

Peripheral blood was drawn into EDTA tubes and centrifuged, after which the plasma fraction was frozen at −80°C until use. Peripheral blood mononuclear cells (PBMCs) were isolated from peripheral blood drawn into sodium heparin tubes by density centrifugation using Histopaque®-1077 (Sigma Aldrich, Saint Louis, MO). PBMCs were washed with RPMI 1640 (Life Technologies, Rockville, MD) supplemented with 10% fetal bovine serum (FBS, Gemini Bio-Products, Woodland, CA), 1% penicillin/streptomycin (Mediatech, Washington, DC), and 2 mM L-glutamine (Mediatech) (hereafter referred to as R10 medium), frozen in small aliquots of FBS with 10% DMSO (Sigma), and stored in a liquid nitrogen cryofreezer until use.

PBMC preparation

Cryopreserved PBMCs were rapidly thawed and washed in R10 medium. Viable PBMCs that excluded trypan blue (Sigma) were counted by direct microscopic visualization using a hemacytometer, pelleted, and then re-suspended at an adequate cell number for subsequent experiments.

HO-1 induction experiments

Cobalt protoporphyrin IX (CoPP) was purchased as a powder from Frontier Scientific (Park City, Utah), dissolved in 0.1 mM NaOH (Sigma), and then titrated to a pH of 7.6. PBMCs were cultured on Upcell™ 96 F MicroWell plates (Nalge Nunc, Rochester, NY), either with saline or 25 μM CoPP in R10 at 37°C for 48 hours. After incubation, adherent cells were harvested by incubating the plates at 25°C for 20 minutes.

Flow cytometry antibody labeling

The monoclonal antibodies (mAbs) used in this study were purchased from Abcam (Cambridge, MA), BD Biosciences (Franklin Lakes, NJ), Beckman Coulter (Indianapolis, IN), BioLegend (San Diego, CA), eBiosciences (San Diego, CA), and Invitrogen (Carlsbad, CA), and are summarized in detail in Additional file 4: Table S1. Briefly, cells were washed in staining buffer containing PBS with 2% FBS and 20 mM EDTA (Sigma) before a 30 minute incubation at 4°C in the presence of a cocktail of mAbs as well as Amine-Aqua Dead Cell Stain (Invitrogen). Afterwards, cells were washed with staining buffer. Intracellular staining with the HO-1 antibody (Abcam) alongside a secondary antibody (Invitrogen) was performed for one hour at 4°C in cells that were fixed and permeabilized in BD Cytofix/Cytoperm, according to the manufacturer's protocol. All cells underwent a final wash prior to fixation in 1% paraformaldehyde (Sigma). Data were acquired on an LSR II flow cytometer (BD) and analyzed using FlowJo software (Treestar, Ashland, OR). Gates for flow cytometric analyses were based on "fluorescence-minus-one" control stains.

Quantitative PCR

For quantitative PCR analysis, PBMCs were harvested after culturing for 48 hours and RNA was isolated using TRIzol® Reagent (Invitrogen, Carlsbad, CA). Total cellular RNA (0.2 µg) was used for cDNA synthesis using Oligo-dT primers and Reverse Transcriptase from Omniscript (Qiagen). Relative expression levels of *HMOX1* mRNA were measured by quantitative RT-PCR using validated Taqman® Gene Expression assay mixes for human *HMOX1* (Hs00157965_m1) and human *HPRT* (Hs99999909_m1) according to the manufacturer's protocol (Applied Biosystems). An AB Step One Plus instrument was used for amplification and detection, and the 2-ΔΔCT calculation was used to measure *HMOX1* gene expression relative to *HPRT* [11].

Statistical analyses

Linear regressions, correlation analyses, ANOVAs, and paired T tests were made across biomarkers of interest using GraphPad Prism v5.0d (Graphpad Software, La Jolla, CA, USA). For flow cytometric expression levels, geometric mean fluorescence intensities (gMFI) were used. $CD4^+$ T cell immune reconstitution was measured by subtracting the value of each patient's $CD4^+$ T cell count (cells/uL) from the early (median 6.4 months) from the late (median 29.3 months) ART timepoint, then dividing by the total number of months spanning that time period.

Additional files

Additional file 1: Figure S1. Three blood myeloid subpopulations were defined by expression of HLA-DR, CD14, CD16, and CD11c: $CD14^{hi}$ $CD16^-$ classical monocytes, $CD14^{dim}CD16^+$ non-classical monocytes, and $CD11c^+$ myeloid dendritic cells (mDCs) (Flow plots from ART patients described in Table 3).

Additional file 2: Figure S2. Antiretroviral therapy is associated with decreased T cell activation. Column statistics were performed by 1-way ANOVA on the % expression of HLA-DR and CD38 on (A) $CD4^+$ T cells and (B) $CD8^+$ T cells.

Additional file 3: Figure S3. Monocyte populations are defined by distinct cell surface receptors. Thawed PBMC samples from Early ART Patients (ART time point 1 in Table 3) (n = 24) were analyzed for cell surface expression of monocyte markers. Plots depict staining intensity (geometric mean fluorescence intensity) of various myeloid markers (HO-1, HLA-DR, CD11b, CD11c, CD33, and CD124) in $CD14^{hi}CD16^-$, $CD14^{dim}CD16^+$, and $CD14^-CD16^-$ cells (column statistics performed by 1-way ANOVA, with asterisks representing the significance to the decimal place of the p value).

Additional file 4: Table S1. Antibodies used for flow cytometry staining.

Competing interests

The authors report no conflict of interest for this study.

Authors' contributions

LS and GMO carried out the immunological studies, acquired and performed the data analyses, and drafted the manuscript. TDB participated in the design of the immunological studies, and provided technical expertise. SGD performed the clinical design of the study. JNM performed the clinical statistical analyses. JMM conceived of the study, and participated in its design and coordination and drafted the manuscript. All authors read and approved the final manuscript.

Acknowledgements

L.S. was supported by a pre-doctoral dissertation California HIV Research Program grant (#D09-SF-313). G.M.O. was supported by NIH Training Grants T32 AI060530 and 2T32AI007641 as well as the Gates Foundation Award # OPP1024421 and the NIH Loan Repayment Program. T.D.B. was a fellow of the Pediatric Scientist Development Program (supported by the American Pediatric Society, the American Academy of Pediatrics, and the March of Dimes) and is supported by NIH/NICHD grant number 1K08HD067295 and the NIH Loan Repayment Program. J.M.M. was supported by NIH Awards U01 AI43641 and R37 AI40312, and is the recipient of the National Institutes of Health Director's Pioneer Award as part of the National Institutes of Health Roadmap for Medical Research (DPI OD00329). The SCOPE cohort was supported by the Centers for AIDS Research at UCSF (PO AI27763), CFAR Network of Integrated Systems (R24 AI067039), the UCSF CTSI (UL1 RR024131), NIAID (RO1 AI087145, K24AI069994, AI-76174, amfAR, and the Ragon Institute. This work was also supported by the AIDS Research Institute at UCSF and the Harvey V. Berneking Living Trust.

Author details

[1]Division of Experimental Medicine, Department of Medicine, University of California, San Francisco, CA 94110, USA. [2]Department of Bioengineering and Therapeutic Sciences, University of California, San Francisco, CA 94110, USA. [3]Division of Hospital Medicine, Department of Medicine, University of California, San Francisco, CA 94110, USA. [4]Division of Neonatology, Department of Pediatrics, University of California, San Francisco, CA 94110, USA. [5]Eli and Edythe Broad Center of Regeneration Medicine and Stem Cell Research, University of California, San Francisco, CA 94110, USA. [6]Positive Health Program, Department of Medicine, University of California, San Francisco, CA 94110, USA. [7]Department of Epidemiology and Biostatistics, University of California, San Francisco, CA 94110, USA.

References

1. Auffray C, Sieweke MH, Geissmann F: **Blood monocytes: development, heterogeneity, and relationship with dendritic cells.** *Annu Rev Immunol* 2009, **27:**669–692.
2. Ziegler-Heitbrock L: **The CD14+ CD16+ blood monocytes: their role in infection and inflammation.** *J Leukoc Biol* 2007, **81:**584–592.
3. Ancuta P, Moses A, Gabuzda D: **Transendothelial migration of CD16+ monocytes in response to fractalkine under constitutive and inflammatory conditions.** *Immunobiology* 2004, **209:**11–20.
4. Szaflarska A, Baj-Krzyworzeka M, Siedlar M, Weglarczyk K, Ruggiero I, Hajto B, Zembala M: **Antitumor response of CD14+/CD16+ monocyte subpopulation.** *Exp Hematol* 2004, **32:**748–755.
5. Smeekens SP, van de Veerdonk FL, Joosten LA, Jacobs L, Jansen T, Williams DL, van der Meer JW, Kullberg BJ, Netea MG: **The classical $CD14^{++}$ $CD16^-$ monocytes, but not the patrolling $CD14^+$ $CD16^+$ monocytes, promote Th17 responses to Candida albicans.** *Eur J Immunol* 2011, **41:**2915–2924.
6. Thieblemont N, Weiss L, Sadeghi HM, Estcourt C, Haeffner-Cavaillon N: **CD14lowCD16high: a cytokine-producing monocyte subset which expands during human immunodeficiency virus infection.** *Eur J Immunol* 1995, **25:**3418–3424.

7. Han J, Wang B, Han N, Zhao Y, Song C, Feng X, Mao Y, Zhang F, Zhao H, Zeng H: **CD14(high)CD16(+) rather than CD14(low)CD16(+) monocytes correlate with disease progression in chronic HIV-infected patients.** *J Acquir Immune Defic Syndr* 2009, **52:**553–559.
8. Chauveau C, Rémy S, Royer PJ, Hill M, Tanguy-Royer S, Hubert FX, Tesson L, Brion R, Beriou G, Gregoire M, Josien R, Cuturi MC, Anegon I: **Heme oxygenase-1 expression inhibits dendritic cell maturation and proinflammatory function but conserves IL-10 expression.** *Blood* 2005, **106:**1694–1702.
9. Burt TD, Seu L, Mold JE, Kappas A, McCune JM: **Naive human T cells are activated and proliferate in response to the heme oxygenase-1 inhibitor tin mesoporphyrin.** *J Immunol* 2010, **185:**5279–5288.
10. Levere RD, Staudinger R, Loewy G, Kappas A, Shibahara S, Abraham NG: **Elevated levels of heme oxygenase-1 activity and mRNA in peripheral blood adherent cells of acquired immunodeficiency syndrome patients.** *Am J Hematol* 1993, **43:**19–23.
11. Seu L, Burt TD, Witte JS, Martin JN, Deeks SG, McCune JM: **Variations in the heme oxygenase-1 microsatellite polymorphism are associated with plasma CD14 and viral load in HIV-infected African-Americans.** *Genes Immun* 2012, **13:**258–267.
12. Ziegler-Heitbrock L, Ancuta P, Crowe S, Dalod M, Grau V, Hart DN, Leenen PJ, Liu YJ, MacPherson G, Randolph GJ, Scherberich J, Schmitz J, Shortman K, Sozzani S, Strobl H, Zembala M, Austyn JM, Lutz MB: **Nomenclature of monocytes and dendritic cells in blood.** *Blood* 2010, **116:**e74–e80.
13. Deeks SG, Kitchen CM, Liu L, Guo H, Gascon R, Narváez AB, Hunt P, Martin JN, Kahn JO, Levy J, McGrath MS, Hecht FM: **Immune activation set point during early HIV infection predicts subsequent CD4+ T-cell changes independent of viral load.** *Blood* 2004, **104:**942–947.
14. Cassol E, Malfeld S, Mahasha P, van der Merwe S, Cassol S, Seebregts C, Alfano M, Poli G, Rossouw T: **Persistent microbial translocation and immune activation in HIV-1-infected South Africans receiving combination antiretroviral therapy.** *J Infect Dis* 2010, **202:**723–733.
15. Shao L, Sperber K: **Impaired regulation of HLA-DR expression in human immunodeficiency virus-infected monocytes.** *Clin Diagn Lab Immunol* 2002, **9:**739–746.
16. Brunialti MK, Martins PS, Barbosa de Carvalho H, Machado FR, Barbosa LM, Salomao R: **TLR2, TLR4, CD14, CD11B, and CD11C expressions on monocytes surface and cytokine production in patients with sepsis, severe sepsis, and septic shock.** *Shock* 2006, **25:**351–357.
17. Hearps AC, Maisa A, Cheng WJ, Angelovich TA, Lichtfuss GF, Palmer CS, Landay AL, Jaworowski A, Crowe SM: **HIV infection induces age-related changes to monocytes and innate immune activation in young men that persist despite combination antiretroviral therapy.** *AIDS* 2012, **26:**843–853.
18. Amirayan-Chevillard N, Tissot-Dupont H, Capo C, Brunet C, Dignat-George F, Obadia Y, Gallais H, Mege JL: **Impact of highly active anti-retroviral therapy (HAART) on cytokine production and monocyte subsets in HIV-infected patients.** *Clin Exp Immunol* 2000, **120:**107–112.
19. Seu L, Ortiz GM, Epling L, Sinclair E, Swainson LA, Bajpai UD, Huang Y, Deeks SG, Hunt PW, Martin JN, McCune JM: **Higher CD27(+)CD8(+) T Cells Percentages during Suppressive Antiretroviral Therapy Predict Greater Subsequent CD4(+) T Cell Recovery in Treated HIV Infection.** *PLoS One* 2013, **8:**e84091.
20. Hunt PW, Martin JN, Sinclair E, Bredt B, Hagos E, Lampiris H, Deeks SG: **T cell activation is associated with lower CD4+ T cell gains in human immunodeficiency virus-infected patients with sustained viral suppression during antiretroviral therapy.** *J Infect Dis* 2003, **187:**1534–1543.
21. Sandler NG, Wand H, Roque A, Law M, Nason MC, Nixon DE, Pedersen C, Ruxrungtham K, Lewin SR, Emery S, Neaton JD, Brenchley JM, Deeks SG, Sereti I, Douek DC, for the INSIGHT SMART Study Group: **Plasma Levels of Soluble CD14 Independently Predict Mortality in HIV Infection.** *J Infect Dis* 2011, **203:**780–790.
22. Appleby LJ, Nausch N, Midzi N, Mduluza T, Allen JE, Mutapi F: **Sources of heterogeneity in human monocyte subsets.** *Immunol Lett* 2013, **152:**32–41.
23. Berg KE, Ljungcrantz I, Andersson L, Bryngelsson C, Hedblad B, Fredrikson GN, Nilsson J, Björkbacka H: **Elevated CD14++CD16- monocytes predict cardiovascular events.** *Circ Cardiovasc Genet* 2012, **5:**122–131.
24. Maldarelli F, Palmer S, King MS, Wiegand A, Polis MA, Mican J, Kovacs JA, Davey RT, Rock-Kress D, Dewar R, Liu S, Metcalf JA, Rehm C, Brun SC, Hanna GJ, Kempf DJ, Coffin JM, Mellors JW: **ART suppresses plasma HIV-1 RNA to a stable set point predicted by pretherapy viremia.** *PLoS Pathog* 2007, **3:**e46.
25. Pakker NG, Notermans DW, De Boer RJ, Roos MT, De Wolf F, Hill A, Leonard JM, Danner SA, Miedema F, Schellekens PT: **Biphasic kinetics of peripheral blood T cells after triple combination therapy in HIV-1 infection: a composite of redistribution and proliferation.** *Nat Med* 1998, **4:**208–214.
26. Jaworowski A, Kamwendo DD, Ellery P, Sonza S, Mwapasa V, Tadesse E, Molyneux ME, Rogerson SJ, Meshnick SR, Crowe SM: **CD16+ monocyte subset preferentially harbors HIV-1 and is expanded in pregnant Malawian women with Plasmodium falciparum malaria and HIV-1 infection.** *J Infect Dis* 2007, **196:**38–42.
27. Favre D, Mold J, Hunt PW, Kanwar B, Loke P, Seu L, Barbour JD, Lowe MM, Jayawardene A, Aweeka F, Huang Y, Douek DC, Brenchley JM, Martin JN, Hecht FM, Deeks SG, McCune JM: **Tryptophan catabolism by indoleamine 2,3-dioxygenase 1 alters the balance of TH17 to regulatory T cells in HIV disease.** *Sci Transl Med* 2010, **2:**32–36.
28. Wagener FA, Volk HD, Willis D, Abraham NG, Soares MP, Adema GJ, Figdor CG: **Different faces of the heme-heme oxygenase system in inflammation.** *Pharmacol Rev* 2003, **55:**551–571.
29. Kapturczak MH, Wasserfall C, Brusko T, Campbell-Thompson M, Ellis TM, Atkinson MA, Agarwal A: **Heme oxygenase-1 modulates early inflammatory responses: evidence from the heme oxygenase-1-deficient mouse.** *Am J Pathol* 2004, **165:**1045–1053.

10

Virological failure of staggered and simultaneous treatment interruption in HIV patients who began Efavirenz-based regimens after allergic reactions to nevirapine

Krittaecho Siripassorn[1*], Weerawat Manosuthi[1], Aranya Pakdee[1], Sunanta Natprom[1], Anuttra Chaovavanich[1], Narongsak Hengphadpanadamrong[1], Khobchok Woratanarat[1], Aroon Lueangniyomkul[1], and Kiat Ruxrungtham[2] on behalf of the Bamrasnaradura study team

Abstract

Objective: The objective of this work was to study the virological outcomes associated with two different types of treatment interruption strategies in patients with allergic reactions to nevirapine (NVP). We compared the virological outcomes of (1) HIV-1-infected patients who discontinued an initial NVP-based regimen because of cutaneous allergic reactions to NVP; different types of interruption strategies were used, and second-line regimen was based on efavirenz (EFV); and (2) HIV-1-infected patients who began an EFV-based regimen as a first-line therapy (controls).

Methods: This retrospective cohort included patients who began an EFV-based regimen, between January 2002 and December 2008, as either an initial regimen or as a subsequent regimen after resolving a cutaneous allergic reaction against an initial NVP-based regimen. The study ended in March 2010. The primary outcome was virological failure, which was defined as either (a) two consecutive plasma HIV-1 RNA levels >400 copies/mL or (b) a plasma HIV-1 RNA level >1,000 copies/mL plus any genotypic resistance mutation.

Results: A total of 559 patients were stratified into three groups: (a) Simultaneous Interruption, in which the subjects simultaneously discontinued all the drugs in an NVP-based regimen following an allergic reaction (n=161); (b) Staggered Interruption, in which the subjects discontinued NVP treatment while continuing nucleoside reverse transcriptase inhibitor (NRTI) backbone therapy for a median of 7 days (n=82); and (c) Control, in which the subjects were naïve to antiretroviral therapy (n=316). The overall median follow-up time was 43 months. Incidence of virological failure in Simultaneous Interruption was 12.9 cases per 1,000 person-years, which trended toward being higher than the incidences in Staggered Interruption (5.4) and Control (6.6). However, differences were not statistically significant.

Conclusions: Among the patients who had an acute allergic reaction to first-line NVP-based therapy and later began an EFV-based regimen, virological outcomes resulting from a staggered interruption of treatment (with a continuation of NRTI backbone therapy for 7 days after discontinuing NVP) did not differ from those of the patients who began an EFV-based regimen as their initial therapy (Control). However, the virological failure of Simultaneous Interruption was possibly higher than those of Control and Staggered Interruption.

Keywords: Nevirapine hypersensitivity or allergy, Efavirenz, Simultaneous interruption, Staggered interruption, Thai

* Correspondence: Krittaecho@yahoo.com
[1]Department of Internal Medicine, Bamrasnaradura Infectious Diseases Institute, 126 Tiwanon Road, Nonthaburi 11000, Thailand
Full list of author information is available at the end of the article

Introduction

Non-nucleoside analog reverse transcriptase inhibitor (NNRTI)-based regimens are currently recommended as a first-line therapy for HIV-1-infected patients because of their virological potency, lower risk of drug interactions and lower cost, as well as the availability of fixed-dose combinations. Nevirapine (NVP) is a first-line NNRTI recommended for antiretroviral-naïve patients, according to the European AIDS Clinical Society (EACS) guidelines [1]. NVP is also an acceptable first-line NNRTI for HIV-1-infected patients, according to the current Department of Health and Human Services (DHHS) guidelines [2]. NVP retains its usefulness in antiretroviral-naïve patients due to its lack of teratogenic effects or central nervous system toxicity and a lower cost than efavirenz (EFV) (a preferred initial NNRTI drug). However, one drawback of NVP is its induction of allergic reactions in approximately 5-14% of users worldwide [3-6]. After discontinuing NVP because of this allergic reaction, these patients may begin using other NNRTIs, such as EFV or etravirine (ETR). Most of these patients continue to take EFV even after the allergic reaction to NVP is resolved because of the lower incidence of rash associated with EFV vs. NVP and the requirement of a single daily dose. A recurrent rash has been described in approximately 12.6% (95% confidence interval 2.7–22.4%) of HIV-1-infected patients who previously experienced an allergic reaction to NVP and then began using EFV [7].

The method of antiretroviral treatment interruption following an allergic reaction to an NNRTI-based regimen is a major consideration. The simultaneous discontinuation of all the drugs in a NNRTI-based regimen would result in a period of functional NNRTI monotherapy; NNRTIs exhibit a longer plasma half-life and a longer duration of detectable levels than nucleoside analog reverse transcriptase inhibitors (NRTIs) [8]. NNRTIs exhibit a low genetic barrier to resistance; a single point mutation may lead to high NVP or EFV resistance [9,10]. As of November 3, 2008, the DHHS guidelines [11] recommend that patients either first halt the use of NNRTIs and then continue using NRTIs for a period of time (i.e., staggered interruption) or switch from an NNRTI-based regimen to a protease inhibitor (PI)-based regimen before discontinuing antiretroviral drugs (ARV). The simultaneous interruption of all the drugs in an NNRTI-based regimen is not recommended because it might induce a resistance mutation. This guideline is based primarily on clinical studies on the prevention of mother-to-child transmission [12-14] and treatment interruption strategies [15].

HIV-1-infected patients with a history of allergic reactions to NVP who plan to begin an EFV-based regimen may later experience different effects from those associated with the prevention of mother-to-child transmission or with treatment interruption strategies. Thus, we conducted a retrospective cohort study to examine the effectiveness of different types of treatment interruption strategies in HIV-1-infected patients who halted an NVP-based regimen because of cutaneous allergic reactions to NVP and later began an EFV-based regimen.

Methods

Study population

This retrospective cohort study was performed at the Bamrasnaradura Infectious Diseases Institute, Ministry of Public Health, Nonthaburi, Thailand. The Simultaneous Interruption group consisted of HIV-1-infected patients who simultaneously discontinued the use of all the drugs in an NVP-based regimen after experiencing a cutaneous allergic reaction to the treatment. The Staggered Interruption group consisted of HIV-1-infected patients who first discontinued the use of NVP after experiencing a cutaneous allergic reaction to an NVP-based regimen but who continued with other NRTIs for several days. The Control group included patients who began an EFV-based regimen as first-line therapy and who were never exposed to NVP. The study end date was March 2010.

A total of 12,803 medical records of HIV-1-infected patients were retrieved from a medical database and reviewed (Figure 1). The inclusion criteria were as follows: (a) documented HIV-1 infection, (b) 18–70 years of age, (c) began an EFV-based regimen as the initial treatment or began an EFV-based regimen after the resolution of a cutaneous allergic reaction to the initial NVP-based regimen, and (d) began an EFV-based regimen between January 2002 and December 2008 at the Bamrasnaradura Infectious Diseases Institute. The exclusion criteria were as follows: (a) previously received a non-HAART regimen, such as a dual-NRTI regimen or a single-dose NVP with zidovudine monotherapy, and (b) a history of diseases or conditions that severely affect either kidney or liver function, such as decompensated liver cirrhosis or end-stage renal disease.

The study was approved by the Ethics Committee for Research in Human Subjects, Department of Disease Control, Ministry of Public Health, Thailand.

Data collection

Data were collected from the medical records of the eligible patients. These data included (a) demographic features, (b) any history of allergic reactions to NVP-based regimens or other drugs, (c) previous and current antiretroviral (ARV) regimens, (d) CD4 cell counts and plasma HIV-1 RNA levels, and (e) both laboratory and clinical adverse events.

Plasma HIV-1 RNA was initially measured using reverse transcriptase polymerase chain reaction (RT-PCR) with a COBAS AMPLICOR HIV-1 MONITOR test, version 1.5 (Roche Molecular Systems, Inc., Branchburg, NJ, USA),

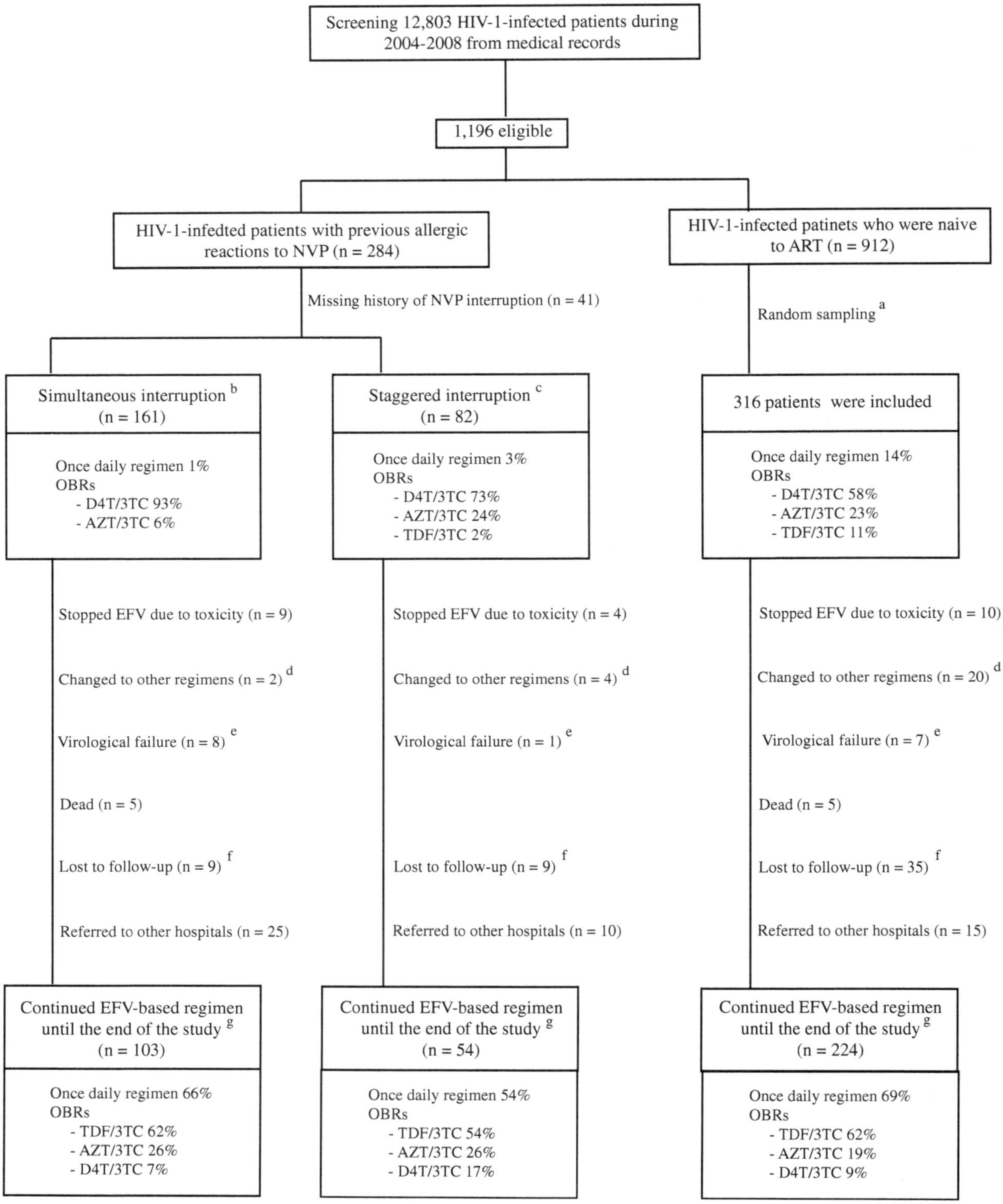

Figure 1 (See legend on next page.)

(See figure on previous page.)
Figure 1 Profile of the study cohort. ART = Antiretroviral therapy; AZT = Zidovudine; D4T = Stavudine; EFV = efavirenz; NVP = Nevirapine; OBRs = optimized background regimens; TDF = tenofovir; 3TC = lamivudine. [a]Random sampling was performed using random numbers. [b]HIV-1-infected patients who simultaneously discontinued all drugs in NVP-based regimens when they experienced allergic reactions to NVP-based regimens. [c]HIV-1-infected patients who discontinued NVP first but continued use of the other NRTIs for a few days when they experienced allergic reactions to NVP-based regimens. [d]This criterion included patients who changed EFV to other NNRTIs or PIs. It did not include patients who only changed or modify NRTIs. [e]Virological failure was defined as either (1) having two consecutive results of plasma HIV-1 RNA >400 copies/ml after 6 month of a EFV-based regimen or (2) having plasma HIV-1 RNA >1,000 copies/ml plus having any genotypic resistance mutation to efavirenz-based regimen. [f]It included either (1) patients who did not have clinical visits for more than 3 months from appointment date or (2) patients who stopped efavirenz-based regimen for more than 3 months. [g]The cohort ended on 31 March 2010.

which detects plasma HIV-1 RNA levels in the range of 50–100,000 copies/ml (ultrasensitive technique) or 400–1,000,000 copies/ml (standard technique). After June 2008, plasma HIV-1 RNA levels were evaluated using real-time PCR with a COBAS® AmpliPrep/COBAS® TaqMan® HIV-1 test (Roche Molecular Systems, Inc.), which can be used to measure plasma HIV-1 RNA levels in the range of 40–10,000,000 copies/ml.

Patients who did not appear for clinical visits for more than 3 months after a missed appointment or who discontinued an EFV-based regimen for more than 3 months were considered lost to follow-up. Patients who halted an EFV-based regimen for fewer than 3 months were classified as having an EFV-based regimen interruption.

We defined an adverse laboratory event as any laboratory result of at least a grade 3, according to the Division of AIDS Table for Grading the Severity of Adult and Pediatric Adverse Events (the DAIDS AE grading table). A clinical adverse event was defined as any clinical adverse event that resulted in the physician changing or modifying the antiretroviral regimen. A patient was allowed to continue participating in the study if the physician only changed or modified the NRTIs used. However, if the physician changed EFV to other NNRTIs or PIs, the patient was discontinued from the study cohort.

Between January 2010 and March 2010, there was a final evaluation of the HIV-1-infected patients who continued an EFV-based regimen through the end of study. The evaluation consisted of the following: (a) a plasma HIV-1 RNA assay, (b) a CD4 cell count, (c) a complete blood count, and (d) blood chemistry tests. Patients were informed about the evaluation if they (a) came to the hospital during this period, (b) were continuing an EFV-based regimen, and (c) did not have the results of any plasma HIV-1 RNA measurements obtained between October 1, 2009 and December 31, 2009. At the end of the study, 381 patients were still participating (Figure 1). Of these, 205 patients were eligible for the final evaluation because 176 patients had undergone plasma HIV-1 RNA assays between October 2009 and December 2009. There were 201 patients (98%) who completed the evaluation and provided written informed consent for the study. The remaining four patients attended the follow-up examination at the hospital, but we were unable to contact them concerning the evaluation and consent form.

Statistical analysis

The primary outcome was virological failure, which was defined as either (a) two consecutive plasma assay results indicating HIV-1 RNA levels >400 copies/mL after 6 months of an EFV-based regimen or (b) a single plasma HIV-1 RNA level >1,000 copies/mL in addition to any genotypic resistance mutation to an EFV-based regimen. These criteria included only virological results obtained after 6 months of an EFV-based regimen. Genotypic resistance mutations were included in the virological criteria to reduce the bias from viral blips and noncompliance.

The secondary outcomes were as follows: (a) the percentage of patients who exhibited virological suppression; (b) the CD4 cell counts; (c) the clinical outcomes of death, major opportunistic infection, immune recovery syndrome, and non-AIDS-associated disease; and (d) adverse laboratory and clinical events.

The relative risk and 95% confidence intervals were calculated to compare the differences in primary outcome among the groups. In addition, stratified analysis models were used to evaluate the effects of confounding factors on the primary outcome.

Virological suppression was defined as either (a) a plasma HIV-1 RNA level <50 copies/ml (based on RT-PCR using the COBAS Amplicor HIV-1 Monitor test, version 1.5) or (b) a plasma HIV-1 RNA level <40 copies/ml (based on real-time PCR using the COBAS® AmpliPrep/COBAS® TaqMan® HIV-1 test).

The baseline characteristics and outcomes were analyzed with (a) a chi-squared test for dichotomous data, (b) the Mann–Whitney test or the Kruskal-Wallis test for continuous data with a non-normal distribution, and (c) an unpaired t-test and a one-way ANOVA for continuous data with a normal distribution. All the reported p-values were two-sided and were considered statistically significant if $p<0.05$. The analyses were performed using SPSS version 14.

Results

Participants and baseline demographic features

Figure 1 presents the profile of the study cohort. There were 559 patients at the beginning of the study (January 2002) and 381 patients at the end of the study (March 2010).

Among the 139 patients who (a) were lost to follow-up (n = 53), (b) were referred to other hospitals (n = 50), (c) experienced a change in therapy from EFV to another ARV (n = 26), and (d) died (n = 10), 104 patients (74.8%) underwent plasma HIV-1 RNA assays within 6 months before they were removed from the cohort. Ninety-five of these patients (91.3%) demonstrated virological suppression.

There were 26 patients in the study (4.7%) whose therapy was changed from EFV to another ARV (another NNRTI or PI) (Figure 1). This group did not include patients who (a) received only changes or modifications to their NRTIs or (b) failed an EFV-based regimen or experienced EFV toxicity. The main reasons for substituting another therapy for EFV were financial issues (35%) and pregnancy (23%).

The baseline demographic features of the patients are summarized in Table 1. The patients in the Staggered Interruption group continued using other NRTIs after discontinuing NVP for a median (IQR) duration of 7 (6, 9) days. The NRTIs that were most commonly used in the Staggered Interruption group were stavudine/lamivudine (d4T/3TC, 73.3%) and zidovudine/lamivudine (AZT/3TC, 23.3%).

Main outcomes

Table 2 summarizes the outcomes of this cohort.

The overall median (IQR) duration of the follow-up period was 43 (22, 66) months. The Simultaneous Interruption group had a significantly longer follow-up period than the other two groups ($p<0.001$).

There were 27 patients who experienced EFV-based regimen interruptions during the study (Table 2). The Simultaneous Interruption group had more documented regimen interruptions than the other two groups ($p = 0.007$). The median (IQR) duration of the EFV-based regimen interruptions was 42 (12, 60) days. Common causes of the regimen interruptions included (a) financial issues (n =7), (b) toxicity (n = 7), and (c) poor compliance with the medication regimen (n = 7). There were 13 patients who discontinued all ARVs during regimen interruptions, whereas the remaining patients switched to other therapies, such as PI- or NVP-based regimens.

The incidence of virological failure was trended toward being higher in the Simultaneous Interruption group than in the other groups (Table 2), but this difference was not

Table 1 Baseline demographic and clinical characteristics of eligible HIV-1-infected patients

	Available data (n)	EFV-based regimens			*p* value[d]
		Simultaneous Interruption[a]	Staggered Interruption[b]	Controls[c]	
Total number, n	559	161	82	316	
Mean age, years (SD)	559	41.8 (8.3)	39.4 (9.4)	43.0 (8.4)	0.003
Female, %	559	39.1	59.8	33.9	<0.001
Mean body weight, kilograms (SD)	556	54.9 (9.2)	54.8 (9.8)	56.9 (12.4)	0.091
History of previous major opportunistic infections, %	556	40.6	35.4	51.9	0.007
History of previous allergic reactions to other drugs (exclude NVP), %	555	32.7	30.9	11.4	<0.001
Median duration of previous NVP-based regimens, days (IQR)	234	14 (11,27)	14 (12, 30)		0.574
Median baseline of CD4 cell count, cells/uL (IQR) [e]	543	69 (24, 140)	90 (26, 167)	47 (13, 132)	0.006
Baseline plasma HIV-1 RNA >100,000 copies/ml, % [e]	258	69.6	77.4	76.0	0.595
Baseline EFV-based regimens					
-Once-daily regimen,%	556	0.6	2.5	13.7	<0.001
-OBRs	559				
D4T/3TC, %		93	73	58	
AZT/3TC, %		6	24	23	
TDF/3TC, %			2	11	

Note: AZT = Zidovudine; D4T = Stavudine; EFV = Efavirenz; IQR = Interquartile range; NVP = Nevirapine; OBRs = Optimized background regimens; SD = Standard deviation; TDF = Tenofovir; 3TC = Lamivudine.

[a]HIV-1-infected patients who simultaneously discontinued all drugs in NVP-based regimens when they experienced allergic reactions to NVP-based regimens.

[b]HIV-1-infected patients who discontinued NVP first but continued use of the other NRTIs for a few days when they experienced allergic reactions to NVP-based regimens.

[c]HIV-1-infected patients who were naïve to antiretroviral therapy and were never exposed to NVP before beginning EFV-based regimens.

[d]*p*-value represents the difference between the three groups (Simultaneous interruption, Staggered interruption, and Control).

[e]These results would be included if they were examined within 6 months before starting EFV-based regimens.

Table 2 Results of treatment outcomes with EFV-based regimens in eligible HIV-1-infected patients (n = 559)

	Available data (n)	EFV-based regimens			
		Simultaneous Interruption[a]	Staggered Interruption[b]	Controls[c]	*p* value[d]
Total number, n	559	161	82	316	
Median duration of EFV-based regimens, months (IQR)	559	57 (27–73)	31 (18–52)	40 (23–65)	<0.001
Once-daily regimen at end of study, %	378	66.0	53.7	69.2	0.097
Documented EFV-based regimen interruption, % [e]	559	9.3	3.7	2.8	0.007
Frequency of plasma HIV-RNA assays	559				
> 2 times/year, %		14.9	32.9	22.2	0.030
1–2 times/year, %		57.1	48.8	60.4	
< 1 time/year, %		28.0	18.3	17.4	
Primary outcome					
Incidence of virological failure, cases per 1,000 person-years	559	12.9	5.4	6.6	
Relative risk of having virological failure when compared to Control group, (95% CI)	559	1.97 (0.62–6.38)	0.83 (0.02–6.43)		
Secondary outcomes					
Virological suppression[g] at 24 (±3) months, % (Per-protocol-analysis)	440	66.9	76.9	68.9	0.411
Median CD4 cell counts at 24 (±3) months, cells/μL (IQR)	327	352 (258–524)	387 (309–458)	340 (237–473)	0.483
Median increase from baseline in CD4 cell counts at 24 (±3) months, cells/μL (IQR)	317	264 (184–374)	292 (220–384)	273 (178–383)	0.647
Major opportunistic infections, %	556	6.83	4.88	5.75	0.812
Paradoxical immune recovery syndrome, %	541	4.55	2.60	2.90	0.603
Malignancy, %	559	1.24	0.00	1.27	0.736
Non-AIDS defining conditions [h], %	559	0.62	0.00	0.32	1.000
Death, %	559	3.10	0.00	1.58	0.206

Note: AZT = Zidovudine; CI = Confidence interval; D4T = Stavudine; EFV = Efavirenz; IQR = Interquartile range; NVP = Nevirapine; OBRs = Optimized background regimens; SD = Standard deviation; TDF = Tenofovir; 3TC = Lamivudine.

[a]HIV-1-infected patients who simultaneously discontinued all drugs in NVP-based regimens when they experienced allergic reactions to NVP-based regimens.

[b]HIV-1-infected patients who discontinued NVP first but continued use of the other NRTIs for a few days when they experienced allergic reactions to NVP-based regimens.

[c]HIV-1-infected patients who were naïve to antiretroviral therapy and were never exposed to NVP before beginning EFV-based regimens.

[d]*p*-value represents the difference between the three groups (Simultaneous interruption, Staggered interruption, and Control).

[e]Patients who halted EFV-based regimens for fewer than 3 months were classified as having an EFV-based regimen interruption and remained in the study.

[f]Virological failure was defined as either (1) having two consecutive results of plasma HIV-1 RNA >400 copies/ml after 6 month of a EFV-based regimen or (2) having plasma HIV-1 RNA >1,000 copies/ml plus having any genotypic resistance mutation to EFV-based regimen.

[g]Virological suppression was defined as having plasma HIV-1 RNA either: (1) having plasma HIV-1 RNA <50 copies/ml (based on RT-PCR using the COBAS Amplicor HIV-1 Monitor Test Ver 1.5, Roche Molecular Systems Inc., Branchburg, NJ, USA),or (2) having plasma HIV-1 RNA <40 copies/ml (based on RT-PCR using the COBAS® AmpliPrep/COBAS® TaqMan® HIV-1 test, Roche Molecular Systems Inc., Branchburg, NJ, USA).

[h]Non-AIDS defining conditions included major cardiovascular, renal and hepatic disease outcomes as defined by the Strategies for Management of Antiretroviral Therapy (SMART) Study Group [16].

statistically significant. The relative risk of virological failure between the Simultaneous Interruption and Control groups was 1.97 (0.62-6.38), p = 0.100. The relative risk between the Simultaneous Interruption and Staggered Interruption groups was 2.38 (0.32–105.75), p = 0.224. The Staggered Interruption group displayed virological outcomes comparable to those of the Control group.

There were imbalances in the three groups' baseline characteristics, such as age, sex, previous history of major opportunistic infections, baseline CD4 cell count, frequency of ARV administration, and history of EFV-based regimen interruptions (Table 1 and Table 2). A stratified analysis was performed to adjust for the effects of these factors on the primary outcome (virological failure). There were no significant differences between the adjusted relative risk ratios and the crude relative risk ratios.

Overall, 12 of the 16 subjects (75%) who experienced virological failure underwent genotypic resistance assays prior to changing to other regimens (Simultaneous Interruption n =6, Staggered Interruption n = 1, and Control n = 5). The mutations detected in these 12 subjects included TAMs (n = 4), M184V mutations (n = 6), and NNRTI-resistance mutations (n = 10). The incidence of NNRTI-resistance mutations in the Simultaneous Interruption group was 8.1 cases/1,000 person-years, which trended toward being higher than the incidences in the

Staggered Interruption (5.4 cases/1000 person-years) and Control (3.74 cases/1000 person-years) groups. However, these differences were not statistically significant. The Y181C and G190A NNRTI-resistance mutations, which are frequently related to the selective effect of NVP [17,18], were identified in only one subject in each of the Staggered Interruption and Simultaneous Interruption groups.

At 24 months after EFV-based regimens, there were 440 patients in the cohort. Virological suppression at 24 (±3) months after receiving EFV-based regimens (per-protocol analysis) was not significantly different among the three groups (p = 0.411) (Table 2). However, there were only 314 patients (71%) who had virological results during this period, and patients who did not have virological results were counted as non-suppressed when we analyzed for virological suppression.

Adverse events of EFV-based regimens

Table 3 presents the adverse events associated with EFV-based regimens among the study cohort. There were 23 patients (4.1%) who were unable to tolerate EFV (Figure 1), mainly due to either (a) EFV-induced central nervous system toxicity (n = 10) or (b) EFV-induced allergic reactions (n = 8).

Discussion

The current guidelines [2,19] recommend the use of a staggered interruption strategy in patients who must interrupt an NNRTI-based regimen. The duration of the use of NRTIs after the discontinuation of the NNRTI regimen ranged from 1 to 3 weeks [2,8,19]. However, the optimal duration has not been determined.

In this study, the patients in the Staggered Interruption group, who continued the use of 2 NRTIs for a median of 7 days after discontinuing NVP, had virological outcomes comparable to those of the Control group (Figure 1 and Table 2). These results are in accordance with a post-study analysis of the Strategies for Management of Antiretroviral Therapy (SMART) trial by Fox et al. [15]. Consequently, it should be appropriate to use a staggered interruption strategy if the NRTIs are to be continued for 7 days.

Among the HIV-infected patients who received an NVP-based regimen for at least 2 weeks, the duration of detectable NVP levels after discontinuation varied from 7 to 21 days [20,21]. Thus, patients who experience acute

Table 3 Adverse events of EFV-based regimens in eligible HIV-1-infected patients (n = 559)

	EFV-based regimens			
	Simultaneous Interruption[a]	Staggered Interruption[b]	Controls[c]	p value[d]
Total number, n	161	82	316	
Significant clinical adverse events[e]				
Lipoatrophy/Lipodystrophy, %	47.2	26.8	31.0	0.001
Mitochondrial toxicity[f], %	2.5	6.1	0.3	0.001
Severe anemia, %	3.1	2.4	2.9	0.957
Renal toxicity, n (%)	1 (0.6%)	0	0	0.435
CNS toxicity, n (%)	4 (2.5%)	2 (2.4%)	5 (1.6%)	0.6293
Allergic reactions to EFV, n (%)	3 (1.9%)	1 (1.2%)	4 (1.3%)	0.816
Allergic reactions to NRTIs, n (%)	1 (0.6%)	1 (1.2%)	5 (1.6%)	0.672
≥ Grade 3 laboratory adverse events[g]				
Diabetes Mellitus[h], %	3.7	2.4	5.7	0.369
Hypertriglyceride[i], %	5.6	2.4	2.9	0.261
Hypercholesterolemia[j], %	8.1	2.4	4.1	0.088
Transaminitis[k], %	4.4	0.0	1.0	0.027

Note: CNS = Central nervous system; EFV = Efavirenz; NRTI = Nucleoside analogue reverse transcriptase inhibitor.
[a]HIV-1-infected patients who simultaneously discontinued all drugs in NVP-based regimens when they experienced allergic reactions to NVP-based regimens.
[b]HIV-1-infected patients who discontinued NVP first but continued use of the other NRTIs for a few days when they experienced allergic reactions to NVP-based regimens.
[c]HIV-1-infected patients who were naïve to antiretroviral therapy and were never exposed to NVP before beginning EFV-based regimens.
[d]p-value represents the difference between the three groups (Simultaneous interruption, Staggered interruption, and Control).
[e] Significant clinical adverse events was defined as clinical events that caused doctors to change or modify antiretroviral therapy.
[f]Mitochondrial toxicity was diagnosed if a patient had both (1) serum lactate ≥ 2 mmol/L, and (2) symptoms caused by NRTI toxicity such as lipoatrophy, peripheral neuropathy, and lactic acidosis.
[g]These events were diagnosed based on the Division of AIDS Table for Grading the Severity of Adult and Pediatric Adverse Events ("DAIDS AE grading table").
[h]Diabetes mellitus defined as a new onset with medication initiation is indicated OR uncontrolled DM despite medication modification.
[i]Triglyceride >750 mg/dL.
[j]Cholesterol >300 mg/dL.
[k]either AST or ALT ≥ 185 u/L.

allergic reactions to an NVP-based regimen may acquire NNRTI-resistant mutations if they simultaneously stop all the drugs in the NVP-based regimen. A simultaneous interruption strategy for discontinuing NNRTI-based regimens is not recommended in the current DHHS guidelines [2]. In this study, there was a higher incidence of virological failure and genotypic resistance mutations to NNRTI in the Simultaneous Interruption group than in the other groups. Thus, a simultaneous interruption strategy is not advisable.

The median follow-up time duration of the Simultaneous Interruption group was significantly longer than those of the other groups ($p<0.001$) (Table 1). This result may have been influenced by a general recommendation in the DHHS guidelines (the November 3, 2008 version) [11] that a staggered interruption strategy should be employed to prevent NNRTI resistance after discontinuing NNRTI-based regimens. In this study, there were 141 (88%) patients in the Simultaneous Interruption group who began an EFV-based regimen prior to November 3, 2008.

The current guidelines recommend that patient plasma HIV-1 RNA levels and CD4 cell counts be monitored regularly, at least twice per year [1,2,22]. Nevertheless, the plasma HIV-1 RNA levels of 21% of the cohort were assayed less than once per year. Thus, the final evaluation was designed to assess the laboratory data of the patients who remained in the cohort through the end of study. The evaluation may have produced a more accurate diagnosis of laboratory-related events and data, such as virological outcomes and laboratory adverse events.

In the beginning of the study, d4T/3TC was commonly administered to our patients (Figure 1) because TDF was not available in our hospital until January 2007.

The low incidence of virological failure may have resulted from the removal from the cohort of patients who were lost to follow-up (e.g., either a documented discontinuation of an EFV-based regimen for more than 3 months or a failure to attend a follow-up examination at the hospital for longer than 3 months after the original appointment date). These patients generally exhibited low compliance with ARV therapy, which is associated with virological failure [23,24].

This study had the following limitations: (a) a retrospective design; (b) a non-randomized design; (c) some incomplete data (including CD4 cell counts, plasma HIV-1 RNA levels, and the results of genotypic resistance assays); (d) a follow-up loss of 9.5%; and (e) the frequent use, in the beginning of the study, of NRTI drugs such as d4T/3TC that are not preferred NRTIs under the current guidelines (1, 2, 22). These limitations should be carefully considered when interpreting the data from this study.

Conclusion

In our cohort of patients who experienced acute allergic reactions to first-line NVP-based therapy and later began an EFV-based regimen, the virological outcomes of the Staggered Interruption group (who continued 2 NRTIs for 7 days after discontinuing NVP) did not differ from those of the Control group (who began an EFV-based regimen as their initial treatment). However, the virological failure in the Simultaneous Interruption group was possibly higher than that in the Staggered Interruption and Control groups.

Abbreviations

ABC: Abacavir; ARV: Antiretroviral; AZT: Zidovudine; DHHS: Department of Health and Human Services; D4T: Stavudine; EACS: European AIDS clinical society; EFV: Efavirenz; ETR: Etravirine; NNRTI: Non-nucleoside analogue reverse transcriptase inhibitor; NRTIs: Nucleoside analogue reverse transcriptase inhibitors; NVP: Nevirapine; PI: Protease inhibitor; SMART: Strategies for management of antiretroviral therapy; TDF: Tenofovir; 3TC: Lamivudine.

Competing interests

Krittaecho Siripassorn received research and/or honoraria/travel grants from Merck, Sharp and Dohme and Bristol-Myers Squibb in the past five years. KiatRuxrungtham received consultancy fees and/or honoraria and travel and/or research grants from Tibotec, F Hoffmann-La Roche, Merck, Sharp and Dohme, Bristol-Myers Squibb, Gilead, Abbott, and Glaxo SmithKline.

Authors' contributions

KR and WM prepared drafts of the report and reviewed and edited the final manuscript. AP and SN screened medical records and contributed important information to the methods section. AC, NH, KW, and AL reviewed medical records and provided information to validate the use of the chosen analytical methods. All authors read and approved the final manuscript.

Acknowledgements

The authors wish to thank the following for their assistance in completing this study: Clinical Research Collaboration Network (CRCN), Thailand and SuthatChottanapund, M.D. (Doctor of Philosophy in Tropical Medicine, Epidemiology Track) contributed to the research methodology, data management and statistical analysis. The Bamrasnaradura study team provided medical records data and included BoonchaiKowadisaiburana, M.D., NatpatuSanguanwongse, M.D., PatamaSutha, M.D., RungrojMahachaiagree, M. D., SomsitTansuphaswadikul, M.D., WannaratAmornnimit, M.D., WisitPrasithsirikul, M.D., and WirojMankhatitham, M.D. The authors thank Elliot Churchill (MS, MA, AMWA Certification) for her assistance in reviewing and making suggestions for improvement of this manuscript.
The study was supported by a grant from The Department of Disease Control, Ministry of Public Health, Thailand.

Author details

[1]Department of Internal Medicine, Bamrasnaradura Infectious Diseases Institute, 126 Tiwanon Road, Nonthaburi 11000, Thailand. [2]Department of Medicine, Faculty of Medicine, Division of Allergy and Clinical Immunology, Chulalongkorn University, Bangkok, Thailand.

References

1. Panel on The European AIDS Clinical Society (EACS): *European guidelines for treatment of HIV infected adults in Europe [version 6.1, November 2012]*. http://www.europeanaidsclinicalsociety.org/images/stories/EACS-Pdf/EacsGuidelines-v6.1-2edition.pdf. Accessed [Jan 25, 2013].
2. Panel on Antiretroviral Guidelines for Adults and Adolescents: *Guidelines for the use of antiretroviral agents in HIV-1-infected adults and adolescents*: Department of Health and Human Services; 2012. Available at http://www.

aidsinfo.nih.gov/contentfiles/lvguidelines/adultandadolescentgl.pdf. Accessed [December 5, 2011].
3. van Griensven J, Zachariah R, Rasschaert F, Mugabo J, Atte EF, Reid T: **Stavudine- and nevirapine-related drug toxicity while on generic fixed-dose antiretroviral treatment: incidence, timing and risk factors in a three-year cohort in kigali, rwanda.** *Trans R Soc Trop Med Hyg* 2010, **104:**148–153.
4. Manosuthi W, Sungkanuparph S, Tansuphaswadikul S, Inthong Y, Prasithsirikul W, Chottanapund S, Mankatitham W, Chimsuntorn S, Sittibusaya C, Moolasart V, *et al*: **Incidence and risk factors of nevirapine-associated skin rashes among HIV-infected patients with CD4 cell counts <250 cells/microL.** *Int J STD AIDS* 2007, **18:**782–786.
5. Antinori A, Baldini F, Girardi E, Cingolani A, Zaccarelli M, Di Giambenedetto S, Barracchini A, De Longis P, Murri R, Tozzi V, *et al:* **Female sex and the use of anti-allergic agents increase the risk of developing cutaneous rash associated with nevirapine therapy.** *AIDS* 2001, **15:**1579–1581.
6. Yozviak JL, Doerfler RE, Woodward WC: **Effectiveness and tolerability of nevirapine, stavudine, and lamivudine in clinical practice.** *HIV Clin Trials* 2001, **2:**474–476.
7. Mehta U, Maartens G: **Is it safe to switch between efavirenz and nevirapine in the event of toxicity?** *Lancet Infect Dis* 2007, **7:**733–738.
8. Taylor S, Boffito M, Khoo S, Smit E, Back D: **Stopping antiretroviral therapy.** *AIDS* 2007, **21:**1673–1682.
9. Johnson VA, Brun-Vezinet F, Clotet B, Gunthard HF, Kuritzkes DR, Pillay D, Schapiro JM, Richman DD: **Update of the drug resistance mutations in HIV-1: December 2009.** *Top HIV Med* 2009, **17:**138–145.
10. Antinori A, Zaccarelli M, Cingolani A, Forbici F, Rizzo MG, Trotta MP, Di Giambenedetto S, Narciso P, Ammassari A, Girardi E, *et al*: **Cross-resistance among nonnucleoside reverse transcriptase inhibitors limits recycling efavirenz after nevirapine failure.** *AIDS Res Hum Retroviruses* 2002, **18:**835–838.
11. Panel on Antiretroviral Guidelines for Adults and Adolescents: *Guidelines for the use of antiretroviral agents in HIV-1-infected adults and adolescents*: Department of Health and Human Services; 2008:1–139. Available at http://www.aidsinfo.nih.gov/ContentFiles/AdultandAdolescentGL.pdf. Accessed January 15, 2009.
12. Arrive E, Newell ML, Ekouevi DK, Chaix ML, Thiebaut R, Masquelier B, Leroy V, Perre PV, Rouzioux C, Dabis F: **Prevalence of resistance to nevirapine in mothers and children after single-dose exposure to prevent vertical transmission of HIV-1: a meta-analysis.** *Int J Epidemiol* 2007, **36:**1009–1021.
13. McIntyre JA, Hopley M, Moodley D, Eklund M, Gray GE, Hall DB, Robinson P, Mayers D, Martinson NA: **Efficacy of short-course AZT plus 3TC to reduce nevirapine resistance in the prevention of mother-to-child HIV transmission: a randomized clinical trial.** *PLoS Med* 2009, **6:**e1000172.
14. Arrive E, Chaix ML, Nerrienet E, Blanche S, Rouzioux C, Coffie PA, Kruy Leang S, McIntyre J, Avit D, Srey VH, *et al*: **Tolerance and viral resistance after single-dose nevirapine with tenofovir and emtricitabine to prevent vertical transmission of HIV-1.** *AIDS* 2009, **23:**825–833.
15. Fox Z, Phillips A, Cohen C, Neuhaus J, Baxter J, Emery S, Hirschel B, Hullsiek KH, Stephan C, Lundgren J: **Viral resuppression and detection of drug resistance following interruption of a suppressive non-nucleoside reverse transcriptase inhibitor-based regimen.** *AIDS* 2008, **22:**2279–2289.
16. El-Sadr WM, Lundgren JD, Neaton JD, Gordin F, Abrams D, Arduino RC, Babiker A, Burman W, Clumeck N, Cohen CJ, *et al*: **CD4+ Count-guided interruption of antiretroviral treatment.** *N Engl J Med* 2006, **355:**2283–2296.
17. Hanna GJ, Johnson VA, Kuritzkes DR, Richman DD, Brown AJ, Savara AV, Hazelwood JD, D'Aquila RT: **Patterns of resistance mutations selected by treatment of human immunodeficiency virus type 1 infection with zidovudine, didanosine, and nevirapine.** *J Infect Dis* 2000, **181:**904–911.
18. Sungkanuparph S, Manosuthi W, Kiertiburanakul S, Piyavong B, Chumpathat N, Chantratita W: **Options for a second-line antiretroviral regimen for HIV type 1-infected patients whose initial regimen of a fixed-dose combination of stavudine, lamivudine, and nevirapine fails.** *Clin Infect Dis* 2007, **44:**447–452.
19. BHIVA Writing Committee: **British HIV association (BHIVA) guidelines for the treatment of HIV-infected adults with antiretroviral therapy (2006).** *HIV Med* 2006, **7:**487–503.
20. Kikaire B, Khoo S, Walker AS, Ssali F, Munderi P, Namale L, Reid A, Gibb DM, Mugyenyi P, Grosskurth H: **Nevirapine clearance from plasma in african adults stopping therapy: a pharmacokinetic substudy.** *AIDS* 2007, **21:**733–737.
21. Mackie NE, Fidler S, Tamm N, Clarke JR, Back D, Weber JN, Taylor GP: **Clinical implications of stopping nevirapine-based antiretroviral therapy: relative pharmacokinetics and avoidance of drug resistance.** *HIV Med* 2004, **5:**180–184.
22. Sungkanuparph S, Techasathit W, Utaipiboon C, Chasombat S, Bhakeecheep S, Leechawengwongs M, Ruxrungtham K, Phanuphak P: **Thai national guidelines for antiretroviral therapy in HIV-1 infected adults and adolescents 2010.** *Asian Biomed* 2010, **4:**515–528.
23. Bangsberg DR: **Less than 95% adherence to nonnucleoside reverse-transcriptase inhibitor therapy can lead to viral suppression.** *Clin Infect Dis* 2006, **43:**939–941.
24. Paterson DL, Swindells S, Mohr J, Brester M, Vergis EN, Squier C, Wagener MM, Singh N: **Adherence to protease inhibitor therapy and outcomes in patients with HIV infection.** *Ann Intern Med* 2000, **133:**21–30.

11

Is the Sexual Behaviour of HIV Patients on Antiretroviral therapy safe or risky in Sub-Saharan Africa?

Asres Berhan[1] and Yifru Berhan[1,2*]

Abstract

Background: Reports on the sexual behavior of people on antiretroviral therapy (ART) are inconsistent. We selected 14 articles that compared the sexual behavior of people with and without ART for this analysis.

Methods: We included both cross-sectional studies that compared different ART-naïve and ART-experienced participants and longitudinal studies examining the behavior of the same individuals pre- and post-ART start. Meta-analyses were performed both stratified by type of study and combined. Outcome variables assessed for association with ART experience were any sexual activity, unprotected sex and having multiple sexual partners. Random-effect models were applied to determine the overall odds ratios. Sub-group analyses and meta-regression analyses were performed to examine sources of heterogeneity among the studies. Sensitivity analysis was also conducted to evaluate the stability of the overall odds ratio in the presence of outliers.

Results: The meta-analysis failed to show a statistically significant association of any sexual activity with ART experience. It did, however, show an overall statistically significant reduction of any unprotected sex, having multiple sexual partners and unprotected sex with HIV negative or unknown HIV status with ART experience. Meta-regression showed no interaction between duration of ART use or recall period of sexual behavior with the sexual activity variables. However, there was an association between the percentage of married or cohabiting participants included in a study and reductions in the practice of unprotected sex with ART.

Conclusion: In general, this meta-analysis demonstrated a significant reduction in risky sexual behavior among people on ART in sub-Saharan Africa. Future studies should investigate the reproducibility and continuity of the observed positive behavioural changes as the duration of ART lasts a decade or more.

Keywords: Antiretroviral therapy, Meta-analysis, Meta-regression, Multiple sexual partners, Unprotected sex, Sub-Saharan Africa

Introduction

Across the globe, the introduction of antiretroviral therapy (ART) has saved millions of life since it was widely introduced in developed countries in 1996 and in sub-Saharan Africa in 2002 [1]. ART contributed to a 19% decline in deaths from HIV infection from 2004 to 2009 [1]. Sub-Saharan region bears 68% of the global HIV burden. By 2009, about 37% of HIV-infected persons in sub-Saharan countries who were eligible for ART were able to access antiretroviral drugs. Just as in developed countries, ART has improved quality of life and survival in sub-Saharan Africa [2-4].

As severely ill HIV patients recover on ART, they feel general wellbeing and their sexual desire is likely to resume. Is the sexual behavior of HIV patients on ART safe or risky? Reports on sexual behaviors of people on ART have been inconsistent; six studies African and non-African countries have shown that patients on ART are more likely to engage in unprotected sex [5-10]; however, other cross sectional and longitudinal studies have reported a decrease in rates of risky sexual behavior after ART [11-15].

* Correspondence: yifrub@yahoo.com
[1]Hawassa University, Hawassa, Ethiopia
[2]Hawassa University College of Medicine and Health Sciences, P.O. Box 1560, Hawassa, Ethiopia

In a systematic review of three articles, Kennedy et al found a significant reduction in sexual risk-taking behaviour among patients on ART in developing countries [16]. One very recent cross-sectional study from Ethiopia showed that more than one third (36.9%) of study participants reported to have unprotected sexual intercourse in three months period prior to data collection [17]. Another cross-sectional study among patients on ART from an informal urban settlement in Kenya found increased rates of inconsistent condom use among women and increased rates of multiple sexual partners among married men [18]. A 2004 meta-analysis of studies from developed countries found that rates of unprotected sex among people on ART were not significantly different from those among HIV-infected people not on ART [19]. It found high rates of unprotected sex, however, among those who believe that they will not transmit HIV while on ART [19].

No previous meta-analysis has been published on the sexual behaviors of people on ART in Sub-Saharan Africa. This meta-analysis and meta-regression was conducted based on studies comparing the sexual behavior of people on ART with HIV-infected people not on ART. We hope this analysis sheds more light on the gradient of risky sexual behaviours among people on ART in Sub-Saharan Africa.

Methods

Search strategy

We conducted a computer search of PubMed, Google Scholar, WHO (HINARI) for articles on risky sexual behavior in relation to ART in sub-Saharan Africa published from January 2000 to October 2011. We obtained article texts either free on-line or from HINARI [20]. Our search terms included "HAART", "Highly active antiretroviral therapy", "ART", "Antiretroviral therapy", "sexual activity", "unprotected sex", "multiple sexual partners and unprotected sex with HIV negative or unknown HIV status", "inconsistent condom use," and the names of Sub-Saharan African countries. We also searched the reference lists of articles identified through the computer search.

Article selection

Articles that fulfilled the following three criteria were included in our meta-analysis: must be published in English, must be conducted in sub-Saharan Africa, and must compare either the sexual behavior of HIV-positive people on ART with that of HIV-positive, ART naïve or the sexual behavior of HIV-positive individuals before ART initiation with the sexual behavior of the same individuals after starting ART.

Our search criteria initially identified 53 complete journal articles on risky sexual behavior of people on ART in sub-Saharan Africa. Based on our inclusion criteria, only 14 of these articles qualified for the meta-analyses. The major reasons for the exclusion of 39 articles were: lack of comparative data on sexual behavior with behavior prior to starting ART or with an ART-naïve people control group; focused solely on knowledge and attitudes without examination of behavior, and review articles that included no data collection. Of the 14 selected articles, six were cross-sectional studies comparing the sexual behaviour of ART naïve with ART experienced people and eight were prospective cohort studies comparing behavior of the same individuals before and after starting ART. General information on the studies included is shown in Table 1.

Data extraction

From the studies that met the inclusion criteria, the following data were abstracted: year of publication, country

Table 1 General information on the studies included, 2011

Reference	Country	Type of study	Type of comparison	Sampled
Wandera B et al. [21]	Uganda	Prospective	Pre-ART vs Post ART	559 ART-naïve
Luchters S et al. [22]	Kenya	Prospective	Pre-ART vs Post ART	234 ART-naïve
Moatti J P et al. [23]	Co ̃te d'Ivoire	Cross-sectional	ART experienced vs. ART naïve	547 ART naïve and 164 ART experienced
Bateganya M et al. [24]	Uganda	Cross-sectional	ART experienced vs. ART naïve	354 ART naïve and 369ART experienced
Pearson C R et al. [25]	Mozambique	Prospective	Pre-ART vs Post ART	277 ART naive
Bunnell R et al. [26]	Uganda	Prospective	Pre-ART vs Post ART	926 ART-naive
Venkatesh K K et al study 1, [27]	South Africa	Prospective	Pre-ART vs Post ART	6263 ART-naive
Eisele T P et al. [28]	South Africa	Cross sectional	ART experienced vs. ART naïve	404 ART naïve and 520 ART experienced
Dia A et al. [29]	Cameroon	Cross-sectional	ART experienced vs. ART naïve	216 ART naïve and 691 ART experienced
Peltzer K et al. [30]	South Africa	Prospective	Pre-ART vs Post ART	735 ART naïve
Sarna A et al. [31]	Kenya	Cross-sectional	ART experienced vs. ART naïve	143 ART naïve and 179 ART experienced
Venkatesh K K et al study2 [32]	South Africa	Cross-sectional	ART experienced vs. ART naïve	247ART-naïve and 1295 ART experienced
Diabate S et al [8]	Co ̃te d'Ivoire	Prospective	Pre-ART vs Post ART	312 ART naïve
McClelland R. S et al. [33]	Kenya	Prospective	Pre-ART vs Post ART	898 ART naïve

where conducted, setting, type of comparison [within individuals (Pre- ART vs. Post- ART) or between individuals (ART naïve vs. ART experienced)], sample size, sexual history (sexually activity, multiple sexual partners, unprotected sex with HIV positive/HIV negative or unknown HIV status, and inconsistent condom use), recall period for sexual activities, duration on ART and proportion of married participants.

Operational definition

In this article, we use the terms "ART-naïve" and "ART-experienced" only with respect to studies comparing behavior among different individuals. We use the terms "pre-ART" and "post-ART" only with respect to studies comparing behavior within the same individuals. We did not attempt to standardize definitions of these terms; we used them as used in each of the articles selected. We use the term "unprotected sex" to mean either sexual activity without the use of a condom or inconsistent condom use with any partner irrespective of HIV serostatus. We use the term "multiple sexual partners" to mean sexual activity with two or more sex partners during the study period. In this analysis, all the study participants were HIV positive. All articles selected for this meta-analysis have got ethical clearance from their respective institution.

Statistical analysis

We used Meta Analyst (Beta 3.13) software [34] and Comprehensive Meta Analysis software [35] to carry out meta-analysis and meta-regression analysis, respectively. We conducted four meta-analyses: on the association of ART experience with any sexual activity, on the association of ART experience with any unprotected sex, on the association of ART experience with having multiple sexual partners and on the association of ART experience with having unprotected sex with partners who were HIV negative or of unknown HIV status. We used the DerSimonian-Laird method (Random-effect model) to calculate the overall odds ratios. To determine the heterogeneity among the studies, it was possible to generate values for Tau^2, Chi-square (Q), I^2 and P-value. For this analysis, when the value of I^2 exceeded 50%, we considered the total variation across the studies to be large and to be due to heterogeneity rather than to chance [36].

In the presence of significant heterogeneity, summary estimates from meta-analyses are believed to be difficult to interpret; and Lijmer et al recommends investigating heterogeneity using subgroup (stratified) analysis and meta-regression analysis [37] Therefore, to examine sources of heterogeneity among the studies, we performed sub-group analyses with Meta Analyst (Beta 3.13) software and meta-regression analysis with Comprehensive Meta Analysis software. Sub-group analysis was carried out at two stages: first, stratifying by type of study (among individuals vs. within individuals); second, combining all studies of both types. Random effects linear meta-regression analysis was performed with three covariates or moderators: duration on ART, recall period for sexual activities and percentage of married participants in the group receiving ART.

Sensitivity analysis was also conducted to see the stability of the overall odds ratio to inclusion of individual studies. For all statistical tests, P-value ≤ 0.05 was considered as statistically significant.

Results

The studies making comparisons among individuals included 5129 participants (1911 ART-naïve participants and 3218 ART–experienced participants). The studies making within-individual comparisons included 1024 participants were included. The participants' duration on ART ranged from 3–36 months (median six months and interquartile range 6–12 months). Figure 1 presents the results of the meta-analysis of any sexual activity in relation to ART experience. Although two studies [23,24] showed a statistically significant increase in sexual activity among ART-experienced as compared with ART-naïve participants, the overall analysis portrayed no association of sexual activity in either of the study types (OR = 1.14; 95% CI, 0.91 to 1.43). However, the proportion of sexually active people was higher among ART-experienced than ART-naïve participants in three of the four studies that made comparisons among individuals [23,24,28].

The within-individual studies were more inconsistent than studies that made comparisons between individuals. Two studies [21,27] found statistically significant decreases in sexual activity post-ART while another two studies [22,25] found increased sexual activity pre-ART.

Sensitivity analysis attested to the stability of the overall odds ratio; it oscillated in the range of 1.07 to 1.21 (changed by ± 0.07 from the overall odds ratio). The test of heterogeneity showed a significant variation among the included studies (Q = 74.7; I^2 = 87.9%), signifying that the variation was due to heterogeneity rather than chance. The impact of duration on ART and recall time on the overall odds ratio was assessed by the random effect meta-regression model. As shown in Table 2, these variables were not found to have a significant effect; the regression coefficient of the log odds ratio of sexual activity was not significantly different from zero in either the analysis of average time while on ART (regression coefficient = –0.016; 95% CI, -0.033 to 0.002; P = 0.078) or the analysis of recall time (regression coefficient = 0.042; 95% CI, -0.020 to 0.104; P = 0.185).

As shown in Figure 2, all studies [21-23,26,27,29-33] but one showed a statistically significant reduction in rates of unprotected sex among people on ART. The divergent study showed a statistically significant increase

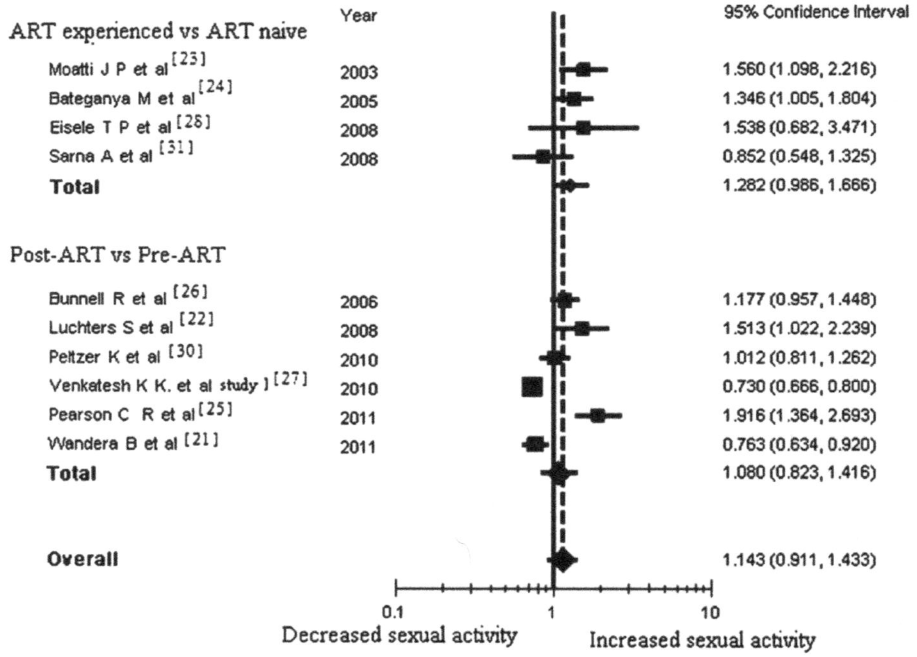

Heterogeneity test				
Tau-Squared	I^2	Q	DF	P-val (Q)
0.105	87.9%	74.685	9.000	0.000

Figure 1 Meta-analysis of the association between antiretroviral therapy experience and any sexual activity; Pooled effect estimate from a random-effects model, 2011.

in unprotected sex among those on ART. The overall odds ratio in the meta-analysis demonstrated a statistically significant reduction in unprotected sex while on ART (OR = 0.437; 95% CI, 0.315 - 0.607). The association appears a bit stronger in the studies comparing rates of unprotected sex among different individuals (OR = 0.414; 95% CI, 0.287 - 0.598). In the sensitivity analysis, the overall odds ratio was very little changed by omitting individual studies (maximum ± 0.06).

The studies included in the meta-analysis of unprotected sex also found to have significant variation due to heterogeneity rather than to chance (Q = 124.4; I^2 = 92.0%). Meta-regression found no statistically significant interaction between unprotected sex and duration on ART (regression coefficient = −0.0328; 95% CI, -0.069 to 0.003; P = 0.076) or between unprotected sex and recall time (regression coefficient = 0.0029; 95% CI, -0.151 to 0.157; P = 0.97). But the meta-regression incorporating six studies [21,22,26,27,30,31] which analyzed the relationship of rates of unprotected sex with the percentage of married or cohabiting participants included in the study demonstrated a significant reduction of unprotected sex

Table 2 Summary of meta-regression analysis findings, 2011

Variable	Regression coefficient	Standard error	95% CI	P-value
Effect of duration on ART on sexual activity	- 0.016	0.009	−0.033, 0.002	0.078
Effect of time of recall on sexual activity	0.042	0.032	−0.020, 0.104	0.185
Effect of time of recall on unprotected sex	0.0029	0.078	−0.151, 0.157	0.97
Effect of duration on ART on unprotected sex	−0.0328	0.018	0.069, 0.003	0.076
Effect of married participants on Unprotected sex	−0.032	0.014	−0.059, -0.004	0.023
Effect of time of recall on multiple sexual partner	0.018	0.047	−0.074, 0.111	0.697
Effect of duration on ART on multiple sexual partners	0.0457	0.037	−0.028, 0.119	0.22
Effect of married participants on multiple sexual partners	0.0313	0.0249	−0.017, 0.080	0.21

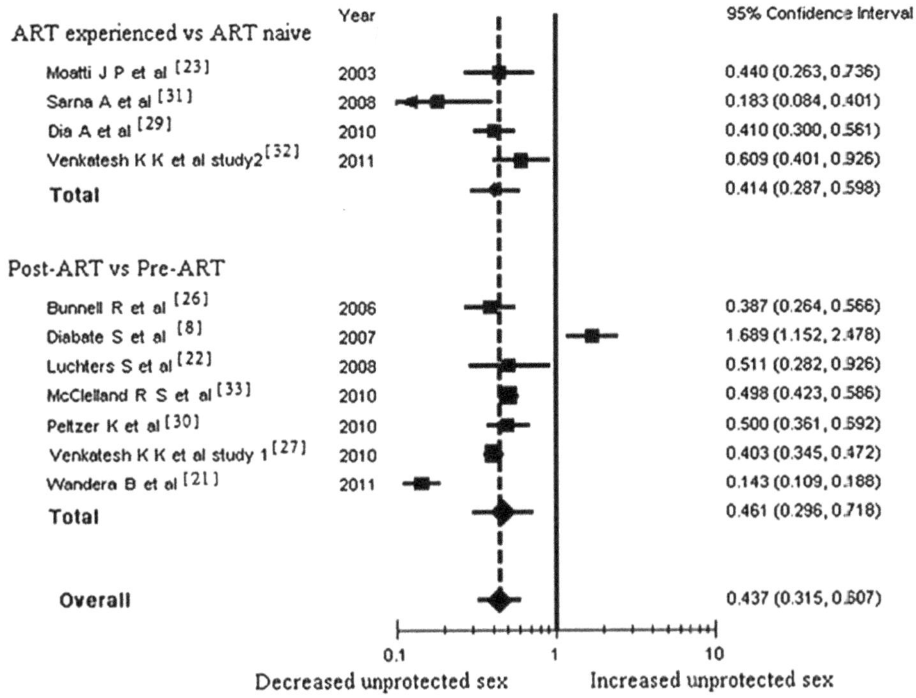

Heterogeneity test				
Tau-Squared	I^2	Q	DF	P-val (Q)
0.263	92.0%	124.355	10.000	0.000

Figure 2 Meta-analysis of the association between antiretroviral therapy experience and any unprotected sex; Pooled effect estimate from a random-effects model, 2011.

as the percentage of married participants increases (regression coefficient = –0.032; 95% CI,-0.059 to –0.004; P = 0.023).

Figure 3 shows the results of the meta-analysis of the relationship of ART experience to rates of multiple sexual partners. The overall odds ratio, including all eight studies which reported this information, indicated that rates of multiple sexual partners were significantly decreased among people on ART (OR = 0.47; 95% CI, 0.248 to 0.888). When considered separately by study type, however, the combined odds ratios were not statistically significant, although two studies of each type [27,31-33] independently showed a statistically significant reduction in rates of multiple sexual partners with ART experience. In other words, rates of multiple sexual partners were not found to be significantly different either when comparing ART-experienced people to ART-naïve people; or when comparing the same individuals' behavior before and after ART initiation. The sensitivity analysis supports the findings of the sub-group analysis; exclusion of Sarna and *et al.* study from the analysis leads to a finding of an insignificant association of ART experience with rates of having multiple sexual partners.

Linear meta-regression analysis showed that neither duration of ART (regression coefficient = 0.0457; 95% CI, -0.028 to 0.119; P = 0.22), recall time (regression coefficient = 0.018; 95% CI, -0.074 to 0.111; P = 0.697) nor percentage of married participants (regression coefficient = 0.0313; 95%CI, -0.017 to 0.080; P = 0.21) were significantly associated with having multiple sexual partners.

Of the 14 studies included, only four [22,25,26,28] reported rates of unprotected sex with HIV-negative or unknown HIV status persons (Figure 4). The meta-analysis of the relationship between ART experience with rates of unprotected sex with HIV negative or unknown HIV serostatus showed a statistically significant reduction among people on ART (OR = 0.55; 95% CI, 0.303 to 0.994).

Discussion

Because of several contradictory reports, the issue of sexual behaviour of people on ART in sub-Saharan Africa still continues to be debatable. This meta-analysis is the first to provide a pooled quantitative estimate of the sexual behavior of people on ART by categorizing and analyzing the studies by type. In other words, the strength of this

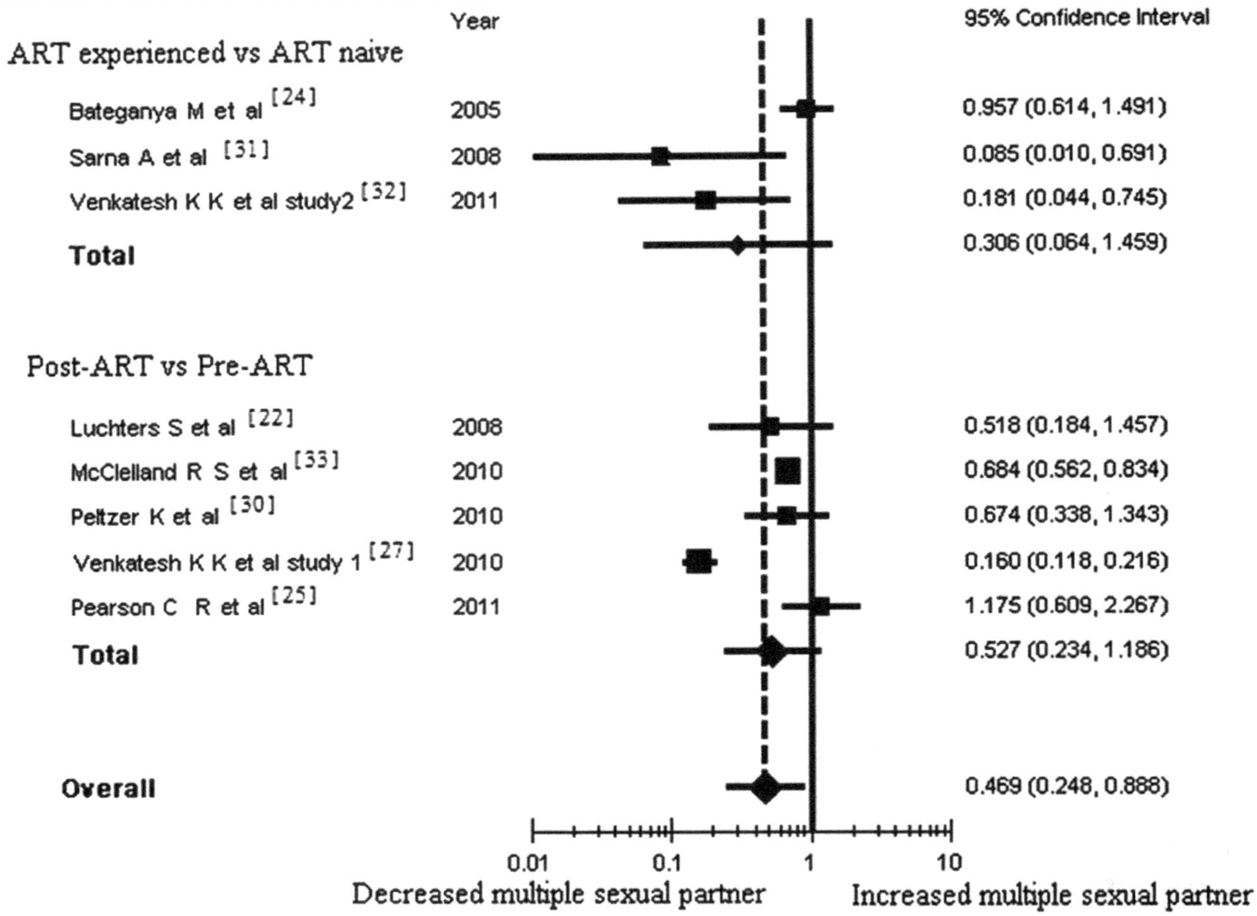

Heterogeneity test				
Tau-Squared	I^2	Q	DF	P-val (Q)
0.658	91.7%	84.391	7.000	0.000

Figure 3 Meta-analysis of the association between antiretroviral therapy experience and having multiple sexual partners; Pooled effect estimate from a random-effects model, 2011.

analysis is that it examined the sexual behavioral change with ART within individuals (pre-ART vs. post-ART study type) and among different individuals (ART-naïve vs. ART-experienced study type), and finally, combining the two study types (HIV-infected people not on ART vs. HIV-infected people on ART). We would expect the within-individual studies to be less affected by confounding variables due to variations between the individuals included than the studies that compared different ART-naïve and ART-experienced individuals. Our analysis also permitted exploration of different dimensions of the sexual behavior of HIV infected patients. Although we found no statistically significant difference in sexual activity among HIV-infected people on ART, six of the 10 studies [22-24,26-28] which reported this variable reported an increase in sexual activity, which is consistent with other report [38]. However, the statistically significant reduction of unprotected sex among those on ART found in both prospective and cross sectional studies is inconsistent with the results of the meta-analysis of studies in developed nations, which found no statistically significant difference in this behavior [19]. Furthermore, this analysis also revealed the reduction in rates of multiple sexual partners and rates of unprotected sex with HIV-negative or unknown HIV status partners by people on ART. This finding may trigger questions as to why risky sexual behavior decreases with ART in sub-Saharan Africa while remaining unchanged in developed nations. One reason

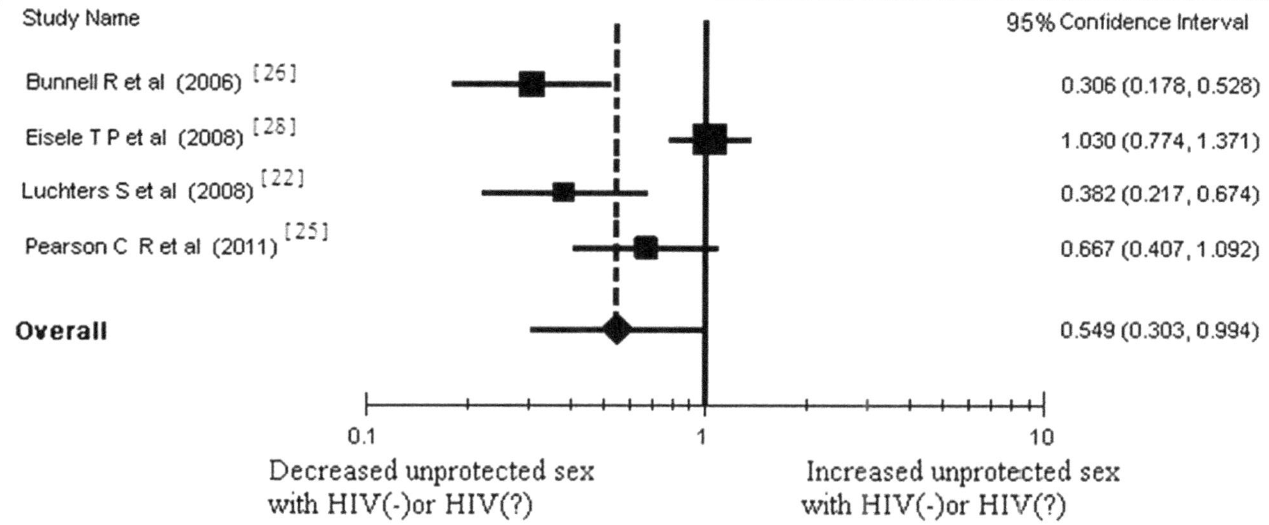

Heterogeneity test				
Tau-Squared	I^2	Q	DF	P-val (Q)
0.308	85.2%	20.256	3.000	0.000

Figure 4 Meta-analysis of the association between antiretroviral therapy (ART) experience and unprotected sex with HIV negative or unknown HIV status partners; Pooled effect estimate from a random-effects model, 2011.

may be that risky sexual practices in sub-Saharan Africa were extremely prevalent at the outset, which we know because sub-Saharan Africa is the region most affected by HIV and because the majority of HIV infections in this region are attributed to unprotected heterosexual intercourse [2,39].

In addition, one may argue that the dramatic improvement in their health after beginning ART may have given HIV patients the hope of living long. Their previous sufferings had been an extremely bad experience; and professionals probably counseled them not to put themselves and their partners at risk of infection with new HIV strains, with HIV strains resistant to antiretroviral drugs and with other sexually transmitted infections. In support of this hypothesis, a qualitative study from Uganda reported that many ART patients were worried about risking their improving health through HIV super-infection and about the risk of resuming sexual practice [40]. The positive behavioral change among ART patients in Sub-Saharan Africa may also be the effect of good adherence to clinic visits, which will provide the chance to refresh their knowledge on HIV and to receive further warnings during every visit. A study conducted in six public HIV clinics has established the association of good ART adherence with decreased risky sexual behaviors [41].

A meta-analysis on adherence to ART in Sub-Saharan Africa and North America found better adherence among Sub-Saharan Africans [42]. The observed good adherence in Sub-Saharan Africa may have contributed as well to avoidance of risky sexual practice. The reported positive behavioral change towards safer sex not only provides HIV patients an advantage in improving the quality of their lives but also reduces their chance of transmitting HIV to their partners and of acquiring new and resistant HIV strains.

There are some studies from Sub-Saharan Africa which report the association of higher rates of unprotected sex with shorter duration of ART therapy (the longer people stay on ART, the lower their rates of unprotected sex) [18,38,43]. However, our meta-regression analysis showed no statistically significant interaction of rates of unprotected sex with duration on ART. This finding also does not support the idea proposed by Womoyi et al, that patients who have just started ART may experience illness which could decrease sexual desire and that as time passes and symptoms of HIV disease are resolved, risky sexual practice could emerge [40].

Our meta-regression also found no significant relationship between sexual activity and the time period over which participants were asked to recall such activity. However, the meta-regression of rates of unprotected sex in relation with the percentage of participants who were married found a significant interaction. The higher the percentage of married participants in a study, the lower the rates of unprotected sex found. This finding would be expected and may explain why the majority of studies included in this analysis found a reduction in unprotected sex, but other reports have not [18].

One limitation of our analysis is that all the primary studies analyzed used interviews to collect data on sexual behavior; this is open to recall bias and social desirability bias [44]. First, in some settings, openly discussing sexual issues may be taboo or interviewees may fear losing value in society. Second, patients on ART, many of whom may have been thoroughly counseled about the consequences of unprotected sex at ART initiation and in subsequent visits, may not feel comfortable reporting truthfully about their subsequent sexual behavior. Another limitation is the lack of data provided by the primary studies. Most of the primary studies failed to include data on stages of HIV disease (such as viral load, CD4 count, clinical condition) and level of medication adherence. Therefore we were unable to analyze the effect of these parameters on sexual behavior of people with and without ART. Many of the primary studies also lacked information on whether married participants had more than one sexual partner. The variation in percentage of married participants in the primary studies does not seem adequate, on its own, to explain variations among the findings. Other sources of heterogeneity, which we did not analyze, could be average age, education level, sex allocation, income, CD4 count and culture of the participants.

In conclusion, the significant reduction in risk taking sexual behavior among people on ART regardless of duration on ART is consistent with several individual studies and a systematic review from developing countries [16,45]. However, it was not possible to identify what contributes to this positive behavioral change, and we are not sure whether the observed behavioral change is sustainable and representative of all sub-Saharan African countries. Recently published non-comparative studies from Sub-Saharan African countries reported that many HIV patients on ART continue to exhibit high risk sexual behavior [10,17,18,46]. As a non-comparative cohort study of people on ART from Uganda showed, risky sexual behaviours were declining before 2004 but thereafter were on the upswing [47]. Although our meta-analysis from comparative primary studies does support some previous research, it is probably premature to conclude that there has been region-wide significant reduction in unprotected sex among people on ART in Sub-Saharan Africa, which were also a concern of other authors [26]. Furthermore, it is known that regardless of ART, men and women have different patterns of sexual activity. However, in this meta-analysis, it was not possible to identify the sexual behaviour differences by men and women; out of eight studies that reported sexual activity, the data set in four was unfit for doing meta-analysis. Therefore, future studies should address the reproducibility of the observed positive behavioral changes in other settings and assess whether they continue as patients stay on ART for a decade or more.

Competing interest

Authors would like to declare that there was no competing interest associated with this manuscript.

Authors' contributions

Both authors (AB and YB) actively involved in designing, articles search, articles selection, and manuscript writing. The contribution of AB was immense in doing the meta-analysis and meta-regression. Both authors read and approved the final manuscript.

Acknowledgment

We would like to thank WHO and publishers for setting up Health Inter Network Access to Research Initiative (HINARI) to enable us to access the full text of articles (included and excluded). We did not receive any financial support for this analysis. But we were energized by Eden Asefa and Dr. Mebrat Deribe to carry out this work. We are also grateful to Dr. Nicole Simmons from John Hopkins University (Baltimore) who reviewed the grammar of the manuscript.

References

1. Joint United Nations Program on HIV/AIDS (UNAIDS): *Report on the global AIDS epidemic.* 2004. http://www.unaids.org/bangkok2004/unaidsglobalreport2004_en.pdf
2. Joint United Nations Program on HIV/AIDS (UNAIDS): *Global Epidemic Report on AIDS.* 2010. www.unaids.org/documents/20101123_GlobalReport_em.pdf
3. Jerene D, Næss A, Lindtjørn B: **Antiretroviral therapy at a district hospital in Ethiopia prevents death and tuberculosis in a cohort of HIV patients.** *AIDS Res Ther* 2006, **3**:10. http://www.aidsrestherapy.com/content/3/1/10
4. Fairall LR, Bachmann MO, Louwagie GMC, Vuuren Cv, Chikobvu P, Steyn D, Staniland GH, Timmerman V, Msimanga M, Seebregts CJ, Boulle A, Nhiwatiwa R, Bateman ED, Zwarenstein MF, Chapman RD: **Effectiveness of Antiretroviral Treatment in a South African Program.** *Arch Intern Med* 2008, **168**(1):86–93.
5. Lightfoot M, Swendeman D, Borus MJR, Comulada WS, Weiss R: **Risk behaviors of youth living with HIV: pre-and post-HAART.** *Am J Health Behav* 2005, **29**(2):162–171.
6. Rice E, Batterham P, Borus MJR: **Unprotected sex among youth living with HIV before and after the advent of highly active antiretroviral therapy.** *Perspect Sex Reprod Health* 2006, **38**(3):162–167.
7. Wilson TE, Gore ME, Greenblatt R, Cohen M, Minkoff H, Silver S, Robison E, Levine A, Gange SJ: **Changes in sexual behavior among HIV-infected women after initiation of HAART.** *Am J Public Health* 2004, **94**(7):1141–1146.
8. Diabate S, Alary M, Koffi CK: **Short-term increase in unsafe sexual behaviour after initiation of HAART in Co^te d'Ivoire.** *AIDS* 2008, **22**(1):154–156.
9. Mei S, Quax R, van de Vijver D, Zhu Y, Sloot PMA: **Increasing risk behaviour can outweigh the benefits of antiretroviral drug treatment on the HIV incidence among men-having-sex-with-men in Amsterdam.** *BMC Infect Dis* 2011, **11**:118. http://www.biomedcentral.com/1471-2334/11/118
10. Olley B: **Higher-risk sexual behaviour among HIV patients receiving antiretroviral treatment in Ibadan, Nigeria.** *Afr J AIDS Res* 2008, **7**(1):71–78.
11. Diamond C, Richardson JL, Milam J, Stoyanoff S, McCutchan JA, Kemper C, Larsen RA, Hollander H, Weismuller P, Bolan R: **Use of and adherence to antiretroviral therapy is associated with decreased sexual risk behavior in HIV clinic patients.** *J Acquir Immune Defic Syndr* 2005, **39**(2):211–218.
12. Bouhnik AD, Moatti JP, Vlahov D, Gallais H, Dellamonica P, Obadia Y: **Highly active antiretroviral treatment does not increase sexual risk behaviour**

among French HIV infected injecting drug users. *J Epidemiol Community Health* 2002, **56**:349–353.

13. Marshall BDL, Milloy MJ, Kerr T, Zhang R, Montaner JSG, Wood E: **No Evidence of Increased Sexual Risk Behaviour after Initiating Antiretroviral Therapy among People who Inject Drugs.** *AIDS* 2010, **24**(14):2271–2278.
14. Bunnel R, Ekwaru JP, Solberg P, Wamai N, Bikaako-Kajura W, Were W, *et al*: **Changes in sexual behaviour and risk of HIV transmission after antiretroviral therapy and prevention interventions in Uganda.** *AIDS* 2006, **20**:85–92.
15. Marcellin F, Bonono C-R, Blanche J, Carrieri MP, Spire B, Koulla-Shiro S, the EVAL study group: **Higher risk of unsafe sex and impaired quality of life among patients not receiving antiretroviral therapy in Cameroon: results from EVAL survey (ANRS 12–116).** *AIDS* 2010, **24**(Suppl 1):S17–S25.
16. Kennedy C, O'Reilly K, Medley A, Sweat M: **The impact of HIV treatment on risk behaviour in developing countries: a systemic review.** *AIDS Care* 2007, **19**(6):707–720.
17. Dessie Y, Gerbaba M, Bedru A, Davey G: **Risky sexual practices and related factors among ART attendees in Addis Ababa public hospitals, Ethiopia: A cross sectional study.** *BMC Public Health* 2011, **11**:422. http://www.biomedcentral.com/1471-2458/11/422
18. Ragnarsson A, Ekström AM, Carter J, Ilako F, Lukhwaro A, Marrone G, Thorson A: **Sexual risk taking among patients on antiretroviral therapy in an urban informal settlement in Kenya: a cross-sectional survey.** *J Int AIDS Soc* 2011, **14**. http://www.jiasociety.org/content/14/1/20
19. Crepaz N, Hart TA, Marks G: **Highly Active Antiretroviral Therapy and Sexual Risk Behavior A Meta-analytic Review.** *JAMA* 2004, **292**:224–236.
20. *Health Inter Network Access to Research Initiative (HINARI)*. http://www.who.int/whalecom0/hinari/eligibility/en/
21. Wandera B, Kamya MR, Castelnuovo B, Kiragga A, Kambugu A, Wanyama JN, Easterbrook P, Sethi AK: **Sexual behaviors over a 3-year period among individuals with advanced HIV/AIDS receiving antiretroviral therapy in an urban HIV clinic in Kampala, Uganda.** *J Acquir Immune Defic Syndr* 2011, **57**:62–68.
22. Luchters S, Sarna A, Geibel S, Chersich MF, Munyao P, Kaai S, Mandaliya KN, Shikely KS, Rutenberg N, Temmerman M: **Safer sexual behaviors after 12 months of antiretroviral treatment in Mombasa, Kenya: A Prospective Cohort.** *AIDS Patient Care STDS* 2008, **22**(7):587–595.
23. Moatti JP, Prudhomme J, Traore DC, Amari AJ, Akribi HAD, Msellati P: **Access to antiretroviral treatment and sexual behaviours of HIV-infected patients aware of their serostatus in Côte d'Ivoire.** *AIDS* 2003, **17**(suppl 3): S69–S77.
24. Bateganya M, Colfax G, Shafer LA, Kityo C, Mugyenyi P, Serwadda D, Mayanja H, Bangsberg D: **Antiretroviral therapy and sexual behavior: a comparative study between antiretroviral-naive and -experienced patients at an urban HIV/AIDS care and research center in Kampala, Uganda.** *AIDS Patient Care STDS* 2005, **19**(11):760–770.
25. Pearson CR, Cassels S, Kurth AE, Montoya P, Micek MA, Gloyd SS: **Change in Sexual Activity 12 Months After ART Initiation Among HIV-Positive Mozambicans.** *AIDS Behav* 2011, **15**:778–787.
26. Bunnell R, Ekwaru JP, Solberg P, Wamai N, Kajura WB, Were W, Coutinho A, Liechty C, Madraa E, Rutherford G, Mermin J: **Changes in sexual behavior and risk of HIV transmission after antiretroviral therapy and prevention interventions in rural Uganda.** *AIDS* 2006, **20**:85–92.
27. Venkatesh KK, de Bruyn G, Lurie MN, Mohapi L, Pronyk P, Moshabela M, Marinda E, Gray GE, Triche EW, Martinson NA: **Decreased sexual risk behavior in the era of HAART among HIV-infected urban and rural South Africans attending primary care clinics.** *AIDS* 2010, **24**:2687–2696.
28. Eisele TP, Mathews C, Chopra M, Brown L, Silvestre E, Daries V, Kendall C: **High Levels of Risk Behavior Among People Living with HIV Initiating and Waiting to Start Antiretroviral Therapy in Cape Town South Africa.** *AIDS Behav* 2008, **12**:570–577.
29. Dia A, Marcellin F, Bonono RC, Boyer S, Bouhnik AD, Protopopescu C, Shiro SK, Carrieri MP, Abe´ C, Spire B: **Prevalence of unsafe sex with one's steady partner either HIV-negative or of unknown HIV status and associated determinants in Cameroon (EVAL ANRS12-116 survey).** *Sex Transm Infect* 2010, **86**:148–154.
30. Peltzer K, Ramlagan S: **Safer sexual behaviours after 1 year of antiretroviral treatment in KwaZulu-Natal, South Africa: a prospective cohort study.** *Sex Health* 2010, **7**:135–141.
31. Sarna A, Luchters SMF, Geibel S, Kaai S, Munyao P, Shikely KS, Mandaliya K, van Dam J, Temmerman M: **Sexual risk behaviour and HAART: a comparative study of HIV-infected persons on HAART and on preventive therapy in Kenya.** *Int J STD AIDS* 2008, **19**:85–89.
32. Venkatesh KK, de Bruyn G, Lurie MN, Modisenyane T, Triche EW, Gray GE, Welte A, Martinson NA: **Sexual risk behaviors among HIV-infected South African men and women with their partners in a primary care program: implications for couples-based prevention.** *AIDS Behav* 2011, doi:10.1007/s10461-011-9941-y (in press).
33. McClelland RS, Graham SM, Richardson BA, Peshu N, Masese LN, Wanje GH, Mandaliya KN, Kurth AE, Jaoko W, Ndinya-Achola JO: **Treatment with Antiretroviral Therapy is Not Associated with Increased Sexual Risk Behaviour in Kenyan Female Sex Workers.** *AIDS* 2010, **24**(6):891–897.
34. Wallace BC, Schmid CH, Lau J, Trikalinos TA: **Meta-analyst: software for meta-analysis of binary, continuous and diagnostic data.** *BMC Med Res Methodol* 2009, **9**(1):80+. http://www.biomedcentral.com/1471-2288/9/80
35. Borenstein M, Hedges L, Higgins J, Rothstein H: *Comprehensive Meta-analysis Version 2*. Englewood NJ: Biostat; 2005.
36. Higgins JPT, Thompson SG, Deeks JJ, Altman DG: **Measuring inconsistency in meta-analyses.** *BMJ* 2003, **327**:557–560.
37. Lijmer JG, Bossuyt PM, Heisterkamp SH: **Exploring sources of heterogeneity in systematic reviews of diagnostic tests.** *Stat Med* 2002, **21**:1525–1537.
38. Eisele TP, Mathews C, Chopra M, Lurie MN, Brown L, Dewing S, Kendall C: **Changes in risk behavior among HIV-positive patients during their first year of antiretroviral therapy in Cape Town South Africa.** *AIDS Behav* 2009, **13**(6):1097–1105.
39. Hargreaves JR, Bonell CP, Boler T, Boccia D, Birdthistle I, Fletcher A, Pronyk PM, Glynn JR: **Systematic review exploring time trends in the association between educational attainment and risk of HIV infection in sub-Saharan Africa.** *AIDS* 2008, **28**(3):403–414.
40. Womoyi J, Mbonye M, Seeley J, Birungi J, Jaffar S: **Changes in sexual desires and behaviours of people living with HIV after initiation of ART: Implications for HIV prevention and health promotion.** *BMC Public Health* 2011, **11**:633. http://www.biomedcentral.com/1471-2458/11/633
41. Diamond C, Richardson JL, Milam J, Stoyanoff S, McCutchan A, Kemper C, Larsen RA, Hollander H, Weismuller P, Bolan R: **Use of and adherence to antiretroviral therapy is associated with decreased sexual risk behavior in HIV clinic patients.** *J Acquir Immune Defic Syndr* 2005, **39**(2):211–218.
42. Mills EJ, Nachega JB, Buchan I, Attaran A, Singh S, Rachlis B, Wu P, Cooper C, Thabane L, Wilson K, Guyatt GH, Bangsberg DR: **Adherence to antiretroviral therapy in Sub-Saharan Africa and North America: A meta-analysis.** *JAMA* 2006, **296**:679–690.
43. Unge C, Sodergard B, Marrone G, Thorson A, Lukhwaro A, Carter J, Ilako F, Ekstrom AM: **Long-term adherence to antiretroviral treatment and program drop-out in a high-risk urban setting in sub-saharan Africa: a prospective cohort study.** *PLoS One* 2010, **5**(10):e13613.
44. Schroder K, Carey MP, Vanable PA: **Methodological challenges in research on sexual risk behaviour: II. Accuracy of self reports.** *Ann Behav Med* 2003, **26**:104–123.
45. Venkatesh KK, Flanigan TP, Mayer KH: **Is expanded treatment preventing new infections? Impact of antiretroviral therapy on sexual risk behaviours in the developing world.** *AIDS* 2011, **25**:1939–1949.
46. Osinde MO, Kaye DK, Kakaire O: **Sexual behaviour and HIV-serodiscordance among HIV patients receiving HAART in rural Uganda.** *J Obstet Gynaecol* 2011, **31**(5):436–440.
47. Shafer LA, Nsubuga RN, White R, Mayanja BN, Chapman R, O'Brien K, der Paal LV, Grosskurth H, Maher D: **Antiretroviral therapy and sexual behaviour in Uganda: a cohort study.** *AIDS* 2011, **25**:671–678.

12

German cohort of HCV mono-infected and HCV/HIV co-infected patients reveals relative under-treatment of co-infected patients

Claudia Beisel, Martin Heuer, Benjamin Otto, Johannes Jochum, Stefan Schmiedel, Sandra Hertling, Olaf Degen, Stefan Lüth, Jan van Lunzen[*†] and Julian Schulze zur Wiesch[†]

Abstract

Background: Current German and European HIV guidelines recommend early evaluation of HCV treatment in all HIV/HCV co-infected patients. However, there are still considerable barriers to initiate HCV therapy in everyday clinical practice. This study evaluates baseline characteristics, "intention-to-treat" pattern and outcome of therapy of HCV/HIV co-infected patients in direct comparison to HCV mono-infected patients in a "real-life" setting.

Methods: A large, single-center cohort of 172 unselected HCV patients seen at the Infectious Diseases Unit at the University Medical Center Hamburg-Eppendorf from 2000–2011, 88 of whom HCV/HIV co-infected, was retrospectively analyzed by chart review with special focus on demographic, clinical and virologic aspects as well as treatment outcome.

Results: Antiviral HCV combination therapy with PEG-interferon plus weight-adapted ribavirin was initiated in 88/172 (52%) patients of the entire cohort and in n = 36 (40%) of all HCV/HIV co-infected patients (group A) compared to n = 52 (61%) of the HCV mono-infected group (group B) (p = 0.006). There were no significant differences of the demographics or severity of the liver disease between the two groups with the exception of slightly higher baseline viral loads in group A. A *sustained virologic response* (SVR) was observed in 50% (n = 18) of all treated HIV/HCV co-infected patients versus 52% (n = 27) of all treated HCV mono-infected patients (p = 0.859). Genotype 1 was the most frequent genotype in both groups (group A: n = 37, group B: n = 49) and the SVR rates for these patients were only slightly lower in the group of co-infected patients (group A: n = 33%, group B: 40% p = 0.626). During the course of treatment HCV/HIV co-infected patients received less ribavirin than mono-infected patients.

Conclusion: Overall, treatment was only initiated in half of the patients of the entire cohort and in an even smaller proportion of HCV/HIV co-infected patients despite comparable outcome (SVR) and similar baseline characteristics. In the light of newer treatment options, greater efforts to remove the barriers to treatment that still exist for a great proportion of patients especially with HIV/HCV co-infection have to be undertaken.

Keywords: HCV/HIV co-infection, Hepatitis C, PEG interferon/ribavirin treatment

Background

In HIV infected patients, liver-related disease has emerged as a leading cause of morbidity and mortality. The prevalence of HCV/HIV co-infection in the HIV population ranges from 10 to up to 50% [1,2]. On the other hand, HIV co-infection may worsen the course of hepatitis C infection, leading to faster progression of liver fibrosis and cirrhosis, liver failure and development of hepatocellular carcinoma (HCC) [3]. Successful treatment of chronic hepatitis C infection has been shown to stop fibrosis progression, prevent liver-associated diseases and mortality of co-infected patients [4]. Therefore, current German and European HIV guidelines recommend early evaluation of all HIV/HCV co-infected patients for possible HCV treatment. In general, HCV genotype, liver fibrosis, IL-28 haplotypes and quantitative HCV RNA are important baseline predictors of SVR [5]. Demographic factors, histological parameters and treatment

* Correspondence: v.lunzen@uke.de
[†]Equal contributors
I. Department of Medicine, Infectious Diseases Unit, University Medical Center Hamburg-Eppendorf, Martinistr. 52, 20246 Hamburg, Germany

related factors can also effect the response to treatment, but in general more than 50% of naïve mono-infected patients will achieve sustained virologic response (SVR) with the current standard therapy (pegylated interferon plus ribavirin) [6,7]. Two large registration trials have shown lower sustained virologic response rates (SVR) for dual therapy in HIV/HCV co-infected patients (~33%) compared to mono-infected patients (47-54%) [8-12]. Higher baseline HCV RNA levels and lower initial ribavirin doses are quoted as possible explanation for the lower SVR seen in co-infected patients [13]. Recent data suggest that higher ribavirin doses are safe and well-tolerated in co-infected patients [14]. Intensified, response guided dual therapy can significantly increase the SVR in co-infected patients [15]. However, less is known about the "real life" treatment outcome of co-infected patients [15].

Great advances have been made with the introduction of the protease inhibitors boceprevir, telaprevir and simeprevir as well as the polymerase inhibitor sofosbuvir that have also been approved for triple therapy in HIV/HCV co-infection [16]. SVR rates of more than 80% have been reported for the triple therapy of naïve patients regardless of the HIV status [16-18].

Despite the unfavorable course of hepatitis C co-infection in HIV positive patients, not all patients are referred to specialists for evaluation for HCV treatment [19]. Furthermore, anti-HCV treatment is only initiated in a subset of all patients for various reasons (e.g. substance abuse, social and psychiatric issues, fear of side effects or drug-drug interactions especially in patients on ART or anticipated low chance of SVR) even in specialized centers [20].

In this "real life" single center study we aimed to summarize the experience and pitfalls of standard dual HCV therapy over the last decade and analyze baseline characteristics, treatment rates and patterns, and outcome of therapy in a German cohort of HCV/HIV co-infected patients. A similar and unselected group of HCV mono-infected patients treated at the same center was evaluated in direct comparison.

Methods

Study population and laboratory markers

88 HIV-seropositive and 84 HIV-seronegative, unpaired, unmatched and unselected treatment-naïve patients with chronic HCV infection were enrolled into this mono-center, retrospective cohort study. All patients presented at the Infectious Diseases Outpatient Clinic of the University Medical Center Hamburg-Eppendorf, Germany in the time period from 2000 – 2011 -before directly acting antivirals (DAA's) became readily available for the treatment of HIV/HCV co-infection. The center is a tertiary care referral center for HIV antiretroviral and HCV antiviral therapy in Germany.

Primary end point of the study was defined as sustained viral response (SVR) by intention-to-treat analysis. Patient charts were analyzed regarding demographics, clinical data (stage of HIV infection; stage of liver fibrosis; therapy regimes and duration; reasons for treatment discontinuation; response to treatment; side effects) as well as laboratory measures such as: HCV genotype; HCV RNA at different time points; HIV RNA; CD4+ T cell count and CD4+/CD8+ ratio at baseline. An assessment of Il28B polymorphisms was not routinely performed

Table 1 Baseline characteristics of patient cohort

Characteristics	Group A: HCV/HIV co-infected patients	Group B: HCV mono-infected patients	p-values
Patients, n	88	84	0.666
Age (y), mean (min./max.)	45 (26/64)	45 (20/72)	0.763
Sex, male/female (%)	66/22 (75/25)	52/32 (61/38)	0.092
Genotype, n (%)			
1	37/88 (42)	49/84 (58)	0.033
2	3/88 (3)	9/84 (10)	0.060
3	25/88 (28)	15/84 (17)	0.102
4	2/88 (2)	5/84 (5)	0.222
Unknwon	21/88 (23)	6/84 (7)	0.003
Liver biopsy, n (%)	17/88 (19)	36/84 (42)	0.001
Fibrosis F3 – F4, n (%)	6/17 (35)	10/36 (27)	0.251
HCV RNA in IU/ml, mean	4 714 165	3 453 862	0.487
(min./max.)	($3/9 \times 10^7$)	($3/3 \times 10^7$)	
HCV RNA > 800 000, n (%)	66/88 (75)	32/84 (38)	0.001
HCV RNA < 800 000, n (%)	22/88 (25)	52/84 (61)	0.001
Alanine transaminase in U/l, mean (min./max.)	78 (3/525)	105 (15/610)	0.098
Start of heptitis C therapy, n (%)	36 (40)	52 (61)	0.006
Liver biopsy, n (%)	10 (27)	27 (51)	0.024
(Fibrosis F3 – F4, n (%)	5 (13)	8 (29)	0.846
HCV RNA in IU/ml, mean	4 799 700	3 222 000	0.530
(min./max.)	($800/9 \times 10^7$)	($3/2 \times 10^7$)	
HCV RNA > 800 000, n (%)	12 (33)	21 (40)	0.502
HCV RNA < 800 000, n (%)	24 (66)	31 (59)	0.502
Alanine transaminase in U/l, mean (min./max.)	94 (29/526)	120 (18/610)	0.321
Duration of therapy in weeks, mean (min./max.)	33 (1/152)	36 (10/128)	0.496
Ribavirin (weight adapted) in mg/week, mean	5764,28	7567,2	0.027
Peg-Interferon-alfa 2a, n (%)	27/36 (75)	41/52 (78)	0.672
Peg-Interferon-alfa 2b, n (%)	0/36 (0)	3/52 (5)	0.143
Non-peg-Interferon, n (%)	3/36 (8)	0/52 (0)	0.034

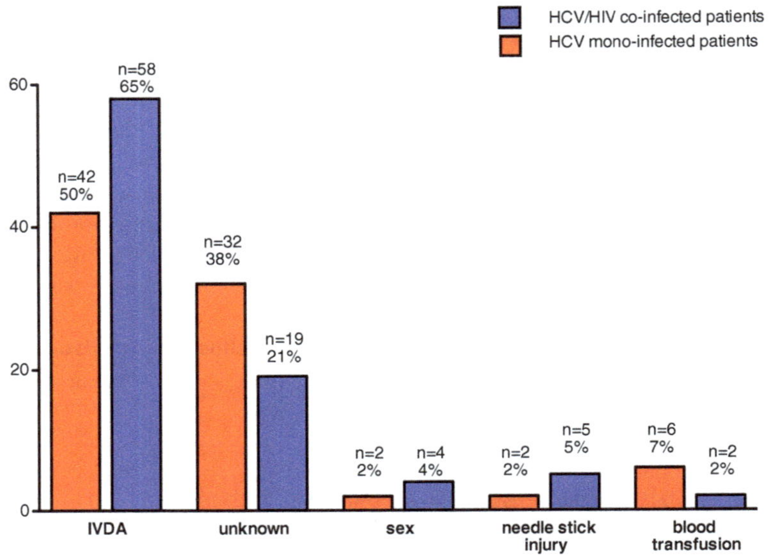

Figure 1 Mode of transmission of hepatitis C Infection.

during this time period as a standard of care procedure [21]. Hemoglobin levels of both groups were compared at different time points to identify the correlation between treatment response and ribavirin dosage as well as to understand whether co-infected patients have a higher risk of developing anemia under HCV therapy [22].

Definitions

SVR was defined as an undetectable HCV RNA, 24 weeks after end of treatment. A rapid virologic response (RVR), defined as an undetectable HCV RNA at week 4 of HCV treatment, and early virologic response (EVR), defined as an undetectable HCV-RNA or ≥2 log reduction of HCV-RNA at week 12 of HCV treatment compared to the baseline viral level. A virologic relapse was defined, if HCV RNA decreased and remained below the limit of detection (<50 IU/mL) during treatment but became detectable after end of treatment. Virologic non-response was defined as RNA level HCV RNA level above the limit of detection throughout treatment or a less than 2 $\log_{10}$ decline in

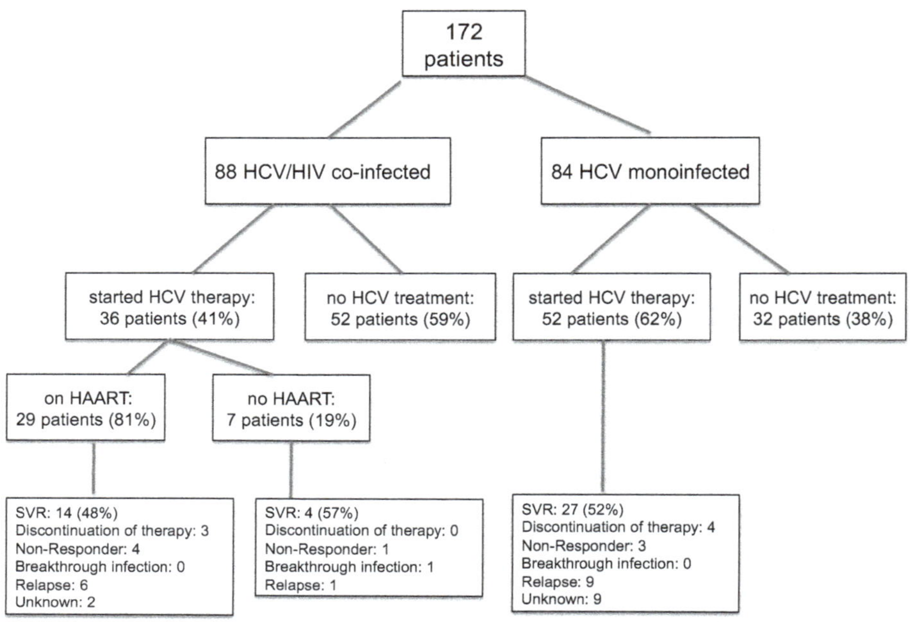

Figure 2 Enrollment, treatment allocation, and follow-up of study participants.

Table 2 Response to HCV therapy

Response to HCV therapy	Group A: HCV/HIV co-infected patients	Group B: HCV mono-infected patients	p-values
SVR all, n (%)	18/36 (50)	27/52 (52)	0.860
RVR, n (%)	9/36 (25)	17/52 (32)	0.440
EVR, n (%)	6/36 (17)	7/52 (13)	0.677
SVR GT 1, n (%)	5/15 (33)	11/27 (40)	0.626
SVR GT 2, n (%)	1/2 (50)	7/8 (87)	0.356
SVR GT 3, n (%)	9/14 (64)	7/12 (58)	0.756
SVR GT 4, n (%)	1/1 (100)	2/4 (50)	0.600
GT unknown, n (%)	2/36 (5)	0/52 (0)	0.809
SVR GT 1 + 4, n (%)	6/16 (37)	13/31 (41)	0.770
SVR GT 2 + 3, n (%)	10/16 (62)	14/20 (70)	0.636
Discontinuation of therapy, n (%)	3/36 (12)	4/52 (7)	0.305
Breakthrough infection, n (%)	1/36 (2)	0/52	0.410
Non-response, n (%)	5/36 (13)	3/52 (5)	0.130
Relapse, n (%)	7/36 (19)	9/52 (17)	0.482
Unknown, n (%)	2/36 (5)	9/52 (17)	0.105
SVR HAART treated patients, n (%)	14/29 (48)	n.a.	n.a.
SVR non-HAART treated patients, n (%)	4/7 (57)	n.a.	n.a.
SVR CD4 Nadir > 200/µl, n (%)	9/18 (50)	n.a.	n.a.
SVR CD4 Nadir < 200/µl, n (%)	9/18 (50)	n.a.	n.a.

HCV RNA from baseline until week 12. The stage of HIV infection was defined according to the Center of Disease Control (CDC) – classification, version 1993 [23].

Statistical analysis

Continuous variables are presented as the mean and standard deviation and categorical parameters are shown as the median and range. The x^2 test and Mann-Withney *U* test were used for analysis of categorical data and of continuous data, respectively. A p value <*0.05* was considered to denote statistical significance. Multiple regression analysis was performed to identify co-variables that might have independently impacted the start of hepatitis C treatment.

Results

Here, we present treatment results of an unsponsored, single-center study of a German cohort of HIV-negative and HIV-infected patients with chronic HCV infection.

We analyzed a total number of 172 treatment-naïve patients with chronic hepatitis C (genotype 1-4) infection. 88 patients were HIV/HCV co-infected (group A), 84 patients were HCV mono-infected (group B) (Table 1).

There were no significant differences or relative shifts of the demographics or genotype distributions.

In both groups rates of advanced fibrosis were low (Fibrosis F3 – F4, n (%): 6 (35) versus 10 (27), p = 0.251), however relative fewer liver biopsies were performed in co-infected patients (p < 0.001) (Table 1). While the mean viral load were similar in both groups, more patients with co-infection (n = 66, 75%) had high viral loads (>800 000 IU/ml) than mono-infected patients (n = 32, 38%) (p < 0.001).

The reported mode of HCV transmission did not differ between groups, with IVDU being the greatest risk factor (Figure 1). The probable mode of HCV transmission was not reported in more patients with mono-infection than co-infection (38% versus 21%) (Table 1).

A total of 36 (40%) HCV/HIV co-infected patients started anti-HCV therapy with standard combination treatment regimen with either PEG-IFN alpha 2a or PEG-IFN alpha 2b (weight adapted) for 48 weeks (genotype 1 and 4) or 24 weeks (genotypes 2 and 3) and weight-adapted ribavirin doses of 800-1400 mg, respectively, compared to n = 52 (61%) of mono-infected patients (p = 0.006). Figure 2 summarizes the allocation of treatment and follow-up.

The safety and tolerability of HCV treatment was generally good in both groups and there were no significant differences in discontinuation of therapy. However, only 2/36 (5%) co-infected patients but 9/52 (17%) mono-infected patients were lost to follow-up (p = 0.105).

Overall, SVR rates were comparable in both groups (group A: 18/36 [50%]; group B: 27/52 [52%] (p = 0.859, ns) (Table 2). There were also no differences detected for any of the genotypes (GT) 1 through 4 (GT1: 5/15 [33%] versus 11/27 [40%], GT2 1/2 [50%] versus 7/8 [87%], GT3 9/14 [64%] versus 7/12 [58%], GT4 1/1 [100%] versus 2/4 [50%]). Notably, we neither observed any significant differences of the early virologic response rates, the relapse rates nor differences of the rate of side effects in either group (Table 2). Of note, ART-naïve patients had similar SVR rates compared with those of ART-treated patients (48% versus 57%, respectively). SVR rates were identical for HIV-positive patients with nadir CD4+ T cell counts of 200/µl and above compared to those under 200/µl (Table 2). However, the numbers in these subgroups were too low to conduct a valid statistical analysis.

We did not find differences in the SVR rates over time in patients treated in the first half in comparison to the second half of the decade (data not shown).

The decrease of hemoglobin levels showed no significant differences during the treatment course in both groups (Figure 3). However, group A received a lower cumulated

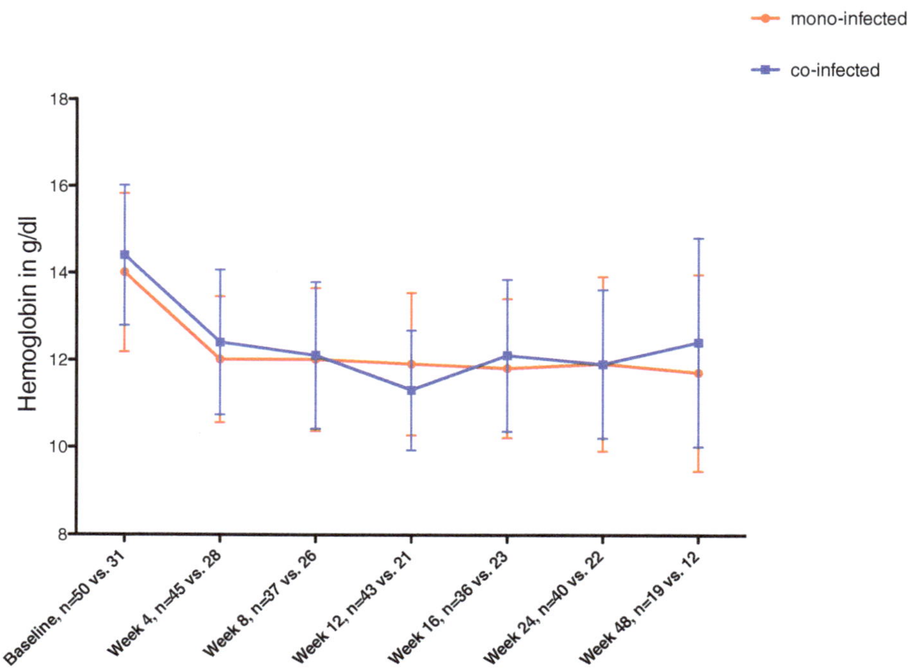

Figure 3 Hemoglobin levels in g/dl of mono-infected (red) versus co-infected (blue) patients during the course of anti-HCV treatment.

dose of weight-adapted ribavirin than group B (5764,2 mg/week versus 7567,2 mg/week; p = 0,027).

We also compared the demographic and clinical characteristics of the mono and co-infected patients who received treatment or were not treated (Tables 3 and 4). Surprisingly, there were few differences between these groups. Indeed, for the mono-infected patients, there was not a single characteristic significantly different (Table 4).

In the group of co-infected patients, there were also few differences between the patients who were treated versus treatment naïve patients. In the univariate analysis advanced age (p = 0.04), high CD4+ T cell counts (absolute p < 0.001, relative p = 0.001), a higher mean CD4+/CD8+ ratio (p = 0.001), lower HIV RNA levels (p = 0.015) and thus a CDC classification A1 – A3 (p = 0.005), were associated with the start of HCV treatment in the group of co-infected patients (Table 3). However, multiple regression analysis could not confirm any of those variables as independent predictors for the initiation of HCV treatment in both groups (data not shown).

80% (n = 29) of the co-infected patients receiving anti-HCV treatment were on concurrent HAART. In contrast, none of the HCV untreated patients with HIV/HCV co-infection were on concurrent HAART.

Discussion

Due to the enhanced risk of rapid progression of liver disease, higher incidence of liver-related complications and higher overall mortality, it is recommended that every HIV/HCV co-infected patient should be evaluated for early HCV treatment [4]. In the present study, we evaluated the treatment decisions and clinical course of HCV/HIV co-infected patients in a real-life treatment setting in a large Northern German university-based cohort in direct comparison to an unselected group of unmatched mono-infected patients treated by the same group of providers.

The first surprising finding is that overall treatment was initiated in only half (88/172) of patients in the entire cohort. Overall SVR was achieved in only 45/88 (51%) of these patients regardless of HIV co-infection status. Our results are in agreement with the results of studies from different parts of the world that show that only a small proportion of the total HCV infected patient population is subjected to treatment and even less are successfully treated [24]. Extrapolating this low number of total successful treatment initiation would have enormous public health consequences [25-27].

This situation might be even worse given the more rapid progression to end stage liver disease in patients co-infected with HCV and HIV [1]. In our current cohort analysis the baseline characteristics of the mono- and co-infected patients with HCV did not differ with regard to stage and severity of liver disease with most patients (group A n = 11; 65% versus group B n = 26; 72%) displaying an early stage of disease (Fibrosis F1- F2). We observed an overall SVR rate of 50% for all genotypes in group A, which is comparable to SVR rates found in randomized clinical trials of peg-INF and ribavirin in

Table 3 Baseline characteristics of HCV/HIV co-infected patients (HCV treated versus untreated)

Characteristics	Group A: HCV/HIV co-infected patients, treated (n = 36)	Group B: HCV/HIV co-infected patients, untreated (n = 52)	p-values
Age, mean (min./max.)	47 (26/64)	45 (27/51)	0.040
Sex, male/female (%)	26/10 (72/28)	40/12 (77/23)	0.617
Genotype, n (%)			
1	15 (42)	22 (42)	0.952
2	2 (6)	1 (2)	0.356
3	14 (39)	11 (21)	0.070
4	1 (2)	1 (2)	0.791
Unknown	4 (11)	17 (33)	0.020
Transmission of HCV, n (%)			
IVDU	21 (58)	37 (71)	0.212
Transfusion	4 (11)	3 (6)	0.363
Needlestick injury	0 (0)	0 (0)	n.a.
Tatoo	0 (0)	0 (0)	n.a.
Sex	1 (3)	3 (6)	0.508
Unknown	10 (28)	9 (17)	0.241
CDC Classification, n (%)			
A1 – A3	13 (36)	10 (19)	0.005
B1 – B3	9 (25)	7 (13)	0.168
C1 – C3	9 (25)	22(42)	0.059
Unknown	5 (13)	14 (25)	0.144
Liver biopsy, n (%)	7/36 (19)	5/52 (9)	0.186
Fibrosis F3 – F4, n (%)	5/7 (71)	1/5 (20)	0.029
HCV RNA in IU/ml, mean (min./max.)	4800 000 (800/9 × 10^7)	4 713 000 (3/6 × 10^7)	0.965
CD4 Count absolute, mean	553,1	396,73	0.001
CD4 Count > 200/μl, n (%)	25 (69)	21 (40)	0.007
CD4 Count < 200/μl, n	2 (3,5)	16 (30)	0.004
CD4 Count unknown, n (%)	7 (19)	15 (28)	0.317
CD4 Count relative, mean	27,9	22,2	0.001
CD4 Nadir in cells/μl, mean	208	194	0.689
CD4/CD8 Ratio, mean	0,67	0,49	0.001
HIV RNA in copy/ml, mean (minimum/maximum)	9 850 (3/16 × 10^4)	71 180 (3/12 × 10^5)	0.015
HIV Treatment, n (%)	29 (36)	0 (0)	n.a.
NRTI, n (%)	20/29 (68)	n.a	n.a.
NNRTI, n (%)	18/29 (62)	n.a	n.a.
PI, n (%)	12/29 (41)	n.a	n.a.
Intregrase Inh., n (%)	2/29 (6)	n.a.	n.a.
Entry Inh., n (%)	0 (0)	n.a.	n.a.

HCV/HIV co-infected patients (27% to 40%) [11,12,28]. However, the SVR rates in mono-infected patients (52%) are slightly lower than those reported by a real-life cohort study of mono-infected patients treated by gastroenterologists at the same institution in the same time span (60,9%) [7]. The reasons for these differences are not clear, but we have to keep in mind that the ID clinic is attending for international patients, who might have different IL-28 haplotypes [7]. Also, it has to be noted that 9/84 of the mono-infected patients were lost to follow-up.

The majority of patients received PEG interferon alpha 2a [29], three patients who were treated early in 2000

Table 4 Baseline characteristics of HCV mono-infected patients (HCV treated versus untreated)

Characteristics	Group A: HCV mono-infected patients, treated (n = 52)	Group B: HCV mono-infected patients, untreated (n = 32)	p-values
Age, mean (min./max.)	44 (22/65)	48 (20/72)	0.112
Sex, male/female (%)	34/18 (65/35)	17/15 (53/47)	0.264
Genotype, n (%)			
1	27 (52)	22 (69)	0.129
2	8 (15)	1 (3)	0.078
3	12 (23)	3 (9)	0.111
4	4 (8)	1 (3)	0.390
Unknown	1 (2)	5 (16)	0.018
Transmission, n (%)			
IVDU	28 (54)	14 (44)	0.369
Transfusion	2 (4)	4 (13)	0.135
Needlestick injury	2 (4)	1 (3)	0.863
Tatoo	2 (4)	0 (0)	0.262
Unknown	18 (35)	13 (41)	0.579
HCV RNA in IU/ml, mean (min./max.)	3 222 000 ($3/2 \times 10^7$)	3 810 000 ($3/3 \times 10^7$)	0.698
Liver biopsy, n (%)	27/52 (51)	9/32 (28)	0.032
Fibrosis F3 – F4, n (%)	8/27 (29)	2/9 (22)	0.209

still received conventional non-pegylated interferon. New direct-acting antiviral agents for hepatitis C genotype 1 infection, such as boceprevir, telaprevir or simeprevir as well as sofosbuvir [17,18,30,31], were not approved yet during the analysed timeperiod.

Despite the satisfactory outcome and an acceptable safety profile, hepatitis C therapy was overall only initiated in half of the patients and even less frequently initiated in HCV/HIV co-infected patients than in HCV mono-infected patients (40% vs. 62%) (p = 0.006) despite the lack of an absolute contraindication according to the chart review in the majority of patients. Reiberger et al. [24] previously also reported a considerable undertreatment of chronic HCV infection in HCV/HIV co-infected patients in a large multicenter study. While our retrospective mono-center study has many limitations that we are aware of, it resembles a "real-life" setting allowing for an evaluation of attitudes towards HCV treatment initiation of the same infectious disease specialists in mono- versus co-infected HCV patients. In our cohort HCV/HIV co-infected patients received less frequently HCV treatment compared to HCV mono-infected patients (p = 0.006) despite being seen by the same specialized ID staff.

Further studies have to look into the reasons of treatment deferral that could range from a potential contra-indication to interferon treatment like depression, anemia or other psychiatric illnesses, or possible objections against treatment initiation because of suspected non adherence and fears from the (co-infected) patient's perspective, as well as relative lower motivation to initiate treatment from the provider perspective because of the fear of inducing severe side effects or the (assumed) lower SVR rates in co-infected patients [32]. Anecdotally, when confronted with the results of the current study the treating ID specialists were surprised by the high SVR rates seen in co-infected patients -especially for the patients that were not on HAART or with lower CD4+ T cell counts. In a follow up study we plan to assess the provider and patient attitudes towards HCV treatment in mono versus co-infected patients by using standardized questionnaires to better understand the barriers to treatment initiation.

Interestingly, in the group of untreated co-infected patients, all patients were HAART naïve. While deferral of HAART treatment might be an indicator for problems of adherence, it is still interesting that only a minority of patients without concurrent HAART regimes received HCV therapy and these patients showed excellent SVR rates. Although guidelines generally recommend selecting patients for HCV treatment whose CD4+ T cell count is high, no study of pegylated interferon plus ribavirin has shown a significant association between CD4+ T cell count less than 350/μl at treatment initiation and SVR to date [33,34]. However, the notion that HCV treatment should only be performed in patients who are on concurrent HAART is a very strong held belief and might be a potential barrier for initiating HCV treatment in HIV co-infection.

Despite comparable rates of development of anemia, HCV/HIV co-infected patients received less ribavirin than mono-infected patients during the course of treatment (5764,3 mg/week versus 7567,2 mg/week; p = 0.027), which may have contributed to the slightly lower SVR rates in co-infected patients (50% versus 52%) [12,15].

It seems that treating physicians are more reluctant to use appropriate weight adapted ribavirin dosages in HCV patients co-infected with HIV. However, this treatment pattern was not warranted since baseline hemoglobin levels were comparable in both patient groups (group A: 14,6 g/dl versus group B: 14,5 g/dl) (Figure 3).

In our analysis, HCV treatment was only initiated in half of the patients of the entire cohort at a University based Infectious Diseases Center. Extrapolating these results for Germany, and taking into account the large proportion of patients who statistically do not clear HCV even after one or several courses of therapy is considered, a great number of HIV/HCV co-infected patients are still in need of efficient antiviral treatment even after one decade of dual combination therapy. Altogether greater efforts to understand and potentially to remove the (provider as well as patient) barriers to evaluation and treatment that still exist for a great proportion of patients have to be undertaken [19,27].

Limitations to our study include the relatively small number of patients, its retrospective design and an unequal proportion of men and women in the study population. For similar reasons we also abstained from performing more elaborate statistical tests like multivariate analysis.

The lack of data on IL28B genotypes is another limitation to the study. A recent study at our center in mono-infected patients showed that our center attends only a small number of patients with Asian or African origin and approximately 20% of patients show a CC haplotype, 60% a C/T haplotype and 20% the T/T haplotype (unpublished data). We would assume similar proportions of Il28B haplotypes in our co-infected patients, however cannot exclude the possibility of higher rates of patients with a T/T haplotype as discussed above.

We conclude that overall HCV treatment was only initiated in half of the cohort and even in a smaller proportion of HCV/HIV co-infected patients despite satisfactory outcome and similar baseline characteristics. In the light of newer treatment options [17,18,30,31], greater efforts to understand the barriers to treatment that still exist for a great proportion of patients have to be undertaken especially in patients co-infected with both viruses. Additionally, further efforts have to be undertaken to implement the national and international HIV and HCV guidelines to real life practice. Larger prospective studies are needed to confirm our findings in view of newer treatment option including directly acting antivirals (DAA) for HCV infection.

Competing interest

The authors declare that they have no competing interests.

Authors' contribution

The work presented here was carried out in collaboration between all authors. JvL and JSzW defined the research theme. CB, MH, JSzW, JvL conceived and designed the study. CB, MH, JJ, JSzW and JvL analyzed the data and interpreted the results. CB and JSzW wrote the first draft. JvL gave important input to the manuscript. BO performed the statistical analysis. SS, SH, OD and SL were involved in patient treatment and patient follow-up. All authors read and approved the final manuscript.

Acknowledgements

We thank the patients for participating in this study. JvL, JSzW and CB get funding by the "Deutsches Zentrum für Infektionsforschung (DZIF)". CB also got funding by the "Deutsche Leberstiftung". JSzW is funded by the DFG (SFB841, A6).

References

1. Rosenthal E, Pialoux G, Bernard N, Pradier C, Rey D, Bentata M, Michelet C, Pol S, Perronne C, Cacoub P: **Liver-related mortality in human-immunodeficiency-virus-infected patients between 1995 and 2003 in the French GERMIVIC Joint Study Group Network (MORTAVIC 2003 Study).** *J Viral Hepat* 2007, **14**:183–188.
2. Bica I, McGovern B, Dhar R, Stone D, McGowan K, Scheib R, Snydman DR: **Increasing mortality due to end-stage liver disease in patients with human immunodeficiency virus infection.** *Clin Infect Dis* 2001, **32**:492–497.
3. Poynard T, Mathurin P, Lai CL, Guyader D, Poupon R, Tainturier MH, Myers RP, Muntenau M, Ratziu V, Manns M, Vogel A, Capron F, Chedid A, Bedossa P: **A comparison of fibrosis progression in chronic liver diseases.** *J Hepatol* 2003, **38**:257–265.
4. Berenguer J, Alvarez-Pellicer J, Martin PM, Lopez-Aldeguer J, Von-Wichmann MA, Quereda C, Mallolas J, Sanz J, Tural C, Bellon JM, Gonzalez-Garcia J: **Sustained virological response to interferon plus ribavirin reduces liver-related complications and mortality in patients coinfected with human immunodeficiency virus and hepatitis C virus.** *Hepatology* 2009, **50**:407–413.
5. Lindh M, Arnholm B, Eilard A, Farkkila M, Hellstrand K, Lagging M, Langeland N, Morch K, Nilsson S, Pedersen C, Buhl MR, Wahlberg T, Wejstal R, Westin J, Norkrans G: **Hepatitis C treatment response kinetics and impact of baseline predictors.** *J Viral Hepat* 2011, **18**:400–407.
6. Kau A, Vermehren J, Sarrazin C: **Treatment predictors of a sustained virologic response in hepatitis B and C.** *J Hepatol* 2008, **49**:634–651.
7. Schulze Zur Wiesch J, Pudelski N, Hoepner L, Supplieth M, Buggisch P, Lohse AW, Luth S: **"Real-Life" comparison of pegylated-interferon 2a versus 2b combination therapy of chronic hepatitis C virus.** *Hepatology* 2011, **53**:1405–1406. author reply 1407.
8. Hadziyannis SJ, Sette H Jr, Morgan TR, Balan V, Diago M, Marcellin P, Ramadori G, Bodenheimer H Jr, Bernstein D, Rizzetto M, Zeuzem S, Pockros PJ, Lin A, Ackrill AM: **Peginterferon-alpha2a and ribavirin combination therapy in chronic hepatitis C: a randomized study of treatment duration and ribavirin dose.** *Ann Intern Med* 2004, **140**:346–355.
9. Manns MP, McHutchison JG, Gordon SC, Rustgi VK, Shiffman M, Reindollar R, Goodman ZD, Koury K, Ling M, Albrecht JK: **Peginterferon alfa-2b plus ribavirin compared with interferon alfa-2b plus ribavirin for initial treatment of chronic hepatitis C: a randomised trial.** *Lancet* 2001, **358**:958–965.
10. Shire NJ, Welge JA, Sherman KE: **Response rates to pegylated interferon and ribavirin in HCV/HIV coinfection: a research synthesis.** *J Viral Hepat* 2007, **14**:239–248.
11. Chung RT, Andersen J, Volberding P, Robbins GK, Liu T, Sherman KE, Peters MG, Koziel MJ, Bhan AK, Alston B, Colquhoun D, Nevin T, Harb G, van der Horst C: **Peginterferon Alfa-2a plus ribavirin versus interferon alfa-2a plus ribavirin for chronic hepatitis C in HIV-coinfected persons.** *N Engl J Med* 2004, **351**:451–459.
12. Torriani FJ, Rodriguez-Torres M, Rockstroh JK, Lissen E, Gonzalez-Garcia J, Lazzarin A, Carosi G, Sasadeusz J, Katlama C, Montaner J, Sette H, Jr Passe S, De Pamphilis J, Duff F, Schrenk UM, Dieterich DT: **Peginterferon Alfa-2a plus ribavirin for chronic hepatitis C virus infection in HIV-infected patients.** *N Engl J Med* 2004, **351**:438–450.
13. Nunez M, Marino A, Miralles C, Berdun MA, Sola J, Hernandez-Burruezo JJ, Galindo MJ, Barreiro P, Martin-Carbonero L, Soriano V: **Baseline serum hepatitis C virus (HCV) RNA level and response at week 4 are the best predictors of relapse after treatment with pegylated interferon plus ribavirin in HIV/HCV-coinfected patients.** *J Acquir Immune Defic Syndr* 2007, **45**:439–444.
14. Jalali Z, Rockstroh JK: **Antiviral drugs and the treatment of hepatitis C.** *Curr HIV/AIDS Rep* 2012, **9**:132–138.
15. Vogel M, Ahlenstiel G, Hintsche B, Fenske S, Trein A, Lutz T, Schurmann D, Stephan C, Khaykin P, Bickel M, Mayr C, Baumgarten A, Buggisch P, Klinker H, John C, Golz J, Staszewski S, Rockstroh JK: **The influence of HAART on the efficacy and safety of pegylated interferon and ribavirin therapy for the treatment of chronic HCV infection in HIV-positive Individuals.** *Eur J Med Res* 2010, **15**:102–111.
16. Sulkowski MS: **HCV therapy in HIV-infected patients.** *Liver Int* 2013, **33**(Suppl 1):63–67.
17. Manns MP, von Hahn T: **Novel therapies for hepatitis C - one pill fits all?** *Nat Rev Drug Discov* 2013, **12**:595–610.
18. Sulkowski MS, Rodriguez-Torres M, Lalezari J, Fessel WJ, Mounzer K, Shuhart M: **All-Oral Therapy With Sofosbuvir Plus Ribavirin For the Treatment of HCV Genotype 1, 2, and 3 Infection in Patients Co-infected With HIV (PHOTON-1).** *Hepatology* 2013, **58**(suppl):313A.
19. Grint D, Peters L, Schwarze-Zander C, Beniowski M, Pradier C, Battegay M, Jevtovic D, Soriano V, Lundgren J, Rockstroh J, Kirk O, Mocroft A: **Temporal**

changes and regional differences in treatment uptake of hepatitis C therapy in EuroSIDA. *HIV Med* 2013, **14**(10):614–623.
20. Fleming CA, Tumilty S, Murray JE, Nunes D: **Challenges in the treatment of patients coinfected with HIV and hepatitis C virus: need for team care.** *Clin Infect Dis* 2005, **40**(Suppl 5):S349–S354.
21. Ge D, Fellay J, Thompson AJ, Simon JS, Shianna KV, Urban TJ, Heinzen EL, Qiu P, Bertelsen AH, Muir AJ, Sulkowski M, McHutchison JG, Goldstein DB: **Genetic variation in IL28B predicts hepatitis C treatment-induced viral clearance.** *Nature* 2009, **461**:399–401.
22. Sulkowski MS, Wasserman R, Brooks L, Ball L, Gish R: **Changes in haemoglobin during interferon alpha-2b plus ribavirin combination therapy for chronic hepatitis C virus infection.** *J Viral Hepat* 2004, **11**:243–250.
23. **AIDS definition update by CDC.** *Am Fam Physician* 1993, **47**:265.
24. Reiberger T, Obermeier M, Payer BA, Baumgarten A, Weitner L, Moll A, Christensen S, Koppe S, Kundi M, Rieger A, Peck-Radosavljevic M: **Considerable under-treatment of chronic HCV infection in HIV patients despite acceptable sustained virological response rates in a real-life setting.** *Antivir Ther* 2011, **16**:815–824.
25. Blackard JT, Sherman KE: **HCV/HIV co-infection: time to re-evaluate the role of HIV in the liver?** *J Viral Hepat* 2008, **15**:323–330.
26. Soriano V, Sulkowski M, Bergin C, Hatzakis A, Cacoub P, Katlama C, Cargnel A, Mauss S, Dieterich D, Moreno S, Ferrari C, Poynard T, Rockstroh J: **Care of patients with chronic hepatitis C and HIV co-infection: recommendations from the HIV-HCV International Panel.** *AIDS* 2002, **16**:813–828.
27. McGowan CE, Monis A, Bacon BR, Mallolas J, Goncales FL, Goulis I, Poordad F, Afdhal N, Zeuzem S, Piratvisuth T, Marcellin P, Fried MW: **A global view of hepatitis C: Physician knowledge, opinions, and perceived barriers to care.** *Hepatology* 2013, **57**(4):1325–1332.
28. Carrat F, Bani-Sadr F, Pol S, Rosenthal E, Lunel-Fabiani F, Benzekri A, Morand P, Goujard C, Pialoux G, Piroth L, Salmon-Ceron D, Degott C, Cacoub P, Perronne C: **Pegylated interferon alfa-2b vs standard interferon alfa-2b, plus ribavirin, for chronic hepatitis C in HIV-infected patients: a randomized controlled trial.** *JAMA* 2004, **292**:2839–2848.
29. Schulze Zur Wiesch J, Lohse AW: **Results of the IDEAL trial: "Mirror, mirror on the wall … which's the fairest peg-interferon of them all?"** *Hepatology* 2009, **50**:2034–2037.
30. Jacobson IM, McHutchison JG, Dusheiko G, Di Bisceglie AM, Reddy KR, Bzowej NH, Marcellin P, Muir AJ, Ferenci P, Flisiak R, George J, Rizzetto M, Shouval D, Sola R, Terg RA, Yoshida EM, Adda N, Bengtsson L, Sankoh AJ, Kieffer TL, George S, Kauffman RS, Zeuzem S: **Telaprevir for previously untreated chronic hepatitis C virus infection.** *N Engl J Med* 2011, **364**:2405–2416.
31. Poordad F, McCone J Jr, Bacon BR, Bruno S, Manns MP, Sulkowski MS, Jacobson IM, Reddy KR, Goodman ZD, Boparai N, DiNubile MJ, Sniukiene V, Brass CA, Albrecht JK, Bronowicki JP: **Boceprevir for untreated chronic HCV genotype 1 infection.** *N Engl J Med* 2011, **364**:1195–1206.
32. Soriano V, Puoti M, Sulkowski M, Cargnel A, Benhamou Y, Peters M, Mauss S, Brau N, Hatzakis A, Pol S, Rockstroh J: **Care of patients coinfected with HIV and hepatitis C virus: 2007 updated recommendations from the HCV-HIV International Panel.** *AIDS* 2007, **21**:1073–1089.
33. Valerio L, Yazdanpanah Y, Poizot-Martin I, Rosenthal E, Marimoutou C, Gastaut JA, Tran A, Dellamonica P, Freedberg KA, Pradier C: **Baseline CD4 cell count and outcome of pegylated interferon plus ribavirin therapy in HIV/hepatitis C virus-coinfected patients.** *J Acquir Immune Defic Syndr* 2008, **47**:50–55.
34. Sulowski M: **Hepatitis C virus-human immunodeficiency virus coinfection.** *Liver Int* 2012, **32**(Suppl 1):129–134.

13

HIV testing practices among New England college health centers

Nilay Patel, Aadia Rana, Alyssa Thomas, John C Barnhart, Timothy P Flanigan, Jacob J van den Berg and Philip A Chan*

Abstract

Background: The prevalence of human immunodeficiency virus (HIV) continues to increase among certain populations including young men who have sex with men (MSM). College campuses represent a potential setting to engage young adults and institute prevention interventions including HIV testing. The purpose of this study was to evaluate testing practices for HIV and other sexually transmitted infections (STIs) on college campuses.

Methods: Medical directors at four-year residential baccalaureate college health centers in New England were surveyed from June, 2011 to September, 2011. Thirty-one interviews were completed regarding experiences with HIV testing, acute HIV infection, other STI testing, and outreach efforts targeting specific at-risk groups such as MSM.

Results: Among schools that responded to the survey, less than five percent of students were tested for HIV at their local college health center in the past academic year (2010–2011). Significant barriers to HIV testing included cost and availability of rapid antibody testing. One-third of college health medical directors reported that their practitioners may not feel comfortable recognizing acute HIV infection.

Conclusions: Improved HIV testing practices are needed on college campuses. Programs should focus on outreach efforts targeting MSM and other at-risk populations.

Keywords: HIV, College, STI, Prevention

Background

The human immunodeficiency virus (HIV) epidemic has continued unabated in the United States with approximately 48,600 new cases per year, prompting a nationwide strategy to increase routine testing, identify new infections, and link HIV-infected individuals to care and treatment [1]. The Centers for Disease Control and Prevention (CDC) estimates that 34% of new HIV infections occurred in individuals aged 15–29 in 2009 [2]. When stratified by transmission category, greater than 60% of new cases of HIV were among men who have sex with men (MSM). While overall incidence has remained stable, HIV rates in those aged 13–29 increased by 21% from 2006 to 2009, with an even more disproportionate 48% increase among young, black MSM [3,4]. A similar epidemiology has been shown among syphilis, with 63% of new infections occurring in MSM and increasing rates in the 15–24 age group during 2004–2008. This suggests a rate of HIV and syphilis incidence that is at least 40 times greater in MSM than other risk groups and mainly in younger individuals [5].

In 2010, there were approximately 12.1 million full-time enrollees in 2,348 four-year colleges and universities throughout the United States [6]. This population is primarily comprised of adolescents and young adults, a group that offers unique challenges for HIV and syphilis prevention. Students are often characterized as being sexually active and having high-risk behaviors, such as multiple sexual partners and inconsistent condom use [7-11]. Students also tend to believe that they are at little to no risk of contracting HIV [12,13]. The age demographic and behaviors of college students place them at risk for infection with HIV and syphilis. Previous studies from colleges in the Southeastern United States demonstrated that a high percentage (>10%) of new infections were among college students [14,15]. These college students tended to be MSM and African American. Students

* Correspondence: PChan@lifespan.org
Alpert Medical School of Brown University, Division of Infectious Diseases, The Miriam Hospital, 1125 North Main Street, Providence, RI 02904, USA

at-risk for infection were found to have perceptions of low personal risk of HIV, believing that HIV dialogue may be detrimental to their relationships [16]. Despite these findings, there have been few public health efforts or follow-up studies to prevent further HIV transmission on college campuses.

In November of 2010, three new cases of acute/recent HIV infection were reported in college students in Rhode Island [17]. These cases, which were diagnosed at local college health centers, suggested there was ongoing transmission in the college community, specifically during the acute phase of HIV when antibody testing can be negative and the risk of transmission is increased [18]. At least one student specifically requested an HIV RNA test (viral load) when his antibody test was negative. Further evaluation of new HIV diagnoses in 2010 in our community revealed a high prevalence of academic students (17%) of which over 70% were MSM and most presented with acute or primary HIV infection (infection within the last six months) [17].

Acute HIV infection is the period of time from infection to the development of antibodies, which is generally two or three weeks but can be as long as several months. Approximately 50 to 80% of individuals with acute HIV infection present with non-specific flu-like symptoms. Standard HIV testing of the serum and oral saliva both involve testing for antibody formation. Thus, an individual with acute HIV infection may have a negative antibody test. Furthermore, acute HIV infection is often misdiagnosed as another viral illness [19]. Medical providers must have a high index of suspicion to diagnose acute HIV infection. The diagnosis is made by testing for HIV RNA (viral load) which must be run at specialized laboratories. Acute HIV infection may comprise a significant number of new infections which are missed by standard antibody tests [18,20].

The prevalence of HIV in the general college population was low in early epidemiological studies [21]. Given the current data suggesting increasing rates in younger populations, evaluation of current testing practices on college campuses is needed to address this shift in demographics. College health services serve as an important source for primary and preventative care for students. Effective HIV and sexually transmitted infection (STI) testing practices and education may prevent further infections both during the college years and later in life. To our knowledge, there is little current data regarding testing practices of HIV and other STIs on college campuses, experiences with acute HIV infection, and the approaches toward addressing sexual healthcare needs in MSM. These issues are critical in designing effective HIV and STI prevention programs on college campuses and addressing the growing epidemic of HIV among younger adults and MSM. This report describes a preliminary survey of college health services in New England regarding their experiences with HIV and STI testing.

Methods

We performed a cross-sectional survey via phone interview on HIV/STI testing practices during the 2010–2011 academic year. The interview was conducted with medical directors at New England college health centers during June to September of 2011. Our sample was restricted to New England's 4-year colleges with non-commuter campuses assuming these schools were more likely to have full-time student health centers with primary health and preventative care services. There were 130 schools that met our inclusion criteria. Characteristics of schools were compiled including size (based on full-time enrollment), private versus public, geographic location, urban versus non-urban, and religious affiliation. Quota sampling was used to identify a representative sample totaling 59 schools based on these characteristics. Recruitment e-mails and letters were sent to medical directors at selected schools. Health centers were subsequently contacted to ask if the medical director was willing to participate. Three attempts were made to contact each school by interviewers.

Categorical questions on the survey were based on the American College Health Association's (ACHA) annual Pap Test and STI Survey which has been extensively piloted in the college setting [8]. These included yes/no questions on whether HIV, syphilis, and other STI testing was offered at the student health center, whether written consent was required, if anonymous testing was available, or if an appointment was needed. Other categorical questions included cost of testing, mode of HIV testing (i.e. rapid versus serum), how results were reported, and how student health centers offer STI testing (routine, on request, specific groups such as MSM, clinical suspicion, etc.). The remaining questions were conducted in a qualitative manner and included open-ended questions about general HIV testing, acute HIV infection, other STI testing, and outreach efforts targeting MSM and other high-risk groups. Questions about gonorrhea and chlamydia were included as a reference to compare HIV and syphilis testing practices against. The study was submitted to the Brown University Institutional Review Board, which deemed it exempt from "human subjects research" as defined in Title 45 CFR Part 46.

Aggregate data was compiled from survey participants. Common themes were highlighted if two or more schools shared similar concerns or ideas in response to open-ended questions. Characteristics of college health centers (school size, private/public status, geographic location, urban/non-urban, and religious affiliation) and categorical response data was analyzed using Fisher's exact test to determine factors associated with HIV testing. Significance was defined as p-values less than 0.05.

Results

A total of 31 medical directors participated in this study (response rate of 52.5%). Among these schools, 58% (18/31) had a full-time enrollment of greater than 5,000 students and 74% (23/31) were private institutions (Table 1). A total of 16% (5/31) reported a religious affiliation, all of which was Catholic. Approximately 55% (17/31) were situated on a non-urban campus. All six states of New England were represented with 10 schools from Massachusetts, seven from Rhode Island, six from Connecticut, four from New Hampshire, three from Vermont, and one from Maine.

HIV testing

Over 90% (28/31) of schools provided some form of HIV antibody testing (Table 2). Among the 28 schools that offered HIV antibody testing, a total of 7,533 tests (Range: 1–1500) were performed during the 2010–2011 academic year. The total full-time enrollment of all participating schools that offered HIV antibody testing was 212,910 students, as reported by the National Center for Education Statistics [6]. This corresponds to a testing rate of 3.54% in the past academic year (95% CI: 3.46-3.62). More than half of health centers tested less than 2.5% of the total student body. During the 2010–2011 academic year, a total of four antibody tests were positive and subsequently confirmed for HIV.

Table 1 Characteristics of colleges and universities (N = 31)

≥ 5,000 students	58% (18/31)
< 5,000 students	42% (13/31)
Connecticut	19% (6/31)
Massachusetts	32% (10/31)
Maine	3% (1/31)
New Hampshire	13% (4/31)
Rhode Island	23% (7/31)
Vermont	10% (3/31)
Public	26% (8/31)
Private	74% (23/31)
Urban	45% (14/31)
Non-Urban	55% (17/31)
Religious Affiliation	16% (5/31)
Nonsectarian	84% (26/31)

Table 2 HIV testing practices at student health centers during the 2010–2011 academic year (N = 31)

HIV antibody testing offered	
Yes	90% (28/31)
No	10% (4/31)
Rapid HIV antibody testing offered	
Yes	38% (10/26)
No	62% (16/26)
Failure of students to receive results	
Never	53% (9/17)
Infrequently	41% (7/17)
Sometimes	6% (1/17)
Number of HIV tests	
Total	7537
Mean (n = 28)	269
Number of positive tests	
Total	4
Cost of HIV testing (no insurance)	
Mean	$26 ($12.50 - $65)
Median	$25
Written consent required	
Yes	43% (12/28)
No	57% (16/28)
Anonymous testing offered	
Yes	21% (6/28)
No	79% (22/28)
Appointment needed	
Yes	68% (19/28)
No	32% (9/28)
Post-exposure prophylaxis (PEP) available	
Yes	34% (10/29)
No	66% (19/29)
Comfortable with recognition of acute HIV infection	
Yes	71% (22/31)
No	29% (9/31)
Diagnosis of acute HIV infection (ever)	
Yes	16% (5/31)
No	84% (26/31)
Viral load testing available	
Yes	70% (21/30)
No	30% (9/30)

No schools had clear guidelines indicating which students should or should not be offered HIV antibody testing. No schools routinely tested all students or provided opt-out testing (practice that includes routine HIV testing unless individual specifically declines).

However, 96% (27/28) of schools which offered HIV antibody testing did so to any student who specifically asked to be tested. All schools offering HIV antibody testing provided testing if a healthcare provider suspected HIV based on clinical presentation or in cases of sexual assault. Most schools offered HIV antibody testing during routine women's health visits, specifically during gynecologic visits or visits to discuss contraception. Three-quarters of schools routinely tested MSM for HIV although many medical directors remarked that the decision about testing is primarily based on self-reported risk behaviors of the individual students.

Of schools that performed HIV antibody testing, 68% (19/28) required an appointment for testing, although nearly all of those requiring appointments stated same-day appointments were available if requested. Urban schools were more likely to require an appointment for HIV testing compared to non-urban schools (79%, 11/14 urban schools required an appointment versus 47%, 8/17 non-urban, p-value = 0.15). Additionally, 90% (25/28) of health centers only provided testing services at the on-campus health center or laboratory. The remaining schools provided either yearly or twice yearly testing at off-campus sites, mostly sponsored by the local campus health center. Written consent for HIV testing was required at one-third of colleges, many of which were in Massachusetts where it is required by state law. Other schools in Connecticut and New Hampshire required written consent as a school policy. Anonymous testing was available at 21% (6/28) of sites. With respect to the type of testing that was offered, 32% (10/31) of respondents stated that rapid antibody testing was available. Schools larger than 5,000 students tended to offer rapid testing more often than did smaller schools (44%, 8/18 schools larger than 5,000 students offered rapid testing versus 15%, 2/13 smaller schools, p-value = 0.18), while schools having a religious affiliation tended not to have rapid testing available compared to nonsectarian schools (0%, 0/5 religious schools offered rapid testing versus 38%, 10/26 nonsectarian schools, p-value = 0.24). Of those schools that did not provide rapid antibody testing, nearly all (91%, 16/18) required students to return to the health center for their results with only one school allowing students to receive results over the phone. Although nine schools did report at least one case of a student not returning for HIV test results during the 2010–2011 academic year, this was a rare occurrence. With respect to cost of testing, 14% (4/28) of schools provided free HIV antibody testing to all students, regardless of insurance status. All of the remaining schools offering testing stated that student insurance covered the cost of the associated appointment and testing but that there was co-pay ranging from $5 to $80. The mean out of pocket expense when not using insurance was $28.78 (median $25) for an HIV antibody test and $90.57 (median $48) for an STI panel covering chlamydia, gonorrhea, and syphilis.

The primary barriers to HIV testing identified by medical directors were financial including cost to students and lack of resources and support services to promote and offer testing. Other barriers included difficulty engaging students and having them present to the health center for testing, "complacent" attitudes about HIV testing, low risk perceptions for HIV infection, stigma, and structural barriers (need for appointments, lack of rapid testing).

Acute HIV infection

Seventy-one percent of medical directors stated their providers are comfortable with the recognition and diagnosis of acute HIV infection, although many directors described a need to provide further training regarding acute HIV infection on campus. Schools with a religious affiliation reported less comfort with the recognition and diagnosis of acute HIV infection when compared with nonsectarian schools (20%, 1/5 affiliated schools versus 81%, 21/26 nonsectarian, p-value < 0.05). A modest 16% (5/31) of schools reported ever diagnosing a case of acute HIV infection, with five schools over four different states in New England.. In total, 58% (18/31) of survey respondents stated their providers had received some training in the recognition and diagnosis of acute HIV infection. This training was primarily in the form of on-campus presentations from faculty at neighboring institutions and was reported as having occurred during training or residency or during in-service presentations more than five years ago. There was a particular need to train providers in differentiating which students needed testing immediately and those that could be safely observed.

Most respondents (67%, 21/31) stated their health center could perform HIV RNA testing for students for whom acute HIV infection was clinically suspected. Schools in urban settings were significantly more likely to offer HIV RNA (viral load) testing than those in non-urban settings (93%, 13/14 urban setting schools offered testing versus 47%, 8/17 non-urban, p-value = 0.02). Urban schools also tended to offer post-exposure prophylaxis (PEP) as compared with non-urban schools (50%, 7/14 urban schools offered PEP versus 18%, 3/17 non-urban, p-value = 0.13).

Testing for other sexually transmitted infections

Ninety-four percent (29/31) of student health centers performed testing for other STIs including gonorrhea, chlamydia and syphilis (Table 3). Ninety-seven percent (28/29) of schools that provided STI testing would perform testing on students who asked for it, who have been sexual assaulted, or when a specific STI was

Table 3 Sexually transmitted infection (STI) testing practices at student health centers (N = 31)

STI testing offered*	
Yes	94% (29/31)
No	6% (2/31)
Cost of STI testing	
Mean	$94 ($0-225)
Median	$56.50
Appointment needed	
Yes	69% (20/29)
No	31% (9/29)
Conduct outreach to high-risk groups	
Yes	71% (22/31)
No	29% (9/31)
Targeted educational resources for LGBT	
Yes	77% (24/31)
No	23% (7/31)
Training on LGBTQ healthcare	
Yes	74% (23/31)
No	26% (8/31)

*Includes gonorrhea, chlamydia, and syphilis testing.
LGBT = Lesbian, gay, bisexual, transgender.

clinically suspected. In contrast to HIV antibody testing, at least 25% (8/29) of schools had clear clinical guidelines about when to perform STI testing. A common example guideline included 'all women who receive Pap smears will have chlamydia and/or gonorrhea testing'. There was less of a consensus about routine testing in men and MSM for STIs. Approximately 62% (18/29) of schools routinely tested MSM for gonorrhea, chlamydia and syphilis, while the other schools tested based on clinical presentation or patient-generated requests.

Ninety-four percent (27/29) of student health centers performed STI testing on-campus and only one school provided urinary gonorrhea and chlamydia testing at a once-yearly, off-campus site. Similar to HIV, 69% (20/29) of schools required an appointment for STI testing. With respect to cost of testing, two schools provided free testing, while 94% (22/29) of schools provided appointments and testing that were covered by student insurance, with a co-pay ranging from $0 to $35.

Targeted outreach

Seventy-seven percent of college health centers had ever conducted training for providers about specific lesbian, gay, bisexual and transgender (LGBT) sexual healthcare needs. Topics included sensitivity training about transgender healthcare concerns, appropriateness of language used by providers in addressing LGBT students, and techniques for gathering a detailed sexual history from LGBT students. A number of directors commented that their training modules may be insufficient, noting there was a particular need to help train providers with sexual history gathering for all students and more specifically for LGBT students.

Seventy-seven percent of college health centers performed some form of targeted outreach to at-risk groups, specifically by reaching out to LGBT groups on their respective campuses. Fewer schools with a religious affiliation tended to conduct outreach compared to nonsectarian schools (40%, 2/5 affiliated schools conducted outreach to high-risk sexual groups versus 77%, 20/26 nonsectarian, p-value = 0.13). The majority of respondents reported that they either handed out brochures and pamphlets to these groups with targeted information, or delivered on-campus presentations about the need to get tested for HIV and STI testing and methods for practicing safer sex. Many health directors described a need for further outreach efforts as well, with at least two directors noting that while they had tried performing targeted outreach, their own efforts were "few and far between". Some individuals also commented that the targeted pamphlets they provide were outdated and weren't "appealing enough to be read by students".

While some providers recognized many LGBT students would benefit from testing more than once a year, they were unclear about which students required more frequent testing. Furthermore, a number of medical directors commented that it was difficult to identify the LGBT students on campus. This was particularly common at schools with a religious affiliation, which noted that perceptions that the health centers were unwelcoming made it difficult to provide targeted outreach efforts. In particular, health centers at religiously affiliated schools reported low HIV risk perception on campus, the inability to distribute condoms, and the inability to conduct sexual health outreach activities as a direct result of the religious affiliation. When asked about outreach to at-risk groups, one medical director responded, "we don't have a high MSM population, this being a Catholic institution," instead the director said the center "focused on inclusivity."

Discussion

HIV testing

Our results reveal that there is widespread undertesting of HIV on college campuses throughout New England. The cumulative testing rates were less than 5% which excludes the 18,303 students at participant schools where HIV testing is not offered. Despite these low testing rates, four cases of HIV were diagnosed at New England college health centers during the

2010–2011 academic year. This is a conservative estimate based on recall bias of the medical directors we interviewed. According to the revised CDC recommendations, HIV screening is recommended for all patients in an opt-out format, particularly in those individuals who have never been tested [22]. The CDC recommends repeat annual testing for those individuals who are at high-risk, including MSM and heterosexual persons who have had more than one sexual partner since their most recent HIV test. These guidelines suggest that college students should be tested at least once for HIV and in many cases annually. This is in contrast to the small minority of college students who report being tested for HIV at least once in their lives. Rates of HIV are increasing among younger MSM and these recommendations should be strongly encouraged on college campuses to ensure MSM participate in HIV testing campaigns.

College health services represent a unique venue to promote HIV testing among students, especially as students make visits to a college health center more than once annually on average. These centers also represent an opportunity to educate students about safe sexual and testing behaviors. Many medical directors commented that students and providers alike have become "complacent" about HIV on college campuses. Directors feel that students' reasons for being HIV tested have morphed from a time in the late 1980's when people feared being infected with HIV to a "routine activity" for a handful of diligent students in the early 2010's. Given the infrequency of reported cases on college campuses, directors describe losing momentum in addressing HIV preventative care on campus.

Acute HIV infection

Acute HIV infection can be difficult to diagnose and requires a high index of suspicion. Many providers are not comfortable recognizing the clinical manifestations of acute HIV infection. This is likely an underestimate given reporting bias. The discomfort with recognizing, and the lack of training and testing for, acute HIV infection represents a number of missed opportunities for HIV diagnosis and prevention. Rates of transmission are higher in patients during the acute phase of HIV when viral loads are highest and many new cases can be attributed to persons during this period [18]. Additionally, individuals who find out they are HIV-infected, subsequently reduce high-risk sexual behaviors following a diagnosis. Medical providers on college campuses should take a sexual history from students presenting with flu-like symptoms. Acute HIV infection should be suspected in the setting of recent (within the last 2–3 weeks) episodes of unprotected sex, especially in MSM and students with multiple or anonymous partners. Students should be counseled that a negative HIV antibody test at this time does not necessarily rule out HIV infection. An HIV RNA (viral load) may be sent to confirm a diagnosis of acute HIV infection. Alternatively, HIV antibody testing may be performed at one month, three month, and six month intervals.

Given that up to 90% of patients may experience some form of acute illness before reaching a latency phase of HIV [18], it is important to increase provider knowledge of acute HIV through training in a variety of healthcare settings, including college health centers. Many directors specifically requested further training regarding acute HIV symptom recognition and testing protocols to help determine which students would benefit from testing.

Barriers to HIV and STI testing

Many college health directors have begun addressing various barriers to HIV, gonorrhea, chlamydia and syphilis testing. These barriers include cost, availability of testing, and the need for appointments versus walk-in testing. The latter has been addressed at some schools by having on-campus testing at sites other than the health centers such as health fairs in the local campus center. This has led to new venues for testing while still providing valuable time for patient education. For HIV testing, some schools have implemented rapid testing which directors uniformly agree is significantly easier and has significantly improved testing practices and education within the clinic, particularly since students no longer need to return for results. Anonymous testing was uncommon at most health centers, though many have attempted to develop confidential testing methods that, for example, do not provide information about the specific laboratory tests performed on laboratory billing invoices. Based on our qualitative results, the clearest variable to cause sudden and dramatic improvements in HIV testing rates was the availability of free HIV testing, regardless of insurance status. Schools that provided free testing had higher total numbers of tests and higher rates of testing as a percentage of the study body population. Due to resource limitations, one school has begun providing free testing only at venues aimed at LGBT groups, due to the increased rate of HIV in this demographic.

Targeted outreach

Outreach efforts at student health centers targeting high-risk sexual groups are encouraging. Many directors highlighted this important need, but also mentioned that their efforts may not be sufficient. Many centers described a need for more LGBT-specific training modules for providers particularly in gathering detailed sexual histories from this subset of patients. Given the recent CDC data showing the HIV epidemic moving into younger MSM populations, providers at student health centers may readily serve as important and existing infrastructure to perform testing. Investment in this training may have widespread benefits in addressing HIV prevention among younger populations in the United States.

Medical directors uniformly agreed that it was important to find venues to engage with LGBT populations, particularly MSM, to discuss their distinct sexual healthcare needs. These comments were often coupled with a desire for clearer guidelines regarding HIV and STI prevention in LGBT populations.

There were a number of limitations to this study. First, the sample size was small (31) and the response rate of the survey was low (52.5%). Although not all schools in the region were captured, the study is the first to start to systematically evaluate HIV and STI testing practices at college health centers in our region. Second, the study was restricted to New England. While demographics of students may change from region to region, college students in New England often represent students from all over the United States. Third, the results were provided by medical directors at their discretion and may be subject to recall bias. It is possible that larger schools with better data systems, staffing and resources that were comfortable with their HIV and STI testing practices were more likely to respond quickly to participation inquiries. The responses of the medical directors may not represent all individuals at the entire health center and should be taken into consideration.

College health services are an integral part of student health on many college campuses. Recent surveillance data suggests an increase in HIV infection in college-aged populations, specifically MSM. Effective HIV prevention programs on college campuses should encourage HIV testing for all college students, with targeted efforts for MSM. Barriers to HIV and STI testing such as cost and availability should be addressed and minimized. Medical providers who provide care to college students should be able to recognize the signs and symptoms of acute HIV infection such as individuals presenting with flu-like symptoms after a high-risk sexual exposure. Student health centers have the potential to provide effective and targeted HIV testing programs on college campuses.

Competing interests

The authors declare that they have no competing interests.

Authors' contributions

NP, AT, TPF, and AR were involved in designing and conducting the study. PAC, JCB, NP, AT, TPF, JJV, and AR were all involved in the analysis of results, writing and editing of the manuscript. All authors read and approved the final manuscript.

Acknowledgements

We would like to acknowledge Dr. Edward Wheeler, MD, Dr. Michele Lally, MD, and Dr. Curt Beckwith, MD, for valuable insight and suggestions during the course of this study. This work was supported by the Lifespan/Tufts/Brown Center for AIDS Research (P30AI042853, PI: Charles Carpenter). Dr. Philip A. Chan is supported by a National Institute of Allergy and Infectious Diseases grant (1K23AI096923-01).

References

1. Centers for Disease Control and Prevention: *HIV Surveillance Report*. 2009.
2. Prejean J, *et al*: **Estimated HIV incidence in the United States, 2006–2009.** *PLoS One* 2009, **6**:e17502.
3. **HIV infection among young black men who have sex with men--Jackson, Mississippi, 2006–2008.** *MMWR Morb Mortal Wkly Rep* 2009, **58**:77–81.
4. **Increase in newly diagnosed HIV infections among young black men who have sex with men--Milwaukee County, Wisconsin, 1999–2008.** *MMWR Morb Mortal Wkly Rep* 2011, **60**:99–102.
5. Pathela P, *et al*: **Men who have sex with men have a 140-fold higher risk for newly diagnosed HIV and syphilis compared with heterosexual men in New York City.** *J Acquir Immune Defic Syndr* 2011, **58**:408–416.
6. *US Department of Education National Center for Education Statistics*. 2011. http://nces.ed.gov.
7. MacDonald NE, *et al*: **High-risk STD/HIV behavior among college students.** *JAMA* 1990, **263**:3155–3159.
8. Smith PD, Roberts CM: **American College Health Association annual Pap test and sexually transmitted infection survey: 2006.** *J Am Coll Health* 2009, **57**:389–394.
9. Adefuye AS, Abiona TC, Balogun JA, Lukobo Durrell M: **HIV sexual risk behaviors and perception of risk among college students: implications for planning interventions.** *BMC Public Health* 2009, **9**:281.
10. Lindley LL, Nicholson TJ, Kerby MB, Lu N: **HIV/STI associated risk behaviors among self-identified lesbian, gay, bisexual, and transgender college students in the United States.** *AIDS Educ Prev* 2003, **15**:413–429.
11. Lewis JE, Malow RM, Ireland SJ: **HIV/AIDS risk in heterosexual college students. A review of a decade of literature.** *J Am Coll Health* 1997, **45**:147–158.
12. Kalichman SC, Nachimson D, Cherry C, Williams E: **AIDS treatment advances and behavioral prevention setbacks: preliminary assessment of reduced perceived threat of HIV-AIDS.** *Health Psychol* 1998, **17**:546–550.
13. Wickman ME, Anderson NLR, Greenberg CS: **The adolescent perception of invincibility and its influence on teen acceptance of health promotion strategies.** *J Pediatr Nurs* 2008, **23**:460–468
14. Hightow LB, *et al*: **The unexpected movement of the HIV epidemic in the Southeastern United States: transmission among college students.** *J Acquir Immune Defic Syndr* 2005, **38**:531–537.
15. Hightow LB, *et al*: **Men who have sex with men and women: a unique risk group for HIV transmission on North Carolina College campuses.** *Sex Transm Dis* 2006, **33**:585–593.
16. Thompson-Robinson M, Richter D, Shegog M: **Perceptions of partner risk and influences on sexual decision-making for HIV prevention among students at historically black colleges and universities.** *J African American Studies*. 2005, **9**:16–28.
17. Chan PA, *et al*: **New HIV infections at Southern New England academic institutions: Implications for prevention.** *AIDS Res Hum Retroviruses* 2012.
18. Pilcher CD, *et al*: **Brief but efficient: acute HIV infection and the sexual transmission of HIV.** *J Infect Dis* 2004, **189**:1785–1792.
19. Schacker T, Collier AC, Hughes J, Shea T, Corey L: **Clinical and epidemiologic features of primary HIV infection.** *Ann Intern Med* 1996, **125**:257–264.
20. Stekler JD, *et al*: **HIV testing in a high-incidence population: is antibody testing alone good enough?** *Clin Infect Dis* 2009, **49**:444–453.
21. Gayle HD, *et al*: **Prevalence of the human immunodeficiency virus among university students.** *N Engl J Med* 1990, **323**:1538–1541.
22. Branson BM, *et al*: **Revised recommendations for HIV testing of adults, adolescents, and pregnant women in health-care settings.** *MMWR Recomm Rep* 2006, **55**:1–17.

14

Virological effectiveness and CD4+ T-cell increase over early and late courses in HIV infected patients on antiretroviral therapy: focus on HCV and anchor class received

Davide Motta[1], Nigritella Brianese[1], Emanuele Focà[1*], Paola Nasta[8], Franco Maggiolo[2], Massimiliano Fabbiani[3], Giuliana Cologni[2], Simona Di Giambenedetto[3], Massimo Di Pietro[4], Nicoletta Ladisa[5], Laura Sighinolfi[6], Silvia Costarelli[7], Filippo Castelnuovo[8] and Carlo Torti[1,9]

Abstract

Background: The aim of this study was to explore the effects of HCV co-infection on virological effectiveness and on CD4+ T-cell recovery in patients with an early and sustained virological response after HAART.

Methods: We performed a longitudinal analysis of 3,262 patients from the MASTER cohort, who started HAART from 2000 to 2008. Patients were stratified into 6 groups by HCV status and type of anchor class. The early virological outcome was the achievement of HIV RNA <500 copies/ml 4–8 months after HAART initiation. Time to virological response was also evaluated by Kaplan-Meier analysis. The main outcome measure of early immunological response was the achievement of CD4+ T-cell increase by ≥100/mm^3 from baseline to month 4–8 in virological responder patients. Late immunological outcome was absolute variation of CD4+ T-cell count with respect to baseline up to month 24. Multivariable analysis (ANCOVA) investigated predictors for this outcome.

Results: The early virological response was higher in HCV Ab-negative than HCV Ab-positive patients prescribed PI/r (92.2% *versus* 88%; $p = 0.01$) or NNRTI (88.5% *versus* 84.7%; $p = 0.06$). HCV Ab-positive serostatus was a significant predictor of a delayed virological suppression independently from other variables, including types of anchor class. Reactivity for HCV antibodies was associated with a lower probability of obtaining ≥100/mm^3 CD4+ increase within 8 months from HAART initiation in patients treated with PI/r (62.2% among HCV Ab-positive patients *versus* 70.9% among HCV Ab-negative patients; $p = 0.003$) and NNRTI (63.7% *versus* 74.7%; $p < 0.001$). Regarding late CD4+ increase, positive HCV Ab appeared to impair immune reconstitution in terms of absolute CD4+ T-cell count increase both in patients treated with PI/r ($p = 0.013$) and in those treated with NNRTI ($p = 0.002$). This was confirmed at a multivariable analysis up to 12 months of follow-up.

Conclusions: In this large cohort, HCV Ab reactivity was associated with an inferior virological outcome and an independent association between HCV Ab-positivity and smaller CD4+ increase was evident up to 12 months of follow-up. Although the difference in CD4+ T-cell count was modest, a stricter follow-up and optimization of HAART strategy appear to be important in HIV patients co-infected by HCV. Moreover, our data support anti-HCV treatment leading to HCV eradication as a means to facilitate the achievement of the viro-immunological goals of HAART.

Keywords: HIV, HCV, HAART

* Correspondence: emanuelefoca@gmail.com
[1]Institute of Infectious and Tropical Diseases, University of Brescia, Brescia, Italy
Full list of author information is available at the end of the article

Introduction

The introduction of highly-active anti-retroviral therapy (HAART) has determined a dramatic improvement in the management of HIV-1 infection, leading to suppression of HIV viraemia and consequent restoration of the immune function. However, viro-immunological effectiveness of HAART may be hampered by other factors [1-4].

In particular, the impact of co-infection with hepatitis C virus (HCV) on treatment response is still controversial despite the large number of published data. In this respect, co-infection with HCV has a potential great relevance because its prevalence is up to 80% in those who acquired HIV through injection drug use [5].

Several studies reported a reduced CD4+ T-cell count recovery in patients with HIV and HCV co-infection with respect to patients with HIV alone [6-13]. This conclusion was further supported by a meta-analysis [14], but was not confirmed by other results [15-17]. Moreover, variable levels of HIV RNA may confound the association of HIV co-infection with CD4+ T-cell count increase. In particular, we need data in patients who obtained early and sustained virological response to minimize the influence of variable levels of HIV replication on the immunological response because the results currently available are inconsistent, with some studies demonstrating a difference [10] and others disproving it [18,19].

Regarding virological response, several studies did not demonstrate any significant associations with HCV status [16,17], however one recent study evaluated time to virological suppression as primary outcome and found that HCV Ab-positivity was associated with a reduced rate of virological suppression at bivariate analysis, but not adjusting for history of intravenous drug use. [20].

The aim of this study was to explore the effects of HCV co-infection on virological effectiveness and on CD4+ T-cell reconstitution in patients with an early and sustained virological response after HAART. Also, stratified analyses were conducted by anchor drug --i.e. the antiretroviral drug added as third component to a backbone of nucleoside reverse transcriptase inhibitors-- to explore whether different drug characteristics may have an effect.

Methods

Design of the study and cohort used

We conducted an analysis on naïve patients enrolled in the Italian MASTER (Management of standardized antiretroviral therapy) cohort who started first line HAART containing protease inhibitors (either boosted by ritonavir - PI/r - or not boosted) or non-nucleoside reverse transcriptase inhibitor (NNRTI) from 1st January 2000 to 31st December 2008. Patients were stratified into 6 groups according to the type of anchor class received (PI, PI/r or NNRTI) and HCV Ab status (positive or negative).

The MASTER cohort is a longitudinal multicenter cohort consisting of a general HIV patient population in nine referral centres throughout Italy (http://www.master-cohort.it). The distinguishing characteristic of this cohort is that data are compiled in a common electronic chart (Health & Notes 3.5®, Healthware S.p.A., Naples, Italy) in use in the participating centres. Data are recorded over a standardized time-scale every 3 months, with merging and data cleaning performed at the coordinating centre every 6 months. Subjects gave written informed consent for participation in the observational cohort, and each site obtained approval by its Ethics Committee.

Study outcomes

Virological outcome

The main virological outcome was the achievement of early virological response, i.e., HIV RNA <500 copies/ml within 8 months from HAART initiation (values included between 4 and 8 months, closest to month 8, were considered). This limit of detection for undetectability was chosen because it was the highest value ever used in the clinical centers participating to the MASTER cohort during the time frame of the study. The main virological outcome was assessed both through intent-to-treat (ITT) and on treatment (OT) analyses. At ITT analysis, all patients were included even if they changed drugs used as anchor (PI or PI/r to NNRTI and *vice-versa*, or PI to PI/r and *vice-versa*); at OT analysis, only patients who did not change class therapy were considered. A logistic model was performed with undetectable HIV RNA as dependent variable and HIV RNA at baseline and HCV Ab reactivity as independent variables.

We also assessed the rate of patients with HIV RNA <500 copies/ml by Kaplan Meier survival curves over a mean length of follow-up of 52 (SD: 33) months.

Possible predictors of time to virological suppression were assessed through Cox regression analysis considering as independent variables either baseline factors (age at HAART initiation, gender, risk factors for HIV acquisition, history of AIDS diagnosis, HIV RNA, HCV Ab status, calendar year at HAART) or time dependent factors (CD4+ T-cell count, type of anchor class). All the variables were input in a multivariate model. The proportional hazards assumption was checked by determining whether plotting the log [−log(survival)] curve against survival time resulted in parallel lines for each covariate. Moreover, scaled Schoenfeld residuals were plotted on functions of time and tested for a non-zero slope.

Immunological outcomes

For the study of early immunological response, we used patients who obtained HIV RNA <500 copies/ml within 8 months from HAART initiation (values included between 4 and 8 months, closest to month 8, were considered) and CD4+ T-cell count was assessed in the same time frame (values closest to month 8 were used). In these patients, two immunological outcomes were evaluated: (i) CD4+ T-cell increase by ≥100/mm^3 from baseline (categorical outcome); (ii) absolute CD4+ T-cell change (continuous outcome). For the categorical outcome, a bivariate logistic analysis was performed with HIV RNA at baseline and HCV Ab status (positive or negative) used as independent variables. For the continuous outcome, ANCOVA model was performed. In this analysis, CD4+ T-cell change from baseline was the dependent variable, HIV RNA value at baseline was the covariate, and HCV Ab reactivity was the fixed effect.

For the study of late immunological response, the same patients were studied until HIV RNA remained undetectable (<500 copies/ml), patients were lost to follow-up (lack of exams for ≥6 months), or died. Moreover, analyses were truncated when <30% patients were under observation to avoid inconsistent results due to an insufficient number of patients under study.

We studied the immunological response as absolute CD4+ T-cell count increase adjusted for CD4+ T-cell count at baseline. First, ANCOVA model was performed in order to assess differences between HCV Ab-positive and HCV Ab-negative patients, stratified by anchor class at month 24 after HAART initiation. In this analysis, baseline CD4+ T-cell count and HCV Ab reactivity were fixed effects. Second, ANCOVA models were used with absolute CD4+ T-cell count increase as dependent variables to assess predictors at months 12 and 24. At this analysis, we considered as possible predictors: age at HAART initiation, gender, risk factors for HIV acquisition, history of AIDS diagnosis, HIV RNA, CD4+ T-cell count, HCV Ab status, calendar year at HAART and type of anchor class.

Additional statistical notes

Descriptive statistics were calculated for quantitative variables (mean, standard deviation – SD, median, minimum and maximum) and qualitative variables (absolute and percent frequencies) as appropriate. Ninety-five percent confidence intervals (95%CI) were calculated for appropriate cases. Variables were compared by means of F test from ANOVA model or χ^2 test in case of quantitative or qualitative variables, respectively.

All analyses have been performed using the statistical software package SAS 9.2 (SAS Inc. Cary, NC). All p value were two-tailed and considered significant if <0.05.

Results

We studied a cohort of 3,262 patients, of whom 863 were positive for HCV Ab. Main characteristics of the population at baseline, stratified into 6 groups by HCV Ab status and type of anchor class (PI, PI/r, NNRTI), are shown in Table 1. In the whole population males were 73%, mean age was 37.2 years at cohort entry and was 39.1 years at HAART initiation. HCV Ab-positive patients were more likely to be younger and IVDU than HCV Ab-negative patients; AIDS events at baseline were more frequent in HCV Ab-negative patients.

Virological analysis (patients stratified by HCV serostatus and classes of anchor drugs)

The early virological response rate was significantly higher in HCV Ab-negative than in HCV Ab-positive patients. The ITT analysis showed that, in the overall population, 87.8% patients achieved virological success. In patients receiving a PI (N = 354), those who did not reach an early virological response were 34/146 (23.3%) among HCV Ab-positive patients *versus* 52/208 (25%) HCV Ab-negative patients ($p = 0.66$); among the 1424 patients treated with PI/r, 44/365 (12%) HCV Ab-positive *versus* 83/1059 (7.8%) HCV Ab-negative patients did not reach the virological response (OR 0.612, 95%CI 0.416 to 0.903, $p = 0.01$); in the NNRTI group (N = 1484) those who did not achieve the virological response were 54/352 (15.3%) HCV Ab-positive *versus* 130/1132 (11.5%) HCV Ab-negative patients (OR 0.717, 95%CI 0.509 to 1.01, $p = 0.06$). Also at OT analysis, significant differences between HCV Ab-positive and HCV Ab-negative patients emerged only in those treated with PI/r (OR 0.582, 95%CI 0.389 to 0.869, $p = 0.01$), and in those treated with NNRTI (OR 0.618, 95%CI 0.419 to 0.912, $p = 0.02$).

Figure 1 (panels "a" and "b") shows the Kaplan-Meier analyses in HCV Ab-negative and in HCV Ab-positive patients for the achievement of virological suppression. Only in patients treated with NNRTI, there was a statistically significant difference for the time to achieve virological response being shorter in HCV Ab-negative patients (log-rank $p = 0.003$). By contrast, no statistically significant differences were found in patients treated with PI and, among patients receiving PI/r, a borderline statistical significance was found in favor of the HCV Ab-negative group (log-rank $p = 0.096$).

Predictors of time to achieve virological suppression

Cox regression analysis was performed in order to explore possible predictors of time to achieve virological suppression (Figure 2). We found that, among the baseline variables, age at HAART initiation (x 10-years older) (HR 1.109, 95%CI 1.065 to 1.155, $p < 0.001$), IVDU as risk factors for HIV acquisition (HR 1.344, 95%CI 1.130 to 1.599, $p = 0.001$), calendar year at HAART (x 1-year more recent) (HR 1.035, 95%CI 1.023 to 1.046, $p < 0.001$), were predictors of shorter time to reach the virological success; instead, HCV Ab-positive status (HR 0.738, 95%CI 0.652 to 0.834, $p < 0.001$) and higher level of HIV RNA (x1 $\log_{10}$

Table 1 Patients' characteristics at baseline

Variable	*HCV Ab+ PI (n = 146)*	*HCV Ab- PI (n = 208)*	*HCV Ab + PI + r (n = 365)*	*HCV Ab- PI + r (n = 1059)*	*HCV Ab + NNRTI (n = 352)*	*HCV Ab- NNRTI (n = 1132)*	*p*
Males [N(%)]	112 (76.7)	148 (71.2)	284 (77.8)	751 (70.9)	257 (73.0)	829 (73.2)	0.163
Age at cohort entry, years [Mean (SD)]	34.3 (8.1)	38.3 (10)	37.2 (9.3)	38.4 (10.6)	34.3 (8.7)	37.2 (10.1)	<0.001
Age at HAART initiation, years [Mean (SD)]	37.8 (6.2)	39.0 (9.6)	41.2 (7.6)	39.5 (10.4)	38.3 (7.3)	38.5 (9.9)	<0.001
Calendar year at HAART [Median (range)]	2001 (2000–2009)	2001 (2000–2009)	2006 (2000–2009)	2006 (2000–2009)	2003 (2000–2009)	2004 (2000–2010)	
Risk factors for HIV acquisition [N(%)]							
Heterosexual	24 (16.4)	122 (58.7)	74 (20.3)	587 (55.4)	79 (22.4)	678 (59.9)	<0.001
MSM	6 (4.1)	56 (26.9)	18 (4.9)	254 (24)	26 (7.4)	316 (27.9)	
IVDU	110 (75.3)	10 (4.8)	228 (62.5)	21 (2)	234 (66.5)	27 (2.4)	
Other/unknown	6 (4.1)	20 (9.6)	45 (12.3)	197 (18.6)	13 (3.7)	111 (9.8)	
AST, IU/L [Mean (SD)]	69.3 (56.4)	44.9 (96.9)	62.1 (54.7)	32.5 (24.2)	58.0 (47.9)	34.0 (28.0)	<0.001
ALT, IU/L [Mean (SD)]	68.9 (61.7)	48.2 (88.5)	70.6 (70.1)	40.9 (45.4)	64.5 (51.4)	38.9 (39.3)	<0.001
Serum creatinine, mg/dL[Mean (SD)]	0.79 (0.26)	1.00 (1.35)	0.84 (0.45)	0.85 (0.43)	0.82 (0.26)	0.87 (0.64)	0.017
Cholesterolaemia, mg/dL [Mean (SD)]	138.3 (40.3)	172.0 (49.7)	150.1 (42.6)	167.1 (46.4)	156.7 (40.3)	165.1 (39.5)	<0.001
Nadir of CD4+ T-cells, cells/mm^3 [Mean (SD)]	143.1 (122.5)	144.8 (140.6)	169.5 (123.6)	169.5 (133.3)	179.3 (115.9)	198.5 (118.8)	<0.001
AIDS diagnosis [N (%)]	43 (29.5)	76 (36.5)	95 (26.0)	314 (29.7)	67 (19.0)	215 (19.0)	<0.001
CD4+ T-cell count, cells/mm^3 [Mean (SD)]	222.4 (220.1)	188.3 (198.4)	210.1 (157.3)	202.5 (175.8)	239.6 (146.5)	233.8 (144.1)	<0.001
HIV-1 RNA, copies/ml [Mean (SD)]	143,968 (178,492)	187,909 (192,419)	208,367 (397,492)	225,939 (529,767)	156,582 (260,891)	191,210 (543,678)	0.116

N: number, SD: standard deviation, PI/r: protease inhibitors boosted by ritonavir, PI: protease inhibitors not boosted by ritonavir NNRTI: non-nucleoside reverse transcriptase inhibitor, IVDU: intravenous drug users, HAART: highly active antiretroviral therapy, MSM: men who have sex with men, AST: Aspartate aminotransferase, ALT: Alanine aminotransferase.

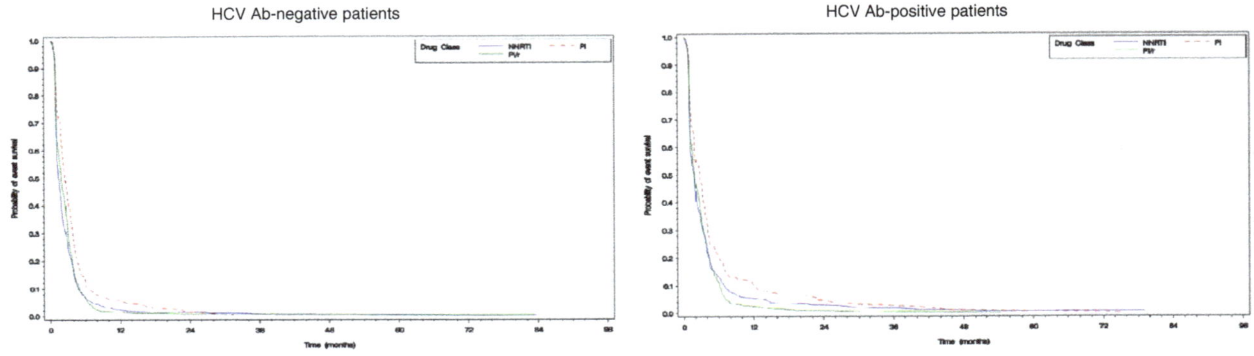

Figure 1 Kaplan Meir analysis of time to virological response. Time to HIV-1 RNA <500 copies/ml in HCV Ab-negative patients (panel a) and HCV Ab-positive patients (panel b) by classes of anchor drugs.

copies/ml) (HR 0.882, 95%CI 0.832 to 0.935, $p < 0.001$) predicted a longer time to obtained the same outcome. Among time-dependent variables, only increasing CD4+ T-cell count was directly associated with time to achieve the virological outcome (HR 1.057, 95%CI 1.047 to 1.066, $p < 0.001$), while type of HAART was not (NNRTI *versus* PI/r, $p = 0.75$; PI *versus* PI/r, $p = 0.08$; others *versus* PI/r, $p = 0.27$).

Immunological analysis (patients stratified by HCV serostatus and classes of anchor drugs)

For the early immunological response, achievement of CD4+ T-cell increase ≥100/mm^3 within 8 months from HAART initiation was evaluated among patients with a virological response. In this analysis, 2,682 patients who had values of CD4+ T-cell count both at baseline and after 4–8 months were considered. Among patients receiving a PI (N = 239) there were not significant differences between mono- and co-infected patients at bivariate analysis (60.8% *versus* 65.5%, $p = 0.35$). Conversely, in the PI/r group (N = 1,220) HCV Ab-positive patients had a lower probability to reach the outcome than HCV Ab-negative patients (62.2% *versus* 70.9%, OR 0.662, 95%CI 0.502 to 0.872, $p = 0.003$). Also, among NNRTI-receiving patients (N = 1,223), CD4+ T-cell count increase ≥100/mm^3 was less likely to be achieved by HCV Ab-positive patients (63.7% *versus* 74.7%, OR 0.595, 95%CI 0.445 to 0.797, $p < 0.001$). A significant difference in CD4+ T-cell count increase was also found in this group at ANCOVA when absolute CD4+ T-cell count increase was analyzed as continuous measure (−36.8/mm^3, 95%CI −53.6 to −20.1, $p < 0.001$).

For the late immunological response, the absolute CD4+ T-cell count for both HCV Ab-negative and HCV Ab-positive patients is depicted in Figure 3. By ANCOVA, at month 24 there was a significant difference between HCV Ab-positive and HCV Ab-negative patients with sustained virological success in terms of absolute CD4+ T-cell count increase both in patients treated with PI/r (mean change [SD]: 248.4 cells/mm^3 [188.6] in HCV Ab-positive patients *versus* 275.5 cells/mm^3 [203.4] in HCV Ab-negative patients; $p = 0.013$) and in those treated with NNRTI containing regimens (mean change [SD]: 211.1 cells/mm^3 [168.3] in HCV Ab-positive patients *versus* 271.0 cells/mm^3 [183.4] in HCV Ab-negative patients; $p = 0.002$).

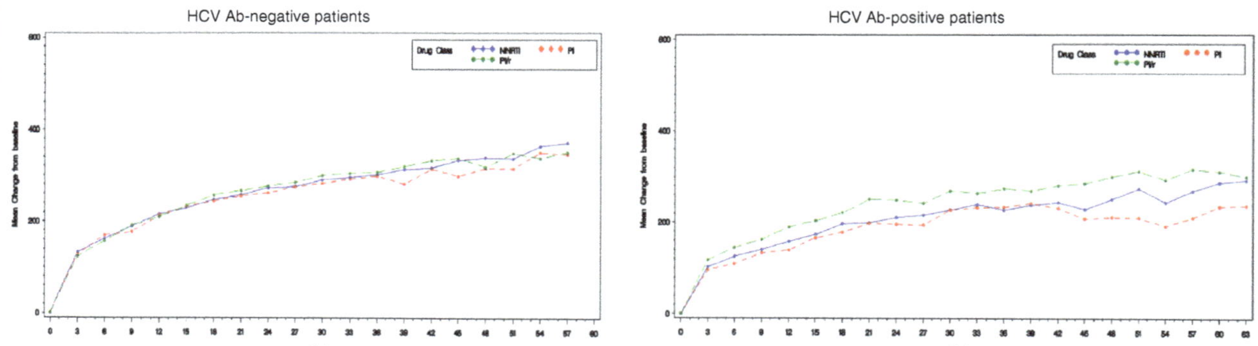

Figure 2 Predictors of time to undetectable HIV RNA (< 500 copies/ml). HAART: highly active antiretroviral therapy, IVDU: intravenous drug users, NNRTI: non-nucleoside reverse transcriptase inhibitor, PI/r: protease inhibitors boosted by ritonavir, PI: protease inhibitors not boosted by ritonavir.

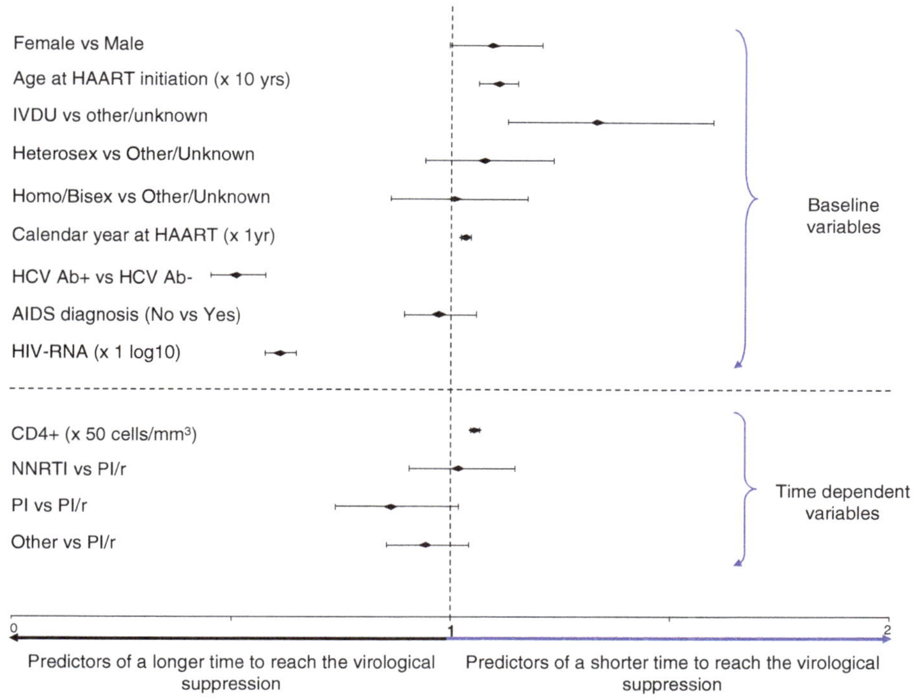

Figure 3 Immune-recovery evaluated as absolute CD4+ T-cell count increase with respect to the baseline. Late immunological outcomes in patients who obtained sustained HIV RNA suppression by year 1: absolute CD4+ T-cell count increase in HCV Ab-negative patients (panel a) and in HCV Ab-positive patients (panel b). Note that for immunological analyses data were cut at month 63 when 30% of the enrolled patients were still under observation.

Predictors of CD4+ T-cell count recovery

Table 2 shows the results of the ANCOVA model performed to investigate possible predictors of CD4+ T-cell recovery at different time-point of the study.

HCV Ab-positive status appeared to predict smaller CD4+ T-cell increase after 12 months of HAART ($p = 0.005$), independently from age at HAART onset, and HIV RNA at baseline, both significant predictors of this outcome ($p = 0.002$ and <0.001, respectively). However, after 24 month of HAART, the impact of HCV Ab status disappeared.

Discussion

In this study, the possible impact of HCV co-infection on viro-immunological effectiveness of different HAART regimens was explored both in the early and in the late follow-up and using both a stratified and a multivariable analysis.

In the overall population we found that 88% patients reached HIV RNA suppression within months 4–8 months from initiation of HAART at ITT analysis. However, percentages differed by HCV co-infection and by anchor class received. In fact, HCV Ab-positive patients obtained HIV

Table 2 Predictors of immune recovery (absolute CD4+ T-cell increase from baseline after HAART)

	12 months		24 months	
Variable	Estimate (SE)	*p*	Estimate (SE)	*p*
Age at HAART initiation [x10-yrs]	−13.6 (3.7)	0.002	−12.0 (5.1)	0.02
AIDS [no vs. yes]	N.S.		25.0 (11.3)	0.03
CD4+ [x50 cells/mm^3]	N.S.		−11.5 (1.6)	<0.001
HIV RNA [x1 log$_{10}$]	−46.8 (5.5)	<0.001	47.1(7.5)	<0.001
HCV + vs HCV-	−38.4 (11.0)	0.005	N.S.	
PI vs PI/r	N.S.		−33.4 (14.8)	<0.02

Results of the ANCOVA models with absolute CD4+ T-cell increase as dependent variable after 12 and 24 months from HAART initiation. Only variables that resulted to be statistically significant in at least one time-point are reported. Models were adjusted for age at HAART onset, gender, risk factors for HIV acquisition, history of AIDS, basal HIV RNA, CD4+ T-cell count, HCV Ab status, calendar year at HAART and type of treatment as anchor (PI/r vs NNRTI or PI).

RNA suppression less likely than HIV mono-infected patients, though this difference was greater in those treated with PI/r (88% *versus* 92.2%) and NNRTI (84.7% *versus* 88.5%) than in those treated with PI (76.7% *versus* 75%). It is possible that this finding reflects a treatment adherence phenomenon. In fact, on one hand, if one assumes that HCV Ab-positivity is a proxy for a negative behavior related to IVDU, with a negative influence on treatment adherence [5,21], the difference in virological suppression would be magnified in patients who received more complex regimens (such as the PI/r most frequently used at the time of the study) [22]. On the other hand, in patients prescribed less potent regimens (such as PI), differences between the two groups could have been diluted. Indeed, the rate of treatment success in these patients was the lowest.

However, when predictors of HIV RNA response were investigated, HCV co-infection appeared to be a negative predictor independently from IVDU, suggesting that the effects of these two variables were not entirely overlapping. This may be due either to HCV co-infection *"per se"* (probably affecting the immune control of HIV replication) or to adherence as unmeasured variable because HCV co-infected patients may have been less adherent to treatment even though they were not IVDU. Further bio-psycho-social investigations are needed to understand the complex relationship between HCV co-infection, the role of adherence behaviors and IVDU as risk factor.

Regarding the other predictors of virological success, the positive impact of aging (possibly reflecting better adherence in older patients) is not new [23,24], as well as the positive impact of more recent calendar years, possibly reflecting a significant improvement in the drug regimens and in the overall standard of care [25,26].

We found a positive impact of higher CD4+ T-cell count as a protective variable for achieving HIV RNA suppression. It is possible that the immune system (either at baseline or reconstituted by HAART) has a role in better controlling HIV replication. If this is the case, our results point to earlier HAART initiation as a means to preserve immune system so that virological suppression is more frequent. But also the lack of virological suppression (or virological suppression in presence of suboptimal adherence [27]), may be a cause rather than a consequence of lower CD4+ count, supporting the importance of a continuing assessment of treatment adherence, especially in HIV/HCV co-infected patients who appear to be disadvantaged.

Regarding the immunological outcomes, reactivity for HCV Ab was associated with a lower probability of obtaining ≥100 CD4+ T-cell count increase within 8 months from HAART initiation and with a smaller CD4+ T-cell count recovery up to 12 months in a multivariable analysis. It has been hypothesized that CD4+ T-cell depletion might result from ongoing cell activation and apoptosis driven by HCV [28] and therefore HCV could lower the CD4+ T-cell recovery through a direct pathogenic effect on lymphocytes even after HAART [29]. Our results, together with this interpretation, suggest that it is important to treat HCV infection aimed at obtaining its eradication, not only with the main goal of treating liver disease but also as a means to improve the viro-immunological outcomes of HAART, especially early upon its inception.

Greub et al. studied a group of 1596 patients (33% of them were HCV Ab-positive) with sustained HIV RNA <400 copies/ml and found that HCV Ab-positive subjects had an impaired CD4+ T-cell recovery in the long term [10]. By contrast, data from Kaufmann's studies did not show any significant difference in CD4+ T-cell recovery when comparing HCV Ab-positive and HCV Ab-negative patients [18]. Our results suggest that, even though HCV infection may have an impact in the short term (either because immune activation has not yet been down-regulated or because HIV RNA is less effectively controlled early upon HAART), a more prolonged undetectability of HIV RNA may eventually counteract the apparent disadvantage occurring in HCV co-infected patients.

The present study suffers from limitations: first, HCV RNA was not considered, therefore patients with HCV Ab-positive but negative HCV RNA may have been included in the analysis, even if patients treated with anti-HCV drugs were excluded with the aim to reduce this possible bias. Second, HCV genotypes were not considered. A small study found that, among 171 HIV/HCV co-infected patients, those infected by HCV genotype 3 had inferior CD4+ T-cell increase after 12 months of follow-up [30]. However data from Antonucci et al. [7] did not find any correlation between HCV genotypes and immune-reconstitution in a cohort of 284 antiretroviral naïve patients. Therefore, further studies are needed to investigate the possible role of HCV genotypes on immune reconstitution in larger cohorts of patients over a longer follow-up. Third, other possible confounders such as severity of liver disease were not measured. Fourth, a <500 copies/ml cut-off for undetectability was considered. It is possible that persistent HIV replication below this cut-off may have had an impact on immune-reconstitution but this effect was not captured in our analysis.

In conclusion, the analysis of virological response suggests that HCV Ab-positive patients need focused interventions to maximize the effectiveness of HAART, especially early upon HAART initiation. Moreover, an higher CD4+ T-cell count predicted better virological control suggesting that preservation of immune functions is important not only to prevent clinical complications but also as a means to better control HIV replication. Thus, earlier HAART initiation is supported, especially in HIV/HCV co-infected subjects whose viro-immunological response may be compromised relative to HIV mono-infected patients. Lastly, it is possible that HCV eradication through specific treatments is beneficial not only for the main goal of treating liver disease but also for the viro-immunological effectiveness of HAART.

Competing interests

Co-authors (CT, NB, EF, PN, FM, GC, SDG, MF, MDP, NL, LS, SC, FC) received grants from several Pharmaceutical Companies for participating to advisory board and scientific conferences but the received supports did not influence the content of this paper. Remaining co-authors: none to declare.

Acknowledgements

This work was partially supported by Janssen Cilag SpA through an unrestricted grant and by NEAT (Network for Excellence in Antiretroviral Treatment) funded by the European Commission (Project number: LSHP-CT-2006-037570).
Statistical analysis was performed by CROS NT (www.cros.it/).
The Italian MASTER Cohort is a large national project involving the major centers providing care to HIV/AIDS patients and includes the following doctors: F. Castelli, G. Carosi, C. Torti, E. Quiros, P. Nasta, G. Paraninfo, E. Focà, Institute of Infectious and Tropical Diseases, University of Brescia, Brescia, Italy; R. Cauda S. Di Giambenedetto, M. Fabbiani, M. Colafigli, Catholic University of Sacred Heart, Rome, Italy; F. Maggiolo Ospedali Riuniti, Bergamo, Italy; A. Scalzini, F. Castelnuovo, I. El Hamad, Spedali Civili di Brescia, Brescia, Italy; F. Mazzotta, S. Locaputo, N. Marino, P. Pierotti M. Di Pietro, C. Blè, F. Vichi, "S. Maria Annunziata" Hospital, Florence, Italy; L. Sighinolfi, "S. Anna" Hospital, Ferrara, Italy; G. Angarano, N. Ladisa, L. Monno, P. Maggi, Policlinico di Bari, Bari, Italy; A. Pan, S. Costarelli, Istituti Ospitalieri, Cremona, Italy; A.Gori, G. Lapadula, M. Airoldi, N Squillace, A.Soria, A. Muscatello, Ospedale S. Gerardo, Monza, Italy; M. Puoti, Ospedale Niguarda Cà Granda Milano, Italy; P. Viale, V. Colangeli, M. Borderi, Policlinico S. Orsola Malpighi, Bologna, Italy.
This work has been presented in part to the "6th IAS Conference on HIV pathogenesis, treatment and prevention", Rome, Italy, 17–20 July 2011, (Abstract TUPE-106).
We would like to thank all patients participating in the MASTER Cohort Study, all doctors and study nurse involved, and the datacentre. We also wish to thank Ms. Francesca Brognoli, Dr. Cristina Minardi for kind technical assistance.

Author details

[1]Institute of Infectious and Tropical Diseases, University of Brescia, Brescia, Italy. [2]Department of Infectious Diseases, Ospedali Riuniti, Bergamo, Italy. [3]Institute of Clinical Infectious Diseases, Catholic University of Sacred Heart, Rome, Italy. [4]Infectious Diseases Clinic, Santa Maria Annunziata Hospital, Florence, Italy. [5]Clinic of Infectious Diseases, Policlinico di Bari, Bari, Italy. [6]Department of Infectious Diseases, S. Anna Hospital, Ferrara, Italy. [7]Department of Infectious Diseases, Istituti Ospitalieri, Cremona, Italy. [8]Spedali Civili di Brescia, Brescia, Italy. [9]Unit of Infectious Diseases, University "Magna Graecia", Catanzaro, Italy.

Authors' contributions

Study concept and design: CT, DM, NB. *Acquisition of data:* CT, DM, NB, EF, PN, FM, GC, SDG, MF, MDP, NL, LS, SC, FC. *Analysis and interpretation of data:* CT, DM, NB, EF. *Drafting of the manuscript:* CT, DM, NB. *Critical revision of the manuscript for important intellectual content:* EF, PN, FM, GC, SDG, MF, MDP, NL, LS, SC, FC. All authors read and approved the final manuscript.

References

1. Furber AS, Maheswaran R, Newell JN, Carroll C: **Is smoking tobacco an independent risk factor for HIV infection and progression to AIDS? A systemic review.** *Sex Transm Infect* 2007, **83**:41–46.
2. Operskalski EA, Kovacs A: **HIV/HCV co-infection: pathogenesis, clinical complications, treatment, and new therapeutic technologies.** *Curr HIV/AIDS Rep* 2011, **8**:12–22.
3. Zellan J, Augenbraun M: **Syphilis in the HIV-infected patient: an update on epidemiology, diagnosis, and management.** *Curr HIV/AIDS Rep* 2004, **1**:142–147.
4. Khan FA, Minion J, Pai M, Royce S, Burman W, Harries AD, Menzies D: **Treatment of active tuberculosis in HIV-coinfected patients: a systematic review and meta-analysis.** *Clin Infect Dis* 2010, **50**:1288–1299.
5. Bollepalli S, Mathieson K, Bay C, Hillier A, Post J, Van Thiel DH, Nadir A: **Prevalence of risk factors for hepatitis C virus in HIV-infected and HIV/hepatitis C virus-coinfected patients.** *Sex Transm Infect* 2007, **34**:367–370.
6. Carlos Martín J, Castilla J, López M, Arranz R, González-Lahoz J, Soriano V: **Impact of chronic hepatitis C on HIV-1 disease progression.** *HIV Clin Trials* 2004, **5**:125–131.
7. Antonucci G, Girardi E, Cozzi-Lepri A, Capobianchi MR, De Luca A, Puoti M, Petrelli E, Carnevale G, Rizzardini G, Grossi PA, Viganò P, Moioli MC, Carletti F, Solmone M, Ippolito G, Monforte AD: **Role of hepatitis C virus (HCV) viremia and HCV genotype in the immune recovery from highly active antiretroviral therapy in a cohort of antiretroviral-naive HIV-infected individuals.** *Clin Infect Dis* 2005, **40**:e101–e109.
8. Braitstein P, Zala C, Yip B, Brinkhof MWG, Moore D, Hogg RS, Montaner JSG: **Immunologic response to antiretroviral therapy in hepatitis C virus-coinfected adults in a population-based HIV/AIDS treatment program.** *J Infect Dis* 2006, **193**:259–268.
9. Carmo RA, Guimarães MDC, Moura AS, Neiva AM, Versiani JB, Lima LV, Freitas LP, Rocha MOC: **The influence of HCV coinfection on clinical, immunological and virological responses to HAART in HIV-patients.** *Braz J Infect Dis* 2008, **12**:173–179.
10. Greub G, Ledergerber B, Battegay M, Grob P, Perrin L, Furrer H, Burgisser P, Erb P, Boggian K, Piffaretti JC, Hirschel B, Janin P, Francioli P, Flepp M, Telenti A: **Clinical progression, survival, and immune recovery during antiretroviral therapy in patients with HIV-1 and hepatitis C virus coinfection: the Swiss HIV Cohort Study.** *Lancet* 2000, **356**:1800–1805.
11. De Luca A, Bugarini R, Lepri AC, Puoti M, Girardi E, Antinori A, Poggio A, Pagano G, Tositti G, Cadeo G, Macor A, Toti M, D'Arminio Monforte A: **Coinfection with hepatitis viruses and outcome of initial antiretroviral regimens in previously naive HIV-infected subjects.** *Arch Intern Med* 2002, **162**:2125–2132.
12. Santin M, Mestre M, Shaw E, Barbera MJ, Casanova A, Niubo J, Bolao F, Podzamczer D, Gudiol F: **Impact of hepatitis C virus coinfection on immune restoration during successful antiretroviral therapy in chronic human immunodeficiency virus type 1 disease.** *Eur J Clin Microbiol Infect Dis* 2008, **27**:65–73.
13. Weis N, Lindhardt BO, Kronborg G, Hansen A-BE, Laursen AL, Christensen PB, Nielsen H, Moller A, Sorensen HT, Obel N: **Impact of hepatitis C virus coinfection on response to highly active antiretroviral therapy and outcome in HIV-infected individuals: a nationwide cohort study.** *Clin Infect Dis* 2006, **42**:1481–1487.
14. Miller MF, Haley C, Koziel MJ, Rowley CF: **Impact of hepatitis C virus on immune restoration in HIV-infected patients who start highly active antiretroviral therapy: a meta-analysis.** *Clin Infect Dis* 2005, **41**:713–720.
15. Peters L, Mocroft A, Soriano V, Rockstroh JK, Losso M, Valerio L, Aldins P, Reiss P, Ledergerber B, Lundgren JD: **Hepatitis C virus coinfection does not influence the CD4 cell recovery in HIV-1-infected patients with maximum virologic suppression.** *J Acquir Immune Defic Syndr* 2009, **50**:457–463.
16. Rockstroh JK, Mocroft A, Soriano V, Tural C, Losso MH, Horban A, Kirk O, Phillips A, Ledergerber B, Lundgren J: **Influence of hepatitis C virus infection on HIV-1 disease progression and response to highly active antiretroviral therapy.** *J Infect Dis* 2005, **192**:992–1002.
17. Sullivan PS, Hanson DL, Teshale EH, Wotring LL, Brooks JT: **Effect of hepatitis C infection on progression of HIV disease and early response to initial antiretroviral therapy.** *AIDS* 2006, **20**:1171–1179.
18. Kaufmann GR, Perrin L, Pantaleo G, Opravil M, Furrer H, Telenti A, Hirschel B, Ledergerber B, Vernazza P, Bernasconi E, Rickenbach M, Egger M, Battegay M: **CD4 T-lymphocyte recovery in individuals with advanced HIV-1 infection receiving potent antiretroviral therapy for 4 years: the Swiss HIV Cohort Study.** *Arch Intern Med* 2003, **163**:2187–2195.
19. Kaufmann GR, Furrer H, Ledergerber B, Perrin L, Opravil M, Vernazza P, Cavassini M, Bernasconi E, Rickenbach M, Hirschel B, Battegay M: **Characteristics, determinants, and clinical relevance of CD4 T cell recovery to <500 cells/microL in HIV type 1-infected individuals receiving potent antiretroviral therapy.** *Clin Infect Dis* 2005, **41**:361–372.

20. Cescon AM, Cooper C, Chan K, Palmer AK, Klein MB, Machouf N, Loutfy MR, Raboud J, Rachlis A, Ding E, Lima VD, Montaner JSG, Rourke SB, Smieja M, Tsoukas C, Hogg RS: **Factors associated with virological suppression among HIV-positive individuals on highly active antiretroviral therapy in a multi-site Canadian cohort.** *HIV Med* 2011, **12**:352–360.
21. Staples CT, Rimland D, Dudas D: **Hepatitis C in the HIV (human immunodeficiency virus) Atlanta V.A. (Veterans Affairs Medical Center) Cohort Study (HAVACS): the effect of coinfection on survival.** *Clin Infect Dis* 1999, **29**:150–154.
22. Goulet JL, Fultz SL, McGinnis KA, Justice AC: **Relative prevalence of comorbidities and treatment contraindications in HIV-mono-infected and HIV/HCV-co-infected veterans.** *AIDS* 2005, **19(Suppl 3)**:S99–S105.
23. Sabin CA, Smith CJ, D' Arminio Monforte A, Battegay M, Gabiano C, Galli L, Geelen S, Gibb D, Guiguet M, Judd A, Leport C, Dabis F, Pantazis N, Porter K, Raffi F, Thorne C, Torti C, Walker S, Warszawski J, Wintergerst U, Chene G, Lundgren J: **Response to combination antiretroviral therapy: variation by age.** *AIDS* 2008, **22**:1463–1473.
24. Greenbaum AH, Wilson LE, Keruly JC, Moore RD, Gebo KA: **Effect of age and HAART regimen on clinical response in an urban cohort of HIV-infected individuals.** *AIDS* 2008, **22**:2331–2339.
25. Sighinolfi L, Torti C, Zeni C, Ghinelli F, Suter F, Maggiolo F, Antinori A, Antonucci G, Castelnuovo F, Ladisa N, Migliorino M, Novati S, De Luca A, Lo Caputo S, Paraninfo G, Tinelli C, Carosi G: **Evolution of antiretroviral prescription and response over a period of 8 years: an Italian multicentre observational prospective cohort study.** *Infection* 2008, **36**:244–249.
26. Prosperi MCF, Cozzi-Lepri A, Antinori A, Cassola G, Torti C, Ursitti MA, Pellizzer GP, Giacometti A, D' Arminio Monforte A, De Luca A: **Favourable evolution of virological and immunological profiles in treated and untreated patients in Italy in the period 1998–2008.** *HIV Med* 2011, **12**:174–182.
27. Podsadecki TJ, Vrijens BC, Tousset EP, Rode RA, Hanna GJ: **"White coat compliance" limits the reliability of therapeutic drug monitoring in HIV-1-infected patients.** *HIV Clin Trials* 2008, **9**:238–246.
28. Núñez M, Soriano V, López M, Ballesteros C, Cascajero A, González-Lahoz J, Benito JM: **Coinfection with hepatitis C virus increases lymphocyte apoptosis in HIV-infected patients.** *Clin Infect Dis* 2006, **43**:1209–1212.
29. Laskus T, Radkowski M, Piasek A, Nowicki M, Horban A, Cianciara J, Rakela J: **Hepatitis C virus in lymphoid cells of patients coinfected with human immunodeficiency virus type 1: evidence of active replication in monocytes/macrophages and lymphocytes.** *J Infect Dis* 2000, **181**:442–448.
30. Seminari E, Tinelli C, Ravasi G, Ripamonti D, Ladisa N, Marino N, Sighinolfi L, Mondello P, Migliorino M, Carosi G, Maserati R: **Hepatitis C infection on immune recovery in HIV-positive patients on successful HAART: the role of genotype 3.** *Curr HIV Res* 2010, **8**:186–193.

15

Impact of tuberculosis on mortality among HIV-infected patients receiving antiretroviral therapy in Uganda

Rong Chu[1,2], Edward J Mills[1,3], Joseph Beyene[1], Eleanor Pullenayegum[1,2], Celestin Bakanda[4], Jean B Nachega[5,6], P J Devereaux[1,7] and Lehana Thabane[1,2*]

Abstract

Background: Tuberculosis (TB) disease affects survival among HIV co-infected patients on antiretroviral therapy (ART). Yet, the magnitude of TB disease on mortality is poorly understood.

Methods: Using a prospective cohort of 22,477 adult patients who initiated ART between August 2000 and June 2009 in Uganda, we assessed the effect of active pulmonary TB disease at the initiation of ART on all-cause mortality using a Cox proportional hazards model. Propensity score (PS) matching was used to control for potential confounding. Stratification and covariate adjustment for PS and not PS-based multivariable Cox models were also performed.

Results: A total of 1,609 (7.52%) patients had active pulmonary TB at the start of ART. TB patients had higher proportions of being male, suffering from AIDS-defining illnesses, having World Health Organization (WHO) disease stage III or IV, and having lower CD4 cell counts at baseline ($p < 0.001$). The percentages of death during follow-up were 10.47% and 6.38% for patients with and without TB, respectively. The hazard ratio (HR) for mortality comparing TB to non-TB patients using 1,686 PS-matched pairs was 1.37 (95% confidence interval [CI]: 1.08 – 1.75), less marked than the crude estimate (HR = 1.74, 95% CI: 1.49 – 2.04). The other PS-based methods and not PS-based multivariable Cox model produced similar results.

Conclusions: After controlling for important confounding variables, HIV patients who had TB at the initiation of ART in Uganda had an approximate 37% increased hazard of overall mortality relative to non-TB patients.

Keywords: Antiretroviral therapy, HIV, Tuberculosis, Propensity score methods, Uganda, Prospective cohort study

Background

The total number of people living with human immunodeficiency virus (HIV) reached 34.0 million (31.6 – 35.2 million) worldwide by the end of 2010, [1] with the majority in Sub-Saharan Africa. One-third of HIV-infected people are estimated to be co-infected with *Mycobacterium tuberculosis* (TB) which can activate or reactivate during the initiation of antiretroviral therapy (ART) due to immune reconstitution inflammatory syndrome (IRIS). However, TB incidence rates vary according to geography and patients' degrees of immunosuppression. The incidence proportion of active TB in HIV-infected patients with latent TB infection is about 10% per year compared to 10% per lifetime for an HIV-uninfected individual [2]. TB is a leading cause of HIV-related death [3]. Recent trial data have shown that early initiation of ART (within two weeks) during TB therapy can improve survival for patients with co-infection [4-6]. Guidelines and policies on joint HIV/TB interventions have been developed to promote synergies between TB and HIV/AIDS prevention and care activities, [7-9] aimed at reducing morbidity and mortality in co-infected patients. On the other hand, joint treatment containing ART and anti-TB drugs may be complicated by overlapping toxicity profiles, complex drug-drug interactions, and IRIS [10-13].

* Correspondence: thabanl@mcmaster.ca
[1]Department of Clinical Epidemiology and Biostatistics, McMaster University, Hamilton, Canada
[2]Biostatistics Unit, 3rd Floor Martha, Room H325, St Joseph's Healthcare Hamilton, 50 Charlton Avenue East, Hamilton, ON L8N 4A6, Canada
Full list of author information is available at the end of the article

To date, the association between active TB and mortality in HIV-infected patients who receive ART is poorly understood, particularly in settings with a relatively lower TB prevalence, such as Eastern Africa [9,13,14]. An observational study from Tororo, Uganda, comprising 1,044 HIV patients showed that TB at the initiation or during follow-up of ART was associated with a 4.7-fold increase in cumulative mortality relative to those without TB [15]. Nevertheless the association of TB disease and mortality was clearly confounded by degree of immunosuppression [15,16]. Several studies in more developed countries suggest incident TB substantially increases the risk of AIDS-related mortality among HIV patients receiving ART [17,18]. A recent meta-analysis suggested little impact of TB on mortality in HIV patients receiving ART [19]. Small numbers of co-infected patients, different procedures of baseline confounding adjustment, and incomplete information on clinical outcomes have led to uncertainty of the impact of active TB on subsequent mortality among co-infected patients on ART and the optimal timing of treatment of both diseases.

Our study involved a large prospective cohort of HIV-infected adult patients in Uganda, and had two objectives: (1) to assess the effect of active pulmonary TB disease at ART initiation on overall survival among HIV patients during ART treatment by adjusting for potential confounders using propensity score (PS) methods, [20-22] and (2) to explore the robustness of the study findings by comparing results from three PS methods (matching on PS, stratifying on PS, adjusting for PS as regression covariate) to conventional (not PS-based) multivariable Cox regression model. These results may help accurately plan TB and HIV/AIDS management activities in HIV patients with TB co-infection.

Methods

Setting, participants and data collection

Our prospective cohort contained HIV-infected patients initiating ART at ten service centres managed by the AIDS Support Organization (TASO) across different settings in Uganda since 2000. Patients received ART from experienced medical staff at TASO clinics, outreach clinics in rural areas, and through community-based treatment programs. Details of the treatment program have been published previously [23]. The standard regimen was two nucleoside reverse transciptase inhibitors and one non-nucleoside reverse transcriptase inhibitor. The current study included adult patients (aged 14 years or older at ART initiation) enrolled between August 2000 and June 2009 (inclusive) as part of an ongoing observational study intended to evaluate the programmatic delivery of services. After ART initiation, patients were scheduled for clinic visits at least every three months. Patients' demographic, clinical, psychosocial, and medication use data were collected by clinicians, and field workers using standardized forms at ART initiation, and each visit.

At the time of data collection, national guidelines in Uganda used three strategies for initiating treatment of TB in a co-infected patient: (1) patient with TB and CD4 cell count < 250 cells/mm^3 or a patient with extra-pulmonary TB or WHO stage IV disease: start TB therapy first and when tolerated (usually within two to six weeks) then introduce ART; (2) pulmonary TB and CD4 250–350 cells/mm^3: start TB therapy for two months then introduce ART, and; (3) pulmonary TB and CD4 > 350 cells/mm^3: defer ART, monitor clinically and also do CD4 cell counts regularly; re-evaluate the patient at eight weeks and the end of TB treatment [24].

Primary outcome, exposure and potential confounding variables

Our primary outcome was time from the initiation of ART to death for any reason after the initiation of ART between August 2000 and June 2009. The primary exposure was active pulmonary TB as evidenced by sputum smear-positive results at the initiation of ART, or suspected TB regardless of sputum results followed up by radiography. Fourteen variables containing clinical and demographic characteristics and medicine history measured at the beginning of ART (baseline), were considered in the study and their roles as potential confounders were investigated. The 14 baseline covariates were gender, age, CD4 count, World Health Organization (WHO) clinical disease stage of HIV/AIDS, presence of AIDS-defining illness, TASO service centre, calendar year of ART initiation, education, marital status, partner sero-status, sexual activity, sexually transmitted infection, history of pneumocystis pneumonia (PCP), and toxoplasmosis. A potential confounder was defined here as a baseline covariate that was likely to associate with the overall survival and baseline disease status of TB. The assessment of association between the covariates and the outcome was primarily based on published literature [25-29]. We also hypothesized the associations between overall survival and some covariates that pertained to the study setting. For example, the variation in political and socioeconomic factors and unmet demand for healthcare workers across the 10 Ugandan study sites were likely to result in difference in patient outcomes [30]. Patient sexual dynamics could potentially affect prevention and treatment for HIV/AIDS in African countries [31-34]. Literature suggested that people with weak immune systems were generally more likely to have active TB disease [35]; and among HIV patients, male gender, low CD4 count, high viral load, severe disease stage, and low socioeconomic status were possible risk factors of active TB disease. We carefully examined the distributions of the 14 covariates between TB and non-TB groups at baseline (see "Statistical analysis" section). We analyzed age and CD4 count as continuous variables, and the other 12 covariates as categorical data coded by a reference level and dummy indicators (Additional file 1).

Statistical analysis

We adopted PS methods to control for confounding, and estimated the causal effect of TB at the initiation of ART on overall survival of HIV patients since their initiation of ART using Cox regression models. We reported the crude and adjusted effects of TB using hazard ratios [HRs]. A patient was censored at the time they were lost to follow-up, or at the end of the study if still alive. PS methods have been increasingly used to control for baseline confounding in observational studies [20-22,36-40]. PS methods are more advantageous than adjusting for multiple covariates simultaneously in a single outcome model when numerous confounders need to be accounted for and the outcome is rare. PS methods provide an easy means to compare distributions of confounding variables between exposure groups within PS-stratified sets. It can be difficult to examine balancing distributions of confounders post-adjustment using the conventional multiple regression methods. We chose Cox regression on PS-matched pairs as the primary method of analysis because empirical evidence suggested PS-matching provides better control for confounding than other PS methods, [41,42] and statistical diagnostic tools for assessing the balance of confounders between PS-matched pairs were readily available [40,43,44]. Specifically, we fit a Cox proportional hazards (PH) model in a dataset containing 1,686 TB cases and 1,686 PS-matched non-TB patients to control for observed potential confounding using a two-step procedure. First, we modeled the relationship between having active TB at baseline and the observed baseline covariates using a logistic regression model ("PS model"). We employed an iterative approach [45] to build the PS model by starting with the 14 observed baseline covariates; we then considered pairwise interactions, and polynomial terms of the continuous variables (age and CD4 cell count) in the PS model. We ultimately included such terms in the model if adding them improved the predictive power of the PS model and its ability to balance covariates between PS-matched pairs. Greater predictive power of the PS model (i.e. how well covariates included in the PS model predict baseline TB disease status) was likely to result in greater balance; the performance of matching was also affected by other factors such as the matching algorithm and associated tuning parameters (e.g. caliper width). We aimed to match each active TB patient to one non-TB patient with the closest logit of the estimated PS, within a caliper of 0.2 of the standard deviation of the logit of the estimated PS [46]. This matching method was shown to lead to optimal estimation of exposure effects in various simulation settings [41,47]. Propensity score is a balancing score, so we assessed PS model adequacy (selection of variables and functional form) based on examining the similarity of the joint distribution of multiple baseline covariates between TB and non-TB patients with the same estimated propensity score [42]. Balance diagnostics of baseline covariates consisted of a series of numerical and graphical measures, including standardized difference, and for continuous covariates, ratio of variance, five-number summaries, quantile-quantile plot, nonparametric density plot, empirical cumulative distribution function and side-by-side boxplot. We repeated the PS modeling – balance diagnostics steps until we were satisfied with the resulting balancing distribution. Second, we fit a stratified Cox PH model to estimate the impact of baseline TB on survival. As outcomes within PS-matched pairs are not independent, we stratified on pairs to controls for within-pair homogeneity, allowing baseline hazard functions to vary across matched strata [45,48]. The appropriateness of the PH assumption was assessed using log-log survival curves.

We applied two other PS methods for confounding control as supportive secondary analyses to assess the robustness of the results of the primary analysis, namely, stratified Cox regression on quintiles of the estimated PS, and a Cox model adjusting for PS and its quadratic and cubic terms as covariates. Conventional (not PS-based) Cox regression directly modeling the effect of TB on overall survival, adjusting for multiple baseline covariates in the same form as included in the final PS model, was also performed.

Complete information was recorded for the study sample on TB status at ART initiation and on all but four baseline covariates, namely, age (8% missing), CD4 count (17.3% missing), sexual activity (17.3% missing) and WHO stage of HIV/AIDS (34.4% missing). Excluding patients with missing data on any of the covariates would have led to a loss of 48% of subjects and 86% of death events. Such exclusions could have affected the stability of statistical models (PS-based or not) due to low event rate and jeopardized the internal validity and generalizability of the study. Therefore, we performed all analyses on five multiple imputation (MI) datasets [49]. We used Markov chain Monte Carlo method assuming multivariate normality to create a monotone missing pattern, followed by separate imputations for the continuous (age, log CD4 count) and categorical (sexual activity and stage of disease) variables using linear and logistic regression models. A number of baseline characteristics (TB status, gender, TASO sites, AIDS status, education level, marital status, partner sero-status, sexually transmitted infection, calendar year of ART initiation, and history of PCP or toxoplasmosis) and follow-up variables (death, regimen switch, patient adherence, and AIDS status post-ART initiation) were included in the imputation procedure. The follow-up variables were assessed after the initiation of ART and before the end of the study (death, lost to follow-up or June 2009, whichever happened first). Patient adherence was assessed at two weeks, two months and thereafter at six months after ART initiation, based on a composite of pharmacy monitored drug possession ratio, pharmacy refill records, and a three day recall report by patients or care givers. TASO calculated the mean adherence to ART for each patient. Adequate clinical adherence was defined as ≥95% (i.e. adherence = yes; Additional file 1) [50,51]. No post-ART variables were included in PS or Cox regression models as they could be causal intermediates between baseline TB status and death, and accounting for them in the models could induce bias. While the same covariates were used to achieve prognostic balance on the five imputed datasets, propensity scores and baseline TB – mortality association were estimated separately for each individual dataset. We then calculated the overall estimate of TB effect, using Rubin's rule [49].

We conducted statistical analyses in SAS version 9.2 (Cary, NC), R 2.14.0 (R Core Development Team) and Stata 10 (College Station, TX).

Ethics approval

University of British Columbia, University of Ottawa, and Mbale Regional Referral Hospital research ethics boards approved this study.

Results

Participant baseline characteristics

The study cohort consisted of 22,477 HIV-infected adult patients aged 14 years or older who started ART between August 2000 and June 2009 (Additional file 2: Figure S1). A total of 1,690 of 22,477 patients (7.52%) had active pulmonary TB disease at the initiation of ART. Table 1 indicates TB patients had lower CD4 counts ($p < 0.001$) and more advanced clinical stages ($p < 0.001$) at the start of ART. TB patients tended to be younger, had higher proportions of male, AIDS-defining illnesses, and a history of PCP ($p < 0.001$). Higher proportions of the TB patients were managed by the Entebbe, Jinja, Tororo and Mulago regional centres, whereas higher proportions of the non-TB patients were observed in Masaka, Mbale, Mbarara, Masindi, and Soroti regions. Summary statistics of the four baseline covariates with missing values was similar in the original and imputed datasets (Additional file 3).

Association between TB at ART initiation and baseline covariates

The final PS model included all 14 baseline covariates, their pairwise interactions with gender and baseline AIDS status (yes or no), and additional quadratic and interaction terms for the continuous variables to improve model fit (Additional file 4). Overall, the PS model predicted baseline TB status well (c statistic = 0.744, p-value = 0.203 for Hosmer and Lemeshow goodness-of-fit test). We were able to match 1,686 of 1,690 baseline TB patients to non-TB patients. PS matching improved the similarity of the distributions of all baseline covariates between TB and non-TB patients and reduced the standardized differences to below 0.1. Table 2 displays the balancing distributions of the baseline covariates for one of the five imputed datasets. Consistent patterns were observed across the imputed datasets. Additional details on specific balance diagnostics of the two continuous covariates are in the appendices (Additional file 5: Figure S2 and Additional file 6: Figure S3).

Association between TB and all-cause mortality

During a median of 21.5 months of follow-up, 1,503 (6.69%) of the 22,477 HIV patients died. The proportions of patients who died with and without TB were 10.47% (median length of follow-up [IQR]: 627.5 days [205–1034]) and 6.38% (median length of follow-up [IQR]: 646 days [306–1045]), respectively, in the original unmatched sample. The proportion of deaths remained higher in the 1,686 PS-matched pairs, with 176 (10.44%; median length of follow-up [IQR]: 629 [205–1036]) and 137 (8.13%; median length of follow-up [IQR]: 659 [286–1023]) deaths in the TB and non-TB groups. An unadjusted Cox model suggested that TB, relative to no TB, increased the hazard of death by 74% (HR = 1.74, 95% CI: 1.49 – 2.04). The HR for all-cause mortality comparing TB to non-TB patients on the 1,686 PS-matched pairs (HR = 1.37, 95% CI: 1.08 – 1.75) was less substantial, indicating TB was associated with a 37% increase in the hazard of death over the course of the study after controlling for potential baseline confounding variables (Table 3). The PS-matched estimate was less precise than the crude due to a decrease of sample size. Kaplan-Meier survival curves for the original sample and PS-matched pairs are displayed in Figures 1 and 2. No violation of the PH assumption was suggested by log-log survival curves.

Additional analyses

Stratifying on PS quintiles and adjusting for PS as a covariate in Cox regression models yielded similar TB effects on survival (PS-stratified HR = 1.36, 95% CI: 1.15-1.60; PS-adjusted HR = 1.34, 95% CI: 1.14 -1.58) (Table 3). Adjusting for multiple baseline covariates simultaneously in the conventional not PS-based Cox model did not alter the association substantially (HR = 1.40, 95% CI: 1.19-1.65). Ratios of the widths of the 95% CIs are presented in Table 3. HR estimates using the alternative adjustment

Table 1 Comparison of baseline and follow-up characteristics between HIV-infected patients with and without co-infection of tuberculosis in the unmatched sample with imputed covariates (for a single multiple imputation dataset)

Characteristics	TB: yes (n = 1690)	TB: no (n = 20787)	P-value	Standardized difference (Ratio of variance for continuous covariate)
Baseline characteristics				
Demographics				
Age (year)				
Mean (SD)	36.87 (8.78)	37.93 (9.48)	<0.0001	−0.117 (0.86)
Min	14	14		
25th percentile	31	31		
50th percentile	36	37		
75th percentile	42	43		
Max	73	93		
Male: n (%)	670 (39.64)	6216 (29.90)	<0.0001	0.206
HIV severity				
CD4 count				
Mean (SD)	143.39 (149.94)	170.82 (172.26)	<0.0001	−0.170 (0.76)
Min	0	0		
25th percentile	45	66		
50th percentile	111	139		
75th percentile	193	208		
Max	1701	1983		
WHO stage: n (%)				
1	43 (2.54)	992 (4.77)	<0.0001	-
2	441 (26.09)	11013 (52.98)		
3	999 (59.11)	7173 (34.51)		
4	207 (12.25)	1609 (7.74)		
AIDS: n (%)	493 (29.17)	3881 (18.67)	<0.0001	0.248
***History of drug use & illnesses*: *n* (%)**				
Pneumocystis pneumonia	28 (1.66)	101 (0.49)	<0.0001	0.114
Toxoplasmosis	11 (0.65)	101 (0.49)	0.3542	0.022
Sexually transmitted infection	341 (20.17)	4353 (20.94)	0.4578	−0.019
***Partner information*: *n* (%)**				
Married poly	125 (7.40)	1801 (8.66)	0.0734	−0.047
Partner sero-positive	417 (24.67)	5801 (27.91)	0.0043	−0.073
Sexually active	1224 (72.43)	15272 (73.47)	0.3508	−0.023
***Other characteristics*: *n* (%)**				
Site				
ENT	378 (22.37)	1950 (9.38)	<0.0001	-
GUL	161 (9.53)	1891 (9.10)		
JIN	276 (16.33)	2586 (12.44)		
MAS	130 (7.69)	2246 (10.80)		
MBL	144 (8.52)	2446 (11.77)		
MBR	116 (6.86)	2641 (12.71)		
MSD	61 (3.61)	1254 (6.03)		
MUL	211 (12.49)	2390 (11.50)		

Table 1 Comparison of baseline and follow-up characteristics between HIV-infected patients with and without co-infection of tuberculosis in the unmatched sample with imputed covariates (for a single multiple imputation dataset) *(Continued)*

SOR	29 (1.72)	1546 (7.44)		
TOR	184 (10.89)	1837 (8.84)		
Education (Higher institute)	58 (3.43)	623 (3.00)	0.3158	0.025
ART start year since 2000				
0	0 (0)	2 (0.01)	<0.0001	-
4	23 (1.36)	946 (4.55)		
5	453 (26.80)	4532 (21.80)		
6	373 (22.07)	3627 (17.45)		
6	507 (30.00)	6715 (32.30)		
8	330 (19.53)	4943 (23.78)		
9	4 (0.24)	22 (0.11)		
Follow-up characteristics				
Death: n (%)	177 (10.47)	1326 (6.38)	<0.0001	0.148
Median (IQR) length of follow-up (days)	627.5 (205–1034)	646 (306–1045)	-	-

Note: For continuous variables, mean and standard deviation for each group, standardized mean difference and ratio of variances between TB and no-TB patients are reported. For categorical variables, frequency and percentage of the specified level, and standardized difference between TB and no-TB patients are reported, unless noted otherwise. *MI* multiple imputation, *SD* standard deviation, *WHO* World Health Organization, *HIV* human immunodeficiency virus, *AIDS* acquired immune deficiency syndromes, *ENT* Entebbe, JIN: Jinja, *MAS* Masaka, *MBL* Mbale, *MBR* Mbarara, *MUL* Mulago, *TOR* Tororo, *GUL* Gulu, *SOR* Soroti, *MSD* Masindi, *IQR* interquantile range.

methods had greater precision relative to the result of the PS-matched analysis, as the latter only utilized data from the matched pairs, a subset of the study sample. The trade-off between accuracy and precision of the PS methods has been noted in previous studies [40,42].

Discussion

This is, to our knowledge, the largest cohort of HIV-infected patients receiving ART in a single African country that has evaluated mortality outcomes in co-infected patients. Descriptive analysis showed that TB patients, compared to non-TB patients, were more likely to be immunosuppressed, have a history of opportunistic infections, and live in particular geographical regions of Uganda. The results of Cox PH analysis using PS matching for confounding control showed that having pulmonary TB disease at the initiation of ART led to a 37% increase in the hazard of all-cause mortality during the follow-up period between 2000 and 2009. Additional analyses using two other PS methods and the conventional (not PS-based) multivariable Cox regression model showed similar results. These analyses may be viewed as sensitivity analyses because different methods use different assumptions and the results seem to remain robust to different ways of adjusting for baseline confounding.

The prevalence of active pulmonary TB at the initiation of ART of 7.52% in the study is consistent with results from a smaller TASO cohort reported from Tororo, Uganda [15]. This indicates that TB is less prevalent in Uganda compared with other African countries, particularly Southern Africa [16]. An open cohort of 7,512 patients receiving ART in South Africa suggested that 15.9% of HIV patients were treated for pulmonary TB at ART initiation between 2004 and 2007. Our finding of a 37% increase in hazard of overall mortality associated with having active TB at ART initiation after controlling for potential baseline confounding is both statistically significant and clinically relevant. This result is different from Westreich et al.'s findings on 7,512 HIV patients in South Africa, indicating pulmonary TB treatment at ART initiation was uncorrelated to the overall survival (HR = 1.06, 95% CI: 0.75-1.49) after adjusting for multiple confounders [16]. While all TB patients in the South Africa study received ART soon after initiation of TB treatment if TB treatment was well tolerated, the current study did not have reliable data on TB treatment at the initiation of ART. Instead the effect of baseline active pulmonary TB disease on mortality was evaluated and active TB patients might or might not have received TB treatment during the course of the study. The difference in baseline exposure between the two studies is likely to be the most important factor explaining the different results and suggests a benefit of starting TB treatment at ART initiation to reduce overall mortality in a co-infected population.

Guidelines on the treatment of TB co-infection with HIV have changed dramatically over the last few years

Table 2 Comparison of baseline and follow-up characteristics between HIV-infected patients with and without co-infection of tuberculosis in propensity score matched pairs with imputed covariates (for a single multiple imputation dataset)

Covariate	TB: yes (n = 1686)	TB: no (n = 1686)	Standardized difference (Ratio of variance for continuous covariate)
Baseline characterstics			
Demographics			
Age (year)			
Mean (SD)	36.89 (8.77)	36.93 (8.87)	−0.005 (0.978)
Min	14	14	
25th percentile	31	31	
50th percentile	36	36	
75th percentile	42	42	
Max	73	77	
Male: n (%)	668 (39.62)	673 (39.92)	−0.006
HIV severity			
CD4 count			
Mean (SD)	143.70 (149.98)	144.34 (139.78)	−0.004 (1.15)
Min	0	0	
25th percentile	45	44	
50th percentile	112	118	
75th percentile	194	196	
Max	1701	1247	
WHO stage: n (%)			
1	43 (2.55)	43 (2.55)	-
2	441 (26.16)	436 (25.86)	
3	996 (59.07)	983 (58.30)	
4	206 (12.22)	224 (13.29)	
AIDS: n (%)	489 (29.00)	479 (28.41)	0.013
***History of drug use & illnesses*: *n* (%)**			
Pneumocystis pneumonia	25 (1.48)	33 (1.96)	−0.037
Toxoplasmosis	11 (0.65)	8 (0.47)	0.024
Sexually transmitted infection	340 (20.17)	339 (20.11)	0.001
***Partner information*: *n* (%)**			
Married poly	125 (7.41)	136 (8.07)	−0.024
Partner sero-positive	417 (24.73)	431 (25.56)	−0.019
Sexually active	1221 (72.42)	1223 (72.54)	−0.003
***Other characteristics*: *n* (%)**			
Site			
ENT	374 (22.18)	378 (22.42)	-
GUL	161 (9.55)	176 (10.43)	
JIN	276 (16.37)	271 (16.07)	
MAS	130 (7.71)	125 (7.41)	
MBL	144 (8.54)	160 (9.49)	
MBR	116 (6.88)	121 (7.18)	
MSD	61 (3.62)	62 (3.68)	
MUL	211 (12.51)	203 (12.04)	

Table 2 Comparison of baseline and follow-up characteristics between HIV-infected patients with and without co-infection of tuberculosis in propensity score matched pairs with imputed covariates (for a single multiple imputation dataset) *(Continued)*

SOR	29 (1.72)	18 (1.07)	
TOR	184 (10.91)	172 (10.20)	
Education (Higher institute)	58 (3.44)	59 (3.50)	−0.003
ART start year since 2000			
4	23 (1.36)	15 (0.89)	-
5	452 (26.81)	428 (25.39)	
6	372 (22.06)	360 (21.35)	
7	505 (29.95)	548 (32.50)	
8	330 (19.57)	330 (19.57)	
9	4 (0.24)	5 (0.30)	
Follow-up characteristics			
Death: n (%)	176 (10.44)	137 (8.13)	0.080
Median (IQR) length of follow-up (days)	629 (205–1036)	659 (286–1023)	-

Note: For continuous variables, mean and standard deviation for each group, standardized mean difference and ratio of variances between TB and no-TB patients are reported. For categorical variables, frequency and percentage of the specified level, and standardized difference between TB and no-TB patients are reported, unless noted otherwise. *MI* multiple imputation, *SD* standard deviation, *WHO* World Health Organization, *HIV* human immunodeficiency virus, *AIDS* acquired immune deficiency syndromes, *ENT* Entebbe, *JIN* Jinja, *MAS* Masaka, *MBL* Mbale, *MBR* Mbarara, *MUL* Mulago, *TOR* Tororo, *GUL* Gulu, *SOR* Soroti, *MSD* Masindi, *IQR* interquantile range.

and may not reflect within-country variability. For example, early guidelines feared drug interactions between TB medication and ART or negative impact on adherence of ART or TB due to pill burden and suggested early treatment for TB disease followed by stabilization with ART. However, more recent evidence from randomized trials [4-6] suggests that starting ART within two weeks of TB treatment to improve survival appears to be well tolerated, and has persuaded guideline makers to recommend co-administration of treatment. In addition, recent data from South Africa found that although IRIS events were associated with slightly lower adherence rates, overall adherence to ART remained high in this co-infected population. The data suggested that concerns about IRIS or drug-drug interactions should not deter clinicians from early ART initiation, but patients developing IRIS events should be monitored closely and potentially targeted for interventions to increase adherence [52]. Other developments are related to the specific setting. Uganda, for example, has a lower national prevalence of co-infection than Southern Africa and has not reported any cases of extensively drug resistant (XDR) TB infections. South Africa, on the other hand, has had an epidemic of XDR co-infections that has resulted in quarantine of some patients and recommendations about interacting with other individuals [53]. National guidelines from Uganda do not match those of South Africa, as discussed earlier.

Limitations of the study emerge from three key sources. First, propensity score methods cannot balance unmeasured confounders in estimating a causal relationship, which is an issue faced by all observational cohorts. Our results may be biased if some unobserved prognostic factors were unbalanced between TB and non-TB groups. While some studies examined the impact of body mass index and anemia on clinical outcomes in co-

Table 3 Effect of tuberculosis (TB) at the initiation of antiretroviral therapy (ART) on overall survival

Method	HR	95% CI	P-value	CI width ratio*
Primary analysis				
Matching on PS	1.37	(1.08, 1.75)	0.011	1
Additional analyses				
Unadjusted Cox regression	1.74	(1.49, 2.04)	<0.001	0.82
Stratified on PS	1.36	(1.15, 1.60)	<0.001	0.66
PS as covariate (linear, quadratic and cubic terms)	1.34	(1.14, 1.58)	<0.001	0.65
Conventional adjusted Cox regression	1.40	(1.19, 1.65)	<0.001	0.69

Results for the propensity score (PS) or covariate-adjusted Cox regression models were aggregated across five multiple imputation datasets using Rubin's rule. *HR* hazard ratio, *CI* confidence interval, *PS* propensity score. * Reference = width of 95% CI for PS-matched estimate.

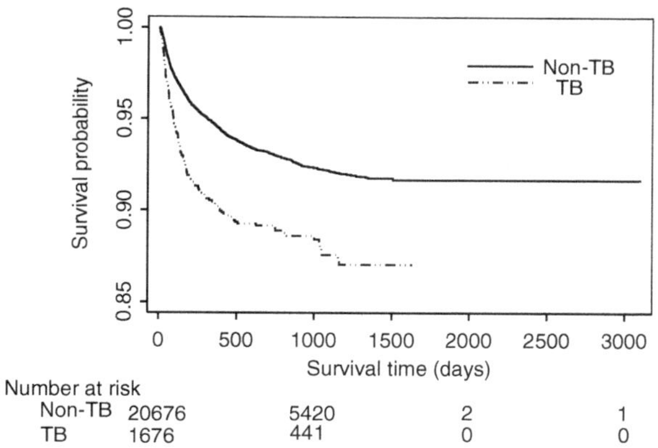

Figure 1 Kaplan–Meier survival curves by baseline TB status in the unmatched study sample.

infected patients [16], such baseline information was unavailable in the current study. More resources need to be dedicated to improve the completeness and accuracy of data collection in HIV patients in underdeveloped regions. Although statistical tools instrumental variable analysis, have been developed to control for bias due to unmeasured confounders [54], strong assumptions are required to ensure estimation accuracy, and such assumptions can be difficult to verify using empirical data. Second, the multiple imputation method employed to impute the missing values for baseline covariates requires missing at random (MAR) assumption (i.e. missingness can be explained by differences in the observed data). Although the current imputation procedure included a number of baseline characteristics and follow-up variables, we could not rule out the existence of additional variables that were highly associated with missingness. The MAR assumption is unverifiable using data collected within a study. Third, our results are predominantly based on adult, HIV-infected, African patients who initiated ART in Uganda, during 2004 to 2009, hence limiting their generalizability. The effect of active pulmonary TB disease on HIV patients in other age or ethnic groups (for instance, children and adolescents) and from different geographic regions should be further investigated.

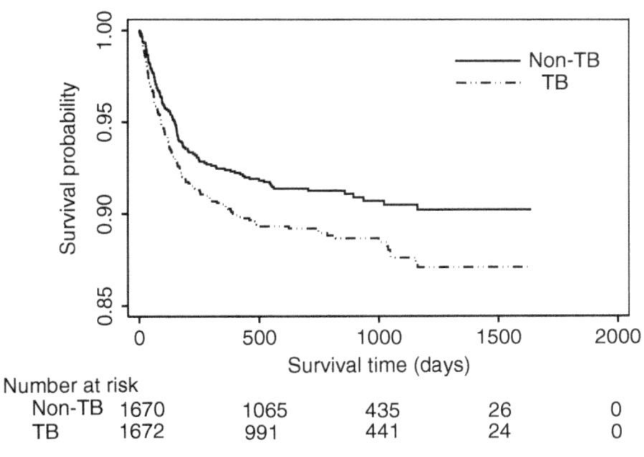

Figure 2 Kaplan–Meier survival curves by baseline TB status in propensity score matched pairs for a single multiple imputation dataset.

Our study shows a 37% increase in the hazard of death among co-infected patients compared with those only infected with HIV. We used pulmonary TB disease as documented through sputum and radiologic confirmation for the diagnosis of TB disease as TASO, along with most AIDS service organizations in Africa, lacked the infrastructure to consistently diagnose extra-pulmonary TB disease. Also, we recognize that sensitivity of sputum smear for diagnosis of pulmonary TB in HIV-infected patients was poor (less than 50%) and thus we followed up patients with suspect TB disease with radiologic examinations regardless of sputum results. Because TB is associated with mortality (as observed in this study), misclassifying actual active TB patients into the non-TB group would attenuate the magnitude of the TB effect on death; as a result the apparent estimates of TB effects on death would be less substantial than the actual effects.

Conclusions

In summary, our current study suggests a moderate increase in the hazard of death associated with having active TB disease at the initiation of ART in HIV-infected patients receiving ART in Uganda. Our finding is complementary to results of the recent SAPIT, [4] CAMELIA, [5] and STRIDE trials [6] that demonstrate improved survival when ART is initiated during TB therapy. The results also validate the WHO guidelines that urge a more aggressive approach to management of both TB and HIV [55].

Additional files

Additional file 1: Coding of baseline covariates and post-ART variables.

Additional file 2: Figure S1. Study flowchart.

Additional file 3: Summary statistics of the four baseline covariates with missing values in the original and imputed datasets.

Additional file 4: Results of the final propensity score (PS) model.

Additional file 5: Figure S2. Distribution of age (in years) at ART initiation in TB and no-TB group in the original sample and PS-matched pairs for a single MI dataset. From top to bottom: quantile-quantile plots, empirical cumulative distribution functions (circles represent TB and triangles represent no-TB), nonparametric density curves (solid line represents TB and dashed line represents no-TB), and side-by-side boxplots.

Additional file 6: Figure S3. Distribution of CD4 cell counts at ART initiation in TB and no-TB group in the original sample and PS matched pairs for a single MI dataset. From top to bottom: quantile-quantile plots, empirical cumulative distribution functions (circles represent TB and triangles represent no-TB), nonparametric density curves (solid line represents TB and dashed line represents no-TB), and side-by-side boxplots.

Abbreviations

TB: Tuberculosis; ART: Antiretroviral therapy; HIV: Human immunodeficiency virus; AIDS: Acquired immune deficiency syndromes; WHO: World Health Organization; TASO: AIDS Support Organization; IRIS: Immune reconstitution inflammatory syndrome; PCP: Pneumocystis pneumonia; PS: Propensity score; HR: Hazard ratio; MI: Multiple imputation; MAR: Missing at random; SD: Standard deviation; CI: Confidence interval; ENT: Entebbe; JIN: Jinja; MAS: Masaka; MBL: Mbale; MBR: Mbarara; MUL: Mulago; TOR: Tororo; GUL: Gulu; SOR: Soroti; MSD: Masindi; IQR: Interquantile range.

Competing interests

The authors declare that they have no competing interest.

Authors' contributions

RC participated in the conception and design of the study, data cleaning and analysis, results interpretation, and drafting and revision of the manuscript. EM participated in the conception and design of the study, data collection, results interpretation, and revision of the manuscript. JB and EP participated in review of statistical methods, results interpretation, and revision of the manuscript. CN participated in data collection from TASO clinics and review of drafts. JBN and PJD participated in results interpretation and revision of the manuscript. LT participated in the conception and design of the study, results interpretation, and revision of the manuscript. All authors read and approved the final manuscript.

Acknowledgements

RC received studentship from Father Sean O'Sullivan Research Centre, St. Joseph's Healthcare Hamilton. RC holds a doctoral research award from the Canadian Institutes of Health Research. This study was supported in part by funds from the CANNeCTIN program.

Author details

[1]Department of Clinical Epidemiology and Biostatistics, McMaster University, Hamilton, Canada. [2]Biostatistics Unit, 3rd Floor Martha, Room H325, St Joseph's Healthcare Hamilton, 50 Charlton Avenue East, Hamilton, ON L8N 4A6, Canada. [3]Faculty of Health Sciences, University of Ottawa, Ottawa, Canada. [4]The AIDS Support Organization (TASO), Kampala, Uganda. [5]Department of Medicine and Centre for Infectious Diseases, Stellenbosch University, Cape Town, South Africa. [6]Departments of Epidemiology and International Health, Johns Hopkins Bloomberg School of Public Health, Baltimore, MD, USA. [7]Hamilton Health Sciences, Population Health Research Institute, Hamilton, Canada.

References

1. World Health Organization: *Global summary of the HIV/AIDS epidemic.* 2009. [http://www.who.int/hiv/data/2009_global_summary.gif] Accessed July 16, 2012.
2. Selwyn PA, Hartel D, Lewis VA, Schoenbaum EE, Vermund SH, Klein RS, Walker AT, Friedland GH: **A prospective study of the risk of tuberculosis among intravenous drug users with human immunodeficiency virus infection.** *N Engl J Med* 1989, **320**(9):545–550.
3. *Centers for Disease Control and Prevention. TB and HIV/AIDS. CDC HIV/AIDS facts.* 2012. [http://www.cdc.gov/hiv/resources/factsheets/PDF/hivtb.pdf] Accessed July 16, 2012.
4. Abdool Karim SS, Naidoo K, Grobler A, Padayatchi N, Baxter C, Gray A, Gengiah T, Nair G, Bamber S, Singh A, Khan M, Pienaar J, El-Sadr W, Friedland G, Abdool Karim Q: **Timing of initiation of antiretroviral drugs during tuberculosis therapy.** *N Engl J Med* 2010, **362**(8):697–706.
5. Blanc FX, Sok T, Laureillard D, Borand L, Rekacewicz C, Nerrienet E, Madec Y, Marcy O, Chan S, Prak N, Kim C, Lak KK, Hak C, Dim B, Sin CI, Sun S, Guillard B, Sar B, Vong S, Fernandez M, Fox L, Delfraissy JF, Goldfeld AE, CAMELIA (ANRS 1295-CIPRA KH001) Study Team: **Earlier versus later start of antiretroviral therapy in HIV-infected adults with tuberculosis.** *N Engl J Med* 2011, **365**(16):1471–1481.
6. Havlir DV, Kendall MA, Ive P, Kumwenda J, Swindells S, Qasba SS, Luetkemeyer AF, Hogg E, Rooney JF, Wu X, Hosseinipour MC, Lalloo U, Veloso VG, Some FF, Kumarasamy N, Padayatchi N, Santos BR, Reid S, Hakim J, Mohapi L, Mugyenyi P, Sanchez J, Lama JR, Pape JW, Sanchez A, Asmelash A, Moko E, Sawe F, Andersen J, Sanne I, AIDS Clinical Trials Group Study A5221: **Timing of antiretroviral therapy for HIV-1 infection and tuberculosis.** *N Engl J Med* 2011, **365**(16):1482–1491.
7. World Health Organization: *Joint HIV/Tuberculosis interventions.* 2012. [http://www.who.int/hiv/topics/tb/tuberculosis/en/] Accessed July 16, 2012.
8. Marks S, Magee E, Robison V: **Reported HIV status of tuberculosis patients—United States, 1993-2005.** *MMWR Morb Mortal Wkly Rep* 2007, **56**(42):1103–1106.
9. Harries AD, Zachariah R, Corbett EL, Lawn SD, Santos-Filho ET, Chimzizi R, Harrington M, Maher D, Williams BG, De Cock KM: **The HIV-associated tuberculosis epidemic–when will we act?** *Lancet* 2010, **375**(9729):1906–1919.
10. Burman WJ, Jones BE: **Treatment of HIV-related tuberculosis in the era of effective antiretroviral therapy.** *Am J Respir Crit Care Med* 2001, **164**(1):7–12.
11. Narita M, Ashkin D, Hollender ES, Pitchenik AE: **Paradoxical worsening of tuberculosis following antiretroviral therapy in patients with AIDS.** *Am J Respir Crit Care Med* 1998, **158**(1):157–161.
12. McIlleron H, Meintjes G, Burman WJ, Maartens G: **Complications of antiretroviral therapy in patients with tuberculosis: drug interactions, toxicity, and immune reconstitution inflammatory syndrome.** *J Infect Dis* 2007, **196**(Suppl 1):S63–S75.
13. Gandhi NR, Nunn P, Dheda K, Schaaf HS, Zignol M, van Soolingen D, Jensen P, Bayona J: **Multidrug-resistant and extensively drug-resistant tuberculosis: a threat to global control of tuberculosis.** *Lancet* 2010, **375**(9728):1830–1843.
14. Lonnroth K, Castro KG, Chakaya JM, Chauhan LS, Floyd K, Glaziou P, Raviglione MC: **Tuberculosis control and elimination 2010–50: cure, care, and social development.** *Lancet* 2010, **375**(9728):1814–1829.
15. Moore D, Liechty C, Ekwaru P, Were W, Mwima G, Solberg P, Rutherford G, Mermin J: **Prevalence, incidence and mortality associated with tuberculosis in HIV-infected patients initiating antiretroviral therapy in rural Uganda.** *AIDS* 2007, **21**(6):713–719.
16. Westreich D, MacPhail P, Van Rie A, Malope-Kgokong B, Ive P, Rubel D, Boulme R, Eron J, Sanne I: **Effect of pulmonary tuberculosis on mortality in patients receiving HAART.** *AIDS* 2009, **23**(6):707–715.
17. Lopez-Gatell H, Cole SR, Hessol NA, French AL, Greenblatt RM, Landesman S, Preston-Martin S, Anastos K: **Effect of tuberculosis on the survival of women infected with human immunodeficiency virus.** *Am J Epidemiol* 2007, **165**(10):1134–1142.
18. Lopez-Gatell H, Cole SR, Margolick JB, Witt MD, Martinson J, Phair JP, Jacobson LP, Multicenter AIDS Cohort Study: **Effect of tuberculosis on the survival of HIV-infected men in a country with low tuberculosis incidence.** *AIDS* 2008, **22**(14):1869–1873.
19. Straetemans M, Bierrenbach AL, Nagelkerke N, Glaziou P, van der Werf MJ: **The effect of tuberculosis on mortality in HIV positive people: a meta-analysis.** *PLoS One* 2010, **5**(12):e15241.
20. Rosenbaum PR, Rubin DB: **The central role of the propensity score in observational studies for causal effects.** *Biometrika* 1983, **70**(1):41–55.
21. Rosenbaum PR, Rubin DB: **Reducing bias in observational studies using subclassification on the propensity score.** *J Am Stat Assoc* 1984, **79**:516–524.
22. Rubin DB: **The design versus the analysis of observational studies for causal effects: parallels with the design of randomized trials.** *Stat Med* 2007, **26**(1):20–36.
23. Bakanda C, Birungi J, Nkoyooyo A, Featherstone A, Cooper CL, Hogg RS, Mills EJ: **Cohort Profile: The TASO-CAN Cohort Collaboration.** *Int J Epidemiol* 2012, **41**(4):946–950. http://ije.oxfordjournals.org/content/41/4/946.
24. Ministry of health: *National Antiretroviral Treatment and Care Guidelines for Adults and Children: Kampala.* Uganda: Earnest Publishers; 2008.
25. Druyts E, Dybul M, Kanters S, Nachega J, Birungi J, Ford N, Thorlund K, Negin J, Lester R, Yaya S, Mills EJ: **Male sex and the risk of mortality among individuals enrolled in antiretroviral therapy programs in Africa: a systematic review and meta-analysis.** *AIDS* 2013, **27**(3):417–425.
26. *AIDS Basics.* ; 2013. [http://aids.gov/hiv-aids-basics/] Accessed June 22, 2013.
27. Vlahov D, Graham N, Hoover D, Flynn C, Bartlett JG, Margolick JB, Lyles CM, Nelson KE, Smith D, Holmberg S, Farzadegan H: **Prognostic indicators for AIDS and infectious disease death in HIV-infected injection drug users: plasma viral load and CD4+ cell count.** *JAMA* 1998, **279**(1):35–40.
28. May M, Sterne JA, Sabin C, Costagliola D, Justice AC, Thiebaut R, Gill J, Phillips A, Reiss P, Hogg R, Ledergerber B, D'Arminio Monforte A, Schmeisser N, Staszewski S, Egger M, Antiretroviral Therapy (ART) Cohort Collaboration: **Prognosis of HIV-1-infected patients up to 5 years after initiation of HAART: collaborative analysis of prospective studies.** *AIDS* 2007, **21**(9):1185–1197.

29. Dheda K, Shean K, Zumla A, Badri M, Streicher EM, Page-Shipp L, Willcox P, John MA, Reubenson G, Govindasamy D, Wong M, Padanilam X, Dziwiecki A, van Helden PD, Siwendu S, Jarand J, Menezes CN, Burns A, Victor T, Warren R, Grobusch MP, van der Walt M, Kvasnovsky C: **Early treatment outcomes and HIV status of patients with extensively drug-resistant tuberculosis in South Africa: a retrospective cohort study.** *Lancet* 2010, **375**(9728):1798–1807.
30. Bakanda C, Birungi J, Mwesigwa R, Zhang W, Hagopian A, Ford N, Mills EJ: **Density of healthcare providers and patient outcomes: evidence from a nationally representative multi-site HIV treatment program in Uganda.** *PLoS One* 2011, **6**(1):e16279.
31. Mills EJ, Beyrer C, Birungi J, Dybul MR: **Engaging men in prevention and care for HIV/AIDS in Africa.** *PLoS Med* 2012, **9**(2):e1001167.
32. Epstein H, Swidler A, Gray R, Reniers G, Parker W, Parkhurst J, Short R, Halperin D: **Measuring concurrent partnerships.** *Lancet* 2010, **375**(9729):1869. author reply 1870.
33. Eyawo O, de Walque D, Ford N, Gakii G, Lester RT, Mills EJ: **HIV status in discordant couples in sub-Saharan Africa: a systematic review and meta-analysis.** *Lancet Infect Dis* 2010, **10**(11):770–777.
34. Padian NS, Manian S: **The concurrency debate: time to put it to rest.** *Lancet* 2011, **378**(9787):203–204.
35. Centers for Disease Control and Prevention: *Basic TB Facts.* 2013. [http://www.cdc.gov/tb/topic/basics/risk.htm] Accessed June 22, 2013.
36. Austin PC: **A critical appraisal of propensity-score matching in the medical literature between 1996 and 2003.** *Stat Med* 2008, **27**(12):2037–2049.
37. Gayat E, Pirracchio R, Resche-Rigon M, Mebazaa A, Mary JY, Porcher R: **Propensity scores in intensive care and anaesthesiology literature: a systematic review.** *Intensive Care Med* 2010, **36**(12):1993–2003.
38. Tleyjeh IM, Kashour T, Zimmerman V, Steckelberg JM, Wilson WR, Baddour LM: **The role of valve surgery in infective endocarditis management: a systematic review of observational studies that included propensity score analysis.** *Am Heart J* 2008, **156**(5):901–909.
39. Guo S, Fraser MW: *Propensity Score Analysis: Statistical Methods and Applications.* Thousand Oaks, CA: SAGE Publications, Inc.; 2010.
40. Austin PC: **Balance diagnostics for comparing the distribution of baseline covariates between treatment groups in propensity-score matched samples.** *Stat Med* 2009, **28**(25):3083–3107.
41. Austin PC: **A Tutorial and Case Study in Propensity Score Analysis: An Application to Estimating the Effect of In-Hospital Smoking Cessation Counseling on Mortality.** *Multivariate Behav Res* 2011, **46**(1):119–151.
42. Austin PC: **An Introduction to Propensity Score Methods for Reducing the Effects of Confounding in Observational Studies.** *Multivariate Behav Res* 2011, **46**(3):399–424.
43. Cohen J: *Statistical power analysis for the behavioural sciences: 2nd ed.* Hillsdale, NJ: Lawrence Erlbaum Associates Publishers; 1988.
44. Ho DE: **Using propensity scores to help design observational studies: application to the tobacco litigation.** *Health sciences and outcomes research methodology* 2001, **2:**169–188.
45. Austin PC, Mamdani MM: **A comparison of propensity score methods: a case-study estimating the effectiveness of post-AMI statin use.** *Stat Med* 2006, **25**(12):2084–2106.
46. Coca-Perraillon M: *Local and global optimal propensity score matching.* Orlando, Florida: Proceedings of the SAS Global Forum 2007; 2007.
47. Austin PC: **Optimal caliper widths for propensity-score matching when estimating differences in means and differences in proportions in observational studies.** *Pharm Stat* 2011, **10**(2):150–161.
48. Cummings P, McKnight B, Greenland S: **Matched cohort methods for injury research.** *Epidemiol Rev* 2003, **25:**43–50.
49. Little RJA, Rubin DB: *Statistical Analysis with Missing Data: 2nd ed.* New Jersey: John Wiley & Sons, Inc.; 2002.
50. Abaasa AM, Todd J, Ekoru K, Kalyango JN, Levin J, Odeke E, Karamagi CA: **Good adherence to HAART and improved survival in a community HIV/AIDS treatment and care programme: the experience of The AIDS Support Organization (TASO), Kampala, Uganda.** *BMC Health Serv Res* 2008, **8:**241-6963-8-241.
51. Kiboneka A, Nyatia RJ, Nabiryo C, Anema A, Cooper CL, Fernandes KA, Montaner JS, Mills EJ: **Combination antiretroviral therapy in population affected by conflict: outcomes from large cohort in northern Uganda.** *BMJ* 2009, **338:**b201.
52. Morroni C, Chaisson R, Goliath R, *et al*: *Influence of IRIS on ART adherence in HIV+ adults.* South Africa: CROI; 2012. Abstract# 941.
53. Gandhi NR, Moll A, Sturm AW, Pawinski R, Govender T, Lalloo U, Zeller K, Andrews J, Friedland G: **Extensively drug-resistant tuberculosis as a cause of death in patients co-infected with tuberculosis and HIV in a rural area of South Africa.** *Lancet* 2006, **368**(9547):1575–1580.
54. Stukel TA, Fisher ES, Wennberg DE, Alter DA, Gottlieb DJ, Vermeulen MJ: **Analysis of observational studies in the presence of treatment selection bias: effects of invasive cardiac management on AMI survival using propensity score and instrumental variable methods.** *JAMA* 2007, **297**(3):278–285.
55. World Health Organization: *Treatment of tuberculosis: guidelines for national programmes: 3rd ed.* Geneva, Switzerland: World Health Organization; 2003.

Prevalence of dyslipidemia among HIV-infected patients using first-line highly active antiretroviral therapy in Southern Ethiopia

Agete Tadewos[1], Zelalem Addis[2*], Henock Ambachew[3] and Sandip Banerjee[4]

Abstract

Background: Data on lipid profile abnormalities among patients receiving highly active antiretroviral treatment in Ethiopia are very limited. The aim of this study was to determine the prevalence of dyslipidemia and characteristics of lipid profiles among patients living with human immunodeficiency virus (HIV) using first-line highly active antiretroviral therapy (HAART) in Southern Ethiopia.

Methods: This cross sectional comparative group study was conducted between March and May 2012, and included 113 HIV infected patients treated for a minimum of one year with first-line HAART regimens that included Efavirenz and Nevirapine (HAART group) and others 113 who had never received HAART (pre-HAART group). Serum lipid profiles were determined after overnight fasting and dyslipidemia was assessed according to the United State National Cholesterol Education program-III guideline. For statistical analysis Chi-square, student's t-test, and logistic regression were used using Statistical Package for Social Sciences (SPSS) Version 20.

Result: Ninety-three (82.3%) of HAART and 87 (76.9%) pre-HAART patients had at least one laboratory abnormality, which is compatible with a diagnosis of dyslipidemia. Total cholesterol ≥ 200 mg/dl occurred in 43.4% of HAART and 15.9% pre-HAART patients (p=<0.0001), whereas HDL-cholesterol below 40 mg/dl occurred in 43.4% and in 63.7% respectively, (p=0.002). The LDL-cholesterol ≥ 130 mg/dl occurred in 33.6% of HAART and 15% pre-HAART patients (p=0.001), while triglycerides ≥ 150 mg/dl occurred in 55.8% and 31.0% respectively, (p=0.001). Receiving of HAART was significantly and positively associated with raised total cholesterol, LDL-cholesterol, and triglycerides. The adjusted odds ratio (95% CI) of HAART-treated vs. pre-HAART was 3.80 (1.34-6.55) for total cholesterol ≥ 200 mg/dl; 2.64 (1.31-5.32) for LDL- cholesterol ≥ 130 mg/dl and 2.50 (1.41-4.42) for triglycerides ≥150 mg/dl.

Conclusion: Use of first-line antiretroviral therapy regimens that contain Efavirenz and Nevirapine were associated with raised total cholesterol, LDL-cholesterol, and triglycerides, an established atherogenic lipid profiles. Lipid profiles should be performed at baseline before commencement of antiretroviral therapy and then periodically through treatment follow-up to monitor any rising trends.

Keywords: Dyslipidemia, HIV/AIDS, Antiretroviral therapy, *Ethiopia*

* Correspondence: zelalemaddis@ymail.com
[2]School of Biomedical and Laboratory Sciences, University of Gondar College of Medicine and Health Science, P.O Box 196, Gondar, Ethiopia
Full list of author information is available at the end of the article

Introduction

In 2011, an estimated 34 million people were living with human immunodeficiency virus /acquired immunodeficiency syndrome (HIV/AIDS) worldwide; of them 22.9 million were living in Sub-Saharan Africa. About 1.2 million people were estimated to be living with HIV in Ethiopia [1].The introduction of highly active antiretroviral therapy (HAART) has led to a marked reduction in AIDS-related morbidity and mortality [2]. Since its introduction patients have started to live longer, however co-morbid problems have been emerged. Dyslipidemia, insulin resistance, and diabetes are some of metabolic complications of long-term use of HAART [3]. The characteristics of dyslipidemia in HIV-infected patients receiving HAART includes, elevated level of total cholesterol (TC), LDL-cholesterol (LDL-c), triglycerides (TG), and decreased HDL-cholesterol (HDL-c), include with severe hypertriglyceridemia in some patients [4]. Some antiretroviral drugs, such as stavudine (d4T) [5], and protease inhibitors (PIs) [6], increase the blood levels of TC, LDL-c, and TGs with variable effects on levels of HDL-c. Nevirapine (NVP) use is associated with increases in LDL-c [7], whereas increases in TC and TG are observed with use of efavirenz (EFV), particularly with longer duration of therapy [8]. Therefore, the use of HAART raises concerning metabolic disorders and cardiovascular risk in HIV infected patients who now present an extended life expectancy [9]. The prevalence of dyslipidemia in resource-limited settings has not been well characterized and current World Health Organization (WHO) antiretroviral therapy (ART) guidelines do not include a recommendation that lipid monitoring should be conducted in patients receiving first-line HAART [10]. In addition, evidences in support of dyslipidemia associated with first-line HAART that include EFV and NVP in Sub-Sahara African countries are scarce [11,12].The aim of the present study was to determine the prevalence of dyslipidemia and characteristics of lipid profiles among people living with HIV infection receiving first-line HAART in Southern Ethiopia.

Methods

Study setting and study population

This was a cross-sectional comparative group study. Subjects were recruited between March 2012 and May 2012 at ART clinic of Hawassa University Referral Hospital. Two groups of participants were selected for this study. The first group included HIV-infected individuals who had been receiving WHO recommended first-line HAART for a minimum of one year (HAART group). Participants used first-line HAART regimens that included nucleoside reverse transcriptase inhibitors (NRTIs): lamivudine (3TC), ZDV, or d4T, and non-nucleoside reverse transcriptase inhibitors (NNRTIs): NVP or EFV. Patients who had had their therapy regimens changed during follow-up were not included. The second group was pre-tested and confirmed HIV-positive individuals who were not yet getting HAART. All participants included were ≥18 years of age and HAART treated group to have a good ART adherence (adherence rate ≥ 95%). A good adherence is defined by missing < 2 dose of 30 doses or < 3 dose of 60 doses; and it was adopted from Ethiopian Federal Ministry of Health, HIV Care/ART follow-up form. Participants receiving lipid altering therapies, pregnant women, known diabetes mellitus patients and renal failures were excluded.

Assessments and measurements

For all participants, data were collected on the socio-demographic informations along with body mass index, medical history including diabetes mellitus, renal failures, use of drugs that alter lipid profiles, and current use of anti-TB drugs. $CD4^+$ lymphocyte count was done by using flow cytometry instrument (Becton Dickinson, CA, USA). Blood sample was collected from each participant after a 12 hour overnight fast and centrifuged at 3000 cycles/ minute, and then serum was obtained for lipid profiles. Fasting serum TC and TG were assayed by enzymatic method (Linear chemicals, Montgat, Spain). Serum HDL-c determined by enzymatic method after a selective precipitation of apolipoprotein containing lipoproteins (very low density lipoprotein, LDL-c, and apolipoprotein a (Lpa) by phosphotungstic acid/$MgCl_2$ (Linear chemicals, Montgat, Spain). LDL-c was assessed by enzymatic method after precipitation of LDL by polyvinyl sulfate (Linear chemicals, Montgat, Spain) and then LDL-c was calculated by subtracting the supernatant cholesterol fractions from the TC of the sample. And also the TC/HDL-c ratio was calculated.

Finally dyslipidemia was defined as TC ≥ 200 mg/dl, HDL-c < 40 mg/dl, LDL-c ≥ 130 mg/dl, TG ≥ 150 mg/dl and TC/HDL-c ratio ≥ 5 by the United States National Cholesterol Education Program, Adult Treatment Panel (NCEP-ATP) III guidelines [13].

Statistical analysis

The estimation of the sample size was based on the difference between proportions and the following parameters were considered: alpha (α) = 5%, beta (β) = 10 % and power = 90%. Concerning dyslipidemia, we considered frequencies of LDL-c ≥130 mg/dl, which was 21% for the group of individuals with HIV/AIDS without HAART treatment [14]; and 40.8% for patients receiving HAART treatment [15]. With these parameters, the sample size calculated was 230 participants (115 pre-HAART and 115 HAART-treated patients).Data entry and Database management was completed using EPI-INFO 2002. Statistical analyses were done using Statistical Package for Social Sciences (SPSS) Version 20. Chi-square test was used to evaluate differences in frequency distribution. Student's t-test was applied to assess differences between two means. Logistic regression was also used to determine the association of independent factors (age, gender, and treatment status, type of treatment, current CD4 counts, and history of smoking, body mass index and current use of anti-TB drugs) with abnormal level of each lipid profile. P-value less than 0.05 considered as statistically significant at 95% confidence interval (CI).

Ethical consideration

The study was approved by the ethical review committee of School of Biomedical and Laboratory Sciences, University of Gondar. All individuals participated in the study provided their informed consent.

Results

General characteristics of study participants

Total number of participants enrolled in the study was 226, with 79 (35%) males and 147 (65%) females. Two groups were studied: the first group 113 HIV-infected patients (38 (33.6%) males, 75 (66.4%) females) were currently receiving HAART treatment; the second group 113 patients (41 (36.3%) males, 72 (63.7%) females) were pre-HAART. The age of individuals who were on HAART was 37.2 ± 8.7 while that of pre-HAART was 33.7 ±8.3 years and the age difference was significantly different (Table 1). First-line HAART regimens were a combinations of 2NRTI and 1NNRTI. All regimens included 3TC. HAART patients had been on treatment for a mean of 49.4 months (standard deviation: 16.5). The number of patients on ZDV/3TC/EFV, and ZDV/3TC/NVP regimens were 22 (19.5%) and 36 (31.8%) respectively, while those on d4T/3TC/EFV, and d4T/3TC/NVP regimens were 24 (21.2%) and 31 (27.4%) respectively. Accordingly, 58 (51.3%) patients were on ZDV, 55 (48.7%) were on d4T, 46 (40.7%) were on EFV, and 67 (59.3%) were on NVP.

Table 1 Characteristics of study population by HAART status in Hawassa, Southern Ethiopia

Variables	HAART group (n=113)	pre-HAART group (n=113)
Gender = Female, n (%)	75 (66.4)	72 (63.7)
Male, n (%)	38 (33.6)	41 (36.3)
Age, (years), mean ± SD	37.2 (8.7)	33.7 (8.3)**
18–30 years, n (%)	26 (23)	49 (43.4)
31–40 years, n (%)	59 (52.2)	47(41.6)
41–50 years, n (%)	21 (18.6)	12 (10.6)
>50 years, n (%)	7 (6.2)	5 (4.4)
BMI (Kg/m^2), mean ± SD	22.3 (4.1)	21.5 (3.9)
<18 Kg/m^2, n (%)	8 (7)	14 (12.4)
18–25 Kg/m^2, n (%)	82 (72.6)	84 (74.3)
>25 Kg/m^2, n (%)	23 (20.4)	15 (13.3)
CD4+ count ($cells/mm^3$), mean ± SD	460 (221)	356 (216.7) ***
< 200 $cells/mm^3$, n (%)	16 (14.2)	29 (25.7)
200–400 $cells/mm^3$, n (%)	32 (28.3)	44 (38.9)
> 400 $cells/mm^3$, n (%)	65 (57.5)	40 (35.4)
Duration of HAART, mean ±SD	49.4 (16.5)	–
12–24 months, n (%)	10 (8.8)	–
24–36 months, n (%)	18 (15.9)	–
36–48 months, n (%)	27 (23.9)	–
48–60 months, n (%)	24 (21.2)	–
> 60 years, n (%)	34 (30.1)	–
Current anti-TB users, n (%)	0	4 (3.5)
Current smoking, n (%)	6 (5.3)	7 (6.2)
Past smoking, n (%)	15 (13.3)	13 (11.5)

BMI, body mass index; HAART, highly active antiretroviral therapy; mo, month; TB, tuberculosis; SD, standard deviation; ** p-value < 0.01; *** p-value < 0.001.

Dyslipidemia and characteristics of lipid profiles

Ninety-three (82.3%) of HAART treated and 87 (76.9%) pre-HAART patients had at least one laboratory abnormality, which is compatible with a diagnosis of dyslipidemia (Figure 1). The prevalence of TC ≥ 200 mg/dl, LDL-c ≥130 mg/dl and TG ≥150 mg/dl were significantly higher in HAART group when compared to pre-HAART group. The prevalence of HDL-c below 40 mg/dl was significantly higher in pre-HAART group when compared to those on HAART. However, there was no significant difference in TC/HDL-c ratio between HAART treated and pre-HAART patients (Table 2).

Dyslipidemia and first-line HAART

No significant difference observed in lipid profile derangements between patients receiving ZDV when compared to those on d4T; and patients treated with EFV when compared to those treated with NVP (Table 3 and Table 4). In addition, no significant difference observed in lipid derangements between HAART treated males and females; however, the proportion of raised LDL-c is slightly higher in females when compared to males (Figure 2).

Dyslipidemia and risk factors

Multivariate analysis was adjusted for potential confounding factors such as age, sex, current history of smoking, past history of smoking, BMI, CD4+cells, current use of anti-TB drugs, and HAART treatment. Receiving of HAART was significantly and positively associated with raised TC, LDL-c, and TG. The adjusted odds ratio (95% CI) of HAART-treated vs. pre-HAART was 3.80 (1.34-6.55) for TC ≥200 mg/dl; 2.64 (1.31-5.32)

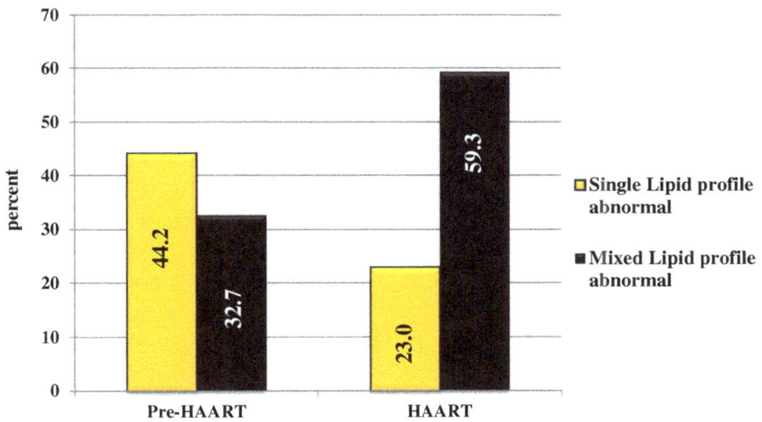

Figure 1 Category of dyslipidemia among study population by HAART status in Hawassa, Southern Ethiopia Number of patients in HAART group was 113 and in pre-HAART group were113; number of patients with single lipid profile abnormal in pre-HAART group and HAART group were respectively, 50 and 26; and number of patients with mixed lipid profiles abnormal in pre-HAART group and HAART group were respectively, 37 and 67; HAART, highly active antiretroviral therapy; (single lipid profile abnormal means only one lipid parameter is abnormal and mixed lipid profile abnormal means more than one lipid parameters abnormal within a single individual).

for LDL-c ≥ 130 mg/dl and 2.50 (1.41-4.42) for TG ≥ 150 mg/dl. However, antiretroviral therapy was not positively associated with decreased of HDL-cholesterol (Table 5).

Univariate and multivariate analysis were also applied to assess independent risk factors for each abnormal lipid profile in the subgroup of 113 HAART treated patients. In these both models, age was the risk factor of raised TC and decreased HDL-c; and BMI was the risk factor of raised TC in HAART treated patients (Table 6).

Table 2 Serum lipid profiles of study population by HAART status in Hawassa, Southern Ethiopia

Parameters	HAART group (n=113)	Pre-HAART group (n=113)
Total cholesterol, mean ± SD	199.6 (51.5)	155.4 (44) ***
< 200mg/dl	64 (56.6%)	95 (84.1%)
≥ 200mg/dl	49 (43.4%)	18 (15.9%) ***
HDL-cholesterol, mean ± SD	43.2 (14.3)	33.3 (12.8) ***
< 40mg/dl	49 (43.4%)	72 (63.7%) **
≥ 40mg/dl	64 (56.6%)	41 (36.3%)
LDL-cholesterol, mean ± SD	119.3 (43)	97.3 (36.2) ***
< 130mg/dl	75 (66.4%)	96 (85%)
≥ 130mg/dl	38 (33.6%)	17 (15.0%) **
Triglycerides, mean ± SD	204 (143)	138 (76) ***
< 150mg/dl	50 (44.2%)	78 (69%)
≥150mg/dl	63 (55.8%)	35 (31.0%) ***
TC/HDL-c ratio, mean ± SD	5.2 (2.4)	5.3 (2.6)
< 5	62 (54.9%)	64 (56.6%)
≥ 5	51 (45.1%)	49 (43.4%)

HAART, highly active antiretroviral therapy; TC, total cholesterol; HDL, high-density lipoprotein; LDL, low- density lipoprotein; SD, standard deviation; ** p-value < 0.01; *** p-value <0.001.

Discussion

The aim of this cross-sectional study carried out in a resource limited East African setting was to assess the prevalence of dyslipidemia (lipid profile derangements) among HIV-infected patients receiving first-line HAART that include NNRTIs. We found that CD4 cell count in the HAART group was significantly different from the pre-HAART group, thus showing the effects of HAART in improving the immunological properties of the subjects.

In the present study, the majority of HAART patients (82.3%) had at least one laboratory abnormality, which is compatible with a diagnosis of dyslipidemia

Table 3 Prevalence of abnormal lipid profiles among patients treated with NRTIs based first-line antiretrovirals in Hawassa, Southern Ethiopia

Lipid profile	ZDV-based n=58 (%)	d4T-based n=55 (%)	*p-value*
TC ≥ 200 mg/dl	25 (43.1)	24 (43.6)	0.95
HDL-c < 40 mg/dl	24 (41.4)	25 (45.4)	0.66
LDL-c ≥ 130 mg/dl	20 (34.5)	18 (32.7)	0.84
TG ≥ 150 mg/dl	32 (55.2)	31 (56.4)	0.41
TC/HDL-c ratio ≥5	24 (41.4)	27 (49.1)	0.89

TC, total cholesterol; HDL-c, high-density lipoprotein cholesterol; LDL-c, low-density lipoprotein cholesterol; TG, triglyceride; ZDV, Zidovudine; d4T, stavudine; p, significance level.

Table 4 Prevalence of abnormal lipid profiles among patients treated with NNRTIs based first-line antiretrovirals in Hawassa, Southern Ethiopia

Lipid profile	EFV-based n=46 (%)	NVP-based n=67 (%)	P value
TC ≥ 200 mg/dl	18 (39.1)	31 (46.3)	0.45
HDL-c < 40 mg/dl	22 (47.8)	27 (40.3)	0.43
LDL-c ≥ 130 mg/dl	14 (30.4)	24 (35.8)	0.55
TG ≥ 150 mg/dl	25 (54.3)	38 (56.7)	0.80
TC/HDL ratio ≥5	22 (47.8)	29 (43.3)	0.63

TC, total cholesterol; HDL-c, high-density lipoprotein cholesterol; LDL-c, low-density lipoprotein cholesterol; TG, triglyceride; EFV, Efavirenz; NVP, Nevirapine; p, significance level.

according to NCEP-ATP III criteria. We found that the proportions of raised TC, LDL-c and TG were significantly higher in HAART group when compared to pre-HAART group. The proportion of HDL-c below 40 mg/dl was significantly higher in the pre-HAART group when compared to those on HAART, thus indicating the effects of HAART treatment in raising the lipid profiles, in addition to the restoration of health. However, there was no significant difference between treated group and non-treated group regarding TC/HDL-c ratio, this because increases in TC were counterbalanced by HDL-c improvement. The described raised lipid profiles (TC, LDL-c and TG), are atherogenic [13,16,17], and suggest a potential risk for the development of cardiovascular diseases in a significant proportion of HIV-infected patients in the near future.

The association between lipid derangements and HAART has been mainly depicted for regimens that contain PIs [6,18]. In addition, NNRTIs derange lipid profiles during therapy [7,8]. However, supportive evidences are very scarce in Sub-Sahara African countries concerning lipid derangements in patients receiving NNRTs including regimens [11,12]. We found that the prevalence of raised TC in HAART group was (43.4%). This prevalence rate is higher than the study reported from a resource poor West African setting [19]. The prevalence rate in this study was 4.5%. However, in this study, the cutoff limit was >210 mg/dl; and this value is higher than that of NCEP-ATP III guidelines, as used in our study. Based on HDL-c cut off value, the prevalence of HDL-c in our treatment group was 43.4%. This is comparable with the prevalence rate reported from Spain [20]. However, it is higher than the prevalence reported from rural South India [21]. The prevalence rate in this study was 24.8%. The prevalence of raised LDL-c in our HAART group was 33.6%. It is similar with the prevalence reported from India [21]. We found that the prevalence of raised TG in HAART group was 55.8%. This is not in line with the prevalence reported from Cameroon [14], Kenya [15], and India [21]. The prevalence rates in these three studies were respectively, 43.5%, 22.5%, and 42.1%. However, there are suggestions that the magnitude of lipid profile derangements induced by first-line HAART could show variation with duration of treatment, across populations and setting.

The reports from rural South India and Brazil indicated that the proportion of lipid profile derangements

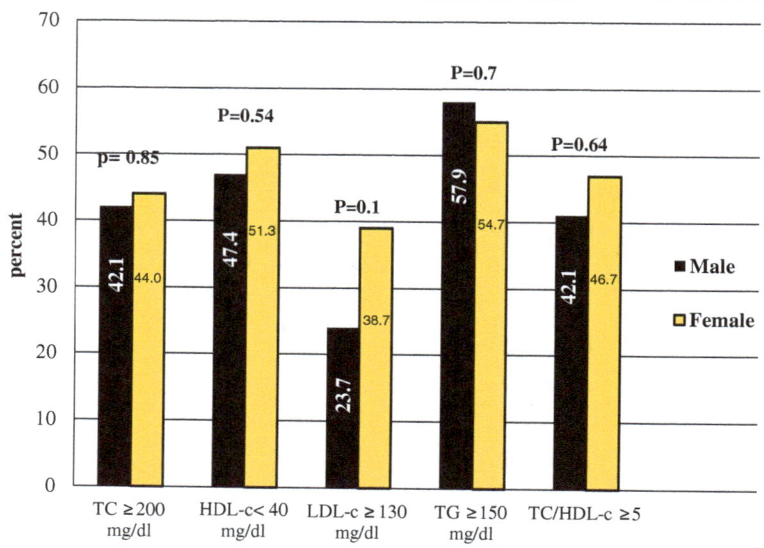

Figure 2 Gender and abnormal lipid profiles among first-line HAART treated patients in Hawassa, Southern Ethiopia. [Males (n=38); females (n=75); TC, total cholesterol; HDL-c, high-density lipoprotein cholesterol; LDL-c, low-density lipoprotein cholesterol; TG, triglyceride].

Table 5 Associations HAART and other variables with dyslipidemia among HIV-infected patients in Hawassa, Southern Ethiopia

Explanatory variable	Outcome	variables		
	TC ≥ 200 mg/dl	HDL< 40 mg/dl	LDL ≥ 130 mg/dl	TG ≥ 150 mg/dl
	AOR (95% CI)	AOR (95% CI)	AOR (95% CI)	AOR (95% CI)
$CD4^+$cells ≥200/mm^3*	1.00	1.00	1.00	1.00
$CD4^+$cells < 200/mm^3	0.91 (0.39-2.10)	1.95 (0.94-4.07)	0.89 (0.37-2.15)	0.87 (0.42-1.80)
P-value	0.82	0.07	0.79	0.71
BMI ≤ 25 Kg/m^2*	1.00	1.00	1.00	1.00
BMI > 25 Kg/m^2	2.96 (1.35-6.49)	0.55 (0.26-1.18)	2.66 (1.17-5.59)	2.82 (1.31-6.07)
P-value	**0.007**	0.13	**0.02**	**0.008**
Gender = Female*	1.00	1.00	1.00	1.00
Male	0.71 (0.32-1.57)	0.73 (0.38-1.42)	0.53 (0.22-1.25)	1.44 (0.74-2.82)
P-value	0.4	0.36	0.15	0.28
Age ≤ 40 years*	1.00	1.00	1.00	1.00
Age > 40 years	3.04 (1.41-6.55)	2.64 (1.23-5.69)	3.28 (1.48-7.30)	1.47 (0.71-3.05)
P-value	**0.004**	**0.01**	**0.004**	0.29
Pre-HAART*	1.00	1.00	1.00	1.00
HAART	3.80 (1.34-7.44)	0.44 (0.25-0.78)	2.64 (1.31-5.32)	2.50 (1.41-4.42)
P-value	**<0.0001**	**0.005**	**0.006**	**0.002**
No smoking*	1.00	1.00	1.00	1.00
Current smoking	0.90 (0.20-4.00)	2.13 (0.57-8.01)	0.32 (0.36-2.82)	0.75 (0.21-2.64)
P-value	0.89	0.26	0.3	0.65
No smoking*	1.00	1.00	1.00	1.00
Past smoking	0.77 (0.25-2.33)	1.46 (0.57-3.75)	0.56 (0.16-1.91)	0.67 (0.26-1.75)
P-value	0.64	0.43	0.35	0.42
No ant-TB drug *	1.00	1.00	1.00	1.00
Ant-TB drug	1.85(0.17-20.51)	NA	1.74(0.1519.82)	NA
P-value	0.62	NA	0.65	NA

HAART, highly active antiretroviral therapy; AOR, adjusted odds ratio; CI, confidence interval; BMI, body mass index; TC, total cholesterol; HDL, high-density lipoprotein cholesterol; LDL, low-density lipoprotein cholesterol; TG, triglyceride; NA, not available; p, significance level; TB, tuberculosis; * Reference category.

were higher among patients received d4T when compared to other NRTIs [21,22]. We found no difference in lipid derangements when patients received d4T compared to those received ZDV. This finding is similar with the reports from Uganda, and Cameroon [11,14]. The randomized trial report of 2 non-nucleosides (2NN) indicated that patients on NVP group had significantly improved HDL-c concentration and had relatively low lipid profile derangements when compared to those on EFV [23]. In line with the reports from rural Uganda [11], Cameroon [14] and India [24], we found no significant difference in lipid profile of patients on EFV compared to those on NVP. In the present study, the raised TC and LDL-c were significantly and positively associated with the use of HAART treatment, and the findings are in line with the study conducted in Cameroon [14].

Limitations of the study

Comprehensive cardiovascular risk stratifications were not assessed in this study. However, the increased risk of cardiovascular diseases associated with described lipid derangements is well known [25-27], and long term use of first-line HAART may have an impact on cardiovascular system. The other limitations were the cross-sectional nature of the study, small number of male participants, and lack of HIV negative controls.

Conclusion

Our study indicates HIV-infected patients receiving WHO-recommended first-line HAART that include Efavirenz and Nevirapine have a high prevalence of lipid profile derangements when compared to those non-treated HIV-infected patients. Uses of first-line HAART regimens are significantly associated with atherogenic

Table 6 Associations of variables with abnormal lipid profiles among first-line HAART treated patients in Hawassa, Southern Ethiopia

Explanatory variables	Outcome	variables		
	TC ≥ 200 mg/dl	HDL-c < 40 mg/dl	LDL-c ≥ 130mg/dl	TG ≥150 mg/dl
BMI > 25kg/m^2				
UOR (95% CI)	3.09 (1.18-8.05)*	0.50 (0.19-1.33)	2.68 (1.05-6.85)*	2.71 (0.98-7.50)
AOR (95% CI)	3.21 (1.16-8.91)*	0.49 (0.17-1.39)	2.44 (0.91-6.51)	2.92 (0.99-8.44)
Gender (male)				
UOR (95% CI)	0.93 (0.42-2.04)	1.28 (0.58-2.80)	0.49 (0.20-1.19)	1.14 (0.52-2.51)
AOR (95% CI)	0.68 (0.23-2.04)	0.69 (0.24-1.96)	0.43 (0.13-1.46)	1.09 (0.40-2.99)
Age > 40 years				
UOR (95% CI)	3.13 (1.28-7.63)*	3.14 (1.29-7.64)*	2.08 (0.86-5.00)	1.97 (0.80-4.84)
AOR (95% CI)	4.43 (1.54-12.72)**	4.22 (1.46-12.16)**	4.28 (1.41-12.97)*	2.12 (0.77-5.82)
HAART ≤ 2 years				
UOR (95% CI)	0.95 (0.24-3.75)	0.35 (0.08-1.49)	1.85 (0.37-9.39)	1.00 (0.26-3.97)
AOR (95% CI)	0.76 (0.16-3.66)	0.30 (0.06-1.47)	1.35 (0.22-8.20)	0.92 (0.21-4.09)
Current smoking				
UOR (95% CI)	0.64 (0.11-3.64)	1.33 (0.26-6.87)	0.38 (0.04-3.36)	0.78 (0.15-4.06)
AOR (95% CI)	0.77 (0.12-5.79)	0.70 (0.10-4.80)	0.51 (0.04-5.82)	0.78 (0.12-5.04)
Past smoking				
UOR (95% CI)	1.17 (0.39-3.47)	1.17 (0.39-3.47)	0.45 (0.12-1.70)	1.22 (0.40-3.70)
AOR (95% CI)	0.82 (0.20-3.34)	0.62 (0.16-2.45)	0.39 (0.08-1.98)	0.88 (0.23-3.40)
d4T				
UOR (95% CI)	1.02 (0.48-2.15)	1.18 (0.56-2.49)	0.92 (0.42-2.02	1.05 (0.50-2.21)
AOR (95% CI)	1.29 (0.57-2.93)	1.41 (0.63-3.16)	1.22 (0.52-2.85)	1.17 (0.53-2.58)
EFV				
UOR(95% CI)	0.75 (0.35-1.60)	1.36 (0.64-2.89)	0.78 (0.35-1.75)	0.91 (0.43-1.93)
AOR (95% CI)	0.77 (0.33-1.79)	1.36 (0.60 3.12)	0.91 (0.37-2.22)	0.97 (0.43-2.18)

HAART, highly active antiretroviral therapy therapy; UOR, un adjusted odds ratio; AOR, adjusted odds ratio; CI, confidence interval; TC, total cholesterol; HDL-c, high-density lipoprotein cholesterol; LDL-c, low- density lipoprotein cholesterol; TG, triglyceride; d4T Stavudine; BMI, body mass index; EFV, Efavirenz; * p-value < 0.05; ** p-value < 0.01. **Reference category:** BMI ≤ 25 Kg/m^2, Females, Age ≤ 40 years, no smoking, Nevirapine group, Zidovudine group; HAART treatment >2years.

lipid profiles. Therefore, the findings indicate that the need to assess lipid profiles at baseline before initiation of HAART treatment and lipid profile monitoring during therapy to monitor any rising trends. Additionally, the results also recommend implementation of well-controlled cohort studies for the evaluation of long-term effects of HAART treatment on lipid profiles.

Abbreviations

2NN: 2 non-nucleosides; AIDS: Acquired immunodeficiency syndrome; HAART: Highly active antiretroviral therapy; ZDV: Zidovudine; d4T: Stavudine; EFV: Efavirenz; ART: Antiretroviral therapy; HDL-c: HDL-cholesterol; 3TC: Lamivudine; HIV: Human immunodeficiency virus; WHO: World Health Organization; LDL-c: LDL-cholesterol; NNRTIs: Non-nucleoside reverse transcriptase inhibitors; NVP: Nevirapine; PIs: Protease inhibitors; TC: Total cholesterol; TG: Triglycerides; SPSS: Statistical package for social sciences; USNCEP-ATP: United States National Cholesterol Education Program, Adult Treatment Panel.

Competing interests

We announce that we have no any competing interests.

Authors' contributions

AT generated and designed the study, performed analysis and interpretation of data including with manuscript drafting, ZA, HA and SB assisted with the design, interpretation of data and the critical appraisal of the manuscript. All authors read and agreed the final manuscript.

Acknowledgements

We want to acknowledge the laboratory technologists and technicians of the Hawassa University referral hospital, ART clinic staffs and advanced clinical monitoring team staffs for their limitless support during data collection. Our gratefulness is also extended to the University of Gondar for financial support, Hawassa University referral Hospital for materials and reagents support; and the HIV/AIDS patients for their voluntarily participation in the study.

Author details

[1]Referral hospital laboratory, Hawassa University College of Medicine and Health Science, Hawassa, Southern Ethiopia. [2]School of Biomedical and Laboratory Sciences, University of Gondar College of Medicine and Health Science, P.O Box 196, Gondar, Ethiopia. [3]Department of Medical laboratory Technology, Hawassa University College of Medicine and Health Science, Hawassa, Southern Ethiopia. [4]Department of Animal and Range, Hawassa University College of Agriculture Sciences, Hawassa, Southern Ethiopia.

References

1. UNAIDS: *AIDS epidemic update 2011*. Geneva: UNAIDS; 2011. http://www.unaids.org/en/dataanalysis/epidemiol. Accessed on 15 Dec 2011.
2. Palella FJ Jr, Delaney KM, Moorman AC, Loveless MO, Fuhrer J, Satten GA, Aschman DJ, Holmberg SD: **Declining morbidity and mortality among patients with advanced human immunodeficiency virus infection.** *N Engl J Med* 1998, **338:**853–860.
3. Cohan GR, HIV-associated metabolic and morphologic abnormality syndrome: **Welcome therapy may have unwelcome effects.** *Postgrad Med* 2000, **107:**141–146.
4. El-Sadr W, Mullin C, Carr A, Gibert C, Rappoport C, Visnegarwala F, Grunfeld C, Raghavan S: **Effects of HIV disease on lipid, glucose and insulin levels: results from a large antiretroviral-naïve cohort.** *HIV Med* 2005, **6:**114–121.
5. Gallant JE, Staszewski S, Pozniak AL, DeJesus E, Suleiman JM, Miller MD, Coakley DF, Lu B, Toole JJ, Cheng AK, 903 Study Group: **Efficacy and safety of tenofovir DF vs stavudine in combination therapy in antiretroviralnaive patients: a 3-year randomized trial.** *JAMA* 2004, **292:**191–201.
6. Anastos K, Lu D, Shi Q, Tien PC, Kaplan RC, Hessol NA, Cole S, Vigen C, Cohen M, Young M, Tien, Phyllis C, Vigen C, Justman J: **Association of serum lipid levels with HIV sero-status, specific antiretroviral agents and treatment regimens.** *J Acquir Immune Defic Syndr* 2007, **459:**34–42.
7. Van der Valk M, Kastelein JJ, Murphy RL, Van Leth F, Katlama C, Horban A, Glesby M, Behrens G, Clotet B, Stellato RK, Molhuizen HO, Reiss P, Atlantic Study Team: **Nevirapine-containing antiretroviral therapy in HIV-1 infected patients results in an antiatherogenic lipid profile.** *AIDS* 2001, **15:**2407–2414.
8. Young J, Weber R, Rickenbach M, Furrer H, Bernasconi E, Hirschel B, Tarr PE, Vernazza P, Battegay M, Bucher HC: **Lipid profiles for antiretroviral-naïve patients starting PI- and NNRTI-based therapy in the Swiss HIV cohort study.** *Antivir Ther* 2005, **10:**585–591.
9. Friis-Moller N, Sabin C, Weber R, Monforte A, El-Sadr W, Reiss P, Thiébaut R, Morfeldt L, De Wit S, Pradier C, Calvo G, Law M, Kirk O, Phillips A, Lundgren J, Bartsch G, Dabis F, Loeliger H, Tressler R, Weller I, Sawitz A, Rickenbach M, Pezzotti P, Krum E, Meester R, Lavignolle V, Sundström B, Fontas E, Torres F, Petoumenos K, *et al*: **Combination antiretroviral therapy and the risk of myocardial infarction.** *N Engl J Med* 2003, **349:**1993–2003.
10. World Health Organization: *Antiretroviral therapy for HIV infection in adults and adolescents 2006 revision*. 2011. http://www.who.int/hiv/pub/arv/adult2010/en/index.html. Accessed on 03 Feb, 2011.
11. Buchacz K, Weidle PJ, Moore D, Were W, Mermin J, Downing R, Kigozi A, Borkowf CB, Ndazima V, Brooks JT: **Changes in lipid profile over 24months among adults on first-line highly active antiretroviral therapy in the home-based AIDS care program in rural Uganda.** *J Acquir Immune Defic Syndr* 2008, **47:**304–311.
12. Zannou DM, Denoeud L, Lacombe K, Amoussou-Guenou D, Bashi J, Akakpo J, Gougounon A, Akondé A, Adé G, Houngbé F, Girard PM: **Incidence of lipodystrophy and metabolic disorders in patients starting non-nucleoside reverse transcriptase inhibitors in Benin.** *Antivir Ther* 2009, **14:**371–380.
13. National Cholesterol Education Program (NCEP): **The third report of the National cholesterol education program (NCEP) expert panel on detection, evaluation, and treatment of high blood cholesterol in adults (adult treatment panel III) final report.** *Circulation* 2002, **106:**3143–3421.
14. Pefura Yone EW, Betyoumin AF, Kengne AP, Folefack FJK, Ngogang J: **First-line antiretroviral therapy and dyslipidemia in people living with HIV-1 in Cameroon: a cross-sectional study.** *AIDS Res Ther* 2011, **8:**33.
15. Manuthu EM, Joshi MD, Lule GN, Karari E: **Prevalence of dyslipidemia and dysglycaemia in HIV infected patients.** *East Afr Med J* 2008, **85:**10–17.
16. Asztalos BF, Schaefer EJ, Horvath KV, Cox CE, Skinner S, Gerrior J, Gorbach SL, Christine Wanke C: **Protease inhibitor-based HAART, HDL, and CHD-risk in HIV-infected patients.** *Atherosclerosis* 2006, **184:**72–77.
17. Sudano I, Spieker LE, Noll G, Corti R, Weber R, Lüscher TF: **Cardiovascular disease in HIV infection.** *Am Heart J* 2006, **151:**1147–1155.
18. Nery MW, Martelli CMT, Turchi MD: **Dyslipidemia in AIDS patients on highly active antiretroviral therapy.** *Braz J Infect Dis* 2011, **15:**151–155.
19. Ogundahunsi O, Oyegunle V, Ogun S, Odusoga O, Daniel O: **HAART and lipid metabolism in a resource poor West African setting.** *Afr J Biomed Res* 2010, **11:**27–31.
20. Bernal E, Masiá M, Padilla S, Gutiérrez F: **High-density lipoprotein cholesterol in HIV-infected patients: evidence for an association with HIV-1 viral load, antiretroviral therapy status, and regimen composition.** *AIDS Patient Care STDS* 2008, **22:**569–575.
21. Kalyanasundaram AP, Jacob SM, Hemalatha R, Sivakumar MR: **Prevalence of Lipodystrophy and Dyslipidemia among Patients with HIV infection on generic ART in Rural South India.** *JIAPAC* 2011, **000:**1–6.
22. Ceccato M, Bonolo P, Souza Neto A, Araújo F, Freitas M: **Antiretroviral therapy-associated dyslipidemia in patients from a reference center in Brazil.** *Braz J Med Biol Res* 2011, **44:**1177–1178.
23. van Leth F, Phanuphak P, Stroes E, Gazzard B, Cahn P, Raffi F, Wood R, Bloch M, Katlama C, Kastelein JJ, Schechter M, Murphy RL, Horban A, Hall DB, Lange JM, Reiss P: **Nevirapine and efavirenz elicit different changes in lipid profiles in antiretroviral therapy-naïve patients infected with HIV-1.** *PLoS Med* 2004, **1:**e19.
24. Padmapriyadarsini C, Ramesh Kumar S, Terrin N, Narendran G, Menon PA, Ramachandran G, Subramanyan S, Venkatesan P, Wanke C, Swaminathan S: **Dyslipidemia among HIV-infected Patients with tuberculosis taking once-daily Nonnucleoside Reverse-Transcriptase Inhibitor–Based Antiretroviral Therapy in India.** *Clin Infect Dis* 2011, **52:**540–546.
25. Grunfeld C: **Dyslipidemia and its Treatment in HIV Infection.** *Top HIV Med* 2010, **18:**112–118.
26. Bozkurt B: **Cardiovascular toxicity with highly active antiretroviral therapy: review of clinical studies.** *Cardiovasc Toxicol* 2004, **4:**243–260.
27. Domingos H, Cunha RV, Paniago AM, Martins DM, Elkhoury EB, Souza AS: **Metabolic effects associated to the highly active antiretroviral therapy (HAART) in AIDS patients.** *Braz J Infect Dis* 2009, **13:**130–136.

Impact of second-line antiretroviral regimens on lipid profiles in an African setting

Zvenyika AR Gomo[1*], James G Hakim[2*], Sarah A Walker[3], Willard Tinago[4], Gibson Mandozana[4], Cissy Kityo[5], Paula Munderi[6], Elly Katabira[7], Andrew Reid[2], Diana M Gibb[3], Charles F Gilks[8] and for the DART Team

Abstract

Background: Increasing numbers of HIV-infected patients in sub-Saharan Africa are exposed to antiretroviral therapy (ART), but there are few data on lipid changes on first-line ART, and even fewer on second-line.

Methods: DART was a randomized trial comparing monitoring strategies in Ugandan/Zimbabwean adults initiating first-line ART and switching to second-line at clinical/immunological failure. We evaluated fasting lipid profiles at second-line initiation and ≥48 weeks subsequently in stored samples from Zimbabwean patients switching before 18 September 2006.

Results: Of 91 patients switched to second-line ART, 65(73%) had fasting samples at switch and ≥48 weeks, 14(15%) died or were lost <48 weeks, 10(11%) interrupted ART for >14 days and 2(2%) had no samples available. 56/65(86%) received ZDV/d4T + 3TC + TDF first-line, 6(9%) ZDV/d4T + 3TC + NVP and 3(5%) ZDV + 3TC with TDF and NVP. Initial second-line regimens were LPV/r + NNRTI in 27(41%), LPV/r + NNRTI + ddI in 33(50%) and LPV/r + TDF + ddI/3TC/ZDV in 6(9%). At second-line initiation median (IQR) TC, LDL-C, HDL-C and TG (mmol/L) were 3.3(2.8-4.0), 1.7(1.3-2.2), 0.7(0.6-0.9) and 1.1(0.8-1.9) respectively. Levels were significantly increased 48 weeks later, by mean (SE) +2.0(0.1), +1.1(0.1), +0.5(0.05) and +0.4(0.2) respectively ($p < 0.001$; TG $p = 0.01$). 3% at switch vs 25% 48 weeks later had TC >5.2 mmol/L; 3% vs 25% LDL-C >3.4 mmol/L and 91% vs 41% HDL-C <1.1 mmol/L ($p < 0.001$). Similar proportions had TG >1.8 mmol/L (0 vs 3%) and TC/HDL-C ≥5 (40% vs 33%) ($p > 0.15$).

Conclusion: Modest lipid elevations were observed in African patients on predominantly LPV/r + NNRTI-based second-line regimens. Routine lipid monitoring during second-line ART regimens may not be warranted in this setting but individual cardiovascular risk assessment should guide practice.

Keywords: Antiretroviral therapy, Lipid profile changes, Protease inhibitors, Non-nucleoside reverse transcriptase inhibitors, African setting

Introduction

HIV infection in sub-Saharan Africa and in particular in Central and Southern Africa continues to exact a heavy burden [1]. The past decade has seen a rapid expansion of antiretroviral therapy (ART) rollout particularly in sub-Saharan Africa [1]. This has resulted in a reduction of mortality and morbidity and improvement in quality of life [1].

With an estimated 9.7 million people in lower and middle income countries on ART by the end of 2012 the adverse consequences of treatment are likely to become increasingly significant. Increasing use of ART has been accompanied by the emergence of a range of complications associated with treatment among which short and long-term cardiovascular complications have been observed [2]. Many of these have been poorly documented in the sub-Saharan African setting.

* Correspondence: zargomo@gmail.com; jhakim@mweb.co.zw
[1]Department of Chemical Pathology, College of Health Sciences, University of Zimbabwe, Avondale, PO Box A178, Harare, Zimbabwe
[2]Department of Medicine, College of Health Sciences, University of Zimbabwe, Avondale, PO Box A178, Harare, Zimbabwe
Full list of author information is available at the end of the article

Hyperlipidaemia is a recognised complication of ART which has an impact on the risk of cardiovascular disease [3-8]. The severity of hyperlipidaemia appears to be associated with the type of ART regimen in use. Many ART regimens result in changes in lipid levels, although protease inhibitor based (PI) regimens have been observed to influence lipid changes to a greater degree than other ART regimens [7,9,10].

There is a paucity of literature documenting lipid changes in HIV infection and during ART in sub-Saharan Africa. A few reports have, however, began to explore lipid and body-shape changes during ART exposure in this setting [11-15]. These reports predominantly focus on first-line ART regimens including in children. Whilst <3% of those on ART are currently receiving second-line, given the substantial numbers currently on first-line, this will increase significantly over the next decade. There is thus an urgent need for more studies that assess lipid changes during the use of various combinations of antiretroviral drugs in Sub-Saharan African patients taking second-line regimens.

This study aimed to conduct preliminary investigations within the DART Trial (Development of Antiretroviral Therapy in Africa) [16], a randomised trial of routine versus clinically driven laboratory monitoring of antiretroviral therapy in adults with HIV infection in Africa. 3,316 ART-naive adults with CD4 < 200 cells/mm^3 from Uganda and Zimbabwe initiated first-line ART with Combivir (co-formulated zidovudine + lamuvudine) plus tenofovir (n = 2469), abacavir (n = 300) or nevirapine (n = 547). WHO ART guidelines [17] defined failure triggered criteria to trigger switch to second-line ART (new/recurrent WHO 4 events in all; CD4 < 100 cells/mm^3 in the 50% randomised to routine laboratory (including CD4) monitoring). In this sub-study we assayed lipids in fasting samples from Zimbabwean participants at switch to second-line ART and ≥48 weeks later. The objective was to determine the magnitude and determinants of lipid changes in patients switched to second-line ART regimens and consider their significance for lipid monitoring recommendations.

Methods

Participants

This is an observational prospective sub-study on participants who switched to lopinavir/ritonavir (LPV/r)-containing second-line ART at clinical failure (WHO 4 event) in those randomised to clinically driven monitoring only (CDM); or at clinical or immunological failure (CD4 < 100 cells/mm^3) in those randomised to laboratory and clinical monitoring (LCM) in the DART trial. Most participants were on LPV/r with a non-nucleoside reverse transcriptase inhibitor (NNRTI) with or without an additional nucleoside reverse transcriptase inhibitor (NRTI) following triple NRTI first-line regimens. Zimbabwean patients were included in the sub-study if they switched to second-line ART before 18 September 2006, allowing 48 weeks follow-up through September 2007, did not interrupt LPV/r-containing ART for >14 days during the first 48 weeks on second-line, and had fasting samples available at switch to second-line and 48 weeks later. Demographic and baseline variables were obtained from the main DART database.

Determination of lipid profiles

Fasting blood samples were collected into 10 ml EDTA tubes after a 10 hour fast (no intake except for water). Plasma was separated at 3000 g for 10 minutes within an hour of collection. The plasma aliquots were stored at -80°C until analysis was performed. Total cholesterol (TC), low density lipoprotein–cholesterol (LDL-C), high density lipoprotein–cholesterol (HDL-C) and triglycerides (TG) were determined on a Beckman Coulter Synchron CX5 analyzer using appropriate Beckman Coulter reagents (Beckman Coulter, Johannesburg, South Africa).[Synchrone CX].

Definitions

Body mass index (BMI) was defined by the formula (body weight in Kg)/(height in m)^2 and categorized as <18.5-underweight, 18.5-24.9-normal, 25.0-29.9-overweight, ≥30.0-obese. To enable comparison with the published literature, criteria from the Third Report of the US National Cholesterol Education Program [18] were used to define abnormal lipid levels as follows: TC ≥5.2 mmol/L, LDL-C ≥3.4 mmol/L, HDL-C ≤1.1, TG ≥1.8 and TC/HDL-C ratio of ≥5 [18]. The Division of AIDS toxicity tables were used to grade lipid toxicity levels [19]. The following abbreviations were used for antiretroviral classes and drugs: nucleoside reverse transcriptase inhibitors (NRTIs), non-nucleoside reverse transcriptase inhibitors (NNRTIs), Protease Inhibitors (PIs), zidovudine (ZDV), lamivudine (3TC), tenofovir (TDF), stavudine (d4T), didanosine (ddI), nevirapine (NVP), efavirenz (EFV), lopinavir/ritonavir (LVP/r).

Statistical analysis

Plasma lipid levels at switch to second-line ART and 48 weeks subsequently were summarised using medians and interquartile ranges, and compared across groups defined by demographic and other characteristics using the Kruskal-Wallis test. Changes in lipid levels between switch to second-line and 48 weeks were compared using paired t-tests. Multivariable linear regression models were used to identify factors independently associated with changes in lipid levels from switch to ≥48 weeks. All models were adjusted for baseline lipid levels. Analyses were performed using STATA 10 (StataCorp, College Station, TX).

Ethical approval

The DART trial (ISCRTN13968779) was approved by the Science and Ethics Committee in Uganda, Medical Research Council in Zimbabwe and Imperial College Research Ethics committee in the United Kingdom. Written informed consent was obtained from each enrolled participant.

Results

Ninety-one DART participants at the Zimbabwe site were switched to second-line ART before 18 September 2006, of whom 65 (71%) had fasting samples at switch and ≥48 weeks later and were included in this sub-study. 26 participants were excluded for the following reasons; 14 (15%) died (no cardiovascular related deaths) or were lost to follow up <48 weeks after switch; 10 (11%) interrupted ART for >14 days; 2 (2%) did not have samples available at both time points. Of the 65 participants included, 34 (52%) were males and 31 (48%) females. The median (IQR) age at switch was 39 (35-44) years, and participants had been on first-line ART for a median (range) 2.2 years (0.9-3.1 years). Characteristics at switch to second-line ART are shown in Table 1. At switch, 16% of participants were underweight according to BMI and an equal proportion, 16%, were overweight or obese. 88% of participants had CD4 counts <100 cells/mm^3.

First-line and second-line ART

56 (86%) of the 65 included participants received ZDV/d4T + 3TC + TDF during first-line ART, 6 (9%) ZDV/d4T + 3TC + NVP, and 3(5%) ZDV + 3TC with TDF and NVP at different stages, mostly due to development of TB or NVP-associated rash. Initial second-line regimens were LPV/r + NNRTI in 27(41%), LPV/r + NNRTI + ddI in 33(50%) and LPV/r + TDF + ddI/3TC/ZDV in 6(9%) participants, reflecting the fact that most patients had received 3NRTI first-line. Of the patients on second-line regimens which included an NNRTI, 9/60 (15%) were on EFV and 51/60 (85%) on NVP. During second-line ART, 5 (8%) patients substituted from NVP to EFV; 1 from ddI to d4T, and 1 from EFV to d4T and back to d4T during the course of pregnancy. Only 4 participants had any time off ART during second-line (2 were for 4 days, 1 for 9 days and 1 for 14 days).

Lipids at switch to second-line ART

At switch to second-line, median (IQR) (mmol/L) plasma fasting lipid concentrations were: TC 3.3 (2.8-4.0), LDL-C 1.7 (1.3-2.2), HDL-C 0.7 (0.6-0.9), TG 1.1 (0.8-1.9), TC/HDL-C ratio 4.6 (4.0-5.6) (Table 1). Using NECP [18] criteria TC was >5.2 mmol/L in 2/65 (3%) participants, LDL-C was >3.4 mmol/L in 2/65 (3%) participants, HDL-C was <1.1 mmol/L in 94% of participants; TC/HDL-C ratio was <5 in 30/65 (60%) participants; and no participant had abnormally raised TG levels.

In the univariate analyses at switch to second-line ART regimens, women had significantly higher TC (+0.8 mmol/L, $p = 0.004$), LDL-C (+0.6 mmol/L, $p = 0.006$) and HDL-C (+0.1 mmol/L, $p = 0.05$). TG levels were not significantly higher (+0.5) mmol/L, $p = 0.80$ in men at switch to second-line ART regimens. There were no statistically significant differences in lipid levels according to age or CD4 count at switch to second-line ART regimens (Table 1); but LDL-C was higher in those with higher BMI at switch ($p = 0.04$), with similar non-significant trends for TC and TG.

Patients who had received ART combinations containing NVP in first-line had higher HDL-C (+0.2 mmol/L, $p = 0.02$) at switch than those who had received ART combinations containing TDF and other NRTIs only (Table 1). Of note there was a statistically significantly higher TC ($p = 0.04$) in patients who had received ZDV/d4T + 3TC + TDF first-line.

Anthropometric, immunologic and lipid profile changes from switch to ≥48 weeks of second-line ART

Fasting lipid profiles (TC, LDL-C, HDL-C, TC/HDL-C ratio and TG) after ≥48 weeks of second-line ART are shown in Table 2; TC, LDL-C and HDL-C remained higher in women persisted, and associations between higher TC, LDL-C and TG and higher BMI strengthened. Lipid levels were significantly increased after ≥48 weeks of second-line ART, by (mean mmol/L) TC +2.0, LDL-C +1.1, HDL-C +0.5 (all $p < 0.001$) and TG +0.40 ($p = 0.01$) (Table 3, Figure 1). The percentage increase in lipid levels after ≥48 weeks of second-line ART was TC 59%, LDL-C 61%, HDL-C 71% and TG 29% (Table 3). There was no significant change in TC/HDL-C ratio, $p = 0.94$ (Table 3).

Comparing switch vs ≥48 weeks of second-line ART, the proportion of participants with TC >5.2 mmol/L was 3% vs 60% respectively, and 3% vs 25% respectively had LDL-C >3.4 mmol/L (both $p < 0.001$). However, as HDL-C also increased, the proportion of participants with HDL-C <1.1 mmol/L decreased after ≥48 weeks of second-line ART from 94% vs 41% ($p < 0.001$). There were no significant changes in the proportion with TG >1.8 mmol/L (0 vs 3% respectively, $p = 0.16$) or TC/HDL-C ratio ≥5 (40% vs 33% respectively, $p = 0.17$). DAIDS toxicity criteria showed a corresponding but small shift to higher grades 3 and 4.

Factors associated with changes in lipid profiles on second-line

We performed multivariable regression analyses including all demographic and clinical factors weakly ($p < 0.20$) associated with a change in at least one lipid variable

Table 1 Demographic data, BMI, CD4 count and plasma lipid levels at initiation of second-line ART (switch from first-line ART)

At switch to second-line	n (%)	TC mean (se)	†P	LDL-C mean (se)	†P	HDL-C mean (se)	†P	TG mean (se)	†P	TC/HDL-C ratio mean (se)	†P
All	65	3.4 (0.1)		1.8 (0.1)		0.7 (0.03)		1.4 (0.1)		4.9 (0.2)	
Sex											
Females	31 (48%)	3.8 (0.2)	0.004	2.1 (0.2)	0.006	0.8 (0.04)	0.05	1.3 (0.1)	0.80	4.9 (0.2)	0.66
Males	34 (52%)	3.0 (0.1)		1.5 (0.1)		0.7 (0.04)		1.8 (0.2)		4.8 (0.3)	
Age (years)											
<35	17 (26%)	3.4 (0.2)	0.61	1.7 (0.2)	0.7	0.8 (0.1)	0.78	1.3 (0.3)	0.10	4.8 (0.4)	0.46
35-44	33 (51%)	3.4 (0.2)		1.9 (0.1)		0.7 (0.1)		1.5 (0.1)		4.9 (0.2)	
≥45	15 (23%)	3.2 (0.4)		1.7 (0.2)		0.7 (0.1)		1.5 (0.3)		4.8 (0.3)	
¥BMI (kg/m^2)											
<18.5	10 (16%)	3.0 (0.3)	0.11	1.6 (0.2)	0.04	0.8 (0.1)	0.33	1.0 (0.3)	0.46	4.2 (0.4)	0.45
18.5-24.9	41 (67%)	3.4 (0.1)		1.8 (0.1)		0.7 (0.1)		1.6 (0.2)		4.9 (0.2)	
25-29.9	8 (13%)	3.4 (0.3)		1.8 (0.2)		0.7 (0.1)		1.4 (0.2)		4.8 (0.2)	
30-39.9	2 (3%)	4.0 (0.1)		2.4 (0.1)		0.7 (0.1)		1.7 (0.9)		5.5 (0.5)	
CD4 cell/mm^3											
<100	57 (88%)	3.3 (0.1)	0.95	1.7 (0.1)	0.47	0.7 (0.02)	0.64	1.5 (0.1)	0.85	4.8 (0.2)	0.73
100-199	6 (9%)	3.9 (0.9)		2.1 (0.6)		0.7 (0.1)		1.4 (0.2)		6.0 (1.0)	
≥200	2 (3%)	4.0 (0.6)		2.2 (0.7)		1.2 (0.1)		0.6 (0.2)		3.5 (0.8)	
ART-during first-line											
ZDV/d4T + 3TC + TDF	56 (86%)	3.4 (0.1)	0.59	1.8 (0.1)	0.30	0.7 (0.03)	0.02	1.5 (0.1)	0.04	5.0 (0.2)	0.09
±ZDV/d4T++NVP	9 (14%)	3.4 (0.2)		1.9 (0.2)		0.9 (0.10)		0.9 (0.1)		4.0 (0.4)	

†P-values for continuous BMI, Age and CD4 vs lipids calculated using Spearman correlation.
¥4 participants with missing weight at initiation of second –line ART.
±Including 3 patients who had substituted NVP- > TDF for hepatotoxicity (2) or anti-TB therapy (1) during first-line.
TC: total cholesterol, LDL-C: low density lipoprotein–cholesterol, HDL-C: high density lipoprotein–cholesterol, TG: triglyceride, BMI: Body mass index. All lipid levels are expressed in mmol/L.

Table 2 BMI, CD4 Count and lipid levels at ≥48 weeks on second-line ART

48 weeks after switch to second-line	n (%)	TC mean (se)	†P	LDL-C mean (se)	†P	HDL-C mean (se)	†P	TG mean (se)	†P	TC/HDL-C ratio mean (se)	†P
All	65	5.4 (0.2)		2.9 (0.1)		1.2 (0.05)		1.9(0.2)		4.9 (0.3)	
Sex											
Females	31 (48%)	5.8 (0.2)	0.03	3.2 (0.2)	0.003	1.3 (0.07)	0.03	1.8 (0.2)	0.71	4.6 (0.2)	0.69
Males	34 (52%)	5.1 (0.2)		2.5 (0.1)		1.1 (0.06)		2.0 (0.2)		5.1 (0.4)	
BMI (kg/m^2)											
<18.5	4 (6%)	4.8 (0.4)	0.04	2.6 (0.5)	0.05	1.2 (0.3)	0.57	1.0 (0.2)	0.003	4.6 (0.9)	0.55
18.5-24.9	36 (56%)	5.2 (0.2)		2.7 (0.2)		1.2 (0.1)		1.5 (0.1)		5.0 (0.4)	
25-29.9	21 (32%)	5.8 (0.3)		3.1 (0.2)		1.2 (0.1)		2.4 (0.3)		4.8 (0.4)	
30-39.9	4 (6%)	5.9 (0.3)		3.1 (0.4)		1.2 (0.4)		2.8 (1.1)		5.0 (1.0)	
CD4 cell/mm^3											
<100	2 (3%)	4.6 (0.9)	0.93	2.6 (0.6)	0.28	1.1 (0.1)	0.10	0.8 (0.02)	0.24	4.2 (1.1)	0.31
100-199	10 (15%)	5.7 (0.2)		3.0 (0.2)		1.4 (0.1)		1.8 (0.5)		4.1 (0.4)	
≥200	53 (82%)	5.4 (0.2)		2.8 (0.1)		1.2 (0.1)		1.9 (0.2)		5.1 (0.3)	

TC: total cholesterol, LDL-C: low density lipoprotein–cholesterol, HDL-C: high density lipoprotein–cholesterol, TG: triglyceride, BMI: Body mass index. All lipid levels are expressed in mmol/L.
†P-values for continuous BMI and CD4 vs. lipids calculated using Spearman correlation.

Table 3 Plasma Lipid levels changes from switch to ≥48 weeks on second-line ART

	Initiation of second-line (mean; sd)	48 weeks later (mean; sd)	Changes (SE)	% Change	P-value
	n = 65	n = 65	n = 65		
TC	3.4 (1.0)	5.4 (1.2)	+2.0 (0.1)	59%	<0.001
LDL-C	1.8 (0.7)	2.8 (0.9)	+1.1 (0.1)	61%	<0.001
HDL-C	0.7 (0.2)	1.2 (0.4)	+0.5 (0.05)	71%	<0.001
TG	1.4 (1.0)	1.9 (1.3)	+0.4 (0.2)	29%	0.01
TC/HDLC-C	4.9 (1.4)	4.9 (2.1)	+0.0 (0.3)	0%	0.94

(TC, LDL-C, HDL-C, TG) at ≥48 weeks on univariable analysis, and adjusting for baseline (switch) values (Table 4). All models thus included sex, age, lipid levels at switch to second-line ART, BMI at ≥48 weeks, and type of second-line regimen (EFV vs NVP vs no NNRTI; ddI vs no ddI). Controlling for baseline lipid levels and other factors, in comparison to men, women had significantly greater increases in LDL-C (+0.5, $p = 0.04$) after ≥48 weeks on second-line ART. Older patients had significantly greater increases in TC (+0.4, $p = 0.02$), LDL-C (+0.3, $p = 0.06$) and HDL-C (+0.1, $p = 0.02$) after ≥48 weeks on second-line ART. There was a trend towards greater TG increases (+0.08 mmol/L, $p = 0.07$) and smaller HDL-C increases (-0.02 mmol/L, $p = 0.08$) in those with higher BMI.

Patients taking LPV/r with NNRTIs appeared to have greater increases in TC, LDL-C and HDL-C than those taking LPV/r with NRTIs (numbers were however small). Those taking EFV appeared to have larger increases in LDL-C (+0.9 mmol/L, $p = 0.03$) than HDL-C (+0.4, $p = 0.02$).

Discussion

This study reports our observations of lipid changes following switch from first-line ART to second-line regimens containing new classes of antiretroviral drugs with a view to making recommendations on lipid level measurement during second-line ART in an African setting. It should be noted that the DART study (DART) was conducted at a time when triple- nucleoside regimens were in vogue and hence second-line regimens contained a combination of boosted-PIs and NNRTI with or without the addition of NRTIs.

It is well established that increased TC, LDL-C, TC/HDL-C ratio and TG are associated with an increased risk of cardiovascular events, while raised HDL-C reduces this risk [18]. These observations have been made in large studies that indicate these associations to hold across all ethnicities [20]. Observations in resource-rich countries show that HIV infection is associated with low serum lipid levels depending on degree of immunosuppression and viraemia [6,7]. Several studies in African settings have made similar observations on patients before ART initiation [21-24]. ART has transformed the lives of HIV infected patients but changes in lipid levels are a recognised complication of ART [6,9,25]. Although the belief is that Africans in sub-Saharan Africa generally have low lipid levels, there is evidence that this is changing in response to many factors including

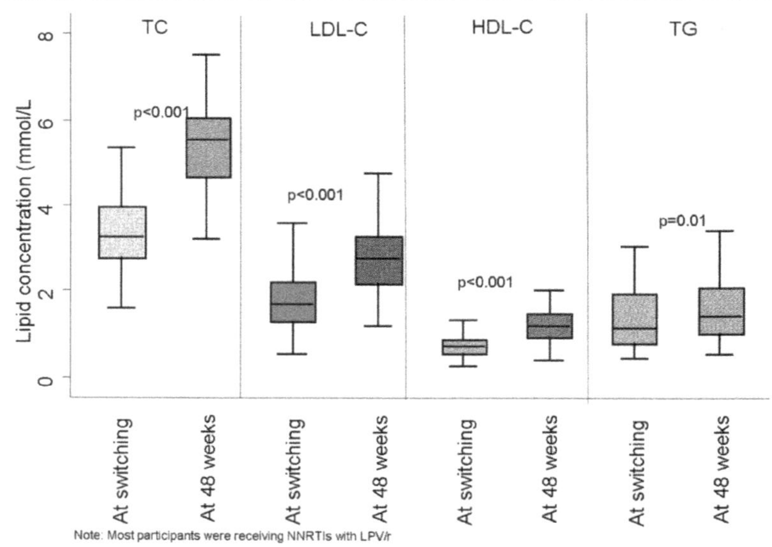

Figure 1 Fasting plasma lipids at switch to second-line and 48 weeks later. Footnote 1: Total Cholesterol (TC), Low-density lipoprotein-cholesterol (LDL-C), High-density lipoprotein-cholesterol (HDL-C) and triglycerides (TG) levels were statistically significantly increased ≥48 weeks on switching to second-line ART regimens ($p < 0.001$).

Table 4 Multivariable linear regression analyses for factors associated with changes in lipid levels from switch to ≥48 weeks on second-line ART

At switch to second- line*	n (%) or median (IQR)	TC effect (se)	P	LDL-C effect (se)	P	HDL-Ceffect (se)	P	TG effect (se)	P
Gender									
Females	32 (48%)	+04 (0.3)	0.14	+0.5 (0.2)	0.04	+0.1 (0.08)	0.26	−0.07 (0.3)	0.81
Age (per 10 year increase)	38 (34-43)	+0.4 (0.2)	0.02	+0.3 (0.1)	0.06	+0.1 (0.06)	0.02	−0.04 (0.2)	0.87
BMI (kg/m^2) per 2 units	21 (17-26)	+0.02 (0.03)	0.47	+0.02 (0.03)	0.41	−0.02 (0.01)	0.08	+0.08 (0.04)§	0.07
NVP	50 (77%)	+1.3 (0.4)	0.004	+0.6 (0.3)	0.10	+0.6 (0.2)	<0.001	+0.4 (0.6)	0.43
EFV	9 (14%)	+1.6 (0.5)	0.003	+0.9 (0.4)	0.03	+0.4 (0.2)	0.02	+0.4 (0.6)	0.57
ddI	34 (52%)	−0.04 (0.3)	0.88	−0.1 (02)	0.54	−0.1 (0.1)	0.21	+0.2 (0.3)	0.54

Al l models are adjusted for baseline lipid level.
§BMI at week 48 (rather than at switch to second-line) as this was a better predictor.
*Reference category: man aged 40 years with BMI 25 at switch, receiving LPV/r plus NRTIs (no NNRTI) without ddI as their second-line regimen.

urbanization with changes in diet, low exercise level and increasing prevalence of hypertension, diabetes and smoking [26].

At baseline (switch to second-line ART after a median of 2.2 years of first-line ART) the TC, LDL-C and TG levels in our study participants were low which is consistent with a low atherogenic risk [18]. The HDL-C levels were however low reflecting a high atherogenic risk. The combination of low TC and low HDL-C resulted in a TC/HDL-C ratio of 4.9 which is reflective of a borderline [18], but relatively high atherogenic risk if one considers the generally low TC and LDL-C levels. After ≥48 weeks of second-line ART predominantly consisting of a combination of PI/r and NNRTI with or without NRTIs there was a marked increase in lipid levels; relative increases of TC 59%, LDL-C 61%, HDL-C 71% and TG 29%. The TC/HDL-C ratio remained unchanged because of the marked increase in HDL-C. Women had a greater increase in LDL-C than men. Older patients had greater increases in TC, LDL-C and HDL-C. Those with higher BMI had greater increases in TG, and smaller increases in HDL-C than those with lower BMI.

In a South African study of 42 patients on an NNRTI-based first-line regimen the TC, LDL-C, HDL-C and TG levels (mean ± standard deviation) following 2.1 years of first-line ART exposure were; 4.75 ± 1.24, 2.65 ± 0.97 and 1.41 ± 0.42 and 1.20 ± 1.18 respectively [13]. In contrast in our patients after 2.2 years of first-line ART (ie at switch to second-line ART); TC, LDL-C and HDL-C levels were lower but TG was higher than in the South African study. The difference could, at least in part, be explained by the lower proportion of women in our study than in the South African study, 48% vs 64% respectively. Indeed there were other important differences between our two studies. Our patients were predominantly on a triple-nucleoside first-line regimen (86%) while the South African patients were all on an NNRTI regimen. However, in a Ugandan study of 374 patients (49% women) who were on a predominantly NNRTI-based first-line regimen (98% on NVP), lipid levels (mmol/L) after 2 years were; 3.91; 2.05; 1.22; 1.35; and 3.4 for TC, LDL-C, HDL-C, TG and TC/HDL-C ratio respectively [14], again TC, LDL-C and HDL-C higher than values at switch to second-line in our Zimbabwean study, but lower than in South Africa. Of note, HDL-C at switch to second-line ART was markedly low in the Zimbabwean study. Interestingly TG levels were more similar in all three studies.

The lipid levels in this Zimbabwean African population are generally low after exposure to a predominantly triple nucleoside first-line ART regimen. The choice of second-line regimens which mostly contained both PI/r and NNRTIs in our study was dictated by first-line exposure. It is therefore not possible to fully ascribe lipid changes to either the PI/r or NNRTI class of antiretroviral drugs, given the small number of patients not receiving NNRTI second-line. PI-based regimens have been associated with elevated lipid levels in several studies [5,9,27], although the setting of such changes is often complex [7]. In a study in Benin a significant increase in TC was observed in a cohort of 88 patients who were on an NNRTI first-line regimen [28]. Several studies have shown that NNRTI based regimens are associated with elevated TC and LDL-C levels [8,9,28] with regimens combining PIs and NNRTIs showing higher degrees of dyslipidaemia [8]. Various members of the PI class have been shown to have varying effects on lipid changes. In a South African study, after 48 weeks of first-line ART, there was a smaller rise in LDL-C level with an Atazanavir based regimen compared to a Nelfinavir based regimen. Indeed in comparison to Nelfinavir, Atazanvir exposure was not associated with clinically relevant increases in TC, LDL-C or TG. Another limitation of our study is that we did not have a sufficient numbers of patients on EFV versus those on NVP to allow comparison of the impact of these two NNRTIs on lipid change. The percentage increases in TC, HDL-C and TG were high, but because of relatively low baseline levels at switch to second-line ART, the levels attained after exposure to second-line ART were modest.

In this study an almost equal number of men and women of similar ages were recruited which gives us the opportunity to compare lipid changes between men and women unlike studies in resource-rich countries which have predominantly studied men. The fact that women had higher lipid levels than men at switch and 48 weeks later is difficult to explain since normally men have higher athrogenic lipids than women [18]. A partial explanation may be the higher BMI in females compared to males. Indeed both men and women had similar degrees of immunosuppression as shown by similar CD4 counts.

Because of the generally low level of lipids in African populations the facilities to perform lipid assays are limited and expensive. It may therefore not be possible to give a recommendation on routine monitoring of lipids, or even how often lipid levels should be monitored in this population. This preliminary study suggests that lipid changes do occur over the short-to-medium term on second-line LPV/r containing regimens, but are generally mild abnormalities, and are at least partially offset (in terms of cardiovascular risk) by increases in HDL-C, furthermore our results are limited by the short follow-up period. The best approach for the time being may, therefore, be to recommend assessment of total atherogenic risk ie risk factors such as smoking, hypertension, diabetes, BMI and family history to guide monitoring for and indeed treatment of lipids in individual patients. We await further studies to provide more general guidelines on the monitoring and management of lipids during ART based on risk factors for cardiovascular disease, and the impact of various classes of antiretroviral drugs or individual agents.

Competing interests

This work was supported by the UK Medical Research Council [grant number G0600344]; the UK Department for International Development (DFID); and the Rockefeller Foundation. GlaxoSmithKline; Gilead and Boehringer-Ingelheim donated first-line drugs for DART, and Abbott provided Kaletra/Aluvia as part of the second-line regimen for DART. The authors declare that they have no competing interest.

Authors' contributions

ZAR, JGH, SAW, DMG and CFG contribute to concept, study design, prepared and edited manuscript. AR, CK, EK and PM were involved in data acquisition and edited manuscript. SAW, WT and GM conducted statistical analysis and data interpretation. All authors read and approved the final manuscript.

Acknowledgements

We thank all the patients and staff from all the centres participating in the DART trial.

MRC/UVRI Uganda Research Unit on AIDS, Entebbe, Uganda: H Grosskurth, P Munderi, G Kabuye, D Nsibambi, R Kasirye, E Zalwango, M Nakazibwe, B Kikaire, G Nassuna, R Massa, K Fadhiru, M Namyalo, A Zalwango, L Generous, P Khauka, N Rutikarayo, W Nakahima, A Mugisha, J Todd, J Levin, S Muyingo, A Ruberantwari, P Kaleebu, D Yirrell, N Ndembi, F Lyagoba, P Hughes, M Aber, A Medina Lara, S Foster, J Amurwon, B Nyanzi Wakholi, K Wangati, B Amuron, D Kajungu, J Nakiyingi, W Omony, K Fadhiru, D Nsibambi, P Khauka.

Joint Clinical Research Centre, Kampala, Uganda: P Mugyenyi, C Kityo, F Ssali, D Tumukunde, T Otim, J Kabanda, H Musana, J Akao, H Kyomugisha, A Byamukama, J Sabiiti, J Komugyena, P Wavamunno, S Mukiibi, A Drasiku, R Byaruhanga, O Labeja, P Katundu, S Tugume, P Awio, A Namazzi, GT Bakeinyaga, H Katabira, D Abaine, J Tukamushaba, W Anywar, W Ojiambo, E Angweng, S Murungi , W Haguma, S Atwiine, J Kigozi, L Namale. A Mukose, G Mulindwa, D Atwiine, A Muhwezi, E Nimwesiga, G Barungi, J Takubwa, S Murungi, D Mwebesa, G Kagina, M Mulindwa, F Ahimbisibwe, P Mwesigwa, S Akuma, C Zawedde, D Nyiraguhirwa, C Tumusiime, L Bagaya, W Namara, J Kigozi, J Karungi, R Kankunda, R Enzama.

University of Zimbabwe, Harare, Zimbabwe: A Latif, J Hakim, V Robertson, A Reid, E Chidziva, R Bulaya-Tembo, G Musoro, F Taziwa, C Chimbetete, L Chakonza, A Mawora, C Muvirimi, G Tinago, P Svovanapasis, M Simango, O Chirema, J Machingura, S Mutsai, M Phiri, T Bafana, M Chirara, L Muchabaiwa, M Muzambi, E Chigwedere, M Pascoe, C Warambwa, E Zengeza, F Mapinge, S Makota, A Jamu, N Ngorima, H Chirairo, S Chitsungo, J Chimanzi, C Maweni, R Warara, M Matongo, S Mudzingwa, M Jangano, K Moyo, L Vere, I Machingura.

Infectious Diseases Institute (formerly the Academic Alliance) Makerere University, Mulago, Uganda: E Katabira, A Ronald, A Kambungu, F Lutwama, I Mambule, A Nanfuka, J Walusimbi, E Nabankema, R Nalumenya, T Namuli, R Kulume, I Namata, L Nyachwo, A Florence, A Kusiima, E Lubwama, R Nairuba, F Oketta, E Buluma, R Waita, H Ojiambo, F Sadik, J Wanyama, P Nabongo, J Oyugi, F Sematala, A Muganzi, C Twijukye, H Byakwaga.

The AIDS Support Organisation (TASO), Uganda: R Ochai, D Muhweezi, A Coutinho, B Etukoit.

Imperial College, London, UK: C Gilks, K Boocock, C Puddephatt, C Grundy, J Bohannon, D Winogron.

MRC Clinical Trials Unit, London, UK: J Darbyshire, DM Gibb, A Burke, D Bray, A Babiker, AS Walker, H Wilkes, M Rauchenberger, S Sheehan, C Spencer-Drake, K Taylor, M Spyer, A Ferrier, B Naidoo, D Dunn, R Goodall.

Independent DART Trial Monitors: R Nanfuka, C Mufuka-Kapuya.

DART Virology Group: P Kaleebu (Co-Chair), D Pillay (Co-Chair), P Awio, M Chirara, D Dunn, DM Gibb, C Gilks, R Goodall, A Kapaata, M Katuramur, F Lyagoba, R Magala, B Magambo, K Mataruka, A McCormick, L Mugarura, T Musunga, M Nabankkema, J Nkalubo, P Nkurunziza, C Parry, V Robertson, M Spyer, D Yirrell.

Trial Steering Committee: I Weller (Chair), A Babiker (Trial Statistician), S Bahendeka, M Bassett, A Chogo Wapakhabulo, J Darbyshire, B Gazzard, C Gilks, H Grosskurth, J Hakim, A Latif, C Mapuchere, O Mugurungi, P Mugyenyi; Observers: C Burke, M Distel, S Jones, E Loeliger, P Naidoo, C Newland, G Pearce, S Rahim, J Rooney, M Smith, W Snowden, J-M Steens.

Data and Safety Monitoring Committee: A Breckenridge (Chair), A McLaren (Chair-deceased), C Hill, J Matenga, A Pozniak, D Serwadda.

Endpoint Review Committee: T Peto (Chair), A Palfreeman, M Borok, E Katabira.

Author details

[1]Department of Chemical Pathology, College of Health Sciences, University of Zimbabwe, Avondale, PO Box A178, Harare, Zimbabwe. [2]Department of Medicine, College of Health Sciences, University of Zimbabwe, Avondale, PO Box A178, Harare, Zimbabwe. [3]MRC Clinical Trials Unit, London, UK. [4]Department of Community Medicine, University of Zimbabwe, Harare, Zimbabwe. [5]Joint Clinical Research Centre, Kampala, Uganda. [6]MRC Programme on AIDS/Uganda Virus Research Institute, Entebbe, Uganda. [7]Infectious Disease Institute, Mulago Hospital, Kampala, Uganda. [8]Imperial College, London, UK.

References

1. UNAIDS: **Global report: UNAIDS Report on the global AIDS epidemic 2013.** UNAIDS/JC2502/1/E. Revised and reissued, November 2013. Available at: http://www.unaids.org/en/media/unaids/contentassets/documents/epidemiology/2013/gr2013/UNAIDS_Global_Report_2013_en.pdf. Accessed 06 January 2013.
2. Luetkemeyer AF, Havlir DV, Currier JS: **Complications of HIV disease and antiretroviral treatment.** *Top HIV Med* 2010, **18:**57–65.
3. Palacios R, Santos J, Ruiz J, Gonzalez M, Valdivielso P, Marquez M, Gonzalez-Santos P: **Short-term lipid changes associated with highly**

active antiretroviral therapy in naive HIV-infected patients. *J Acquir Immune Defic Syndr* 2003, **34**:249–251.
4. Carr A, Samaras K, Burton S, Law M, Freund J, Chisholm DJ, Cooper DA: A syndrome of peripheral lipodystrophy, hyperlipidaemia and insulin resistance in patients receiving HIV protease inhibitors. *AIDS* 1998, **12**:F51–F58.
5. Carr A, Samaras K, Thorisdottir A, Kaufmann GR, Chisholm DJ, Cooper DA: Diagnosis, prediction, and natural course of HIV-1 protease-inhibitor-associated lipodystrophy, hyperlipidaemia, and diabetes mellitus: a cohort study. *Lancet* 1999, **353**:2093–2099.
6. Riddler SA, Smit E, Cole SR, Li R, Chmiel JS, Dobs A, Palella F, Visscher B, Evans R, Kingsley LA: Impact of HIV infection and HAART on serum lipids in men. *JAMA* 2003, **289**:2978–2982.
7. Aberg JA: Cardiovascular complications in HIV management: past, present, and future. *J Acquir Immune Defic Syndr* 2009, **50**:54–64.
8. Friis-Moller N, Weber R, Reiss P, Thiebaut R, Kirk O, d'Arminio Monforte A, Pradier C, Morfeldt L, Mateu S, Law M, El-Sadr W, De Wit S, Sabin CA, Phillips AN, Lundgren JD, DAD Study Group: Cardiovascular disease risk factors in HIV patients–association with antiretroviral therapy. Results from the DAD study. *AIDS* 2003, **17**:1179–1193.
9. Fontas E, van Leth F, Sabin CA, Friis-Moller N, Rickenbach M, d'Arminio Monforte A, Kirk O, Dupon M, Morfeldt L, Mateu S, Petoumenos K, El-Sadr W, de Wit S, Lundgren JD, Pradier C, Reiss P, DAD Study Group: Lipid profiles in HIV-infected patients receiving combination antiretroviral therapy: are different antiretroviral drugs associated with different lipid profiles? *J Infect Dis* 2004, **189**:1056–1074.
10. Mulligan K, Grunfeld C, Tai VW, Algren H, Pang M, Chernoff DN, Lo JC, Schambelan M: Hyperlipidemia and insulin resistance are induced by protease inhibitors independent of changes in body composition in patients with HIV infection. *J Acquir Immune Defic Syndr* 2000, **23**:35–43.
11. Arpadi S, Shiau S, Strehlau R, Martens L, Patel F, Coovadia A, Abrams EJ, Kuhn L: Metabolic abnormalities and body composition of HIV-infected children on Lopinavir or Nevirapine-based antiretroviral therapy. *Arch Dis Child* 2013, **98**:258–264.
12. Armstrong C, Liu E, Okuma J, Spiegelman D, Guerino C, Njelekela M, Grinspoon S, Fawzi W, Hawkins C: Dyslipidemia in an HIV-positive antiretroviral treatment-naive population in Dar es Salaam, Tanzania. *J Acquir Immune Defic Syndr* 2011, **57**:141–145.
13. George JA, Venter WD, Van Deventer HE, Crowther NJ: A longitudinal study of the changes in body fat and metabolic parameters in a South African population of HIV-positive patients receiving an antiretroviral therapeutic regimen containing stavudine. *AIDS Res Hum Retroviruses* 2009, **25**:771–781.
14. Buchacz K, Weidle PJ, Moore D, Were W, Mermin J, Downing R, Kigozi A, Borkowf CB, Ndazima V, Brooks JT: Changes in lipid profile over 24 months among adults on first-line highly active antiretroviral therapy in the home-based AIDS care program in rural Uganda. *J Acquir Immune Defic Syndr* 2008, **47**:304–311.
15. Piloya T, Bakeera-Kitaka S, Kekitiinwa A, Kamya MR: Lipodystrophy among HIV-infected children and adolescents on highly active antiretroviral therapy in Uganda: a cross sectional study. *J Int AIDS Soc* 2012, **15**:17427.
16. Mugyenyi P, Walker AS, Hakim J, Munderi P, Gibb DM, Kityo C, Reid A, Grosskurth H, Darbyshire JH, Ssali F, Bray D, Katabira E, Babiker AG, Gilks CF, Grosskurth H, Munderi P, DART Trial Team: Routine versus clinically driven laboratory monitoring of HIV antiretroviral therapy in Africa (DART): a randomised non-inferiority trial. *Lancet* 2010, **375**:123–131.
17. WHO: Antiretroviral therapy for HIV infection in adults and adolescents in resource-limited settings: towards universal access. In *Recommendations for a Public Health Approach.* Available at: http://www.who.int/hiv/pub/guidelines/artadultguidelines.pdf?ua=1. Accessed 17 February 2008.
18. NECP Expert Panel on Detection Ea, Treatment of High Blood Cholesterol in Adults: Third report of the National Cholesterol Education Program (NCEP) expert panel on detection, evaluation, and treatment of high blood cholesterol in adults (adult treatment panel iii) final report. *Circulation* 2002, **106**:3143.
19. DAIDS: The Division of AIDS (DAIDS) Standardized Toxicity Table for Grading Severity of Adult Adverse Experiences. Available at: http://rsc.tech-res.com/document/safetyandpharmacovigilance/table_for_grading_severity_of_adult_pediatric_adverse_events.pdf. Accessed August 1992.
20. Yusuf S, Hawken S, Ounpuu S, Dans T, Avezum A, Lanas F, McQueen M, Budaj A, Pais P, Varigos J, Lisheng L: Effect of potentially modifiable risk factors associated with myocardial infarction in 52 countries (the INTERHEART study): case-control study. *Lancet* 2004, **364**:937–952.
21. Salami AK, Akande AA, Olokoba AB: Serum lipids and glucose abnormalities in HIV/AIDS patients on antiretroviral therapies. *West Afr J Med* 2009, **28**:10–15.
22. Nguemaim NF, Mbuagbaw J, Nkoa T, Alemnji G, Teto G, Fanhi TC, Asonganyi T, Same-Ekobo A: Serum lipid profile in highly active antiretroviral therapy-naive HIV-infected patients in Cameroon: a case-control study. *HIV Med* 2010, **11**:353–359.
23. Adewole OO, Eze S, Betiku Y, Anteyi E, Wada I, Ajuwon Z, Erhabor G: Lipid profile in HIV/AIDS patients in Nigeria. *Afr Health Sci* 2010, **10**:144–149.
24. Fourie CM, Van Rooyen JM, Kruger A, Schutte AE: Lipid abnormalities in a never-treated HIV-1 subtype C-infected African population. *Lipids* 2010, **45**:73–80.
25. Grover SA, Coupal L, Gilmore N, Mukherjee J: Impact of dyslipidemia associated with Highly Active Antiretroviral Therapy (HAART) on cardiovascular risk and life expectancy. *Am J Cardiol* 2005, **95**:586–591.
26. Vorster HH, Venter CS, Wissing MP, Margetts BM: The nutrition and health transition in the North West Province of South Africa: a review of the THUSA (Transition and Health during Urbanisation of South Africans) study. *Public Health Nutr* 2005, **8**:480–490.
27. Stein JH, Komarow L, Cotter BR, Currier JS, Dube MP, Fichtenbaum CJ, Gerschenson M, Mitchell CK, Murphy RL, Squires K, Parker RA, Torriani FJ: Lipoprotein Changes in HIV-Infected Antiretroviral-Naive Individuals after Starting Antiretroviral Therapy: ACTG Study A5152s Stein: Lipoprotein Changes on Antiretroviral Therapy. *J Clin Lipidol* 2008, **2**:464–471.
28. Zannou DM, Denoeud L, Lacombe K, Amoussou-Guenou D, Bashi J, Akakpo J, Gougounon A, Akonde A, Ade G, Houngbe F, Girard PM: Incidence of lipodystrophy and metabolic disorders in patients starting non-nucleoside reverse transcriptase inhibitors in Benin. *Antivir Ther* 2009, **14**:371–380.

18

Partner notification in the context of HIV: an interest-analysis

Amos K Laar[1*], Debra A DeBruin[2] and Susan Craddock[3]

Abstract

Codes of confidentiality play an essential role in the intimate discourses in many learned professions. Codes with various prescriptions exist. The Hippocratic Oath for example, prescribes rewards to the secret keeper, for keeping secret what ought to be kept secret, and punishments for failing. In public health practice, partner notification, arguably is one endeavor that tests the durability of this secret keeping doctrine of the health professional. We present an interest-analysis of partner notification in the context of HIV service rendition. Using principles-based analysis, the interests of the individual, the state/public health, and the bioethicist's are discussed. The public health interests in partner notification, which are usually backed by state statutes and evidence, are premised on the theory that partners are entitled to knowledge. This theory posits that knowledge empowers individuals to avoid continuing risks; knowledge of infection allows for early treatment; and that knowledgeable partners can adapt their behavior to prevent further transmission of infection to others. However, persons infected with HIV often have counter interests. For instance, an infected person may desire to maintain the privacy of their health status from unnecessary disclosure because of the negative impacts of disclosure, or because notification without a matching access to HIV prevention and treatment services is detrimental. The interest of the bioethicist in this matter is to facilitate a resolution of these conflicted interests. Our analysis concludes that governmental interests are not absolute in comparison with the interests of the individual. We reiterate that any effort to morally balance the benefits of partner notification with its burdens ought to first recognize the multivalent nature of the interests at play.

Keywords: HIV, partner notification, interest-analysis, principles-based analysis

Introduction

One of the things that learned professions such as law, the clergy, medicine, and even public health have in common is codes of confidentiality. These codes ensure the sanctity of the intimate conversations that characterize them. In public health practice for example, client-provider confidentiality, has been treasured for ages [1]. The earliest explicit codification of confidentiality in the context of medicine is attributed to Hippocrates of Cos (460 BC – 370 BC). Titled "Oath of Hippocrates" the code prescribes rewards to the secret keeper, for living up to his obligations and punishments for those who do not (see extract below):

> *"Whatsoever in the course of practice I see or hear (or even outside my practice in social intercourse) that ought never to be published abroad, I will not divulge, but consider such things to be holy secrets. "Now if I keep this oath and break it not, may I enjoy honor, in my life and art, among all men for all time; but if I transgress and forswear myself, may the opposite befall me..."* [2].

Millennia upon millennia, medical oaths continue to agree fundamentally with the tenets of the Hippocratic ethics. This is not to say that professionals' obligation to keep the secrets of their clients has been polemics-free. Alan Brandt in his *"No Magic Bullet, the social history of venereal diseases in the United States ..."* animates the vehemence with which physicians within the United States (US), and those from across the Atlantic debated the issue of partner notification [3]. Brandt recounts the various medical, military, and public health responses

* Correspondence: alaar@ug.edu.gh
[1]Department of Population, Family, & Reproductive Health, School of Public Health, University of Ghana, Accra, Ghana
Full list of author information is available at the end of the article

that have arisen over the years – including the incarceration of prostitutes during World War I to the establishment of the extensively debated premarital blood tests. Of note, Brandt calls for the destabilization of the naturalness with which efforts that combat sexually transmissible infections have centered on punishment for sexual misconduct.

Introduced for syphilis and then extended to include gonorrhea in the 1930s and 1940s [3,4], partner notification is now considered useful for a wide range of sexually transmissible infections (STIs) [5]. Partner notification is currently defined as the process whereby the sexual partner(s) of a case (an index patient) is/(are) identified and informed of their exposure, then invited to testing, counseling and, where necessary, treatment [6,7]. As a term, "partner notification" has undergone some metamorphoses in the past decade and-a-half. Prior to 1998, guidelines of the US Centers for Disease Control and Prevention (CDC) contained "contact tracing" or "partner notification". These terms were dropped in 1998 for "partner counseling and referral services" [8]. The current CDC guidelines use "partner services" [6]. Related terminologies in current use include "expedited partner therapy", "privilege to warn" "duty to warn" and "duty to disclose". While many academics consider these as equivalent activities, public health practitioners consider them to be vastly different in most respects except for the principal goal [9]. Each has unique logistic and substantive issues. For instance, partner notification as is currently defined, requires that only sexual partners be notified that they have been in contact with a sexually transmissible infection. It is a confidential process: details of the index cases are known only to the health professionals treating them and are not divulged either to sexual partners or to disease notification systems. Contact tracing entails all the health care's actions taken to trace and actively and systematically contact all the partners/contacts indicated by the index person as having had relationships with him/her at risk. Bayer and Toomey discriminate between contact tracing and duty to warn [10]. They note that the moral "duty to warn", arose out of the clinical setting in which the physician knew the identity of the person deemed to be at risk. This approach provided a warrant for disclosure to endangered persons without the consent of the patient and could involve the revelation of the identity of the "threatening" party (the index patient). Bayer and Toomey lament that confusion regarding the approaches has led many to mischaracterize processes that are fundamentally voluntary as mandatory, and processes that respect confidentiality as invasive of privacy.

We note, however, that the terminology of partner notification differs between countries; it is used interchangeably with contract tracing in such countries as the United Kingdom and Australia. The global guidelines from the World Health Organization (WHO) [11] use partner notification. The WHO and the Joint United Nations Programme on HIV/AIDS (UNAIDS) recommend that partner notification be done on a voluntary basis [12]. Where partner notification has to be done without consent, the UNAIDS provides clear guidelines [13] such as: (i) The HIV-positive person in question has been thoroughly counselled; (ii) Counseling of the HIV-positive person has failed to achieve appropriate behavioral changes; (iii) The HIV-positive person has refused to notify, or consent to the notification of his/her partner(s); (iv) A real risk of HIV transmission to the partner(s) exists; (v) The HIV-positive person is given reasonable advance notice; (vi) The identity of the HIV-positive person is concealed from the partner(s), if this is possible in practice; (vii) Follow-up is provided to ensure support to those involved, as necessary.

As illustrative examples, we summarize below the global outlook of partner notification using relevant resources from the US, Europe, as well as the WHO global guidelines. These guidelines provide background and basis for the roll out of partner notification services globally. First, a technical report commissioned by the European Centre for Disease Prevention and Control (ECDC) details the public health benefits and context for partner notification within Europe [5]. The report notes that, some countries have wide-ranging legal obligations to enforce partner notification, others have laws that are not enforced; and there are countries in the region with no such laws at all. There are laws or regulations in eleven European countries that make partner notification compulsory for the healthcare provider, the patient or both [5].

Second, the CDC recommendations for partner services for Human Immunodeficiency Virus (HIV) infection and three other STIs (syphilis, gonorrhea, and chlamydial infection) provide implementation guidance in the United States [6]. As used in the recommendations, "partner services" is broad, with partner notification as a critical component. Functions of partner services include prevention counseling, HIV and STD testing, treatment or linkage to medical care, linkage or referral to other services.

Third, the WHO in April 2012 issued guidance on couples HIV testing and counseling including antiretroviral therapy (ART) for treatment and prevention in sero-discordant couples [11]. Partner notification is a prominent feature of the guidelines.

Beyond this background, we present a review of the principles and goals of partner notification, partner notification methods and approaches, and the data behind partner notification.

Review

We constructed searches with relevant key words in *OvidMedline,* and *Embase.* These were supplemented with 'unrestricted searches" in Google Scholar. Citations of retrieved resources were also perused for additional resources. A careful study of these and other resources provided the background data for our analysis. The first search in OvidMedline with key words [HIV infections, partner notification or contact tracing, privacy] spanned the period 1946 to week 4 of September 2013 and yield 83 records. These were manually reviewed and reduced to 27. A related search in the same database replaced partner notification or contact tracing, with partner service or expedited partner therapy and yielded 27 records that were manually reviewed and reduced to six. A third search in Embase using same key words yield two resources. Both were relevant.

Principles and goals of partner notification

Cognizant of the hypothesis that secrecy nurtures disease by providing an environment conducive to the spread of infection, Gostin and Hodge [14] note that one of the earliest recorded public health strategies for STI prevention was to pierce the veil of secrecy surrounding these hidden diseases by notifying sexual partners of infected patients. This was supported by the moral theory that sexual partners could take precautions and seek medical treatment if the risk of infection was disclosed. Once the risks of infection were identified, the incidence of STD infection would decline suggestively as infected persons reduced behaviors that placed them at risk for disease [12]. The following principles as set out in all partner notification guidelines, serve as the foundation for providing partner notification services: Such services ought to be client-centered, confidential, voluntary, free, evidence-based, comprehensive and integrative, culturally, and developmentally appropriate, accessible and available to all [5,6].

Every partner notification program seeks to maximize access to HIV prevention services by providing all infected persons (index patients) with support to ensure that the partners are confidentially informed of their exposure, tested, and linked to medical care. At the community level, partner notification seeks to reduce future rates of transmission in line with the current treatment as prevention arguments [15-17]. By linking partners to care and reducing their viral load, the community viral load/level of infectiousness is reduced [18-22]. Also, by identifying persons with previously undiagnosed HIV infection through partner notification and linking them to medical care services, and possibly to ART, partner notification services help reduce transmission within the community.

Partner notification methods and approaches

Conventionally, four strategies have been used in implementing partner notification: provider referral, self-referral, contract referral, and dual referral.

Provider referral notification involves a partner being notified of their possible exposure by a health professional who has been specifically trained to locate and notify partners. The healthcare worker then links the partners to medical, prevention, and support services while protecting the confidentiality of the index patient.

In a patient referral, the index patient takes responsibility for informing their sexual partner(s) of their possible exposure to an STI and for referring them to services. Introduced in the 1970s in response to high levels of gonococcal infection [23], patient referral has since been widely used for a wide range of STIs [5,6,24].

Contract referral notification involves index patients selecting specific partners they prefer to notify and agreeing to a specific time frame in which they will do so. Patients agree that if they do not notify the selected partners within the established time frame, the provider will notify the partners. Dual referral notification involves an index patient and the provider (or third party) jointly notifying a partner of exposure [5]. The data in support of partner notification are summarized below.

The data behind partner notification' in the context of HIV

Credible data exist in support of partner notification's role in HIV prevention-care cascade. We present some of these data. In the US for example, when syphilis prevalence peaked in 1990, partner notification among other national public health interventions contributed to its reduction and, later, elimination [25]. The efforts were adjudged to be cost efficient [25,26]. Also, evaluation of 10 years of data from the New York program for notification and referral services for gonorrhea, as well as of other program data showed a reduction in gonorrhea prevalence [27,28].

Other calls for the implementation of partner notification exist. For instance, it is argued that, of the approximately 1–1.2 million persons living with HIV infection in the United States, 25% are not aware of their infection; transmission from persons not aware of their infection accounts for 54%-70% of new infections [29,30]. A case is therefore made for partner notification given that it effectively identifies persons with previously undiagnosed HIV infection [31].

We present now the interests and counter interests in partner notification.

The interests in partner notification

Partner notification as a public health intervention, is implemented by governments to, among other reasons, reduce the incidence of new cases of STIs in individuals and in the community [5]. However, such interests of the government sometimes conflict with those of the individual. Two cases in the United States, the Jew Ho v. Williamson (1900) and Jacobson v. Massachusetts (1905) speak to such conflicting interests in public health practice. In his distillation of Jacobson v. Massachusetts, Gostin notes that governmental interests, though grounded firmly in statutory directives such as the police power[a], are not absolute [32]. Gostin clarifies that police powers cannot be exercised in a manner that violates the constitutional rights of individuals.

Resolution of these conflicted interests may call for legal jurisprudence, intervention by ethicists/bioethicists, or both. "Interest Analysis" has been applied in the past to resolve related conflicting interests [33,34]. Coined by Brainerd Currie in 1963, and popularized by Gostin and Hodge [14], interest analysis, as we will apply in this paper will entail a disinterested analysis of the various interests in partner notification, and not in legal jurisprudence. The interests at play here are the interests of the index patient, the interests of partner, and the interest of the public health profession/al. These interests are discussed.

Public health interests in partner notification

The public health interests of partner notification are justified in a number of ways. First, such interests are premised on the theory that partners are entitled to knowledge. This theory posits that "knowledge empowers individuals to avoid continuing risks; knowledge of infection allows for early treatment; and that knowledgeable partners can adapt their behavior to prevent further transmission of infection to others" [14,35]. Available evidence shows that people are less likely to have unprotected sex once they are aware of their HIV status [36,37]. Additionally, equipping public health officials with knowledge helps to prevent infection of and/or to treat sexual partners – control the spread of STI and its attendant consequences in the general public [35,36]. A review by Christie and Kendall show that prevalence of HIV among identified contacts ranges from 15% to 30%, with the majority of contacts being unaware of their possible exposure. Their conclusions concur with afore cited works [25-28] that, that partner notification is an effective public health intervention [38]. Thus partner notification programs offer substantial benefits to three principal groups: persons infected with HIV, their partners, and the community [6]. Presented this way, public health interest may be viewed as coinciding with those of the index patient, the interests of his/her partner, and the interests of the community as a whole.

Individual level interests

While governmental interests in partner notification may be equated to the interest of all, persons infected with HIV have individualized or counter interests [14]. For instance, an infected person may desire to maintain the privacy of their health status from unnecessary disclosure because of the negative impacts of disclosure (done consensually or otherwise). Emotional or physical abuse by or against the index patient, domestic violence of a physical or psychological nature as well as dissolution of a long-standing relationship [39,40] have been associated with partner notification. Theresa Yuricic [41] writes about how stigma particularly within the African-American community potentially decreases the efficacy of partner notification laws in this population. Disclosure of HIV status she notes can result in social stigma among their family and friends. Yuricic further discusses how disclosure makes them vulnerable to discrimination in employment, housing, and insurance [41]. Angela Nicoletti [42] enumerates other interests including fear of losing family support. Negative impacts of partner notification on infant feeding have been recording in Ghana [43]. It may thus seem reasonable, given these potential and real negative implications on the index patient, to respect their interests when systems or health personnel are unable to assure their security. In this regard, screening for likelihood of violence and/or other serious negative consequences on the index patient ought to be an important part of the partner notification process.

The bioethicist's interests in partner notification

The interest of the bioethicist in this matter is to facilitate a moral resolution of the conflicted interests. S/he is interested in providing nuanced answers to such questions as whether or not index patients or healthcare providers have a moral duty to inform partners of their exposure risk, whether or not the healthcare provider's relationship with the index patient takes priority over the obligation to protect others from the patient's infection, or just how important is the partner's right to know that he or she may be at risk? These are not ordinary questions. Gostin and Hodge [14] note that while the law provides its own answers to these questions, ethical reasoning or moral resolution is important. The fundamental conceptual problem is the difficulty in telling which of the claims (the index patient's or the partner's) should take precedence. Our analysis draws on Kass and Gielen's [14,44] as well as Gostin and Hodge's [14] earlier works. Like Kass and Gielen, we believe that principles-based analysis may help in the bioethicist's search for answers to the above questions.

Partner notification and the principle of beneficence

To Tom L. Beauchamp, and James Franklin Childress, beneficence means that persons have the responsibility to do good for others, to prevent harm to others, or, at the very least, to avoid directly harming others [45]. In the context of partner notification, promoting beneficence would mean carefully balancing the harms and benefits of partner notification – balancing the various interests. Without a doubt, any effort that seeks to prevent new HIV infections is pregnant with beneficence. An important question that earlier commentators have asked is: "how ethically effective partner notification programs are in achieving this goal" [44]. To provide a reasonable response as to the extent partner notification programs satisfy the principle of beneficence, Kass and Gielen [44] suggest a set of five assumptions all of which need to be met. These are:

1. The index patients must know and be willing to disclose the names of their contacts, and it must be possible to locate the contacts;
2. a significant proportion of the persons contacted must not have known already that they had been exposed to HIV, and they must have been practicing unsafe practices before and be willing to change to safer practices now;
3. A significant proportion of the persons contacted must be willing to be tested;
4. Some number of those found to be HIV-infected will not have known already that they were infected;
5. Some number of persons found to be HIV-infected must have been practicing unsafe practices before being contacted who will change to safer practices after being informed of their potential exposure.

We suggest a sixth assumption – partners who willingly accept to be tested when found to be HIV+ would have unfettered access to HIV treatment and prevention services for self and other partners. We note however, that arguments in support of this newly introduced assumption, needs to be nuanced by discussions on the ethical tensions associated with HIV treatment commodity allocation dynamics. For instance in settings where ARVs are very scarce, arguments concerning whether or not it is ethical to divert scarce ARVs from PLHIV who meet both the implicit adherence and the explicit medical eligibility criteria to others who do not. In support of the former, Elliot Marseille and colleagues argue forcefully for the supremacy of prevention over treatment even when it means denying treatment to medically eligible PLHIV [46]. Brock and Wikler [47] also argue that 'the strongest moral imperative directs us to give priority to saving the most lives even if this means lowering the priority given to the goal of universal access to treatment, to provide maximum protection from HIV infection'. Macklin and Cowan on the contrary argue that it will be unethical to 'deliberately watch patients with treatable AIDS worsen and die, if medications for treatment are diverted to for this purpose [48].

The extent to which Kass and Gielen's assumptions were met then or now is unknown. There are no published studies evaluating partner notification programs on the terms stated above. Studies whose findings could qualify as near approximations suggest that partners who were notified were significantly more likely to modify their sexual behavior and to avoid intercourse than those who had not been notified [49,50]. Other studies show that partners believe their chances for preserving their individual health rely in substantial part on notification of risk [17,37]. It follows, they argue, that universal notification is a plus to preserving and promoting public health. Yet, many infected persons, particularly women, counter these observations by documenting the costs of partner notification in the form of domestic violence and abuse [37,39,40].

Determining the balance between these competing interests is not easy. In its current application, partner notification may not represent a proper balance – "beneficence-wise". This paper's stance based on a conditional consequentialist reasoning supports the roll out of partner notification. In line with current arguments for treatment as prevention (TasP) and pre-exposure prophylaxis (PrEP), partner notification should have an additional condition of ensuring that index patients and their notified partners have access to HIV treatment and prevention commodities. The second condition (which entails prior screening for possible partner abuse) is inked in the latest guidelines by the CDC [6].

Partner notification and the principle of justice

Justice, according to Beauchamp and Childress, requires that people be treated fairly [45]. That is restrictions cannot be imposed on, or benefits provided to, one person or one group of people when another similarly-situated person or group is treated differently without adequate justification [45]. Any partner notification program that mirrors the above is morally indefensible. For instance, programs that prioritize men who have sex with men (MSM), female sex workers, or index patients suspected to have concurrent multiple sex partners or selectively notifies their partners should have a sound scientific justification. Such sound justifications would include for example, evidence showing that the group is significantly at greater risk of transmitting or acquiring the infection – in the case of MSM and sex workers. In that case disproportionate benefits/risks will not be unjust.

Per evidence [6,11], partner notification policies may be said to be just, but not necessarily practicable or fair implementation-wise. Pottker-Fishel's analysis of legal cases, state statutes and other literature shows that many states' statutes on partner notification are ineffective and burdensome, placing too much responsibility on health care providers [51]. There are also other studies that suggest that physicians may execute their responsibilities with regard to partner notification inconsistently depending on the demographics of their HIV-infected patients. For instance, findings of a national survey of US physicians that assessed among others partner management, and clinical practices for STIs including HIV show that variables such as gender, race, and sexual orientation would influence a decision to maintain or to violate patient confidentiality [52].

From the female index patient's perspective, partner notification programs while beneficial for women who are HIV-negative, may be harmful for HIV-positive women (costs such as domestic violence and other abuses have been discussed in this paper). Some commentators have argued that since uninfected women stand to benefit more from the implementation of partner notification programs than infected women, partner notification may be unjust. Second, given that women are at greater risk of heterosexual transmission than are men, it may be argued that heterosexual women are more likely than heterosexual men to benefit from partner notification. These are relevant justice questions. We nevertheless, believe that the disproportionate benefits in these instances are not unjust, as they are also disproportionate risks.

Partner notification and the principle of respect for autonomy

The third bioethical principle of respect for autonomy, means that people must be respected as autonomous agents who have the right to make decisions for themselves without interference from others [45]. Some commentators have argued that, this principle creates a moral right to decide whether, when, and to whom one should release personal information. On the one hand, if this principle is followed to the letter, and in the context of partner notification, an index patient in his/her quest to preserve his/her privacy can simply choose not to disclose his/her partners' names. On the other hand, a partner's normative claim about invasion of autonomy is also reasonable. Partners, according to Gostin and Hodge [14] can appeal to autonomy in claiming a right to know. Partners could argue that they cannot make rational, or autonomous choices in the absence of relevant information. Indeed, Sarah Conly's recent work titled *"Against Autonomy: Justifying Coercive Paternalism"* [53] would seem to favor the partner's claim. The autonomous index patient's right to engage in behaviors of his/her choosing does not extend to behaviors that can result in serious harm to partner(s). On the basis of these, an index patient may have no legitimate moral claim to maintain his/her confidentiality when doing so has a real potential to harm (HIV infection and its associated consequences in this case).

Conclusions

This review notes that, partner notification is grounded in credible evidence, and is sound in public health standings, but has multivalent ethical tensions and interests. Our analysis shows that while governmental interests are based on evidence and in some instances backed by state statutes, they are not absolute in comparison with the interests of the index patient. By all means, the autonomy of the index patient should be respected and so should the interest of his/her partners, and the community's at large. Against this backdrop, we reiterate that any effort to morally balance the benefits of partner notification with its burdens ought to first recognize the multivalent nature of the interests at play.

Abbreviations

ART: Antiretroviral therapy; CDC: United States Centers for Disease Control and Prevention; ECDC: European Centre for Disease Prevention and Control; HIV: Human Immunodeficiency Virus; PEP: Post-exposure prophylaxis; PrEP: Pre-exposure prophylaxis; STIs: Sexually transmissible infections; TasP: Treatment as prevention; UNAIDS: The Joint United Nations Programme on HIV/AIDS; WHO: World Health Organization..

Competing interests

The authors declare that they have no competing interests.

Authors' contributions

AL conceived the original idea for the paper, discussed the idea with DAD and SC and obtained inputs. AL drafted the first version manuscript. DAD and SC contributed to the drafting and subsequent revisions of the manuscript. All authors read and approved the final version of the manuscript.

Acknowledgments

We acknowledge the contribution of Del Reed, of the Health Sciences Libraries, University of Minnesota Twin Cities Campus. Del constructed the search strategies, and conducted the literature searches.

Author details

[1]Department of Population, Family, & Reproductive Health, School of Public Health, University of Ghana, Accra, Ghana. [2]Center for Bioethics, University of Minnesota, Minneapolis, USA. [3]Department of Gender, Women, and Sexuality Studies, University of Minnesota, Minneapolis, USA.

References

1. Epstein R, Thomas JC, Rutecki GW. Please don't say anything: partner notification and the patient-physician relationship. Virtual Mentor. 2003;5. doi: 10.1001/virtualmentor.2003.5.11.ccas2-0311
2. The hippocratic oath. BMJ. 1998;317:1110.
3. Brandt AM. No magic bullet: a social history of venereal disease in the United States since 1880. New York, New York, USA: Oxford University Press; 1987. p. 304
4. Harrison LW. Anti-venereal measures in Denmark and Sweden. Br J Vener Dis. 1939;15:1–17.
5. ECDC: European Centre for Disease Prevention and Control. Public health benefits of partner notification for sexually transmitted infections and HIV. Stockholm: ECDC: European Centre for Disease Prevention and Control; 2013. p. 132.
6. CDC: Recommendations for partner services programs for HIV infection, syphilis, gonorrhea, and chlamydial infection. MMWR Recommendations and reports: Morbidity and mortality weekly report Recommendations and reports/Centers for Disease Control. Atlanta Georgia, USA: Centers for Disease Control and Prevention (CDC); 2008.
7. Hogben M. Partner notification for sexually transmitted diseases. Clinical infectious diseases : an official publication of the Infectious Diseases Society of America. 2007;44 Suppl 3:S160–74.
8. CDC. HIV partner counseling and referral services guidance. Atlanta, GA: US Department of Health and Human Services; 1998.
9. Bruckman D. Contact Tracing. In: Loue S, editor. Mental Health Practitioner's Guide to HIV/AIDS. New York, NY, USA: Springer New York; 2013. p. 159–64.
10. Bayer R, Toomey KE. HIV prevention and the two faces of partner notification. Am J Public Health. 1992;82(8):1158–64.
11. WHO. Guidance on couples HIV testing and counselling including antiretroviral therapy for treatment and prevention in serodiscordant couples: recommendations for a public health approach. Geneva, Switzerland: WHO; 2012.
12. Gable L, Gostin L, Hodge J, Gamharter K, Van-Puymbroeck R. Legal aspects of HIV/AIDS: a guide for policy and law reform. Washington, DC: The World Bank; 2007.
13. UNAIDS: Office of the United Nations High Commissioner for Human Rights and the Joint United Nations Programme on HIV/AIDS. International guidelines on HIV/AIDS and human rights: 2006 consolidated version. Geneva, Switzerland: UNAIDS; 2006.
14. Gostin LO, Hodge JG. Piercing the veil of secrecy in HIV/AIDS and other sexually transmitted diseases: theories of privacy and disclosure in partner notification. Duke J Gend Law Policy. 1998;5:9–88.
15. Delva W, Eaton JW, Meng F, Fraser C, White RG, Vickerman P, et al. HIV treatment as prevention: optimising the impact of expanded HIV treatment Programmes. PLos Med. 2012;9:e1001258.
16. Lyles CM, Kay LS, Crepaz N, Herbst JH, Passin WF, Kim AS, et al. Best-evidence interventions: findings from a systematic review of HIV behavioral interventions for US populations at high risk, 2000–2004. Am J Public Health. 2007;97:133–43.
17. Passin WF, Kim AS, Hutchinson AB, Crepaz N, Herbst JH, Lyles CM. A systematic review of HIV partner counseling and referral services: client and provider attitudes, preferences, practices, and experiences. Sex Transm Dis. 2006;33:320–8.
18. He N, Duan S, Ding Y, Rou K, McGoogan JM, Jia M, et al. Antiretroviral therapy reduces HIV transmission in discordant couples in rural Yunnan, China. PLoS One. 2013;8:e77981.
19. Cohen MS, Chen YQ, McCauley M, Gamble T, Hosseinipour MC, Kumarasamy N, et al. Prevention of HIV-1 infection with early antiretroviral therapy. N Engl J Med. 2011;365:493–505.
20. Paquette D, Schanzer D, Guo H, Gale-Rowe M, Wong T. The impact of HIV treatment as prevention in the presence of other prevention strategies: Lessons learned from a review of mathematical models set in resource-rich countries. Prev Med. 2013;58:1–8.
21. Quinn TC, Wawer MJ, Sewankambo N, Serwadda D, Li C, Wabwire-Mangen F, et al. Viral load and heterosexual transmission of human immunodeficiency virus type 1. Rakai Project Study Group. N Engl J Med. 2000;342:921–9.
22. Cohen J. Breakthrough of the year. HIV treatment as prevention Science. 2011;334:1628.
23. Potterat JJ, Rothenberg R. The case-finding effectiveness of self-referral system for gonorrhea: a preliminary report. American journal of public health. 1977;67:174–6.
24. Steen R, Soliman C, Bucyana S, Dallabetta G. Partner referral as a component of integrated sexually transmitted disease services in two Rwandan towns. Genitourinary medicine. 1996;72:56–9.
25. Peterman TA, Toomey KE, Dicker LW, Zaidi AA, Wroten JE, Carolina J. Partner notification for syphilis: a randomized, controlled trial of three approaches. Sexually transmitted diseases. 1997;24:511–8.
26. Cohen DA, Wu S-Y, Farley TA. Comparing the cost-effectiveness of HIV prevention interventions. J Acquir Immune Defic Syndr. 2004;37:1404–14.
27. Du P, Coles FB, Gerber T, McNutt L-A. Effects of partner notification on reducing gonorrhea incidence rate. Sex Transm Dis. 2007;34:189–94.
28. Han Y, Coles FB, Muse A, Hipp S. Assessment of a geographically targeted field intervention on gonorrhea incidence in two New York State counties. Sex Transm Dis. 1999;26:296–302.
29. Glynn M, Rhodes P. Estimated HIV prevalence in the United States at the end of 2003. In: Proceedings of National HIV Prevention Conference. Atlanta, GA, June 12-15, 2005.
30. Marks G, Crepaz N, Janssen RS. Estimating sexual transmission of HIV from persons aware and unaware that they are infected with the virus in the USA. AIDS. 2006;20:1447–50.
31. Task Force on Community Preventive S. Recommendations to increase testing and identification of HIV-positive individuals through partner counseling and referral services. Am J Prev Med. 2007;33(2 Suppl):S88.
32. Gostin LO. Jacobson v Massachusetts at 100 years: Police power and civil liberties in tension. American Journal of Public Health. 2005;95:576–81.
33. Brilmayer L. Interest Analysis and the Myth of Legislative Intent. Michigan Law Review. 1980;78:392–431.
34. Kay HH. Currie's interest analysis in the 21st Century: losing the battle, but winning the war. Willamette Law Rev. 2001;37:123–132.
35. Hogben M, McNally T, McPheeters M, Hutchinson AB. The effectiveness of HIV partner counseling and referral services in increasing identification of HIV-positive individuals a systematic review. American journal of preventive medicine. 2007;33:S89–100.
36. Cowan FM, French R, Johnson AM. The role and effectiveness of partner notification in STD control: a review. Genitourinary medicine. 1996;72:247–52.
37. Kissinger PJ, Niccolai LM, Magnus M, Farley TA, Maher JE, Richardson-Alston G, et al. Partner notification for HIV and syphilis: effects on sexual behaviors and relationship stability. Sex Transm Dis. 2003;30:75–82.
38. Christie TKS, Kendall P. The science of partner notification: A review of the available evidence Issue. BCMJ. 2003;45(3):124–7.
39. Koenig LJ, Moore J. Women, violence, and HIV: a critical evaluation with implications for HIV services. Maternal and child health journal. 2000;4:103–9.
40. Koenig LJ, Whitaker DJ, Royce RA, Wilson TE, Callahan MR, Fernandez MI. Violence during pregnancy among women with or at risk for HIV infection. American journal of public health. 2002;92:367–70.
41. Yuricic T. Examination of Partner Notification Laws: What does Partner Notification Mean for HIV/AIDS in the African-American Community, An. Southern Region Black Law Students Association Law J. 2009;3:121–42.
42. Nicoletti A. Perspectives on pediatric and adolescent gynecology from the allied health professional. Journal of pediatric and adolescent gynecology. 2002;15:57.
43. Laar AK, Ampofo WK, Tuakli JM, Quakyi IA. Infant feeding choices and experiences of HIV-positive mothers from two Ghanaian districts. Journal of AIDS and HIV Research. 2009;1:23–33.
44. Kass NE, Gielen AC. The ethics of contact tracing programs and their implications for women. Duke journal of gender law & policy. 1998;5:89–102.
45. Beauchamp TL, Childress JF. Principles of Biomedical Ethics. New York, New York, USA: Oxford University Press; 1994.
46. Marseille E, Hofmann PB, Kahn JG. HIV prevention before HAART in sub-Saharan Africa. Lancet. 2002;359:1851–6.
47. Brock W, Wikler D. Ethical challenges in long-term funding for HIV/AIDS. Health Aff (Millwood). 2009;28:1666–76.
48. Macklin R, Cowan E. Given financial constraints, it would be unethical to divert antiretroviral drugs from treatment to prevention. Health Aff (Millwood). 2012;31:1537–44.
49. Andrus JK. Partner Notification: Can It Control Epidemic Syphilis? Annals of Internal Medicine. 1990;112:539.
50. Wykoff RF, Heath Jr CW, Hollis SL, Leonard ST, Quiller CB, Jones JL, et al. Contact tracing to identify human immunodeficiency virus infection in a rural community. JAMA. 1988;259(24):3563–6.

51. Pottker-Fishel CG. Improper bedside manner: why state partner notification laws are ineffective in controlling the proliferation of HIV. Health Matrix Clevel. 2007;17:147–79.
52. St Lawrence JS, Montaño DE, Kasprzyk D, Phillips WR, Armstrong K, Leichliter JS. STD screening, testing, case reporting, and clinical and partner notification practices: a national survey of US physicians. Am J Public Health. 2002;92:1784–8.
53. Conly S: Against autonomy: justifying coercive paternalism. Cambridge, United Kingdom: Cambridge University Press; 2013:216.

HIV Encephalopathy: pediatric case series description and insights from the clinic coalface

Kirsten A Donald[1*], Kathleen G Walker[2], Tracy Kilborn[3], Henri Carrara[4], Nelleke G Langerak[5], Brian Eley[6] and Jo M Wilmshurst[2]

Abstract

Background: The Human Immune Deficiency Virus (HIV) can manifest neurologically in both adults and children. Early invasion of the central nervous system by the virus, affecting the developing brain, is believed to result in the most common primary HIV-related neurological complication, HIV Encephalopathy (HIVE). In countries such as South Africa where many children have not been initiated on antiretroviral treatment early, HIVE remains a significant clinical problem.

Methods: Children were selected from a clinic for children with neurologic complications of HIV, located at the Red Cross War Memorial Children's Hospital, South Africa 2008–2012. Eligible subjects fulfilled the following inclusion criteria: aged 6 months-13 years; positive diagnosis of HIV infection, vertically infected and HIVE as defined by CDC criteria. Each participant was prospectively assessed by a Pediatric Neurologist using a standardized proforma which collated relevant details of background, clinical and immunological status.

Results: The median age of the 87 children was 64 months (interquartile range 27–95 months). All except one child were on antiretroviral treatment, 45% had commenced treatment <12 months of age. Delayed early motor milestones were reported in 80% and delayed early speech in 75% of children in whom we had the information. Twenty percent had a history of one or more seizures and 41% had a history of behavior problems. Forty-eight percent had microcephaly and 63% a spastic diplegia. CD4 percentages followed a normal distribution with mean of 30.3% (SD 8.69). Viral loads were undetectable (<log 1.6) in 70% of the children. Brain imaging was performed on 56% with 71% of those imaged demonstrating at least one abnormality, most commonly white matter volume loss or signal abnormality.

Conclusions: Amongst the cohort of children referred to this clinic, the diagnosis of HIVE was unrecognized in the general medical services, even in its most severe form. Developmental delay and school failure were major presenting problems. Co-morbidities are a frequent finding and should be sought actively in order to optimize management and promote best possible outcomes for this vulnerable group of children.

Keywords: HIV encephalopathy, Children, MRI, Brain, Developmental delay

Background

According to the World Health Organization, approximately 3.4 million children worldwide are suffering from Human immunodeficiency Virus (HIV) or Acquired immune deficiency syndrome (AIDS) with >90% of them residing in sub-Saharan Africa [1-3]. There are an estimated 300,000 HIV-infected children in South Africa not yet receiving antiretroviral therapy (ART), with an estimated 48,000 new infections among children annually [2,3]. The greatest proportion of these figures represent vertically acquired HIV, which includes infection in utero, at time of delivery and from breast milk [2].

The Western Cape, where the study was completed, commenced its public sector prevention of mother-to-child transmission (PMTCT) intervention programme in 2001. The initial PMTCT programme was based on the HIVNET 012 nevirapine (NVP) regimen, and provision of milk powder for all infants of mothers who elected to formula-feed their offspring for the first 6 months of life.

* Correspondence: kirsty.donald@uct.ac.za
[1]Division of Developmental Pediatrics, Department of Pediatrics and Child Health, University of Cape Town and Red Cross War Memorial Children's Hospital, Cape Town, South Africa
Full list of author information is available at the end of the article

Universal coverage of the PMTCT programme in the province was reached at the beginning of 2003. In mid-2004 an intensified PMTCT programme was introduced based on the CD4 count of all HIV-infected pregnant women. Those women with CD4 count ≤ 200 cells/μL were commenced on antiretroviral therapy (ART), while those with a CD4 count >200 cells/μL were commenced on zidovudine prophylaxis at 34–36 weeks gestation, and during labour administered a single dose of NVP. All infants born to HIV-infected mothers received a single dose of NVP at birth plus a 7-day course of AZT [4]. Between 2004 and 2013 this programme underwent several revisions including progressive liberalization of the criteria used to initiate ART in pregnant women, introduction of 6 week infant testing (previously 14 weeks), introduction of extended NVP prophylaxis for all HIV-exposed infants, promotion of breastfeeding, and the withdrawal of free-formula milk in 2012 [5].

HIV can have neurological manifestations in both adults and children. Early invasion of the central nervous system (CNS) by the virus, affecting the developing fetal and infant brain, is believed to result in the most common primary HIV-related CNS complication, HIV Encephalopathy (HIVE) [6]. In non-treated children prevalence reports have ranged from 20 to 60% [7-14]. HIVE refers to the disease, damage or malfunction of the brain caused by HIV-1. Static HIVE is an unchanging type of encephalopathy, whereas, progressive HIVE is associated with neuroregression. This complication can be present before significant immunosuppression has developed, however its presence in a child infected with HIV constitutes an AIDS-defining illness, [15] reflecting the severity of the disease. According to the Center for Disease Control (CDC), encephalopathy must include criteria in at least one of the following areas for at least 2 months in the absence of a concurrent illness: a) failure to attain or loss of developmental milestones or loss of intellectual ability, b) impaired brain growth or acquired microcephaly and/or c) acquired symmetric motor deficit [15].

While substantial numbers of children have benefitted from antiretroviral treatment (ART), significant barriers to early ART initiation continue to exist, compared to adults infected with HIV. This places untreated children at risk, particularly of central nervous system (CNS) sequelae. HIV-1 invades the developing CNS earlier and with greater severity than observed in adults [7-14]. In addition patients on ART may remain vulnerable to the effects of HIV on the brain because the CNS may be a reservoir for persistent viral replication [16].

Reported specific neurodevelopmental delays in young children associated with HIVE include delays in acquiring early motor and language skills [6,17,18]. These have included general gross motor skills and development co-ordination, muscle tone and deep tendon reflexes. In older children specific cognitive deficits, impaired motor skills and decreased language ability are also reported. Cognitive deficits include verbal and memory impairment and difficulty with visual-spatial integration and executive function [19,20].

Neuroimaging studies using more recently available quantitative magnetic resonance imaging (MRI) techniques are contributing to improved understanding of the underlying neurobiology of the primary effects of HIV on the developing brain. In a study by Ackermann *et al.*, the findings of white matter signal abnormalities in a significant proportion of the brains of young children (mean age: 31.4 months) initiated on ART under 3 months of age, may indicate that infiltration of the CNS by HIV occurs at an extremely early stage of infection [21]. These abnormalities are much more subtle than the global cerebral atrophy and or basal ganglia calcifications which are more typically described in the context of children with HIV encephalopathy (HIVE) [22]. In addition, two recent studies have reported subtle white matter microstructural abnormalities [23] and neurochemical abnormalities [24] in relatively well older children. In particular, Hoare *et al.* reported an association between poor performance on tests of executive function and attention with reduced white matter integrity in the corpus callosum in "slow-progressor" children who were considered too well to require ART. These white matter changes represent a variable combination of diffuse myelin loss, astroglial proliferation, and infiltration by mono and multinucleated macrophages [25]. Methods such as those described above, which can detect more subtle changes in especially white matter integrity, may be key in the investigation of both the timing and natural history of neurological complications of HIV. However, despite this emerging literature there remains a paucity of data from low and middle income countries (LMIC) where the utility of these investigations in a clinical context with high burden of disease, but limited resources and consequent different standard of care remains inadequately explored.

HIVE was found to be the most common primary neurological disorder of HIV infected children diagnosed in the HIV Neurology clinic at Red Cross War Memorial Children's Hospital and in this report we aimed to describe this group of children in order to better understand their profile as well as identify challenges and opportunities for improved management in the clinical context.

Methods

Study population

This paper offers a descriptive profile of HIV infected children referred to a dedicated HIV-Neurology Clinic in

Cape Town, South Africa and diagnosed with HIVE. The overall purpose of this clinic is to screen children identified by clinicians to be at risk for neurologic complications of HIV. Children are evaluated, investigated and a formal neurologic diagnosis given where appropriate. Following this there is a formulation of on-going care plans for these children. As part of the service a database has been collected to help understand the neurologic disease spectrum and demographics of our population group. The health system in South Africa is three-tiered such that the majority of children on ARTs receive treatment at a primary level, where access to neuro-imaging and neuro-cognitive testing is not available. Red Cross War Memorial Children's Hospital is a tertiary level service with access to these facilities. Referrals to the HIV-Neuro clinic come from primary, secondary and tertiary levels. In addition to the specific neurologic conditions such as epilepsy and the complications of secondary CNS infections (primarily tuberculous and other bacterial meningitides), reasons for referral to this clinic include general concerns about developmental delay, particularly delay in onset of walking beyond 2 years, learning difficulties and behavior problems such as memory loss, hyperactivity, poor concentration and not referred as HIVE *per se*.

Children were selected from this clinic over the period 2008–2012. Eligible subjects were those who had attended the HIV Neurology clinic at least once and who fulfilled the following inclusion criteria: aged between 6 months and 13 years; positive diagnosis of HIV infection (includes initial and confirmatory tests), vertical transmission and HIVE as defined by CDC criteria. Children were excluded when they had a history of: an uncontrolled medical condition, such as the presence of an identified CNS condition (other than HIV), CNS infections e.g. Tuberculous Meningitis; drug or alcohol exposure in pregnancy; history of a head injury with loss of consciousness greater than 5 min or any radiological evidence of skull fracture; history of perinatal complications such as hypoxic ischemic encephalopathy or neonatal jaundice requiring exchange transfusion, or neurodevelopmental and or neuroregressive or genetic disorder not attributed to HIV.

Data collection

Each participant was prospectively assessed by a medical specialist (KD or KW) using a standardized proforma which collated relevant details of background, clinical and immunological status information. Background information was collected from the care-giver at the time of assessment, though if supplementary information was available in the medical folder this was also included. Details included source of referral, age, sex, birth history (antenatal, birth complication, gestation and birth weight), past medical, early developmental history and a history of caregivers. In addition, care-givers were asked about the child's home environment and schooling situation. This information was based on caregiver recall, although with respect to identifying age of achieving milestones a timeline follow-back approach was used to achieve best possible recall.

Clinical assessments performed included anthropometry (height, weight, head circumference (OFC)), full neurological and physical examination (indications of spastic diplegia and or long tract signs, microcephaly, peripheral neuropathy, visual and hearing impairment and child's mood). In addition, immunological results collected consisted of most recent CD4 and viral load counts. Due to the disparate facilities from which the children had received their primary ART, information on immunological status at time of HIV diagnosis and ART commencement was available on too few children to include in the analysis.

Children selected for this study were also referred for either Computer Tomography (CT) or Magnetic resonance imaging (MRI) of the brain using the standard clinical neuroimaging protocol used at the hospital. These images were analyzed and reported by a Pediatric Neuroradiogist (TK) at Red Cross War Memorial Children's Hospital. Informed consent is part of the protocol for MRI acquisition in young children. Due to the difficult socio-economic environments from which HIV infected children in South Africa generally come, as well as the high burden of medical appointments they are required to attend, failure to attend hospital appointments (particularly when the visit is not directly related to the management of HIV itself) is extremely common. This was the most common reason for children not having neuroimaging.

Collected information was anonymized and entered onto a password protected database in a private office. Ethical approval was obtained from the University of Cape Town Human Research Ethics committee (UCT HREC 126/2011).

Statistical analysis

Background information, results of clinical assessments, immunological and imaging findings were analyzed by using Stata version 12 (Stata Corp LP, 4905 Lakeway Drive, College Station, Texas 77845 USA). All continuous data was assessed for normality using the Shapiro Wilk test, and parametric or non-parametric summary measures were reported as appropriate.

To determine if there was significant association between the age of starting ART and physical findings of microcephaly and spastic diplegia, the statistician compared the median age at ART commencement with two groups (positive or negative diagnosis) using the Wilcoxon rank-sum (Mann–Whitney test). This analysis was also repeated for testing the relationship between current immunological status and these physical findings.

In addition, analysis was done to determine whether there was an association between imaging abnormalities described in the cohort and the HIVE-defining physical findings of microcephaly and spastic diplegia, age at ART commencement and current immunological status. For each association prevalence ratios were estimated by using generalized linear regression.

Statistical significance level was set at $p < 0.05$.

Results

Study cohort background information

The algorithm as presented in Figure 1 provides an overview of the number of children identified, selected and included for proforma assessment and neuroimaging procedures. During the study period 145 children were seen in the HIV Neurology clinic, of which 87 children fulfilled the criteria for eligibility (HIVE) and were included in this study. The remaining 58 children had other neurological complications of HIV such as cerebrovascular events, severe epilepsy or a background of other complicating medical factors (especially opportunistic CNS infections, perinatal complications and history of maternal substance use in pregnancy) which excluded an isolated diagnosis of HIVE. Only children who were diagnosed with HIVE were included in the analysis. Twenty nine of the 87 children were referred from primary health care clinics, 35 from secondary level hospitals and 23 from other clinics or wards at RCWMCH. Analysis of carer consistency showed 11 had consistent care with 2 parents, 38 had consistent care with one parent and 37 had had multiple carers during this time (which may have included a parent during some of that time).

Table 1 provides an overview of the background information of the HIVE study cohort. The median age of the children was 64 months interquartile range (IQR) of 27 to 95 months, with the majority aged between 2–9 years (87%). All except one child were on ART at time of first assessment, and 38 children (45%) had first received ART before the age of 12 months. Of the 87 children included, 85 were referred to the clinic as a result of concern regarding their failure to attain early developmental milestones, school failure or behavioral problems, but were not formally diagnosed with HIVE prior to being seen at the HIV-Neurology clinic.

With regards to the early milestones, delayed walking was reported in 60/75 children (80%) and delayed early

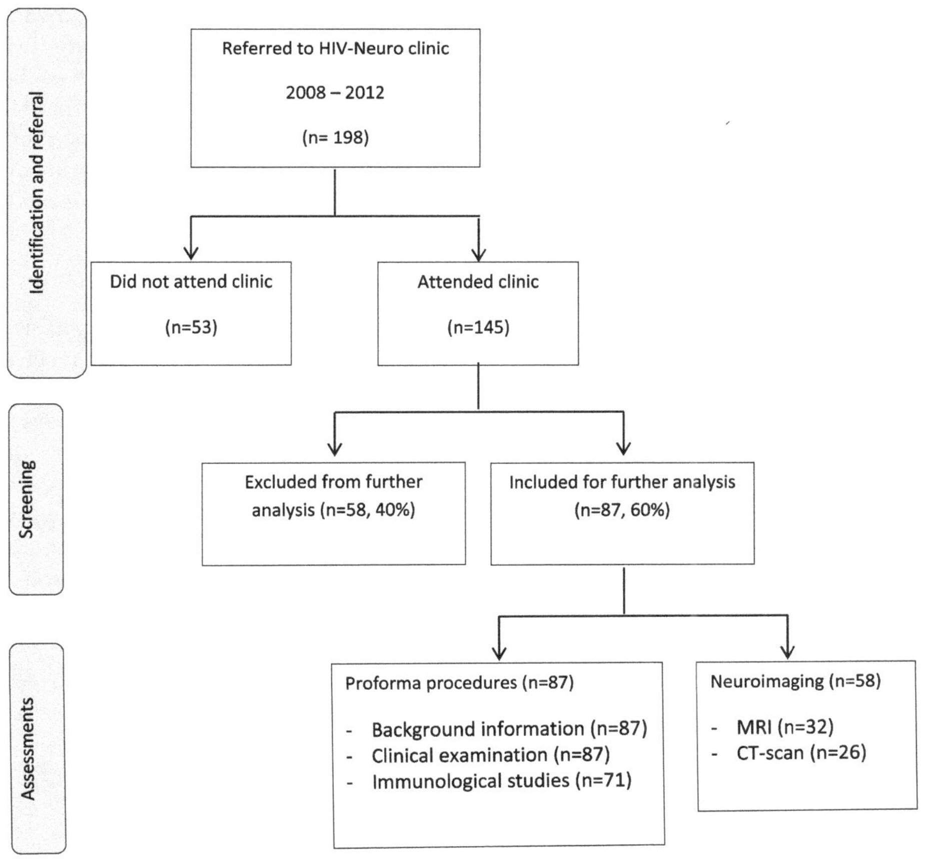

Figure 1 Study algorithm.

Table 1 Background information for children with HIVE

Variable (total number of assessments)	Subjects n	%
Gender (n = 87)		
Male	51	59
Female	36	41
Age group at examination (n = 87)		
<2 years	16	18
2 – 4 years	24	28
5 – 9 years	36	41
10 – 14 years	11	13
Age at ART commencement (n = 87)		
<12 months	38	44
12 – 36months	33	38
>36 months	14	16
Not reported	2	2
Developmental milestone walking (n = 75)		
On time	15	20
Delayed (>18 months)	60	80
Not old enough to tell	5	N/A
Not reported	7	N/A
Developmental milestone talking (n = 72)		
On time	18	25
Delayed (>18 months)	54	75
Not old enough to tell	4	N/A
Not reported	11	N/A
Home environment (n = 87)		
home	49	56
Institution, orphanage, foster home	13	15
bio foster (adopted by family member)	20	23
other foster	4	5
Not reported	1	1
School (n = 87)		
Mainstream pre-school	32	37
Mainstream school	35	40
Special school/care center	4	5
None	7	8
Not reported	9	10
Repeating grades		
Yes	37	43
No	27	31
Not reported	23	26

speech in 54/72 children (75%). Of the 81 children from whom a medical history was available 17 children (20%) had a history of one or more seizure and 14 (17%) had already been assigned a formal diagnosis of attention deficit hyperactivity disorder by their treating doctor when they were referred to the clinic. In addition, 33 children (41%) had a history of behavior problems as reported by their parents. Sixty-seven (86%) children were attending a mainstream educational facility at the time of assessment and more than half of the children of school-going age (57%) had had to repeat a school-year or was not age appropriate for their current school grade. All participants were of low socioeconomic status and 37 (43%) of them were living in a foster or adopted home environment.

Clinical information

Anthropometric measures weight, height and head circumference were at least 2 standard deviations below that expected for age in more than half of the study-cohort. Of the 87 children who underwent physical exam, 42 children (48%) presented with microcephaly (head circumference <2standard deviations from the age norms on WHO growth charts), 55 (63%) with spastic diplegia. Thirty-three children (37%) had active ear disease (chronic otitis media). Clinical findings are detailed in Table 2.

Immunological status

Recent CD4 count (percentage) and viral loads (log value) were available for 70 and 71 children with HIVE respectively. All the children about whom we had immunological information were on ART at the time of assessment. CD4 percentages followed a normal distribution with mean of 30.3% (SD 8.69). Viral loads were undetectable (<log 1.6) in 50 (70%) of the children. The mean viral load was log 2.07 (IQR 1.3-2.3).

Neuroimaging

Brain imaging was successfully performed on 49 of the 87 (56%) children. Five children received both MRI and CT scans (their findings are aggregated) and 4 children failed their scan and so their findings are not reported, making up the total of 58 scans recorded in Figure 1. Fourteen children had normal scans, while 35 (71%) presented with at least one abnormality, six children with a combination of two abnormalities, two children with three abnormalities and three children with four abnormalities. Table 3 gives an overview of the CT and MRI imaging findings reported in the HIVE study-cohort and Figures 2 and 3 show examples of the most common neuroimaging findings.

Associations with microcephaly and spastic diplegia

There was no statistically significant difference in age at starting ART between those with and without microcephaly ($p = 0.4$, Wilkoxon rank-sum (Mann–Whitney test), $z = -0.87$). Similarly for spastic diplegia, there was

Table 2 Clinical findings for children with HIVE

Variable	Subjects	
	n	%
Weight		
Normal	43	49
3rd – 10th centile	16	18
<3rd centile	28	32
Height		
Normal	24	28
3rd – 10th centile	20	23
<3rd centile	26	30
Not recorded	17	20
Physical exam		
Spastic diplegia/long tract signs	55	63
Microcephaly	42	48
Learning Difficulties	6	7
Peripheral Neuropathy	1	1
Visual impairment	1	1
Hearing impairment	2	2
Ears		
Normal	36	41
Acute otitis media	7	8
Chronic suppurative otitis media	26	30
not examined/recorded	16	18

no statistically significant difference in age at starting ART between those with and without spastic diplegia, although this approached significance ($p = 0.06$, Wilkoxon rank-sum (Mann–Whitney test), $z = 1.83$).There was no increased relative risk for a particular imaging abnormality with this group. Neither recent CD4 percentage values nor the presence/absence of detectable viral load correlated with the presence of particular neuroimaging findings in our cohort.

Table 3 Neuroimaging findings

Variable	Subjects	
	n	%
Imaging		
Global Atrophy	10	20
Basal Ganglia Calcifications	4	8
White Matter Signal Change	9	18
White Matter Volume Loss	12	24
Grey Matter Volume Loss	4	8
Thinning of Corpus Callosum	9	18
Other	6	12
Normal	14	29

Discussion

This study describes the clinical, immunological and imaging features of a clinical group of 87 children with HIVE attending a dedicated referral clinic for children with neurologic complications of HIV infection. Current figures clearly demonstrate the major burden of childhood HIV is carried by countries in sub-Saharan Africa. It is apparent that even in South Africa where the roll-out of ART to both HIV infected children and adults, has improved the outlook for children, HIVE remains a problem in clinical practice.

We established that amongst the cohort of children referred to us, the specific diagnosis of HIVE is frequently unrecognized in general medical services, even in its most severe form. Postulated reasons for this include busy clinics where the time taken to do a full neurology examination is difficult to find, or where clinicians, though recognizing the problem, referred the children for more detailed assessment in order to exclude other causes of the neurology problems in this group. Pediatric services and in particular more specialized neurology services are particularly under-represented across the African continent [26]. This implies that the milder forms are probably being missed in overburdened health systems such as that in South Africa and other resource-limited countries.

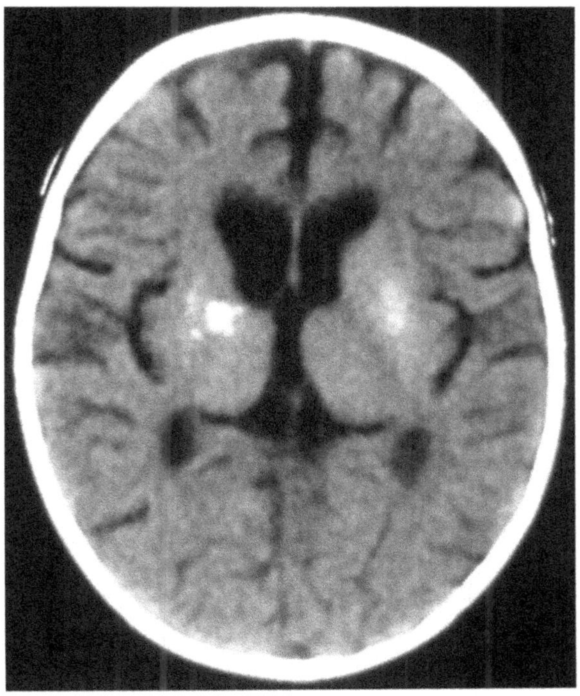

Figure 2 Axial CT Brain showing bilateral basal ganglia calcification and cerebral shrinkage in a 1year old child with HIVE.

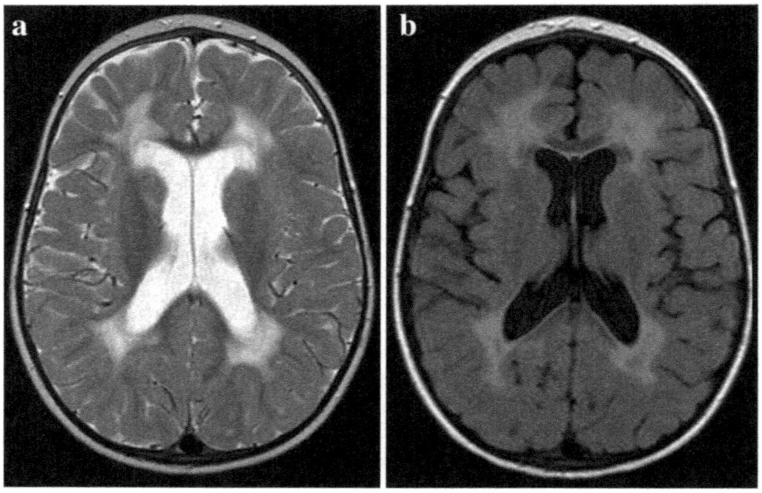

Figure 3 Axial T2 (a) and FLAIR (b) images of an HIV-positive child showing bilateral symmetrical high signal in the periventricular white matter with normal basal ganglia. Prominence of the cerebral sulci implies volume loss.

The reported prevalence of neurodevelopmental delays in HIV-infected children varies between 8 to >60% depending on the measures used and clinical populations [10,11,17,19,27,28]. Evidence is emerging that even children started on effective ART at a very young age, may demonstrate adverse neurologic outcomes in later childhood [18,20,21]. The presence of a history of delayed early motor and language milestones in the vast majority of this cohort is to be expected as their diagnosis preselects them into a severely affected group. However, this history of these delays suggest that the CNS damage in these children was present from early infancy and that despite almost uniformly good viral control at time of assessment, the residual effects of the virus on the developing neurological system is likely to be long-lasting.

Although with formal neuropsychological testing some of the children excluded from the diagnosis of HIVE in this cohort might have met criteria for the diagnosis, there will remain a group whose overall cognitive performance falls within the normal range (or within 2 SDs of the norm), but who have specific learning difficulties. Evidence for this spectrum of subtler neurocognitive effects is described in even completely asymptomatic children [23]. The concept of a "milder" form of neurocognitive disturbances in HIV infected children such as the adult condition of HIV-associated neurocognitive disorder (HAND) is recognized but is yet to achieve a consensus definition in children and adolescents. This condition may have significant effects in functional terms on the learning potential of the child (especially at school). This is a critical discourse, as it is likely to be important in informing treatment guidelines for these children especially in contexts where access to treatment may depend on clinical criteria. Although our older children did not consistently undergo formal neuropsychological testing, a significant proportion of these children were repeating grades at school. This can be regarded as a manifestation of functional neurocognitive compromise.

Co-morbidities were found to be significant management issues in this group of children with HIVE. Twenty percent had suffered one or more seizures, 40% had reported behavior problems with 18% a formal diagnosis of ADHD and 39% had active ear disease. Relatively "minor" conditions such as recurrent ear infections, which are inadequately managed, can affect a child's hearing. Even mild hearing loss in this complex disorder where a child may have additional cognitive and or learning difficulties, could have serious long-term effects on their school outcome and future economic potential. High prevalence of behavior problems amongst other groups of children with chronic medical conditions is well described. HIV integration into the frontal cortex and connecting structures of the CNS are suggested as possible mechanisms for specific behavioral manifestations in this group [29,30]. The figure reported here is in keeping with some of the chronic physically disabling conditions such as Duchenne muscular dystrophy and other neuromuscular conditions (41%) where one may expect there to be a higher prevalence [31]. The high prevalence of co-morbidities in this group highlights the importance of actively enquiring after and managing these aspects of the child's medical profile.

Although a definitive clinical or imaging predictor for HIVE has not been defined, risk factors associated with HIVE include maternal and child immune status, high CSF and plasma viral load, high circulating monocytes, timing of infection, route of transmission, and availability of early treatment [2,27,28]. This previously reported literature has implicated high viral loads as a predictor for HIVE. Over two thirds of our group had undetectable viral loads at time of assessment so this made it a largely unhelpful variable to use in our group. Information on peak viral loads or viral loads at the time of diagnosis prior to ART initiation may have been more helpful in this analysis. Of interest there was no statistically significant association between age at starting ART and the presence of microcephaly, though the association between age at starting ART and spastic diplegia approached significance in this group. Children manifesting spastic diplegia as their neurological criterion for HIVE are likely to represent the severe end of the spectrum of the disorder and the trend towards association with delayed ART in this group is consistent with studies which have demonstrated poorer neurological outcomes in children with deferred ART initiation [18].

Imaging findings described in HIVE have focused on a number of characteristics. These include Computer Tomography (CT) findings of generalized atrophy, ventriculomegaly, and basal ganglia calcification [32-35]. Although these are the most commonly reported signs of HIVE on CT scan; they appear not to be that common in absolute terms amongst children with HIVE and may represent the severe end of the spectrum of the disorder. Magnetic Resonance Imaging (MRI) studies have shown white matter microstructural changes amongst HIV-infected, but not encephalopathic children [23,35]. Neuroimaging changes in the brains of HIV-infected children could represent important indicators of disease. A study showed correlations between changes in the corpus callosum and significant reduced executive function and attention tests, as well as relations between changes in superior longitudinal fasiculus and reduced functional performance [23]. On the other hand, in another older study, 76% of asymptomatic HIV-positive children were found to have at least one abnormality of global atrophy as well as more specific white matter changes on brain CT scan [32]. Very few of these studies have correlated the neuroimaging findings with neurological findings in the children they describe. In our cohort, clinical neuroimaging sequences, even in an experienced specialist unit did not correlate usefully with physical findings. A large proportion of scans (29%) were completely normal despite all the children having abnormal neurological findings suggestive of upper motor neuron pathology (microcephaly and or spastic diplegia). It is probable that more sophisticated MRI techniques such as diffusion tensor imaging would be able to identify abnormalities in white matter integrity at a microstructural level, however this is not likely to represent a practical clinical approach in our setting in the foreseeable future.

Introduction of ART is associated with prolonged survival rates of children suffering from HIV by promoting a broad spectrum of general and specific health measures including normal growth and development, improved immunity, reduced risk of and vulnerability to infections [36,37]. Its essential role in the effective management of the disease is now undisputed. ART is also associated with dramatically decreased the prevalence of HIVE in the United States from 35-50% to less than 2% [2,38]. Furthermore, early initiation of ART results in improved neurodevelopmental outcomes compared to deferred initiation [18]. However, in resource-limited contexts such as South Africa, where ART is not always easily accessible and treatment is frequently delayed beyond infancy, HIVE remains an important and frequently undiagnosed clinical problem.

Limitations of our study include relatively small sample size and cross-sectional study design. All data was captured from a data-base of a working clinic at a tertiary centre in South Africa. The vast majority of HIV infected children are primarily treated at primary level health institutions which are staffed by medical officers and not pediatricians or sub-specialists in neurology, child psychiatry or developmental pediatrics and where the burden of attending to the immediate life-threatening medical issues are likely to result in only the severe developmental or behavioral issues being identified. As a result, the relatively small number of children in this report is likely to represent superficial evidence of a much larger under-recognized problem. Another significant limitation includes the fact that behavioral history and psychosocial information was collected via carer report rather than standardized testing and represents the reality of what even a specialized clinic is able to offer in the clinical setting in the present environment. However, both clinicians who assessed the children are experienced in addressing this scope of problem and the time-line follow-back method was used to optimize parental recall where appropriate. In addition, the lack of formal neurocognitive evaluations on the older age group of children presenting to the clinic means that the diagnosis of HIVE was made on one of the two physical CDC criteria. As such this group of 87 children most likely represents the more severe end of the HIVE spectrum (i.e. all the children with a diagnosis of HIVE had an abnormal neurological examination, making analysis for clinical predictors very difficult). The lack of useful clinical associations between physical findings and immunological or imaging findings is not entirely surprising given the cross-sectional study design and particular cohort.

Conclusion

The assessment of this group of children revealed some useful insights for clinical practice. Regular anthropometric measurements including height and head circumference should be recorded in order to identify children at risk of growth failure as well as making the diagnosis of HIVE where appropriate. Structural neuroimaging may not be helpful in the day-to-day management of a significant group of children with HIVE. It is however, useful in excluding secondary conditions where indicated, especially where long tract signs are present such as spastic diplegia. School failure is a major problem in this group and in a society where HIV remains highly stigmatizing and the school is frequently not aware of the child's diagnosis, many parents are reluctant to seek help for their child's learning problems. Co-morbidities are a frequent finding in the South African setting and need to be sought actively in order to optimize management and promote best possible educational outcomes for this vulnerable group of children.

Recently circulated national guidelines for the initiation of ART in South Africa now recommends blanket treatment for the <60 month age group (with older children needing to meet clinical or immunological criteria). However, until this year, official national policy only recommended immediate treatment for infants under 12 months of age [39]. As a result there is still a large pool of children who would not have been included in the blanket ART initiation group and who remain untreated and vulnerable to the effects of the virus on the developing central nervous system. This study highlights that in order to improve the quality of life of these children earlier diagnosis of neurological risk at primary health care levels is needed.

Competing interests

The authors declare that they have no competing interests.

Authors' contributions

KD and KW conceived of the research and collected the data, KD was also involved in the analysis and was the primary author of the paper, JW assisted with study design and write up. BE provided support for analysis strategy and contributed to write up. HC contributed to analysis strategy and analysis. TK analyzed neuroimaging and contributed to write up. NL assisted with analysis and contributed to write up. All authors read and approved the final manuscript.

Acknowledgements

This study was conducted without external funding sources, but the authors would like to thank the clinic staff at the Division of Paediatric Neurology and all the children and families who are included in this study.

Author details

[1]Division of Developmental Pediatrics, Department of Pediatrics and Child Health, University of Cape Town and Red Cross War Memorial Children's Hospital, Cape Town, South Africa. [2]Division of Pediatric Neurology, Department of Pediatrics and Child Health, University of Cape Town and Red Cross War Memorial Children's Hospital, Cape Town, South Africa. [3]Department of Pediatric Radiology, Red Cross War Memorial Children's Hospital, Cape Town, South Africa. [4]Department of Public Health and Family Medicine, University of Cape Town, Cape Town, South Africa. [5]Department of Neurosurgery, University of Cape Town, Cape Town, South Africa. [6]Division of Pediatric Infectious Diseases, Department of Pediatrics and Child Health, University of Cape Town and Red Cross War Memorial Children's Hospital, Cape Town, South Africa.

References

1. Tindyebwa D, Kayita J, Musoke P, Eley B, Nduati R, Tumwesigye N, et al. Handbook on Paediatric AIDS in Africa. 2nd ed. Kampala: African Network for the Care of Children Affected by AIDS (ANECCA); 2011.
2. UNAIDS. Together we will end AIDS. 2012. p. 1–140.
3. WHO, UNAIDS, UNICEF. Global HIV/AIDS Response-Progress Report 2011. 2011. p. 1–219.
4. Eley B. Addressing the paediatric HIV epidemic: a perspective from the Western Cape Region of South Africa. Trans R Soc Trop Med Hyg. 2006;100:19–23.
5. Western Cape Department of Health: Revision of the protocol for the prevention of mother-to-child transmission of HIV. 2007, Circular No: H127/2007
6. Van Rie A, Harrington PR, Dow A, Robertson K. Neurologic and neurodevelopmental manifestations of pediatric HIV/AIDS: a global perspective. Eur J Paediatr Neurol. 2007;11(1):1–9.
7. Lobato MN, Caldwell MB, Ng P, Oxtoby MJ. Encephalopathy in children with perinatally acquired human immunodeficiency virus infection. Pediatric spectrum of disease clinical consortium. J Pediatr. 1995;126(5 Pt 1):710–5.
8. Tahan TT, Bruck I, Burger M, Cruz CR. Neurological profile and neurodevelopment of 88 children infected with HIV and 84 seroreverter children followed from 1995 to 2002. Braz J Infect Dis. 2006;10(5):322–6.
9. Blanche S, Rouzioux C, Moscato ML, Veber F, Mayaux MJ, Jacomet C, et al. A prospective study of infants born to women seropositive for human immunodeficiency virus type 1. HIV infection in newborns french collaborative study group. N Engl J Med. 1989;320(25):1643–8.
10. Bruck I, Tahan TT, Cruz CR, Martins LT, Antoniuk SA, Rodrigues M, et al. Developmental milestones of vertically HIV infected and seroreverters children: follow up of 83 children. Arq Neuropsiquiatr. 2001;59(3-B):691–5.
11. Chase C, Ware J, Hittelman J, Blasini I, Llorente A, Anisfeld E, et al. Early cognitive and motor development among infants born to women infected with human immunodeficiency virus. Pediatrics. 2000;106(2):e25.
12. Englund JA, Baker CJ, Raskino C, McKinney RE, Lifschitz MH, Petrie B, et al. Clinical and laboratory characteristics of a large cohort of symptomatic, human immunodeficiency virus-infected infants and children. AIDS Clinical trials group protocol 152 study team. Pediatr Infect Dis J. 1996;15(11):1025–36.
13. Epstein LG, Sharer LR, Oleske JM, Connor EM, Goudsmit J, Bagdon L, et al. Neurologic manifestations of human immunodeficiency virus infection in children. Pediatrics. 1986;78(4):678–87.
14. Foster CJ, Biggs RL, Melvin D, Walters MD, Tudor-Williams G, Lyall EG. Neurodevelopmental outcomes in children with HIV infection under 3 years of age. Dev Med Child Neurol. 2006;48(8):677–82.
15. CDC: 1994 revised classification system for HIV infection in children less than 13 years of age. CDC 1994, 443(RR12):1–10.
16. Thomas SA. Anti-HIV drug distribution to the central nervous system. Curr Pharm Des. 2004;10(12):1313–24.
17. Van Rie A, Mupuala A, Dow A. Impact of the HIV/AIDS epidemic on the neurodevelopment of preschool-aged children in Kinshasa. Democratic Republic of the Congo. Pediatrics. 2008;122(1):e123–8.
18. Laughton B, Cornell M, Grove D, Kidd M, Springer P, Dobbels E, et al. Early antiretroviral therapy improves neurodevelopmental outcomes in infants. AIDS. 2012;26(13):1685.
19. Abubakar A, Van Baar A, Van de Vijver FJ, Holding P, Newton CR. Paediatric HIV and neurodevelopment in sub-Saharan Africa: a systematic review. Trop Med Int Health. 2008;13(7):880–7.
20. Laughton B, Cornell M, Boivin M, Van Rie A: Neurodevelopment in perinatally HIV-infected children: a concern for adolescence. J Int AIDS Soc. 2013 Jun 18;16:18603. doi: 10.7448/IAS.16.1.18603. Review. PMID: 23782482.
21. Ackermann C, Andronikou SF, Laughton BF, Kidd MF, Dobbels EF, Innes S FAU, et al. White Matter Signal Abnormalities in Children with suspected HIV-Related Neurologic Disease on Early Combination Antiretroviral Therapy. Pediatr Infect Dis J JID - 8701858 EDAT- 2014/03/07 06:00 MHDA- 2014/03/07 06:00 CRDT- 2014/03/06 06:00 AID - 10.1097/INF.0000000000000288 doi] PST - aheadofprint 0305.
22. Hoare J, Ransford GL, Phillips N, Amos T, Donald K, Stein DJ. Metab Brain Dis. 2014 Jun;29(2):221-9. doi: 10.1007/s11011-013-9456-5. Epub 2013 Dec 12. PMID: 24338026
23. Hoare J, Fouche JP, Spottiswoode B, Donald K, Philipps N, Bezuidenhout H, et al. A diffusion tensor imaging and neurocognitive study of HIV-positive children who are HAART-naïve "slow progressors". J Neurovirol. 2012;18:205–12.
24. Prado PC, Escorsi-Rosset S, Cervi M, Santos A. Image evaluation of HIV encephalopathy: a multimodal approach using quantitative MR techniques. Neuroradiology. 2011;53(11):899–908.

25. Gray L, Sterjovski J, Churchill M, Ellery P, Nasr N, Lewin SR, et al. Uncoupling coreceptor usage of human immunodeficiency virus type 1 (HIV-1) from macrophage tropism reveals biological properties of CCR5-restricted HIV-1 isolates from patients with acquired immunodeficiency syndrome. Virology. 2005;337(2):384–98.
26. Wilmshurst JM, Cross JH, Newton C, Kakooza AM, Wammanda RD, Mallewa M, et al. Children with epilepsy in Africa: recommendations from the international child neurology association/African child neurology association workshop. J Child Neurol. 2013;28(5):633–44.
27. Msellati P, Lepage P, Hitimana D, Van Goethem C, Van de Perre P, Dabis F. Neurodevelopmental testing of children born to human immunodeficiency virus type 1 seropositive and seronegative mothers: a prospective cohort study in Kigali, Rwanda. Pediatrics. 1993;92(6):843–8.
28. Le Doaré K, Bland R, Newell M. Neurodevelopment in children born to HIV-infected mothers by infection and treatment status. Pediatrics. 2012;130(5):e1326–44.
29. Joska JA, Hoare J, Stein DJ, Flisher AJ. The neurobiology of HIV dementia: implications for practice in South Africa. AfrJPsychiatry (South Africa). 2011;14(1):17–22.
30. Gadow KD, Angelidou K, Chernoff M, Williams PL, Heston J, Hodge J, et al. Longitudinal study of emerging mental health concerns in youth perinatally infected with HIV and peer comparisons. J Dev Behav Pediatr. 2012;33(6):456–68.
31. Darke J, Bushby K, Le Couteur A. Survey of behaviour problems in children with neuromuscular diseases. Eur J Paed Neurol. 2006;10:129–34.
32. Kieck JR, Andronikou S. Usefulness of neuro-imaging for the diagnosis of HIV encephalopathy in children. S Afr Med J. 2004;94(8):628–30.
33. King SM, Edwards V, Blaser S, Smith ML, Rieder M, Read SE. Evaluation of the role of routine serial cranial computed tomography in the management of children with human immunodeficiency virus infection. Pediatr AIDS HIV Infect. 1997;8(1):15–22.
34. Safriel YI, Haller JO, Lefton DR, Obedian R. Imaging of the brain in the HIV-positive child. Pediatr Radiol. 2000;30(11):725–32.
35. Tucker KA, Robertson KR, Lin W, Smith JK, An H, Chen Y, et al. Neuroimaging in human immunodeficiency virus infection. J Neuroimmunol. 2004;157(1–2):153–62.
36. Blanche S, Newell ML, Mayaux MJ, Dunn DT, Teglas JP, Rouzioux C, et al. Morbidity and mortality in European children vertically infected by HIV-1. The French pediatric HIV infection study group and European collaborative study. J Acquir Immune Defic Syndr Hum Retrovirol. 1997;14(5):442–50.
37. Brodt HR, Kamps BS, Gute P, Knupp B, Staszewski S, Helm EB. Changing incidence of AIDS-defining illnesses in the era of antiretroviral combination therapy. AIDS. 1997;11(14):1731–8.
38. Patel K, Ming X, Williams PL, Robertson K, Oleske J, Saege GR: Impact of HAART and CNS-penetrating antiretroviral regimens on HIV-encephalopathy among perinatally infected children and adolescents. AIDS. 2009 Sep 10;23 (14):1893-901. doi: 10.1097/QAD.0b013e32832dc041.
39. National Department of Health, South Africa: Guidelines for the Management of HIV in Children 2nd Edition 2010. 2010.

20

Increased mortality after a first myocardial infarction in human immunodeficiency virus-infected patients

David Carballo[1*], Cécile Delhumeau[2], Sebastian Carballo[3], Caroline Bähler[4], Dragona Radovanovic[4], Bernard Hirschel[2], Olivier Clerc[5], Enos Bernasconi[6], Dominique Fasel[7], Patrick Schmid[8], Alexia Cusini[9], Jan Fehr[10], Paul Erne[11], Pierre-Fréderic Keller[1,12], Bruno Ledergerber[10], and Alexandra Calmy[2] for the Swiss HIV Cohort Study and AMIS registry

Abstract

Aims: HIV infection may be associated with an increased recurrence rate of myocardial infarction. Our aim was to determine whether HIV infection is a risk factor for worse outcomes in patients with coronaray artery disease.

Methods: We compared data aggregated from two ongoing cohorts: (i) the Acute Myocardial Infarction in Switzerland (AMIS) registry, which includes patients with acute myocardial infarction (AMI), and (ii) the Swiss HIV Cohort Study (SHCS), a prospective registry of HIV-positive (HIV+) patients. We included all patients who survived an incident AMI occurring on or after 1st January 2005. Our primary outcome measure was all-cause mortality at one year; secondary outcomes included AMI recurrence and cardiovascular-related hospitalisations. Comparisons used Cox and logistic regression analyses, respectively.

Results: There were 133 HIV+, (SHCS) and 5,328 HIV-negative [HIV-] (AMIS) individuals with incident AMI. In the SHCS and AMIS registries, patients were predominantly male (72% and 85% male, respectively), with a median age of 51 years (interquartile range [IQR] 46–57) and 64 years (IQR 55–74), respectively. Nearly all (90%) of HIV+ individuals were on successful antiretroviral therapy. During the first year of follow-up, 5 (3.6%) HIV+ and 135 (2.5%) HIV- individuals died. At one year, HIV+ status after adjustment for age, sex, calendar year of AMI, smoking status, hypertension and diabetes was associated with a higher risk of death (HR 4.42, 95% CI 1.73-11.27). There were no significant differences in recurrent AMIs (4 [3.0%] HIV+ and 146 [3.0%] HIV- individuals, OR 1.16, 95% CI 0.41-3.27) or in hospitalization rates (OR 0.68 [95% CI 0.42-1.11]).

Conclusions: HIV infection was associated with a significantly increased risk of all-cause mortality one year after incident AMI.

Keywords: Coronary artery disease, Myocardial infarction, HIV infection, Fatal outcome

Introduction

Coronary artery disease (CAD) has a higher prevalence and earlier onset in HIV-positive (HIV+) individuals [1]. In the era of combined antiretrovial therapy, serious non-AIDS complications (e.g., malignancies, liver disease, renal failure and major cardiovascular events) have been associated with a mortality risk twice that of AIDS-related events [2,3]. Specifically, data over a median follow-up period of 5.9 years from the HIV+ US Veteran Aging Cohort demonstrated a higher rate of incident acute myocardial infarction (AMI) among HIV+ compared to HIV- veterans (hazard ratio [HR] 1.48, 95% CI 1.27-1.72) [4]. Among patients followed by the Swiss HIV Cohort Study (SCHS), 6% of deaths were related to coronary artery disease (CAD) [5]. CAD progression has been linked to both internal and external causes of inflammation and endothelial stress [6,7]. Other studies have reported that HIV infection has worse outcomes in patients with CAD. In addition to the increased prevalence and earlier onset of incident AMI observed in HIV+ patients, this infection may also be associated

* Correspondence: david.carballo@hcuge.ch
[1]Department of Cardiology, University Hospital, Geneva, Switzerland
Full list of author information is available at the end of the article

with worse outcomes in those known to have CAD, such as recurrence of myocardial infarction or the need for coronary revascularization procedures [8-12].

These observations remain controversial, however, as they derive from small studies with heterogeneous inclusion criteria and substantial variation in the enrolled patients' CAD therapy. Indeed, a recent prospective study revealed no differences in clinical outcome in incident AMI after one year of follow up between HIV+ and HIV- patients [13]. To further address this issue we used data pooled from two major nationwide cohorts in a nested cohort study to compare rates of all-cause mortality, recurrent AMI and cardiovascular-related hospitalization after one year of follow-up between populations of HIV+ and HIV- individuals hospitalised in Switzerland for an initial AMI.

Methods

In a nested cohort study we compared clinical outcomes among adults in the Acute Myocardial Infarction in Switzerland (AMIS) registry and the Swiss HIV Cohort Study (SHCS).

The Swiss HIV Cohort Study (SHCS)

The SHCS (www.SHCS.ch) has been enrolling HIV+ individuals aged 16 years or older in Switzerland since 1988; as of December 2011, a total of 17,349 persons were included [14]. All local ethics committees have approved the study; written informed consent is obtained from all participants. Participants receive care at outpatient clinics or physicians' offices, where the following data are collected every six months: vital signs, a structured questionnaire with information on sociodemographic characteristics, illicit drug use, smoking status, co-morbidities and concomitant medications. In addition, a defined set of laboratory tests is performed including complete blood count, liver function tests, a lipid panel, hepatitis virus markers, CD4 cell counts and HIV viral load. Any laboratory results from intervening visits are also collected.

We included all SHCS participants who [1] were aged 18 years or older and [2] had HIV infection confirmed by enzyme-linked immunoabsorbent assay (ELISA) and Western blot who [3] experienced an incident AMI after registration in the SHCS between January 2005 and December 2011. Patients with a history of prior AMI were formally excluded. Diagnosis of myocardial infarction required either electrocardiographic evidence of ST-elevation (ST-elevation myocardial infarction (STEMI)) or non-ST-elevation myocardial infarction (NSTEMI) per ESC/ACC/AHA guidelines and in accordance with the Universal Definition of Myocardial Infarction [15-17]. Information on follow-up events (death, readmission) occurring within the first year after incident AMI was collected in a specific case report form sent to each affiliated SHCS centre.

The Acute Myocardial Infarction in Switzerland (AMIS) registry

AMIS is a nationwide prospective registry with a 12-month follow-up of patients with AMI admitted to 81 hospitals (ranging from community institutions to large tertiary-care facilities) in Switzerland (www.amis-plus.ch) [18-20]. Data are collected via a standardized electronic or paper-based questionnaire and stored centrally at the Institute of Social and Preventive Medicine of the University of Zurich, then validated for plausibility and consistency. Use of the registry was approved by the Over-Regional Ethics Committee for clinical studies, the Swiss Board for Data Security and all cantonal ethics commissions [21].

From this parent cohort, we selected all HIV- men and women aged 18 years old and above who experienced an incident AMI after registration in AMIS between January 2005 and December 2011 [15-17]. Patients with a history of prior AMI were formally excluded. Diagnostic criteria used for AMI in this group were identical to those used in SCHS patients. The selected cut-off inclusion date was January 2005 coinciding with the generalised introduction of drug-eluting coronary artery stents into clinical practice [22,23]. AMI diagnoses were all validated after review of primary source data.

Statistical analysis

Study endpoints

The primary endpoint was all-cause mortality; the secondary endpoint included a second AMI event or hospital readmission, all within one year of follow-up after the incident AMI. The diagnostic criteria used to define all cause mortality, AMI recurrence and hospital readmission was identical in both cohorts. Cardiovascular-related hospitalization was defined as a hospitalization event for reinfarction (STEMI/NSTEMI), unstable angina, need for coronary revascularization or stroke/TIA.

Descriptive analysis Baseline demographic, clinical, laboratory and cardiac risk factor data were summarized according to HIV status using medians (interquartile range [IQR]) and the Wilcoxon rank-sum test for quantitative variables; percentages and chi-squared test for qualitative variables.

The use of platelet inhibitor recipients, antihypertensive drugs and lipid lowering drugs were extracted according to the following criteria: a) for patients registered in the SHCS: beginning these medications before the first AMI episode and until 6 month after the event; b) for patients registered in the AMIS registry: taking these as regular medication when the first AMI episode occurred or at hospital discharge.

Modelling "Time to event" was defined as the time between the hospitalization date for the incident AMI and the date of death, cohort dropout or one year follow-up. Observation time was stopped at the time of the telephone interview when this was shorter that one year. The Kaplan-Meier method was used to calculate survival rate. Survival comparisons between groups were made using the log-rank test with an alpha threshold of 5 %. We developed three scenarios for deceased AMIS patients for whom information on exact date of death was lacking and for whom only the hospital discharge date and one-year follow-up call date were available: a) all deaths were assumed to have occured midway between the date of hospital discharge and the date of the one-year follow-up phone call ("average scenario"; noted $HR_{average}$ in result section); b) all deaths were assumed to have occured on the date of hospital discharge ("worst scenario"; noted HR_{worst}); and c) all deaths were assumed to have occured on the date of the one-year follow-up phone call ("best scenario"; noted HR_{best}).

Hazard ratios were estimated to assess the association of HIV status with the occurrence of death using Cox proportional hazard models. For recurrent AMI and hospital readmission, logistic regression analysis with estimation of odds ratios (OR) on cumulative event information at one year was performed as specific dates were not reported in the AMIS registry. To identify potential confounding risk factors, analyses were first adjusted for gender, age and calendar year of AMI (M1). In addition, we performed 3 additional models adjusted for gender, age and calendar year of AMI to assess the specific contribution of smoking status (M2), hypertension (M3), and diabetes (M4), or the combination of smoking status, hypertension and diabetes (M5) on each of the 3 endpoints of interest. Due to an important number of missing values for the variables cholesterol (20%) and BMI (10%) and the small number of events, it was not feasible to employ more complex models, e.g., further adjustment for cardiovascular treatment, cholesterol, BMI or HIV-related variables. Statistical analyses were performed using Stata Release 12.0 (StataCorp, College Station, Texas, USA).

Results

Baseline characteristics

A total of 133 HIV+ and 5,328 HIV- individuals with incident AMI were enrolled (Figure 1). Compared with HIV – individuals, those who were HIV + were more often male (85.0% versus 72.2%, respectively ($p = 0.001$) and younger (median age 51 [IQR 46–57] years versus 64 years [IQR 55–74] ($p < 0.0001$) (Table 1).

Currently in the SHCS, over 80% of patients are receiving at least three antiretroviral drugs and 56% are treated with either cardiovascular or anti-diabetic drugs [24]. One hundred and forty HIV+ individuals were identified; 105 were already included in the D:A:D cohort

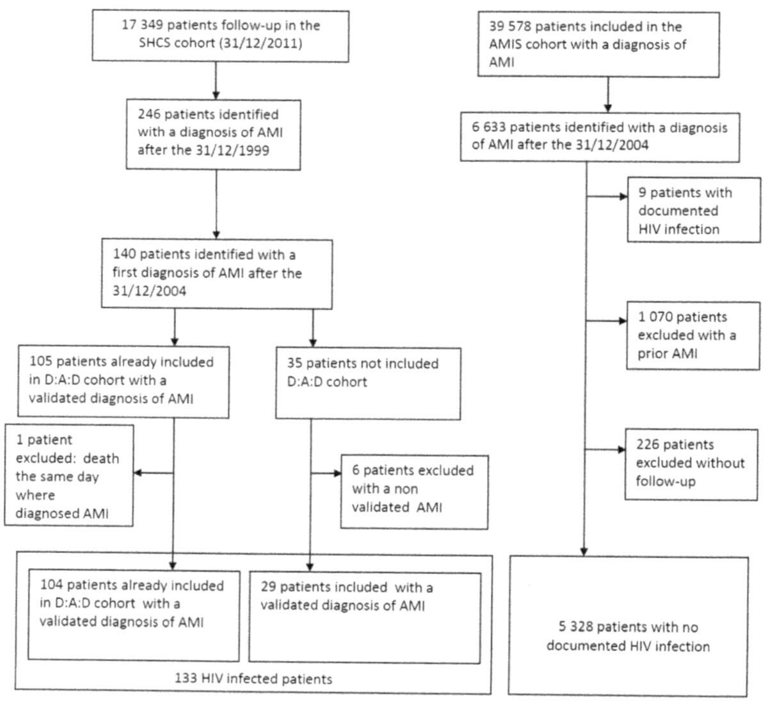

Figure 1 Study flow chart.

Table 1 Baseline characteristics of 133 HIV-positive subjects from the SHCS and 5328 HIV-negative subjects from the AMIS registry at the time of their first myocardial infarction

	SHCS		AMIS registry		
	HIV-positive subjects		HIV-negative subjects		
	Total		Total		P_values[a]
Age, year	133	51 (46–57)	5328	64 (55–74)	**<0.0001**
Men	133	113 (85.0)	5328	3845 (72.2)	**0.001**
Weight (kg)	121	71 (63–71)	5167	78 (69–88)	**<0.0001**
Height (cm)	133	174 (169–178)	4803	171 (165–176)	**0.0003**
Body Mass Index (kg/m^2)	121	23. (21.6–26.1)	4801	26.5 (24.2–29.4)	**<0.0001**
Blood pressure					
Systolic (mmHg)	119	132 (120–149)	5273	140 (120–160)	**0.0034**
Diastolic (mmHg)	119	75 (83–90)	5270	81 (71–94)	0.9015
Other cardiovascular risk factors					
Smoking history	132		5094		**<0.0001**
- Active smokers		77 (58.3)		2009 (39.4)	
- Former smokers		23 (17.5)		1311 (25.7)	
- Non smokers		32 (24.2)		1774 (34.8)	
Family history of CAD[b]	133	18 (13.5)	4717	1571 (33.3)	**<0.0001**
Hypertension	133	32 (24.1)	5323	3231 (60.7)	**<0.0001**
Diabetes mellitus	133	18 (13.5)	4734	739 (15 6)	0.569
Biological parameters					
Glycemia (mmol/l)	116	5.3 (4.7–6.0)	4920	7.1 (6.1–8.8)	**<0.0001**
Total cholesterol (mmol/l)	120	5.4 (4.5–6.3)	4078	5.4 (4.6–6.2)	0.952
HDL cholesterol (mmol/l)	120	1.1 (0.9–1.3)	3720	1.2 (1.0–1.5)	**0.005**
Serum creatinine (umol/l)	121	80 (69–93)	5158	81 (69–94)	0.779
Discharge AMI diagnosis	110		5328		**0.025**
STEMI		53 (48.2)		3135 (58.8)	
NSTEMI		57 (51.8)		2193 (41.2)	
Current cardiovascular treatments					
Platelets inhibitor recipients	133	120 (90.2)	5326	5169 (97.0)	**<0.0001**
Antihypertensive drugs	133	107 (80.5)	5327	4735 (88.9)	**0.002**
Lipid lowering drugs	133	115 (86.5)	5325	5028 (94.4)	**<0.0001**

Data are no. (%) of subjects or median (interquartile range).
[a]Wilcoxon rank-sum test for quantitative variables and chi square test for qualitative variable [b]CAD: coronary artery disease.

(Data Collection on Adverse Events of Anti-HIV Drugs, www.chip.dk/DAD) [25] and had received a diagnosis of AMI according to the criteria described above; one of them was excluded because he died on the day of his first AMI. Thirty five patients were not included in the D:A:D cohort; 29 of these had their diagnosis confirmed by an experienced cardiologist based on available medical records. A total of 133 patients from the SHCS parent cohort were thus eligible for inclusion (Figure 1).

Between January 1, 2005, and December 31, 2011, a total of 6,633 patients with a diagnosis of AMI (STEMI, NSTEMI) were enrolled in the AMIS cohort. Of these, 5,328 were eligible for study inclusion, whilst 1,305 patients were excluded: by cross-checking each participant in both cohorts regarding demographic similarities such as age, sex, and geographic location we were able to identify 9 patients in the AMIS registry who corresponded to patients in the SHCS cohort and who were therefore HIV+. These patients were excluded to have two distinct patient cohorts, one including exclusively HIV+ and one only HIV- individuals. Furthermore 1,070 did not have a first episode of AMI, and 226 did not have complete follow-up (Figure 1).

Cardiovascular risk factors varied by HIV status. Compared with HIV - individuals, HIV + had a lower median

BMI (23.8 kg/m^2 [IQR 21.6-26.1] versus 26.5 kg/m^2 [IQR 24.2-29.4] ($p < 0.0001$), lower systolic (but not diastolic) blood pressure (132 mmHg [IQR 120–149] versus 140 mmHg [IQR 120–160)] ($p = 0.0034$), higher likelihood of being active smokers (58.3% versus 39.4%, $p < 0.0001$), lower likelihood of being former smokers (17.5% versus 25.7%, $p < 0.0001$) and be more likely to be hypertensive or have a family history of CAD (24.1% versus 60.7%, $p < 0.0001$ and 13.5% versus 33.3%, $p < 0.0001$, respectively). Prevalence of diabetes mellitus was similar in the two groups. Among the HIV- AMIS population, 58.8% (3,135/5,328) received a discharge diagnosis of STEMI and the remaining 41.2% a diagnosis of NSTEMI, while among HIV+ individuals, 48.2% (53/110) were diagnosed with STEMI and the remaining 51.8% with NSTEMI. Serum glucose and high density lipoprotein (HDL) cholesterol were lower in HIV+ persons (5.3 mmol/l [IQR 4.7-6.0] versus 7.1 mmol/l [IQR 6.1-8.8], $p < 0.0001$) and 1.1 mmol/l [IQR 0.9-1.3] versus 1.2 mmol/l [IQR 1.0-1.5], $p = 0.005$, respectively). There were no significant differences between groups for total cholesterol and serum creatinine values. HIV - individuals were more likely to be treated with anti-platelet, antihypertensive or lipid lowering drugs after a first AMI than were HIV + patients ($p < 0.0001$ for anti-platelets and lipid-lowering drugs and $p = 0.002$ for anti-hypertensive drug).

Among the HIV+ group 49 patients (46%) were men who have sex with men (MSM) and 20 (15%) were intravenous drug users (IVDU). The median time from HIV diagnosis was 12 years (IQR 8–18) and a similarly long history of antiretroviral treatment (median 11.5 years); 120 (90%) were on antiretroviral therapy (ART) at study entry, with lengthy exposure to both nucleoside reverse transcriptase inhibitors (NRTIs; median10.9 years) and protease inhibitors (PIs; median 5.6 years). Ninety-five (77%) had viral loads below the detection level of 40 copies/ml; median CD4 count was 462 cells/mm^3 (IQR 347–701; see Table 2).

Table 2 HIV parameters at first AMI episode

	SHCS	
	HIV-positive subjects	
	N	Total
Transmission risk category	133	
Heterosexual intercourse		42 (32)
Injection drug use		20 (15)
Men-who-have-sex-with-men		61 (46)
Other/unknown		10 (7)
Time since HIV diagnosis (years)	124	12 (8–18)
Patients with viral load <40 copies per mL	123	95 (77)
CD4 cell count per mm3	129	462 (347–701)
Antiretroviral treatment at the first episode of AMI		
Antiretroviral naïve	133	1 (1)
Not naïve, but not currently on antiretroviral drugs	133	12 (7)
On antiretroviral drugs	133	120 (90)
Antiretroviral regimen containing abacavir	120	51 (43)
Exposure to antiretroviral treatments (previous and current)		
Patients on PI (previous or current)	132	113 (85.6)
Median duration of PI therapy (years)	113	5.6 (3.5–9.4)
Patients under NNRTI (previous or current)	132	88 (86)
Median duration of NNRTI therapy (years)	88	3.5 (0.6–5.9)
Patients on NRTI (previous or current)	132	126 (95)
Median duration of NRTI therapy (years)	126	(6.7–15.1)

Data are no. (%) of subjects or median (interquartile range). PI, protease inhibitors; NNRTI, non-nucleoside reverse-transcriptase inhibitors; NRTI, nucleoside reverse-transcriptase inhibitors.

One-year survival

Median follow-up duration for HIV- subjects was 392 days (IQR 375–414); for 4,953 (93%) of the patients we obtained follow-up by telephone call at 12 ± 3 months; for 92 (2%) it was before 9 months and for 283 (5%) it was beyond 15 months. In the HIV+ group, 128 (96%) patients had a follow-up of at least 12 months, while 5 were lost to follow-up. The exact date of death was known for all but 51 of the deceased HIV- individuals; data regarding repeat AMI and hospital readmission was missing for 394/5,328 (7.4%) and 349/5,328 (6.6%) patients, respectively.

Deaths occurred during the first year of follow-up in five (3.6%) of the HIV+ and 135 (2.5%) of the HIV- individuals; the cause of death was cardiac-related in three of the five HIV+ individuals, and in 44 of 61 HIV- individuals (Table 3). Kaplan Meier estimations of death probability at one year according to HIV status were not significantly different (3.8% vs 2.6%, $p = 0.374$, data not shown). However, at one year, HIV status adjusted for age, sex, calendar year of AMI, smoking status, hypertension and diabetes predicted patients' survival (Table 3): HIV+ individuals with a first episode of AMI had a higher risk of death than their HIV- counterparts (HR 4.42, 95% CI 1.73-11.27). For the 51 deceased HIV- individuals with missing information on the exact date of the event, we conducted a sensitivity analysis to assess whether assigning the unknown date of death to the day of the one-year follow-up phone call or to the day of hospital discharge or would change the estimated risk and found the results were similar (HR_{best} 5.14, 95% CI 1.99-13.27 versus HR_{worse} 4.43, 95% CI 1.74-11.30, respectively).

HIV status remained a significant determinant of the occurrence of death at one year in distinct models integrating smoking status (M3), hypertension (M4), or

Table 3 Death, AMI recurrence, and re-hospitalization for cardiovascular reasons at 1-year follow-up

	SHCS		AMIS registry		M0	M1	M2	M3	M4	M5
	HIV-positive subjects		HIV-negative subjects							
	N Total	N (%)	N Total	N (%)	Crude HR or OR (95% CI)	Age, gender, calendar year Adjusted HR or OR (95% CI)	Age, gender, calendar year, smoking status Adjusted HR or OR (95% CI)	Age, gender, calendar year, hypertension Adjusted HR or OR (95% CI)	Age, gender, calendar year, diabetes Adjusted HR or OR (95% CI)	Age, gender, calendar year, smoking status, hypertension, diabetes Adjusted HR or OR (95% CI)
Deaths:										
- Cardiovascular death		3 (60.0)		44 (32.6)						
- Non-cardiovascular death		2 (40.0)		17 (12.6)						
- Unknown		0 (0)		74 (54.8)						
Total death	133	5 (3.6)	5328	135 (2.5)	1.50 (0.61; 3.65)	4.56 (1.80; 11.57)*	4.53 (1.78; 11.51)*	4.86 (1.91; 12.34)*	4.27 (1.69; 10.82)*	4.42 (1.73; 11.27)*
Recurrent AMI	133	4 (3.0)	4934	146 (3.0)	1.02 (0.37; 2.79)	1.20 (0.43; 3.34)	1.22 (0.44; 3.41)	1.23 (0.44; 3.44)	1.15 (0.41; 3.21)	1.16 (0.41; 3.27)
Re-hospitalization for cardiovascular reasons during the first year following the AMI	133	20 (15.0)	4979	1078 (21.6)	0.64 (0.40; 1.04)	0.66 (0.41; 1.08)	0.67 (0.41; 1.08)	0.69 (0.43; 1.13)	0.65 (0.40; 1.06)	0.68 (0.42; 1.11)
Total	133	20 (15.0)	5328	1199 (22.5)						

M1: Cox proportional hazard regression or logistic regression adjusted for gender, age and calendar year of AMI; **M2:** Cox proportional hazard regression or logistic regression adjusted for gender, age, calendar year of AMI. and smoking status; **M3:** Cox proportional hazard regression or logistic regression adjusted for gender, age, calendar year of AMI and hypertension; **M4:** Cox proportional hazard regression or logistic regression adjusted for gender, age, calendar year of AMI and diabetes; **M5:** Cox proportional hazard regression or logistic regression adjusted for gender, age, calendar year of AMI, smoking status, hypertension and diabetes;
*$p < 0.05$.
HR, hazard ratio; OR, odds ratio.

diabetes (M5) with HRs in similar range in the 3 models (HR 4.53, 95% CI 4.58-11.51, HR 4.86, 95% CI 1.91-12.34, and HR 4.27, 95% CI 1.69-10.82 respectively).

One-year clinical outcome

Recurrent AMI was noted in four (3.0%) HIV+ and 146 (3.0%) HIV- individuals. When adjusted for age, sex, calendar year of AMI, smoking status, hypertension and diabetes, there was no statistically significant difference between groups (M5, Table 3: OR 1.16; 95% CI 0.41-3.27). Hospitalization for cardiovascular-related events occurred in 20 (15%) HIV+ and 1,078 (21.6%) HIV- individuals. However, when adjusted for age, sex, calendar year of AMI, smoking status, hypertension and diabetes, this difference was not statistically significant (M5, Table 3, OR 0.68; 95% CI 0.42; 1.11).

Discussion

In this retrospective nested cohort study we observed that deaths from all causes at one year after incident AMI were nearly 5 times more frequent among HIV+ than HIV- individuals. There was however no statistically significant difference in the risk of recurrent AMI or hospital readmissions in this group. HIV remains a significant risk factor predicting survival after a first incident AMI in this population, after adjustment for several classical risks factors.

Several other studies have examined cardiovascular outcomes in HIV-infected persons. Matezky et al. found that 24 HIV+ individuals who were age- and sex-matched with HIV- controls had a higher rate of reinfarction, recurrent cardiovascular events and revascularization independently of the type of their ART [9]. Another case–control study by Hsue et al. reported a higher rate of coronary restenosis after percutaneous coronary intervention in HIV+ compared to HIV- persons [10]. Boccara et al. reported long-term follow-up (median 41 months) from a case–control study comparing 27 HIV+ persons to 54 HIV- patients undergoing coronary artery bypass. Short-term outcomes (post-operative death, AMI, stroke, mediastinitis and reintervention) at 30 days were similar; however, the rate of occurrence of a first major cardiac event (MACE) was higher in the HIV+ group. This difference was largely attributable to the need for repeat PCI revascularisation of the native coronary arteries [11]. The same group confirmed these results in a more recent publication assessing one-year prognosis of 103 HIV+ and 195 HIV- patients after the occurrence of an acute coronary syndrome (ACS): despite similar angiographic features of coronary artery disease in both groups, recurrent ACS was 6 times more frequent in the HIV+ group [13]. Lorgis et al. Reported that after acute myocardial infarction, HIV status influences long-term risk, although th eshort-term risk is comparable to uninfected patients [26]. A recent meta-analysis of 11 studies including a total of 2,442 patients concluded that HIV+ patients admitted for ACS face a substantial short-term risk of death and a significant long-term risk of coronary revasculization and myocardial infarction, especially if receiving protease inhibitors [27].

Combining these results with our own findings suggests a higher risk of adverse outcomes after a first acute coronary event in HIV+ patients. During a certain era, this may have been in part due to lower revascularization procedure rates for HIV+ patients receiving AMI care, although there is has been an observed trend towards better access [12]. Indeed, an analysis by D:A:D investigators demonstrated an increased use of invasive cardiologic procedures post-AMI when comparing time periods between 1999 and 2002 and between 2009 and 2011. Thus the decreased mortality rate between these two periods (26.4% down to 8.2 %) may be in part due to the use of more efficient medical interventions, rather than in changes in patient characteristics [4,28]. The same trends have been observed in the AMIS Plus population between 1997 and 2011 [29]. Parcea et al. reported a 50% higher relative risk in hospital mortality from an AMI event in HIV+ individuals and observed that common related procedures (including left cardiac catheterization, coronary arteriography, and angiography of the left heart) occurred at significantly lower rates among HIV+ subjects [10].

Of note, the overall mortality rate reported by D:A:D investigators is higher than we found in our study [28]: in D:A:D, the short-term (one-month) mortality was as high as 20%, and over 33 months of follow-up a repeat AMI occured in 10% of the patients. A secular trend time period bias may partly explained this difference, as we only included patients with enrollment after 2005.

Indeed, HIV+ patients have a high-risk cardiovascular profile, largely due to the high prevalence of smokers, there being 60% among the SCHS particpants. Although our analyses were partially adjusted for confounding, the baseline characteristics of participants in the two cohorts differed significantly with respect to weight, BMI and systolic blood pressure: all of which were elevated in the AMIS HIV- group. A recent study showed that HIV infection is associated with a 50% increased risk of AMI beyond that explained by recognized Framingham cardiovascular risk factors, even in patients with sustained viral load suppression [30]. Cruz et al. reported that HIV+ AMI patients were younger and more often lacking in traditional cardiovascular risk factors than their HIV- counterparts [31]. In our cohort, patients from the SHCS were significantly younger and had lower rates of hypertension and diabetes mellitus ($p < 0.0001$). Even patients with sustained viral load suppression are at increased risk of incident AMI, raising the question of whether they may benefit from additional HIV specific prevention strategies such as earlier ART treatment. In the meantime, clinicians should continue to emphasize risk-factor modification strategies that have been proven effective, such as smoking cessation.

Residual HIV replication may possibly explain the increased cardiovascular risk and poorer outcome in HIV+ individuals. Findings from a recent nested case–control study suggest that CD4 T-cell nadir and a high current CD8 T-cell count are associated with an increased risk of AMI in HIV+ individuals [5]. Measures of subclinical coronary atherosclerosis using CT angiography showed a greater prevalence and greater extent of non-calcified plaque and stable calcified plaques in HIV+ men compared to HIV- men [32]. Interestingly, immune activation sCD163, a monocyte activation marker, is associated with subclinical disease (identified as low attenuation plaques) after adjustment for traditional CVD risks factors [33]. This might open new paths for interventions to reduce the risk of AMI in HIV+ patients.

Given that the number of cardiovascular procedures increased overtime, the number of patients in the D:A:D analysis receiving lipid-lowering drugs (44%), antiplatelet therapy (52%) or angiotensin-converting enzyme inhibitors (27%) was low, notwithstanding that these are standard of care in post-AMI management [28]. Our study confirmed that the prescription of standard post MI treatments at the time of AMI was surprisingly low, although better that the numbers reported in the D:A:D cohort, when compared to patients with no documented HIV infection in Switzerland. Boccara et al. already hypothesized that cardiologists may manage HIV-infected patients less aggressively due to the unknown prognosis of HIV infection itself. They observed that HIV- individuals were more likely to have recurrent revascularization guided by silent ischemia, partly explained by the higher use of stress testing found in this population [12]. Optimal dosing of drugs other than those specific for post-AMI treatment is also problematic in the general population; Arnold et al. found that after an AMI, nearly 85% of patients were discharged on beta-blocker doses that were substantially below the established effective dose, while 66% were discharged on insufficient doses of statins and ACE inhibitors [34].

In addition, drug-drug interactions involving cytochromes P450 (the metabolic pathway of many antiretrovirals, mainly boosted protease inhibitors) with inhibitors of the ADP-P2Y12 platelet receptors may lead to deleterious adverse effects: P2Y12 inhibitors such as prasugrel are not adequately bio-activated and thus are not effective [35]. Adverse events related to agents such as clopidogrel have also been well documented [36]. In summary, hypothetical reasons for worse short-term outcomes in HIV+ patients include less frequently use required cathterization procedures [10], ongoing HIV replication and inflammation [5], drug-drug interactions [29], and asymptomatic coronary disease at younger ages [31] leading to a late diagnosis of CAD.

Our study has several limitations. We did not have an exact date of the events of interest for some AMIS patients, although our "three scenarios" sensitivity analyses covering the worst- through best-case survival scenarios were consistent. The coding of the variable for hospitalization and co-medications was different in the two databases, complicating precise comparisons between the SHCS and the AMIS registry. We observed a tendency for fewer hospitalizations in AMIS patients, but this may be due to a reporting bias and misclassification in the SCHS, which documents hospitalizations with a higher degree of precision. These limitations also made a composite endpoint analysis difficult. Furthermore, because of a limited number of confirmed cardiovascular related deaths and a limited number of patients with recurrent AMI, expanding the model to further adjust for cardiovascular treatments, BMI or HIV-related variables, was not feasible.

Conclusions

This study comparing clinical outcomes in individuals registered in two prospective national registries demonstrates an increased risk of death one year after initial AMI in HIV+ patients. These findings warrant further, long-term assessment, as HIV-infected individuals are increasing in prevalence and could benefit from better-informed cardiac risk stratification as well as targeted secondary prevention measures.

Competing interests

The authors declare that they have no competing interests.

Authors' contributions

AC and DC designed the study. CD and BL performed the statistical analyses. AC and DC wrote the first draft of the manuscript. All authors contributed to the interpretation of the results and to the final version of the manuscript. AC, DC and CD had full access to all of the data in the study and take responsibility for the integrity of the data and the accuracy of the data analysis. All authors read and approved the final manuscript.

Acknowledgements

We thank Angela Huttner, Rosemary Sudan and Benjamin Lipsky for their review of the manuscript.

We thank all patients, doctors and nurses associated with the Swiss HIV Cohort Study (SHCS). The SHCS is supported by the Swiss National Science Foundation (grant number 33CS30_134277). The members of the Swiss HIV Cohort Study are: Aubert V, Barth J, Battegay M, Bernasconi E, Böni J, Bucher HC, Burton-Jeangros C, Calmy A, Cavassini M, Egger M, Elzi L, Fehr J, Fellay J, Francioli P, Furrer H (Chairman of the Clinical and Laboratory Committee), Fux CA, Gorgievski M, Günthard H (President of the SHCS), Haerry D (deputy of "Positive Council"), Hasse B, Hirsch HH, Hirschel B, Hösli I, Kahlert C, Kaiser L, Keiser O, Kind C, Klimkait T, Kovari H, Ledergerber B, Martinetti G, Martinez de Tejada B, Metzner K, Müller N, Nadal D, Pantaleo G, Rauch A (Chairman of the Scientific Board), Regenass S, Rickenbach M (Head of Data Center), Rudin C (Chairman of the Mother & Child Substudy), Schmid P, Schultze D, Schöni-Affolter F, Schüpbach J, Speck R, Taffé P, Tarr P, Telenti A, Trkola A, Vernazza P, Weber R, Yerly S.

Author details

[1]Department of Cardiology, University Hospital, Geneva, Switzerland. [2]HIV Metabolic Clinic, University Hospital, Geneva, Switzerland. [3]General Internal Medicine, University Hospital, Geneva, Switzerland. [4]AMIS Plus Data Center, Institute of Social and Preventive Medicine, University of Zurich, Zurich, Switzerland. [5]Infectious Diseases, University Hospital Center, Lausanne, Switzerland. [6]Infectious Diseases, Regional Hospital, Lugano, Switzerland. [7]HIV Unit, Infectious diseases, University Hospital, Basel, Switzerland. [8]Infectious Diseases, University Hospital, Sankt Gallen, Switzerland. [9]Infectious Diseases, University Hospital, Bern, Switzerland. [10]Division of Infectious Diseases and Hospital Epidemiology, University Hospital, Zürich, University of Zurich, Zürich, Switzerland. [11]Cardiology Department, Peripherique Hospital, Lucern, Switzerland. [12]Centre médical Ziggurat, Rue du Jura 11, 2900 Porrentruy, Switzerland.

References

1. Lang S, Mary-Krause M, Cotte L, Gilquin J, Partisani M, Simon A, et al. Increased risk of myocardial infarction in HIV-infected patients in France, relative to the general population. AIDS. 2010;24(8):1228–30.
2. Berry SA, Fleishman JA, Moore RD, Gebo KA. Trends in reasons for hospitalization in a multisite United States cohort of persons living with HIV, 2001–2008. J Acquir Immune Defic Syndr. 2012;59(4):368–75.
3. Neuhaus J, Angus B, Kowalska JD, La Rosa A, Sampson J, Wentworth D, et al. Risk of all-cause mortality associated with nonfatal AIDS and serious non-AIDS events among adults infected with HIV. AIDS. 2010;24(5):697–706.
4. Petoumenos K E-SW, d'Armino Monforte A. Increased risk of cardiovascular disease with age in men: A comparison of D:A:D with HIV cardiovascular disease risk equations. In: 20th Conference on Retroviruses and Opportunistic Infections 2013; Atlanta.
5. Weber R, Ruppik M, Rickenbach M, Spoerri A, Furrer H, Battegay M, et al. Decreasing mortality and changing patterns of causes of death in the Swiss HIV Cohort Study. HIV Med. 2013;14(4):195–207.
6. Lang S, Mary-Krause M, Simon A, Partisani M, Gilquin J, Cotte L, et al. HIV replication and immune status are independent predictors of the risk of myocardial infarction in HIV-infected individuals. Clin Infect Dis. 2012;55(4):600–7.
7. Calmy A, Gayet-Ageron A, Montecucco F, Nguyen A, Mach F, Burger F, et al. HIV increases markers of cardiovascular risk: results from a randomized, treatment interruption trial. AIDS. 2009;23(8):929–39.
8. Boccara F. Cardiovascular complications and atherosclerotic manifestations in the HIV-infected population: type, incidence and associated risk factors. AIDS. 2008;22 Suppl 3:S19–26.
9. Matetzky S, Domingo M, Kar S, Noc M, Shah PK, Kaul S, et al. Acute myocardial infarction in human immunodeficiency virus-infected patients. Arch Intern Med. 2003;163(4):457–60.
10. Hsue PY, Giri K, Erickson S, MacGregor JS, Younes N, Shergill A, et al. Clinical features of acute coronary syndromes in patients with human immunodeficiency virus infection. Circulation. 2004;109(3):316–9.
11. Boccara F, Teiger E, Cohen A, Ederhy S, Janower S, Odi G, et al. Percutaneous coronary intervention in HIV infected patients: immediate results and long term prognosis. Heart. 2006;92(4):543–4.
12. Pearce D, Ani C, Espinosa-Silva Y, Clark R, Fatima K, Rahman M, et al. Comparison of in-hospital mortality from acute myocardial infarction in HIV sero-positive versus sero-negative individuals. Am J Cardiol. 2012;110(8):1078–84.
13. Boccara F, Mary-Krause M, Teiger E, Lang S, Lim P, Wahbi K, et al. Acute coronary syndrome in human immunodeficiency virus-infected patients: characteristics and 1 year prognosis. Eur Heart J. 2011;32(1):41–50.
14. Schoeni-Affolter F, Ledergerber B, Rickenbach M, Rudin C, Gunthard HF, Telenti A, et al. Cohort profile: the Swiss HIV Cohort study. Int J Epidemiol. 2010;39(5):1179–89.
15. Thygesen K, Alpert JS, White HD. Universal definition of myocardial infarction. Eur Heart J. 2007;28(20):2525–38.
16. Yusuf S, Dagenais G, Pogue J, Bosch J, Sleight P. Vitamin E supplementation and cardiovascular events in high-risk patients. The Heart Outcomes Prevention Evaluation Study Investigators. N Engl J Med. 2000;342(3):154–60.
17. Jialal I, Devaraj S. Vitamin E supplementation and cardiovascular events in high-risk patients. N Engl J Med. 2000;342(25):1917–8.
18. Radovanovic D, Erne P. AMIS Plus: Swiss registry of acute coronary syndrome. Heart. 2010;96(12):917–21.
19. Radovanovic D, Urban P, Simon R, Schmidli M, Maggiorini M, Rickli H, et al. Outcome of patients with acute coronary syndrome in hospitals of different sizes. A report from the AMIS Plus Registry. Swiss Med Wkly. 2010;140(21–22):314–22.
20. Jeger RV, Radovanovic D, Hunziker PR, Pfisterer ME, Stauffer JC, Erne P, et al. Ten-year trends in the incidence and treatment of cardiogenic shock. Ann Intern Med. 2008;149(9):618–26.
21. McNamara RL. Cardiovascular registry research comes of age. Heart. 2010;96(12):908–10.
22. Serruys PW, Kutryk MJ, Ong AT. Coronary-artery stents. N Engl J Med. 2006;354(5):483–95.
23. Serruys PW, Degertekin M, Tanabe K, Abizaid A, Sousa JE, Colombo A, et al. Intravascular ultrasound findings in the multicenter, randomized, double-blind RAVEL (RAndomized study with the sirolimus-eluting VElocity balloon-expandable stent in the treatment of patients with de novo native coronary artery Lesions) trial. Circulation. 2002;106(7):798–803.
24. Marzolini C, Back D, Weber R, Furrer H, Cavassini M, Calmy A, et al. Ageing with HIV: medication use and risk for potential drug-drug interactions. J Antimicrob Chemother. 2011;66(9):2107–11.
25. Friis-Moller N, Sabin CA, Weber R, d'Arminio Monforte A, El-Sadr WM, Reiss P, et al. Combination antiretroviral therapy and the risk of myocardial infarction. N Engl J Med. 2003;349(21):1993–2003.
26. Lorgis L, Cottenet J, Molins G, Benzenine E, Zeller M, Aube H, et al. Outcomes after acute myocardial infarction in HIV-infected patients: analysis of data from a French nationwide hospital medical information database. Circulation. 2013;127(17):1767–1774.
27. D'Ascenzo F, Cerrato E, Biondi-Zoccai G, Moretti C, Omede P, Sciuto F, et al. Acute coronary syndromes in human immunodeficiency virus patients: a meta-analysis investigating adverse event rates and the role of antiretroviral therapy. Eur Heart J. 2012;33(7):875–80.
28. Sabin C, Ryom L, Law M. Improvements in short-term mortality following myocardial infarction: the Data Collection on Adverse Events of Anti-HIV Drugs Study. Abstract 748, In: 20th Conference on Retroviruses and Opportunistic Infections 2013; Atlanta.
29. Radovanovic D, Nallamothu BK, Seifert B, Bertel O, Eberli F, Urban P, et al. Temporal trends in treatment of ST-elevation myocardial infarction among men and women in Switzerland between 1997 and 2011. Eur Heart J Acute Cardiovasc Care. 2013;1(3):183–91.
30. Freiberg MS, Chang CC, Kuller LH, Skanderson M, Lowy E, Kraemer KL, et al. HIV infection and the risk of acute myocardial infarction. JAMA Intern Med. 2013;173(8):614–22.
31. Cruz M. Emergency medical service utilization and reperfusion times among HIV+ individuals presenting with ST-elevation myocardial infarction. In: 20th Conference on Retroviruses and Opportunistic Infections 2013; Atlanta.
32. Post W, Jacobson L, Li X. Age and Noncalcified coronary plaque in the Multicenter AIDS Cohort Study. 20th Conference on Retroviruses and Opportunistic Infections. March 3-6, 2013. Atlanta. Abstract 62
33. Subramanian S, Tawakol A, Burdo TH, Abbara S, Wei J, Vijayakumar J, et al. Arterial inflammation in patients with HIV. JAMA. 2012;308(4):379–86.
34. Arnold SV, Spertus JA, Masoudi FA, Daugherty SL, Maddox TM, Li Y, et al. Beyond medication prescription as performance measures: optimal secondary prevention medication dosing after acute myocardial infarction. J Am Coll Cardiol. 2013;62(19):1791–801.
35. Daali Y, Ancrenaz V, Bosilkovska M, Dayer P, Desmeules J. Ritonavir inhibits the two main prasugrel bioactivation pathways in vitro: a potential drug-drug interaction in HIV patients. Metabolism. 2011;60(11):1584–9.
36. Combescure C, Fontana P, Mallouk N, Berdague P, Labruyere C, Barazer I, et al. Clinical implications of clopidogrel non-response in cardiovascular patients: a systematic review and meta-analysis. J Thromb Haemost. 2010;8(5):923–33.

Cytochrome P450 2B6 genetic variants are associated with plasma nevirapine levels and clinical response in HIV-1 infected Kenyan women

Margaret Ngwono Oluka[1*], Faith Apolot Okalebo[1], Anastasia Nkatha Guantai[1], R Scott McClelland[2] and Susan M Graham[2]

Abstract

Background: Polymorphisms in cytochrome P450 2B6 (CYP2B6) affect the steady state plasma concentration of nevirapine. CYP2B6 516G>T and 983T>C are common in African populations, but data on their influence on plasma nevirapine concentration and clinical response in African women are limited. We investigated the impact of CYP 516G>T and 983T>C on plasma nevirapine concentration and clinical outcomes in a prospective cohort study of HIV-infected Kenyan women.

Methods: Study subjects were 66 HIV-1-seropositive women taking nevirapine-based antiretroviral therapy. Plasma collected at week 12 was analyzed for nevirapine concentration by high performance liquid chromatography. Baseline samples were genotyped for CYP2B6 516G>T and 983T>C single nucleotide polymorphisms by real-time polymerase chain reaction. CD4 cell count, plasma viral load, and genotypic drug resistance in plasma and genital secretions were assessed at baseline and during follow up. We evaluated the effect of each genotype on plasma nevirapine concentration at week 12 and on change in CD4 cell count at months 3, 6 and 12. Associations between plasma nevirapine concentration and clinical outcomes were analyzed by logistic or linear regression.

Results: Women with CYP2B6 516TT genotype (n=9) had higher mean nevirapine plasma levels (14.33 μg/mL) compared to those with heterozygous 516GT (9.18 μg/mL; n=25) and wild- type 516GG (7.95 μg/mL; n=32) genotypes (P=0.01). Women heterozygous for the CYP2B6 983TC genotype (n=13) had higher mean nevirapine plasma levels (12.94 μg/mL), compared to women with the homozygous 983TT (8.35 μg/mL; n=53) genotype (P=0.007). In Generalized Estimating Equation analysis, plasma nevirapine levels predicted greater change in CD4 cell count after ART initiation (adjusted beta 119.4 cells/μL, 95% CI, 27.3–211.5 cells/μL, *P*=0.01). The CYP2B6 983TT genotype also predicted greater change in CD4 cell count (adjusted beta 68.6 cells/μL, 95% CI, 3.9–133.4 cells/μL, *P*=0.04). We found no associations between CYP2B6 genotypes and virologic response or toxicity.

Conclusions: CYP2B6 516G>T and CYP2B6 983T>C genotypes were strongly associated with plasma nevirapine concentration, which predicted immunologic response in women on nevirapine-based antiretroviral therapy. These data support continued work on the potential utility of human genetic testing to inform nevirapine dosage optimization for individual patients.

Keywords: CYP2B6, Pharmacogenetics, Nevirapine, HIV infection, Antiretroviral therapy, Women

* Correspondence: olukamarga@yahoo.com
[1]Department of Pharmacology and Pharmacognosy, University of Nairobi, P.O. BOX 19498, Nairobi 00202, Kenya
Full list of author information is available at the end of the article

Background

Sub-Saharan Africa remains severely affected by HIV, accounting for 69% of people living with HIV worldwide [1]. The HIV epidemic in Kenya disproportionately affects women, with prevalence (8.0%) nearly twice that of men (4.3%) [2]. This difference is reflected in the large number of women accessing HIV care and treatment with antiretroviral drugs [3]. Over 70% of patients on first-line antiretroviral therapy (ART) in Kenya take a nevirapine-based regimen [3,4]. This is due to its relatively low cost, manageable pill burden and excellent efficacy [5]. However, the use of nevirapine is limited by a potentially fatal immune-mediated hypersensitivity reaction that manifests as hepatotoxicity, fever, and/or skin rash,[6] and by a fragile genetic barrier to the development of drug resistance [7]. Furthermore, not all patients treated with nevirapine experience optimal response. The etiology of sub-optimal response is multi-factorial and may include differences in adherence, gender, concomitant medications and genes responsible for drug metabolism [8,9].

Nevirapine undergoes oxidative metabolism primarily by cytochrome P450 3A4 (CYP3A4) and 2B6 (CYP2B6), with a minor contribution by 3A5 (CYP3A5) [10,11]. CYP2B6 metabolic activity is subject to the influence of several genetic polymorphisms, as well as strong inhibitors and inducers, contributing to highly variable plasma drug exposure [12-14]. CYP2B6 genetic polymorphisms may be more important in African populations. For example, the single nucleotide polymorphism (SNP) CYP2B6 516G>T (rs3745274), which reduces hepatic CYP2B6 protein expression and activity [15], occurs more frequently in African populations than in Caucasian and Asian populations [16-18]. Moreover, CYP2B6 983T>C (rs28399499), which is a null allele [12], is absent in Caucasians but has a prevalence of 4%–11% in African populations [18,19].

Nevirapine exhibits large inter-individual variability in its pharmacokinetics [20], contributing to variable outcomes among HIV-infected patients. Sub-therapeutic plasma concentrations are associated with treatment failure and the emergence of antiretroviral drug resistance, whereas supra-therapeutic concentrations are associated with toxicity [21]. Several studies have evaluated associations between CYP2B6 516G>T and CYP2B6 983T>C SNPs and steady-state plasma nevirapine levels [22-24]. However, prospective studies evaluating the influence of CYP2B6 polymorphisms on clinical response among HIV-infected African women taking nevirapine-based ART are lacking.

In the present study, we investigated the impact of CYP2B6 516G>T and CYP2B6 983T>C genetic variants on plasma nevirapine levels and clinical outcomes including change in CD4 cell count, plasma viral load (PVL), and the incidence of antiretroviral resistance mutations and adverse reactions.

Results

Baseline characteristics and plasma nevirapine levels

Sixty-nine of the 73 women screened met the inclusion criteria and were tested for CYP2B6 genotypes. Four women who had not been prescribed a nevirapine-based regimen for at least 12 weeks were excluded from analysis. Baseline characteristics of study participants at ART initiation are shown in Table 1. The median age at ART initiation was 36 (inter-quartile range [IQR] 32–40) and the median CD4 count was 126 cells/μL (IQR 79–154 cells/μL). Abnormal alanine aminotransferase (ALT) levels and skin rash were each present in 11 (16%) of the women at baseline. No baseline plasma or genital drug resistance was detected.

Sixty-six of the 69 women in this study had detectable nevirapine levels at week 12. Three women who had undetectable levels were assumed to be non-adherent and were excluded from further analysis. Steady-state plasma nevirapine levels were characterized by wide inter-individual variability, ranging from 1.68 μg/mL to 23.12 μg/mL (median 9.14 μg/mL, IQR 5.98–2.46 μg/mL). No significant correlation was found between $\log_{10}$-transformed plasma nevirapine levels and age (P=0.78) or body mass index (BMI, P=0.19).

Frequency of CYP2B6 genotypes

For the CYP2B6 516G>T SNP, the frequency of the T variant allele was 31.2% (95% CI, 23.6%–39.6%). The number of subjects with GG, GT and TT genotypes were 35 (50.7%), 25 (36.2%), and 9 (13.0%), respectively. For the CYP2B6 983T>C SNP, the frequency of the C variant allele was 10.1% (95% CI, 5.7%–16.4%). Most

Table 1 Baseline characteristics of study participants at initiation of nevirapine-based antiretroviral therapy

Characteristic	Median (IQR) or N (%)
Age (yrs)	36 (32–40)
Weight (kg)	65 (54 – 70)
BMI (kg/m^2)	25.0 (22.3 – 28.2)
CD4 cell count (cells/μL)	126 (79 – 154)
Plasma viral load ($\log_{10}$ copies/mL)	5.54 (5.17 – 5.90)
Cervical viral load ($\log_{10}$ copies/mL)	4.04 (3.42 – 4.60)
ALT levels (>ULN)	11 (15.9)
Skin rash	11 (15.9)
Plasma resistance (present)	0
Genital resistance (present)	0
ART regimen: d4T/3TC/NVP	69 (100)

BMI = body mass index, ALT = alanine aminotransferase, ULN = upper limit of normal, ART = antiretroviral therapy, NVP = nevirapine, d4T = stavudine, 3TC = lamivudine.

individuals (55 or 79.9%) had the homozygous wild type TT genotype, whereas 14 women (20.3%) had the heterozygous mutant TC genotype and none had the homozygous mutant CC genotype. CYP2B6 516G>T polymorphism met Hardy-Weinberg (HW) equilibrium expectations (*P*=0.26). HW equilibrium could not be tested for CYP2B6 983T>C, because the homozygous mutant was not detected in this population. There was no evidence of linkage disequilibrium between rs3745274 and rs28399499 (Fisher's exact *P*=0.45). In terms of inferred phenotypes, 26 (37.7%) individuals were predicted to be extensive metabolizers, 31 (44.9%) to be intermediate metabolizers, and 12 (17.4%) to be slow metabolizers.

CYP2B6 516G>T and 983T>C genotypes and plasma nevirapine levels

Among the 66 women with detectable plasma nevirapine levels, CYP2B6 516G>T and 983T>C SNPs were associated with higher mean plasma nevirapine levels at week 12 (Table 2). A gene-dose effect was evident in the distribution of plasma nevirapine levels among CYP2B6 516G>T and CYP2B6 983T>C genotypes. Mean plasma nevirapine levels were higher among individuals who were homozygous for the mutation (CYP2B6 516TT, 14.33 μg/mL) and in those who were heterozygous for the mutation (CYP2B6 516GT, 9.18 μg/mL) compared to those with the wild-type (CYP2B6 516GG, 7.95 μg/mL, *P*=0.01 across groups). A similar trend was observed for CYP2B6 983T>C, with mean plasma nevirapine levels being higher among individuals expressing the heterozygous genotype (CYP2B6 983TC, 12.94 μg/mL) compared to those with the homozygous wild-type (983TT, 8.35 μg/mL, *P*=0.01 across groups). With regard to the phenotypes, mean plasma nevirapine levels were higher among individuals classified as slow metabolizers (14.76 μg/mL, $P <$ 0.01 compared to extensive metabolizers) and among individuals classified as intermediate metabolizers (9.34 μg/mL, *P*=0.02 compared to extensive metabolizers). The relationships between $\log_{10}$-transformed plasma nevirapine concentrations and CYP2B6 genotypes or phenotypes are summarized in Figures 1a, b and c.

Table 2 CYP2B6 516G>T and 983T>C genotypes and plasma nevirapine concentrations

CYP2B6	N (%)	Plasma nevirapine concentration (μg/mL), geometric mean (95% CI)	P value
CYP2B6 516G>T			
GG	32 (48.5)	7.95 (6.59-9.60)	
GT	25 (37.9)	9.18 (7.52-11.20)	
TT	9 (13.0)	14.33 (9.94-20.67)	
TOTAL	66		0.01*
CYP2B6 983T>C			
TT	53 (80.3)	8.35 (7.33-9.64)	
TC	13 (19.7)	12.94 (10.11-16.56)	
CC	0		
TOTAL	66		0.007*
Phenotypes			
Extensive metabolizers	24 (36.4)	6.92 (5.70-8.41)	
Intermediate metabolizers	30 (45.5)	9.34 (7.78-11.20)	0.02†
Slow metabolizers	12 (18.2)	14.76 (11.38-19.19)	<0.0001†
TOTAL	66		

*Comparison across groups using Stata's *qtlsnp* command.
†ANOVA comparing either intermediate or slow metabolizers to extensive metabolizers (reference category).

Plasma nevirapine levels predicted greater change in CD4 cell count

Higher plasma nevirapine levels were significantly correlated with greater change in CD4 cell count from baseline to month 3 (*P*=0.02) and month 6 (*P*=0.02), but not month 12 (*P*=0.07). In Generalized Estimating Equation (GEE) analysis with adjustment for baseline CD4 cell count, month since ART initiation, and time-updated adherence by pill count, plasma nevirapine levels predicted greater change in CD4 cell count after ART initiation (adjusted beta 119.4 cells/μL, 95% CI, 27.3 to 211.5 cells/μL, *P*=0.01).

CYP2B6 983T>C genotype was associated with greater change in CD4 cell count

There was no difference in CD4 cell count at baseline between the two CYP2B6 983T>C genotype groups (mean 120 for TC, mean 123 for TT, p=0.88). Using Stata's *qtlsnp* command, CYP2B6 983T>C genotypes were associated with mean change in CD4 cell count at month 3 (*P*=0.01), month 6 (*P*=0.02) and month 12 (*P*=0.02). In GEE analysis with adjustment for baseline CD4 cell count, month since ART initiation, and time-updated adherence by pill count, the TT genotype predicted greater change in CD4 cell count (adjusted beta 68.6 cells/μL, 95% CI, 3.9 to 133.4 cells/μL, *P*=0.04) during follow-up (Table 3). Adjustment for $\log_{10}$-transformed plasma nevirapine level diminished this effect, as shown in the last column of Table 3.

There were no differences between baseline CD4 cell count for the three CYP2B6 516G>T genotype groups (mean 127 for GG, 108 for GT, and 142 for TT, p= 0.26). Interestingly, CYP2B6 516G>T genotypes had

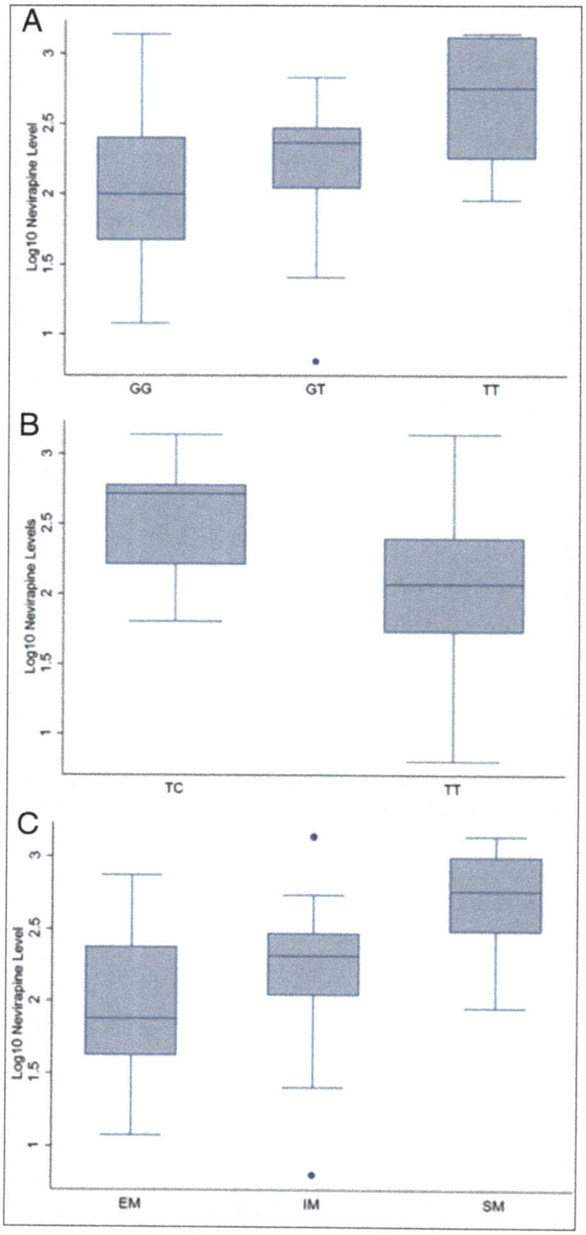

Figure 1 Differences in $\log_{10}$-transformed plasma nevirapine levels by genotype. Panel A, Log_{10}-transformed plasma nevirapine levels for each CYP2B6 516G>T genotype: GG, GT, and TT. Panel B, Log_{10}-transformed plasma nevirapine levels for each CYP2B6 983T>C genotype: TC and TT. Panel C, Log_{10}-transformed plasma nevirapine levels for each CYP2B6 phenotype (predicted from CYP2B6 516G>T and 983T>C genotypes). EM = extensive metabolizer, IM = intermediate metabolizer, SM = slow metabolizer.

no significant effect on the mean change in CD4 cell count at month 3 (P=0.86), month 6 (P=0.61), or month 12 (P=0.54) in this population. This lack of effect was confirmed in a GEE model (results not shown).

No correlation between plasma nevirapine levels and virologic response

There were no correlations between plasma nevirapine levels and change in PVL at month 3 (P=0.95), month 6 (P=0.53), or month 12 (P=0.81). In GEE analysis with adjustment for baseline PVL, month since ART initiation, and time-updated adherence by pill count, no association between plasma nevirapine levels and change in PVL was found (data not shown). *T* test comparisons showed no associations between plasma nevirapine levels and viral suppresion at month 3 (P= 0.38), month 6 (P=0.59), or month 12 (P=0.45). In GEE analysis with adjustment for baseline PVL, month since ART initiation, and time-updated adherence by pill count, there was no association between plasma nevirapine levels and viral suppression (data not shown).

Genotypic resistance was not detected in plasma or genital secretions of study participants at baseline. During follow-up, four (5.8%) and three (4.4%) women developed genotypic resistance in plasma and in genital secretions, respectively. Plasma nevirapine levels were not associated with resistance in either plasma (odds ratio [OR] 0.55, 95% CI 0.004–81.94, P=0.81) or genital tract secretions (OR 3.94, 95% CI 0.006–2497.02, P= 0.68). Adjustment for baseline CD4 cell count and adherence or for baseline PVL and adherence did not change these findings.

Plasma nevirapine levels did not predict hepatotoxicity or skin rash

Of the 69 study participants, 11 (15.9%) had abnormal ALT levels at baseline which persisted through follow-up. Of the 58 women who had normal ALT levels at baseline, 14 (24.1%) had abnormal ALT levels that developed during follow-up. Plasma nevirapine levels were not significantly associated with the development of hepatotoxicity during follow-up, despite an increased odds (OR 5.35, 95% CI 0.27–106.01, P=0.27). Adjustment for adherence, hepatitis B, and baseline CD4 count did not change this result (adjusted odds ratio [aOR] 2.88, 95% CI 0.13–62.95, P=0.50). No correlation was found between plasma nevirapine levels and maximum ALT levels recorded during ART (ρ=0.129, P=0.30, Figure 2). Eleven (15.9%) of the 69 study participants had a skin rash at baseline that persisted over the follow-up period. Of the 58 women with no skin rash at baseline, 27 (46.6%) developed skin rash during follow-up. Plasma nevirapine levels were not associated with a new skin rash (OR 0.36, 95% CI 0.03–3.88, P=0.40). Adjustment for adherence and baseline CD4 count did not change these results (aOR 0.44, 95% CI 0.03–5.97, P=0.54).

Table 3 CYP2B6 983T>C genotype and change in CD4 cell count over the 12-month follow-up period

Variable	Unadjusted beta	P value	Adjusted beta*	P value	Adjusted beta†	P value
CYP2B6 983T>C						
TT genotype	reference		reference		reference	
TC genotype	68.2 (3.3 to 133.0)	0.039	68.6 (3.9 to 133.4)	0.038	57.6 (−4.6 to 119.8)	0.069
Baseline CD4 count	0.0 (−0.4 to 0.5)	0.920	0.0 (−0.4 to 0.4)	0.831	0.1 (−0.3 to 0.5)	0.595
Months since ART initiation	3.3 (0.8 to 5.8)	0.010	3.4 (1.0 to 5.8)	0.005	3.6 (1.1 to 6.0)	0.004
Pill count adherence	0.3 (−1.6 to 2.1)	0.768	0.8 (−1.0 to 2.5)	0.384	0.7 (−1.4 to 2.8)	0.521
Log_{10}-tranformed nevirapine levels	115.3 (26.6 to 204.1)	0.011			85.9 (10.6 to 161.3)	0.025

*Adjusted for all factors included in model.
†With added adjustment for log_{10} plasma nevirapine levels.

Discussion

This prospective study analyzed the association between CYP2B6 516G>T and CYP2B6 983T>C genotypes, plasma nevirapine levels, and clinical response in a well-characterized cohort of HIV-1-positive Kenyan women on first-line nevirapine-based ART. The prevalence of CYP2B6 516T and CYP2B6 983C variants in this population was similar to that reported for other African populations and Kenyan ethnic groups [17,18]. We observed a significant association between both CYP2B6 516G>T and CYP2B6 983T>T genotypes and higher plasma nevirapine concentrations. In addition, plasma nevirapine levels significantly predicted change in CD4 cell counts after ART initiation. Furthermore, CYP2B6 983TC heterozygosity was associated with greater increase in CD4 cell count over the 12-month follow-up period.

CYP2B6 983T>C occurs predominantly in African subjects, with allele frequencies of 4% to 11% [19,20]. Homozygosity for the mutant allele CYP2B6 983 CC was not detected in this population, in concurrence with a previous study [25]. However, heterozygosity for the mutation CYP2B6 983TC was associated with higher plasma nevirapine levels in our study, with heterozygous TC individuals having levels 55% higher than those with the wild type TT. This effect is noteworthy for its magnitude, especially when compared to the smaller effect observed for CYP2B6 516GT (16%). The CYP2B6 983T>C (rs28399499) SNP results in the variant protein CYP2B6*18 with an I328T as the only amino acid change. Its expression *in vitro* results in no detectable protein or activity [26], and it has been designated as a null allele [12]. This null status could explain the greater impact of CYP2B6 983TC compared to the CYP2B6 516GT. In agreement with our results, other studies have reported that CYP2B6 983TC heterozygosity leads to reduction in nevirapine clearance [27,28].

We also made an observation that heterozygosity for CYP2B6 983TC was significantly associated with greater increase in CD4 cell count during follow-up. This observation could be attributed to the fact that CYP2B6

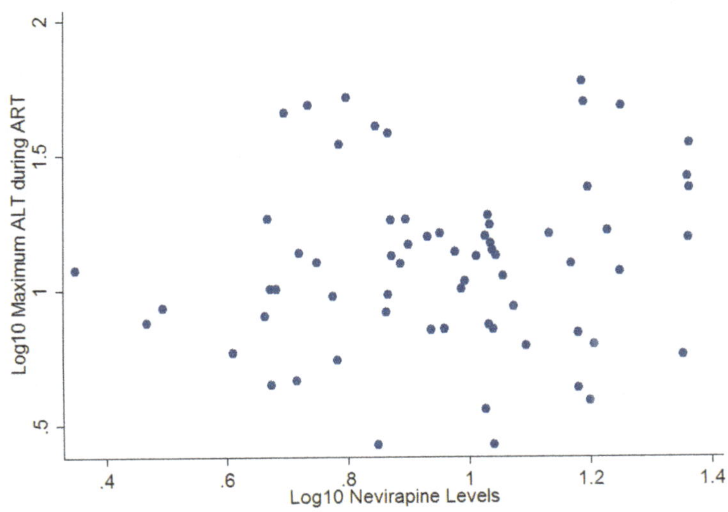

Figure 2 Scatterplot of log_{10}-transformed plasma nevirapine levels and log_{10}-transformed maximum ALT levels during ART.

983TC was associated with higher plasma nevirapine levels, which in turn were associated with greater increase in CD4 cell count, particularly in the early months of ART. In fact, from our multivariable analysis, the addition of plasma nevirapine levels to the model weakened the association between genotype and change in CD4 cell count, providing evidence of at least partial mediation of this association by nevirapine levels.

Previous studies evaluating the impact of CYP2B6 genotypes on clinical outcomes have reported varied results. A study by Haas et al. [29] reported no association between CYP2B6 516G>T genotypes and change in CD4 cell count, in concurrence with our findings. However, in a HIV-1-positive pediatric cohort, CYP2B6 516TT genotype was associated with greater increase in CD4 cell count percentage at week 12, compared to those with the GT and GG genotypes (9.0% vs. 5.0% vs. 3.2% increases, respectively) [30]. More recent studies report a significant association between the CYP2B6 516 T allele, UGT2B7*2, higher efavirenz plasma levels and change in CD4 cell count in HIV-1 positive African patients in Tanzania and Ethiopia [31]. These studies did not include testing for CYP2B6 983T>C. Hence, our study is the first to report a significant association between CYP2B6 983TC heterozygosity and greater increase in CD4 cell count in an African population.

It is unclear why nevirapine concentrations would influence CD4 cell recovery but not have a detectable effect on viral load reduction or suppression. At least one study of patients with virologic suppression on nevirapine has highlighted nevirapine's ability to penetrate reservoir sites and achieve high intracellular concentrations, leading to extremely low levels of viral replication [32]. It is possible that penetration into reservoir sites varied by genotype in this study, leading to an impact on CD4 T cell recovery that was independent of the effect on plasma viral load. Alternatively, because most women achieved virologic suppression and there were no differences in baseline plasma viral load prior to ART initiation, there may have been a floor effect on change in plasma viral load that reduced our power to detect differences by genotype. In contrast, our study participants initiated therapy with very low CD4 counts which increased during ART and reached no ceiling during the 12 months of follow-up. We may, therefore, have had more power to detect differences in CD4 cell recovery. A third explanation is that some other genetic trait linked to the CYP2B6 983T>C phenotype somehow influences CD4 T cell recovery. This is a potential area of investigation, should our results be confirmed in other studies.

A major strength of our study was its design as a prospective study in a well-characterized cohort in which clinical outcomes were carefully measured and recorded. Our study also had a number of limitations. First, suboptimal adherence could have contributed to the observed wide inter-patient variability in plasma nevirapine levels. Second, plasma nevirapine levels could also be under the influence of other drug metabolism and membrane transporter genes which were not studied in our cohort. Third, we do not have information on nutritional status, herbal remedies, or medications obtained outside the research clinic that may have influenced immune response. Fourth, our sample size and duration of follow-up were limited, and we may have failed to detect smaller differences in some outcomes. Despite these limitations, we were able to identify several clinical correlates that were associated with participant genotypes.

Conclusions

In conclusion, we have found in this study that CYP2B6 516G>T and 983T>C genotypes are associated with higher plasma nevirapine exposure in HIV-1 infected Kenyan women, and that higher plasma nevirapine levels and the CYP2B6 983TC genotype were associated with better immunologic response. In this study, neither plasma nevirapine levels nor CYP2B6 genotypes were significantly associated with toxicity or with the emergence of plasma or genital resistance. However, our follow-up time was limited and the incidence of both toxicity and drug resistance was fairly low. We recommend further studies to confirm the role of CYP2B6 genotypes and other relevant genes in the pharmacokinetics and clinical response to nevirapine in HIV-1-positive African women.

Methods

Study population and design

The study was nested within an ongoing prospective cohort study investigating the impact of ART on HIV-1 infectivity in female sex workers in Mombasa, Kenya [33,34]. At the time of this study, ART was initiated for women with CD4 counts ≤200 cells/μL or an AIDS defining illness [35]. Pregnant women were excluded and instead referred to programs offering ART for the prevention of mother to child transmission. Women requiring rifampicin-containing treatment for active tuberculosis were prescribed efavirenz or a triple non-nucleoside reverse transcriptase inhibitor regimen, according to WHO guidance at the time [35]. All women were prescribed co-trimoxazole prophylaxis, unless contraindicated.

The standard ART regimen included nevirapine 200 mg daily for 14 days, then 200 mg twice daily [35]. The NRTI backbone included stavudine or zidovudine plus lamivudine at standard doses [35]. Adherence was promoted by directly observed administration of one of the two daily doses to the women on weekdays during their first month of ART. Pill box organizers and a monthly support group were also used to enhance adherence, which was monitored at each visit by pill count and a validated visual analogue scale [36]. Fluconazole, which can impact nevirapine levels, was prescribed for only one woman in this study, starting at the month 6 visit.

Clinical response to treatment was monitored, including self-reported symptoms and physical examination (including rash). Laboratory testing, including regular testing of CD4 cell count, hemoglobin, ALT, creatinine, and plasma and genital viral load, were performed on stored samples from baseline, month 3, month 6, and month 12 [33,34]. Samples with detectable HIV-1 ribonucleic acid (RNA) after treatment initiation were evaluated for antiretroviral resistance mutations.

All HIV-1-seropositive women who initiated nevirapine-based ART between May 2005 and September 2007 and had stored peripheral blood mononuclear cells (PBMCs) and plasma collected at week 12 of ART were included in this study. Women in the parent ART cohort gave consent at enrollment for long-term storage of samples and for additional studies including genetic testing. The present study was approved as a protocol modification by the University of Washington Human Subjects Research Committee and Kenya Medical Research Institute's Ethics and Research Committee.

Determination of plasma nevirapine levels

Blood plasma collected 10–14 weeks after ART initiation was used for the determination of plasma nevirapine concentrations. Blood collection was not timed in relation to medication dosing, since this pharmacological study was a secondary use of stored samples and data. However, most women attended clinic in the morning, and are likely to have been sampled between 2 and 4 hours after pill ingestion, at an optimal sampling time for nevirapine [37]. Plasma nevirapine concentrations were quantified using a reversed phase high performance liquid chromatographic method adapted from the method of Minzi and Ngaimisi [38]. Calibration curves obtained for nevirapine-spiked plasma samples were linear, with correlation coefficients (r^2) in the range of 0.993–0.996 and a limit of quantitation of 0.86 μg/mL. The intra-day and inter-day precision (CV%) ranged from 6.08–7.96 and 4.72–7.32, respectively. Intra-day and inter-day accuracy (RD%) ranged from 3.47–5.51 and 2.00–8.10, respectively. The mean recovery for low, medium and high concentrations of nevirapine was in the range of 96–110%.

DNA preparation and genotyping procedures

DNA was extracted from PBMCs using the QIAamp DNA blood mini-kit (Qiagen GmbH, Hilden, Germany) according to the manufacturer's protocol. The extracted DNA was quantified using a UV spectrophotometer ND-1000 (NanoDrop Technologies, Wilmington, DE, USA) at 260 nm and normalized to a concentration of 20 ng/mL. Genotyping was carried out on an ABI 7500 Fast Sequence Detection System (Applied Biosystems, Foster City, CA, USA). SNPs were analyzed using the validated Taqman Genotyping Assays purchased from Applied Biosystems for CYP2B6 516G>T (rs3745274; assay ID C_7817765_60) and CYP2B6 983T>C (rs28399499; assay ID C_60732328_20), according to the manufacturer's instructions.

Definitions

CYP2B6 516G>T and 983T>C genotypes were described as homozygous wild type for the G or T alleles (516GG or 983TT), heterozygous (516GT or 983TC), or homozygous mutated (516TT, 983CC). CYP2B6 metabolic phenotypes were inferred from composite CYP2B6 genotypes as previously described [22]. Those with no variant alleles at either positions (516GG or 983TT) were classified as "extensive metabolizers." The term "intermediate metabolizers" described those with a single variant allele at either position, but not both. The term "slow metabolizers" described those with two variant alleles (516TT, 983CC, or 516GT with 983TC).

Changes in CD4 cell count and PVL were assessed at months 3, 6, and 12. Viral suppression was defined as <100 copies HIV-1 RNA per mL of plasma. Hepatotoxicity potentially attributable to ART was defined as a normal ALT at baseline with an elevation above the upper limit of normal during treatment. A possible ART-related skin rash was defined as no rash at baseline followed by rash during treatment. Plasma or genital drug resistance was defined as identification of drug resistance mutations in plasma or genital secretions before or during treatment.

Data analysis

The prevalence of each genetic variant was estimated from the total number of copies of individual alleles divided by the number of all alleles in the study population. Deviation of genotypes from HW equilibrium expectation was estimated using Stata's *hwsnp* command, which calculates an exact HW significance probability. Prevalence estimates were reported with exact binomial confidence intervals. Steady-state plasma nevirapine levels were tested for normality by the Shapiro-Wilk test, and subsequently $\log_{10}$-transformed due to lack of normality. All averages are hence presented as the geometric mean. Women with undetectable levels of nevirapine were excluded from analysis, because it was assumed that they were non-adherent to treatment.

One-way analysis of variance was used to determine whether there were significant differences in continuous variables across genotype or phenotypes groups. The effects of each genotype or phenotype on plasma nevirapine levels at week 12 and on change in CD4 cell count at month 3, 6 and 12 were evaluated using Stata's *qtlsnp* command, which assumes a co-dominant genetic model and tests for an additive effect, a dominant effect and that both effects are equal to zero (this last comparison is equivalent to comparing means across the three possible genotypes and phenotypes). We also modeled the relationship between plasma nevirapine levels and post-ART outcomes including change in CD4 count, plasma viral load, and viral suppression using GEE models with a logit or identify link, independent correlation matrix, and robust standard error estimates. We adjusted these models for month since ART initiation, time-updated adherence by pill count, and either baseline CD4 count or plasma viral load, as appropriate. To determine whether plasma nevirapine levels acted as a mediator in the association between CYP2B6 983T>C genotype and change in CD4 cell count, the effect of adding $\log_{10}$-transformed plasma nevirapine levels to multivariable modeling was also evaluated by GEE analysis.

The correlation between $\log_{10}$-transformed plasma nevirapine levels and age, BMI, change in CD4 cell count, and change in $\log_{10}$-transformed PVL at months 3, 6 and 12 was evaluated with the Pearson's test for correlation. An independent *t* test was used to compare $\log_{10}$-transformed nevirapine levels in women with suppressed versus unsuppressed PVL. Logistic regression was used to test for associations between $\log_{10}$-transformed plasma nevirapine levels and the development of ALT elevation, skin rash, or plasma or genital drug resistance after treatment initiation. The modeled binary outcomes were adjusted for potential confounding factors appropriate to the outcome being evaluated. In the analysis of hepatotoxicity, the presence of hepatitis B infection was included in the model as a potential effect modifier. Data were analyzed using Stata version 11.2 (Stata Corp, College Station, Texas, USA).

Abbreviations

ALT: Alanine aminotransferase; AOR: Adjusted odds ratio; ART: Antiretroviral therapy; BMI: Body mass index; CI: Confidence intervals; CYP2B6: Cytochrome P450 2B6; CYP3A4: Cytochrome P450 3A4; CYP3A5: Cytochrome P450 3A5; GEE: Generalized estimating equation; HW: Hardy-Weinberg; IQR: Inter-quartile range; OR: Odds ratio; PBMC: Peripheral blood mononuclear cells; PVL: Plasma viral load; RNA: Ribonucleic acid; SNP: Single nucleotide polymorphism.

Competing Interests

All authors report no competing interests.

Authors' contributions

RSM conceived the study. SMG led the clinical fieldwork. MNO and FAO conducted plasma nevirapine and genetic testing, with oversight by ANG. SMG conducted the analysis. MNO and SMG drafted the manuscript. All authors provided input and approved the final manuscript.

Acknowledgements

We thank the research staff, particularly Daniel Juma Siminyu (Department of Pharmacology and Pharmacognosy, University of Nairobi) and Godfrey Anyona (Government Chemists) for their contributions towards drug level analysis, the Mombasa Municipal Council for clinical space, and the Coast Provincial General Hospital for laboratory space. Special thanks go to our study participants. This work was supported by the University of Washington's Royalty Research Fund and by National Institutes of Health (NIH) [AI-58698, AI-38518, and AI-069990 to SMG]. Additional support for the Mombasa Field Site was provided by the University of Washington Center for AIDS Research, an NIH-funded program [P30 AI027757].

Author details

[1]Department of Pharmacology and Pharmacognosy, University of Nairobi, P.O. BOX 19498, Nairobi 00202, Kenya. [2]Departments of Medicine, Global Health, and Epidemiology, University of Washington, Seattle, USA and Institute of Tropical and Infectious Diseases, University of Nairobi, Nairobi, Kenya.

References

1. Joint United Nations Programme on HIV/AIDS. UNAIDS Report on the Global AIDS Epidemic. Geneva: World Health Organization; 2013.
2. National AIDS and STI Control Programme. Kenya AIDS Indicator Survey 2012: Preliminary Report. Nairobi: Ministry of Health; 2013.
3. National AIDS Control Council and National AIDS and STI Control Programme. Kenya AIDS Epidemic Update. Nairobi: Ministry of Health; 2012.
4. Braitstein P, Ayuo P, Mwangi A, Wools-Kaloustian K, Musick B, Siika A, et al. Sustainability of first-line antiretroviral regimens: findings from a large HIV treatment program in western Kenya. J Acquir Immune Defic Syndr. 2010;53:254–9.
5. Foreman C, Gazzard B, Johnson M, Sharott P, Collins S. Maintaining cost-effective access to antiretroviral drug therapy through a collaborative approach to drug procurement, consensus treatment guidelines and regular audit: the experience of London HIV commissioners and providers. Sex Transm Infect. 2012;88:112–5.
6. Dong BJ, Zheng Y, Hughes MD, Frymoyer A, Verotta D, Lizak P, et al. Nevirapine pharmacokinetics and risk of rash and hepatitis among HIV-infected sub-Saharan African women. AIDS. 2012;26:833–41.
7. Ngo-Giang-Huong N, Jourdain G, Amzal B, Sang-a-gad P, Lertkoonalak R, Eiamsirikit N, et al. Resistance patterns selected by nevirapine vs efavirenz in HIV-infected patients failing first-line antiretroviral treatment: a Bayesian analysis. PLoS One. 2011;6:e27427.
8. Darwich L, Esteve A, Ruiz L, Bellido R, Clotet B, Martinez-Picado J. Variability in the plasma concentration of efavirenz and nevirapine is associated with genotypic resistance after treatment interruption. Antivir Ther. 2008;13:945–51.
9. Khienprasit N, Chaiwarith R, Sirisanthana T, Supparatpinyo K. Incidence and risk factors of antiretroviral treatment failure in treatment-naïve HIV-infected patients at Chiang Mai University Hospital, Thailand. AIDS Res Ther. 2011;8:42.
10. Riska P, Lamson M, MacGregor T, Sabo J, Hattox S, Pav J, et al. Disposition and biotransformation of the antiretroviral drug nevirapine in humans. Drug Metab Dispos. 1999;27:895–901.
11. Erickson DA, Mather G, Trager WF, Levy RH, Keirns JJ. Characterization of the in vitro biotransformation of the HIV-1 reverse transcriptase inhibitor nevirapine by human hepatic cytochromes P-450. Drug Metab Dispos. 1999;27:1488–95.
12. Klein K, Lang T, Saussele T, Barbosa-Sicard E, Schunck WH, Eichelbaum M, et al. Genetic variability of CYP2B6 in populations of African and Asian origin: allele frequencies, novel functional variants, and possible implications for anti-HIV therapy with efavirenz. Pharmacogenet Genomics. 2005;15:861–73.
13. Ngaimisi E, Mugusi S, Minzi OM, Sasi P, Riedel KD, Suda A, et al. Long-term efavirenz autoinduction and its effect on plasma exposure in HIV patients. Clin Pharmacol Ther. 2010;88:676–84.
14. Habtewold A, Amogne W, Makonnen E, Yimer G, Riedel KD, Ueda N, et al. Long-term effect of efavirenz autoinduction on plasma/peripheral blood mononuclear cell drug exposure and CD4 count is influenced by UGT2B7 and CYP2B6 genotypes among HIV patients. J Antimicrob Chemother. 2011;66:2350–61.
15. Lang T, Klein K, Fischer J, Nüssler AK, Neuhaus P, Hofmann U, et al. Extensive genetic polymorphism in the human CYP2B6 gene with impact on expression and function in human liver. Pharmacogenetics. 2001;11:399–415.

16. Haas DW, Ribaudo HJ, Kim RB, Tierney C, Wilkinson GR, Gulick RM, et al. Pharmacogenetics of Efavirenz and central nervous system side effects: an adult AIDS clinical trials group study. AIDS. 2004;18:2391–400.
17. Matimba A, Oluka MN, Ebeshi BU, Sayi J, Bolaji OO, Guantai AN, et al. Establishment of a biobank and pharmacogenetics database of African populations. Eur J Hum Genet. 2008;16:780–3.
18. Li J, Menard V, Benish RL, Jurevic RJ, Guillemette C, Stoneking M, et al. Worldwide variation in human drug-metabolism enzyme genes CYP2B6 and UGT2B7: implications for HIV/AIDS treatment. Pharmacogenomics. 2012;13:555–70.
19. Mehlotra RK, Bockarie MJ, Zimmerman PA. CYP2B6 983T>C polymorphism is prevalent in West Africa but absent in Papua New Guinea: implications for HIV/AIDS treatment. Br J Clin Pharmacol. 2007;64:391–5.
20. Dahri K, Ensom MH. Efavirenz and nevirapine in HIV-1 infection: is there a role for clinical pharmacokinetic monitoring? Clin Pharmacokinet. 2007;46:109–32.
21. Duong M, Buisson M, Peytavin G, Kohli E, Piroth L, Martha B, et al. Low trough plasma concentrations of nevirapine associated with virologic rebounds in HIV-infected patients who switched from protease inhibitors. Ann Pharmacother. 2005;39:603–9.
22. Haas DW, Gebretsadik T, Mayo G, Menon UN, Acosta EP, Shintani A, et al. Associations between CYP2B6 polymorphisms and pharmacokinetics after a single dose of nevirapine or efavirenz in African Americans. J Infect Dis. 2009;199:872–80.
23. Gozalo C, Gérard L, Loiseau P, Morand-Joubert L, Peytavin G, Molina JM, et al. ANRS 081 Study Group. Pharmacogenetics of toxicity, plasma trough concentration and treatment outcome with nevirapine-containing regimen in anti-retroviral-naïve HIV-infected adults: an exploratory study of the TRIANON ANRS 081 trial. Basic Clin Pharmacol Toxicol. 2011;109:513–20.
24. Heil SG, van der Ende ME, Schenk PW, van der Heiden I, Lindemans J, Burger D, et al. Associations between ABCB1, CYP2A6, CYP2B6, CYP2D6, and CYP3A5 alleles in relation to efavirenz and nevirapine pharmacokinetics in HIV-infected individuals. Ther Drug Monit. 2012;34:153–9.
25. Mahungu T, Smith C, Turner F, Egan D, Youle M, Johnson M, et al. Cytochrome P450 2B6 516G–>T is associated with plasma concentrations of nevirapine at both 200 mg twice daily and 400 mg once daily in an ethnically diverse population. HIV Med. 2009;10:310–7.
26. Honda M, Muroi Y, Tamaki Y, Saigusa D, Suzuki N, Tomioka Y, et al. Functional characterization of CYP2B6 allelic variants in demethylation of antimalarial artemether. Drug Metab Dispos. 2011;39:1860–5.
27. Wyen C, Hendra H, Vogel M, Hoffmann C, Knechten H, Brockmeyer NH, et al. German Competence Network for HIV/AIDS. Impact of CYP2B6 983T>C polymorphism on non-nucleoside reverse transcriptase inhibitor plasma concentrations in HIV-infected patients. J Antimicrob Chemother. 2008;61:914–8.
28. Schipani A, Wyen C, Mahungu T, Hendra H, Egan D, Siccardi M, et al. Integration of population pharmacokinetics and pharmacogenetics: an aid to optimal nevirapine dose selection in HIV-infected individuals. J Antimicrob Chemother. 2011;66:1332–9.
29. Haas DW, Smeaton LM, Shafer RW, Robbins GK, Morse GD, Labbe L, et al. Pharmacogenetics of long-term responses to antiretroviral regimens containing Efavirenz and/or Nelfinavir: an adult aids clinical trials group study. J Infect Dis. 2005;192:1931–42.
30. Saitoh A, Sarles E, Capparelli E, Aweeka F, Kovacs A, Burchett SK, et al. CYP2B6 genetic variants are associated with nevirapine pharmacokinetics and clinical response in HIV-1-infected children. AIDS. 2007;21:2191–9.
31. Ngaimisi E, Habtewold A, Minzi O, Makonnen E, Mugusi S, Amogne W, et al. Importance of ethnicity, CYP2B6 and ABCB1 genotype for efavirenz pharmacokinetics and treatment outcomes: a parallel-group prospective cohort study in two sub-Saharan Africa populations. PLoS One. 2013;8:e67946.
32. Haïm-Boukobza S, Morand-Joubert L, Flandre P, Valin N, Fourati S, Sayon S, et al. Higher efficacy of nevirapine than efavirenz to achieve HIV-1 plasma viral load below 1 copy/ml. AIDS. 2011;25:341–4.
33. Graham SM, Masese L, Gitau R, Jalalian-Lechak Z, Richardson BA, Peshu N, et al. Antiretroviral adherence and development of drug resistance are the strongest predictors of genital HIV-1 shedding among women initiating treatment. J Infec Dis. 2010;202:1538–42.
34. Graham SM, Jalalian-Lechak Z, Shafi J, Chohan V, Deya RW, Jaoko W, et al. Antiretroviral treatment interruptions predict female genital shedding of genotypically resistant HIV-1 RNA. J Acquir Immune Defic Syndr. 2012;60:511–8.
35. National AIDS and STI Control Programme. Guidelines for Antiretroviral Therapy in Kenya. 3rd ed. Nairobi: Ministry of Health; 2005.
36. Oyugi JH, Byakika-Tusiime J, Charlebois ED, Kityo C, Mugerwa R, Mugyenyi P, et al. Multiple validated measures of adherence indicate high levels of adherence to generic HIV antiretroviral therapy in a resource-limited setting. J Acquir Immune Defic Syndr. 2004;36:1100–2.
37. Veldkamp AI, van Heeswijk RP, Mulder JW, Meenhorst PL, Hoetelmans RM, Lange JM, et al. Limited sampling strategies for the estimation of the systemic exposure to the HIV-1 non-nucleoside reverse transcriptase inhibitor nevirapine. Ther Drug Monit. 2001;23:606–11.
38. Minzi OMS, Ngaimisi E. Bioanalytical method for determination of nevirapine in-vivo in resource constrained laboratories. J Chem Pharm Res. 2010;2:431–9.

The development of drug resistance mutations K103N Y181C and G190A in long term Nevirapine-containing antiviral therapy

Yuncong Wang[1,2], Hui Xing[2*], Lingjie Liao[2], Zhe Wang[3], Bin Su[4], Quanbi Zhao[2], Yi Feng[2], Pengfei Ma[2], Jia Liu[3], Jianjun Wu[4], Yuhua Ruan[2] and Yiming Shao[2]

Abstract

Objective: We built a cohort study of HIV patients taking long-term first-line Antiretroviral Therapy in 2003. In this assay, we focused on the development of primary drug resistance mutations against Non-Nucleoside Reverse Transcriptase Inhibitor (NNRTI), K103N, Y181C and G190A.

Method: The cohort study was built in Henan province, China. We used Single Genome Amplification (SGA) to analyze the frequency of K103N, Y181C and G190A in serial plasma samples of three individual patients. We also performed standard genotype HIV drug resistance assay in 204 patients of this cohort study to analyze the frequency of these mutations.

Result: In the SGA sequences, the K103N decreased and vanished, while the frequency of Y181C and G190A increased in individual patient receiving long-term Antiretroviral Therapy (ART). In the sequences of standard genotype HIV drug resistance assay, the frequency of K103N, Y181C and G190A had the similar pattern with that in SGA sequences. Among these patients, the viral suppression were still sufficient after receiving ART for 72 months, and 78.6% (160/204) patients could have their CD4 count over than 200cells/ul.

Conclusion: In some patients, first-line ART had the possibility to provide sufficient treatment effect for over than 72 months, but in long-term treatment, the dominant NNRTI drug resistance mutation K103N could reduced, while the proportion of variants with mutation Y181C or G190A may increased. This result was not similar with that in vitro study, which state that variant with K103N or Y181C had an equal viral fitness with wild type.

Keywords: K103N, Y181C, G190A Navirapine (NVP), Antiviral therapy, Cohort study

Background

Antiretroviral therapy (ART) in China started in 2003 [1], at the end of 2011, over 350,000 HIV-infected patients were receiving ART [2]. Chinese national treatment guidelines for ART is: (1) CD4 cell count, 350/mm^3 (increased from 200/mm^3 in 2008); (2) total lymphocyte count, 1,200/mm^3; or (3) World Health Organization (WHO) stage III or IV disease [3]. The first-line regimen included two kinds of Nucleoside Reverse Transcriptase Inhibitors (NRTI) and one kind of Non-Nucleoside Reverse Transcriptase Inhibitor (NNRTI) [4]. Because of very limited antiretroviral drug formulations and lack of adequate laboratory monitoring of ART patients, most patients who initiated ART during the early phase of the free ART program had to stay on the same regimen for a long period of time (maximum for 112 months in my research). For this fact, the research on the development of drug resistance mutations in long-term ART became more and more necessary.

NNRTIs is a crucial component of Chinese ART, it exhibit a longer plasma half-life and a longer duration of detectable levels than nucleoside analog reverse transcriptase inhibitors (NRTIs) [5]. Nevirapine (NVP) is an acceptable first-line NNRTI for HIV-1-infected patients [6] and is known as the most common NNRTI used in

* Correspondence: xingh@chinaaids.cn
[2]State Key Laboratory for Infectious Disease Prevention and Control, National Center for AIDS/STD Control and Prevention, Chinese Center for Disease Control and Prevention, Collaborative Innovation Center for Diagnosis and Treatment of Infectious Diseases, Beijing, China
Full list of author information is available at the end of the article

the ART regimens of China. In our research, all patients took NVP as NNRTI in their regimens, and were never been stopped and changed.

NVP is a potent NNRTI to fight against HIV, but it has two drawbacks: one, it could cause allergic reactions in approximately 5-14% of users worldwide [7-9], another one is that NVP has a low genetic barrier; a single mutation can lead to a high-level drug resistance against NVP [10,11]. Among the NNRTI drug mutation, K103N, Y181C and G190A are the most common mutation associated with resistance to NVP [12,13]. Even in the patients before ART, Low frequencies of K103N and Y181C are significantly associated with an increased risk of virologic failure [14]. In vitro study, K103N, Y181C and G190A could not provide significant fitness reduction to HIV viruses, variant with these mutations had similar viral replication fitness with the wild type variant [15,16]. In the past, consider the low fitness reduction and high-level resistance of NNRTI associated mutations, researchers seldom paid attention to the NNRTIs resistant profiles resulting from therapy failure, because a single NNRTI treatment failure always means the second NNRTI therapy failure [17,18], and in countries with rich ART resources, patients with NNRTI drug resistance mutations would switch to new regimen but in China, a country with limited antiretroviral drugs, patients had to took same NNRTI drug for long time, so the understanding of the development of NNRTI associated mutations became very necessary.

In this essay, we retrospectively studied the development of K103N, Y181C and G190A in long-term ART.

Method

Study population

National Center for AIDS/STD Control and Prevention built an observational cohort study enrolled 339 patients from Queshan County, Henan Province from December 2003 to December 2004. Patients who were 18 years of age or older and started ART between 2003 and 2004 were included. All patients agreed to participate in the study through informed consent. Patients were followed every 6 months up to 11 November 2012. Due to stopping ART, death or losing to follow-up. By the end of 2012, among these 339 patients, 75 patients died for AIDS associated diseases, 34 patients stopped ART, and 26 patients lost to follow-up, so we had 204 patients for this study.

204 patients in this cohort study were all treated with AZT/ddI/NVP (AZT, 300 mg 2 times/day; ddI, 200 mg 2 times/day; NVP, 200 mg, 2 times/day). Treatment adherence was assessed by questionnaire in each follow-up. The number of patients who had over 95% adherence in each follow-up showed no significant difference ($p > 0.05$).

Sample collection was approved and done by Henan CDC. In each follow-up, Neibor Joining phylogenetic analysis was performed to confirm that the longitudinal samples were from the same patient, and all the information of patients and the results of drug resistance assays were all well stored by China CDC. All patients took Nevirapine (NVP) as the NNRTI in regimen from the initial time and have never been changed (Table 1).

To assess the ART outcome, the date of virologic failure was defined as the first recorded date of plasma viral load of more than 5000 copies/ml after 6 months of treatment, as the 2010 WHO guideline on antiretroviral therapy for HIV infection in adults and adolescents (WHO. Antiretroviral therapy for HIV infection in adults and adolescents: recommendations for a public health approach. 2010). Similarly, the date of immunologic failure was also defined by WHO criteria as the earliest date of any one of the following after 6 months of treatment: posttreatment CD4+ cell count falling to or below baseline $CD4^+$ cell count; 50% decrease from peak $CD4^+$ cell count; or two consecutive $CD4^+$ cell counts of less than 100 cells/ml or last $CD4^+$ cell count of less than 100 cells/ml. Baseline $CD4^+$ cell count was defined as the last pretreatment count within 6 months of treatment. If no pretreatment $CD4^+$ cell count was done, the earliest count within 1 month of starting treatment was used for the baseline value.

Table 1 Characteristics of HIV-infected study population on antiretroviral cohort study Henan Province, central China

Characteristics	N (%) N = 339
Sex	
Male	143 (42.2)
Female	194 (57.8)
Median age at inclusion	39 (25–64)
Education	
Primary school or less	218 (64.2)
Middle school or more	119 (35.8)
Marital status	
Married or living with partner	287 (84.6)
Single, divorced or widowed	52 (15.4)
Occupation	
Farmer	327 (96.5)
Other	12 (3.5)
Risk exposure	
Former plasma donor	327 (96.5)
Sexual transmitted	7 (2.1)
Unknown	5 (1.4)
Original combination antiretroviral regimen	
Zidovudine, didanosine, nevirapine	288 (85.0)
Stavudine, didanosine, nevirapine	51 (15.0)
Stopped cART	34 (10.0)
Patients replacing ddI to 3TC	117 (34.5)

In this study, we used plasma specimens of four time points: treatment for 6–18 months; 30-42 months; 54-67 months and 75-102 months. Among the 204 patients, we select 3 patients for Single Genome Amplification (SGA). The criteria was (1) at least 6 time points; (2) no stopping and restarting ART, (3) the results of CD4 count and viral load were all available.

Laboratory methods

Standard genotype HIV drug resistance assay was performed on the specimens in the four time points mentioned above. SGA were performed in 3 patients. They were all performed in the National center for HIV/STD diseases control and prevention, China CDC. In each follow-up, viral load assays were performed by M2000 Biosystem (Abbott Company, USA). The CD4 cell count for all patients were performed by FACSalibur flow cytometer (BD Company, USA).

Viral RNA extraction and standard genotyping

Viral RNA were extracted from plasma samples using QIAamp Viral RNA Mini Kit (QIAGEN company). We used nested RT-PCR process to get a 1.3 kb (2253–3553) fragment of pol gene, the fragment includes Protease amino acid codons 1–99 and Reverse transcriptase amino acid codons 1–300. The sequences of primers for the first round RT-PCR process could be seen below: MAW265′-TTGG AAATGTGGAAAGGAAGGAC-3 and RT215′-CTGTAT TTCTGCTATTAAGTCTTTTGATGGG-3′. PCR temperature was 50°C, 30 min for reverse transcription, 94°C, 10 min for preheat, followed by 94°C, 30 s; 55°C, 30 s; 72°C, 2 min 30 s, 30 cycles. 72°C 10 min for final amplification. In the second round, we got a 1.3 kb fragment using primer RT205′-CTGCCAGTTCTAGCTCTGCTTC-3′ and PRO15′-CAGAGCCAACAGCCCCACCA-3′. PCR temperature was 94°C,10 min for preheat, followed by 94°C, 30 s; 55°C, 30 s; 72°C, 2 min 30 s, 30 cycles. 72°C 10 min for final amplification.

Single genome amplification (SGA)

RNA was extracted from plasma specimens by QIAamp Viral RNA Mini kit (Qiagen, Germany), and was reverse transcript to cDNA by SuperScriptIII protocol according to the manufacturer's instructions (Invitrogen Life-Technologies, USA). We then dilute cDNA to a moderate concentration in 96-well plates, such that fewer than 29 PCRs yielded an amplification product. According to probability theory, once less than 30% PCR reactions get positive results in 96-well plates, it has more than 80% to get each sequence amplified from a single genome [19,20].

We used 3730 Sequencer (ABI company, USA) to get sequences from all the positive amplification products, and use Sequencher (4.10.1) to clean and edit sequence data. In an individual sequence, if there is no ambiguous base pair, it was confirmed that this sequence amplified from a single genome. Finally, we got about 20 such single genome sequences for each time point.

Data analysis (Ka/Ks Ratio of NNRTI associated mutations)

Ka/Ks ratio is a tool to characterize selection pressure of observed amino acid mutations over observed synonymous mutations, the ratio of the number of non-synonymous substitutions per non-synonymous site (Ka) to the number of synonymous substitutions per synonymous site (Ks) [21]. Ka/Ks ratio was used as an indicator of selective pressure acting on a protein-coding gene. A Ka/Ks value of 1 indicates neutral selection, which means amino acid changes are neither being selected for nor against. A Ka/Ks value of < 1 means negative selection pressure. That is, most amino acid changes are baneful and are selected against. The positive selection (Ka/Ks > 1) is much rare, indicating that amino acid changes are favored and may be useful [22].

The concept of correlated mutations is one of the basic ideas in evolutionary biology. The amino acid substitution rates are expected to be limited by functional constraints. Given the functional constraints operating on gene, a mutation in one position can be compensated by an additional mutation. Then mutation patterns can be formed by correlated mutations responsible for specific conditions. Here, we used conditional Ka/Ks ratio (cKa/Ks), which is a metric to measure the effects of mutations at one site on the selection pressure for mutations at another site.

We conducted cKa/Ks ratio analysis on two dataset, one is RT gene sequences of 204 patients using standard HIV genotype sequencing, the other one is RT gene sequences of three patients using Single Genome Amplification. In the two dataset, we had two time points, one was receiving ART for 12 months (10–14 months), and the other time point was receiving ART for over 60 months (56–73 months).

In dataset one, because it is nearly impossible to get gene sequence from plasma samples with suppressed viral load, there were 75 sequences for the first time point, and 74 for the second time point, in dataset two, we had 99 sequences for the first time point and 109 for the second time point. All the cKa/Ks analysis was done by R Language, using the package CorMut (1.2.0, Zhenpeng Li).

Ethics approval

Chinese Center for Disease Control and Prevention research ethics boards approved this study.

Result

General information

Because of transferring to another clinic center, immigrating to other town, not all the 204 patients participated in four follow-ups of this cohort study. There were 184, 148,

200 and 182 patients participated in each follow-up respectively.

The median treatment duration [M(P25 ~ P75)] of the 204 patients was 86.4 months (77.6-98.0 mo). There were 46 patients receiving ART for over 100 months (22.5%). Among the 204 patients, the main age range was 30–45 years (56.4%), maximum for 63, minimum for 24. Male female ratio was 0.6:1.

The frequency of K103N, Y181C and G190A in SGA

The frequencies of three primary NNRTI drug resistance mutations, K103N, Y181C and G190A, fluctuated during long-term ART. More specifically, K103N decreased, while Y181C and G190A showed increasing trend (Table 2).

In the patient HENDRC593, the frequency of K103N showed a decreasing trend, especially from 44.8 months, the K103N vanished in SGA sequences. On the contrary, G190A showed a dramatic increasing trend from the initiation of ART.

In patients ANHDRC106, after taking ART for 23.9 months, K103N and Y181C became dominant mutations (100%), while the frequency of G190A was 10%. In the follow-up time points, K103N showed a decreasing trend and G190A showed an increasing trend, while Y181C maintained dominant.

In patients HENDRC622, K103N showed a decreasing trend from 20.5 to 61.5 months, while G190A kept 100% in quasispecies. The Y181C increased slightly from 0.0% to 31.6% from receiving ART for 44.7 months to 61.5 months

The research of Jiong Wang [23] stated that mutation K101E + G190S replicate better with NNRTI drug. Here we showed the frequency of K101E in each time points. It is interesting that the frequency of K101E changed with G190A. In patient HENDRC593, the frequency of K101E increased from 64.7% to 100% in 49.9 months, while the frequency of G190A increased exactly from 64.7% to 100% in 49.9 months. In patient ANHDRC106, the frequency of K101E increased from 0% to 100% in 46.4 months, while the frequency of G190A increased from 10% to maximum 84.6% in 46.4 months. In patients HENDRC622, the frequency of G190A kept in 100% in nearly all time points, while the frequency of K101E kept under 30%.

Standard genotyping: the frequency of K103N, Y181C and G190A in long-term cohort study

All drug resistance assays were done by 20 December 2012. All the 204 patients took NVP from the initiation of ART treatment and never changed to another NNRTI drug. We collected the treatment and drug resistance results in 4 time points of the 204 patients: 1.ART for 6-18 months; 2. ART for 30-42 months; 3. ART for 54-67 months; 4. ART for 72-102 months. Then we calculated and analyzed the frequency of K103N, Y181C and

Table 2 NNRTI mutations and treatment information for three individual patients in SGA

ART duration	Patient ID	Viral load	CD4 count	K103N	G190A	Y181C	K101E	SGA quantity
20.5	HENDRC593	500	498	6 (35.3)	11 (64.7)	6 (35.3)	11 (64.7)	17
27.5		500	691	8 (42.1)	11 (57.9)	8 (42.1)	11 (57.9)	19
38.9		2976	770	4 (26.7)	11 (73.3)	7 (46.7)	11 (73.3)	15
44.8		91000	655	3 (15.8)	16 (84.2)	5 (26.3)	16 (84.2)	19
49.9		120000	595	0 (0.0)	23 (100.0)	2 (8.7)	23 (100.0)	23
61.5		52000	696	0 (0.0)	16 (94.1)	5 (29.4)	16 (94.1)	17
76.1		170000	551	0 (0.0)	20 (100.0)	9 (45.0)	18 (90.0)	20
23.9	ANHDRC0106	44730	222	10 (100.0)	1 (10.0)	10 (100.0)	0 (0.0)	10
30.1		159000	196	5 (41.7)	3 (25.0)	12 (100.0)	7 (58.3)	12
35.5		94700	255	5 (33.3)	3 (20.0)	15 (100.0)	10 (66.7)	15
42.6		379000	153	3 (21.4)	3 (21.4)	14 (100.0)	11 (78.6)	14
46.4		17600	294	0 (0.0)	11 (84.6)	13 (100.0)	13 (100.0)	13
52.6		33100	256	1 (7.1)	10 (71.4)	14 (100.0)	13 (92.9)	14
20.5	HENDRC622	2076000	104	10 (83.3)	10 (83.3)	0 (0.0)	2 (16.7)	12
27.4		7263	164	14 (93.3)	15 (100.0)	0 (0.0)	1 (6.7)	15
33.0		17160	142	12 (75.0)	16 (100.0)	0 (0.0)	4 (25.0)	16
44.7		13160	138	9 (81.8)	11 (100.0)	0 (0.0)	2 (18.2)	11
49.9		66000	176	9 (90.0)	10 (100.0)	1 (10.0)	1 (10.0)	10
56.8		81000	130	4 (22.2)	18 (100.0)	2 (11.1)	5 (27.8)	18
61.5		39000	181	8 (42.1)	19 (100.0)	6 (31.6)	1 (5.3)	19

G190A in the four time points (Figure 1). Frequency of K103N showed a decreasing trend while both the frequency of Y181C and G190A showed an increasing trend. Specifically, the frequency of K103N had a negative correlation with treatment duration, and mutation G190A had positive correlation with treatment duration. The frequency of mutation Y181C and treatment duration did not show significant correlation.

We also analyzed the frequency of K101E in 204 patients, but here we showed the correlated rate of K101E and G190A in four time points, they were 3/9, 4/16, 7/23, 10/27 (about 30%).

Treatment effect in long-term Nevirapine-contain ART

At the time point of receiving ART for 6–18 months, 84.8% patients had their CD4 cells counts over 200 cells/ml. At the time point of receiving ART for over 72 months, there were still 78.6% (143/182) patients had their CD4 counts over 200 cells/ml.

For viral load, there were 39.1% patients failed to suppress their viral load in initial period (6–18 months). After receiving ART for over 72 months, 44.5% patients failed to suppress their viral load; it indicated that the first-line ART had the possibility to provide treatment effect in 55.5% patients (Table 3).

Besides the 204 patients, we had three patients performed SGA experiments, all of them had received ART for over 50 months, the maximum one is 76.1 months. After long-term ART, the viral load were failed to be suppressed sufficiently, but the CD4 count were kept steady and were similar with the initial time of ART. The long-term ART appeared to postpone the development of HIV virus.

The correlated mutations with K103N, Y181C and G190A (result of cKa/Ks ratio)

In the result of cKa/Ks analysis all positively correlated mutations (cKa/Ks > 1) were listed here in Tables 4 and 5, mutations with cKa/Ks smaller than 1 were not included in the tables. Mutations in Position 1 were the condition mutations, mutations in Position 2 were the accessory mutations that were favored by ART with mutations in Position 1. It showed that M41L, D67N, T69D, K70R, and K219R were the most common NRTI mutations that

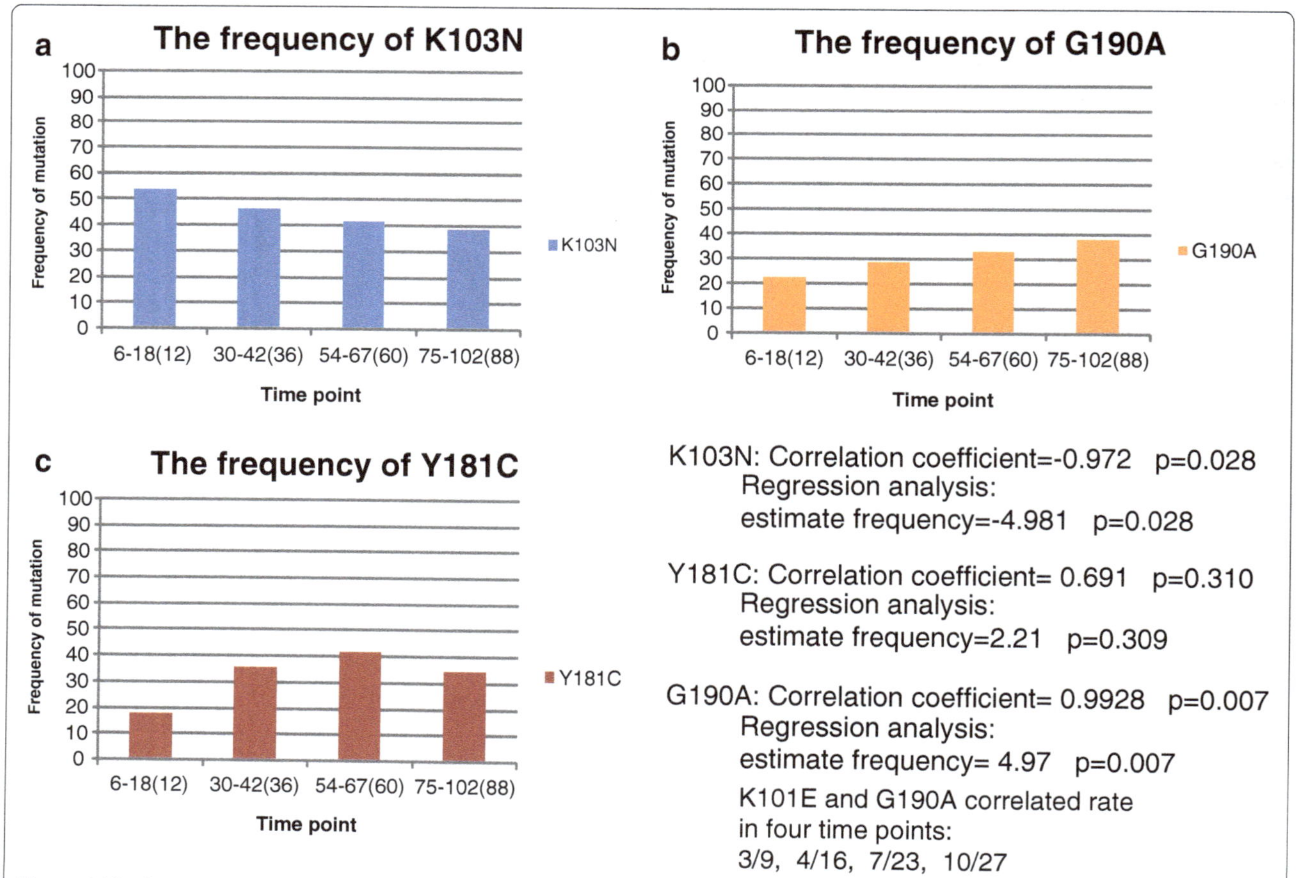

Figure 1 The frequencies of three NNRTI drug resistance mutations in long-term ART treatment. **a**. the frequency of K103N with treatment duration; **b**. the frequency of G190A with treatment duration; **c**. the frequency of Y181C with treatment duration.

Table 3 Treatment effect of long-term ART in 204 patients

Treatment duration(months)	Number of patients	Patients with CD4 > 200 cells/μl	Patients with VL > LDL	Patients with NNRTIdr and CD4 > 200 cells/μl	Patients with NNRTIdr
6-18	184	156 (84.8%)	72 (39.1%)	34 (77.3%)	44
30-42	148	114 (77.0%)	95 (64.2%)	43 (76.8%)	56
54-67	200	147 (73.5%)	105 (52.5%)	49 (70.0%)	70
72-102	182	143 (78.6%)	81 (44.5%)	56 (77.8%)	72

notes:1. The number in this table refer to the number of certain patients, while proportions are in brackets.
2. VL refer to viral load,LDL refer to the lowest detectable viral load of certain method.

associated with the three NNRTI mutations, K103N, Y181C and G190A. In NNRTI mutations besides K103N, Y181C and G190A themselves, H221Y was the most common NNRTI mutations associated with the three NNRTI mutations.

Among K103N, Y181C and G190A, some correlations could be found, but they were not always positively correlated, the correlated mutations network changed with the time of ART. For example, in standard genotype sequencing dataset when receiving ART for 12 months Y181C, G190A and H221Y were positively correlated with K103N, but when receiving ART for over 60 months, Y181C and H221Y were positively correlated with K103N, while G190A was not.

Besides the mutations conferring drug resistance effect, there were a number of accessory mutations or compensatory mutations that correlated with the three NNRTI mutations, more specifically, 5 mutations for G190A in 12 months 14 ones for K103N, and 9 for Y181C. In the dataset of receiving ART for over 60 months, there were 35 mutations that correlated with G190A, 20 mutations for K103N, and 26 mutations for Y181C. It indicated that with the ART extended, more accessory mutations would emerged.

Table 4 Correlated mutations in standard genotype sequencing dataset

	Position1	Mutation type	Position2	Ckaks	Lod
ART for 12 months	K103N	NRTI	M41L	1.5	7.05
		NNRTI	Y181C	1.29	5.17
			G190A	1.6	5.22
			H221Y	5	2.87
	Y181C	NRTI	None	None	None
		NNRTI	H221Y	6	3.45
	G190A	NRTI	None	None	None
		NNRTI	K103S	3	Inf
ART for over 60 months	K103N	NRTI	T69N	1.33	2.39
			K70R	1.17	3.32
		NNRTI	Y181C	1.27	7.16
			H221Y	2.75	5.5
	Y181C	NRTI	D67N	1.8	3.77
			T69N	2.5	5.85
			K70R	5	4.95
		NNRTI	K103N	2	15.78
			H221Y	4	6.05
	G190A	NRTI	D67N	4.8	3.52
			T69N	4	5.71
			K70R	3	3.52
		NNRTI	K101E	6	3.52
			Y181C	1.5	4.11
			K103S	10	Inf

Discussion

This research was based on a cohort study including 204 patients taking first-line ART therapy since early stage infection. By the end of 2012, the median treatment duration was 86.4 months (77.6-98.0 months), including 46 patients received ART for over 100 months (22.5%). In our research, after the ART treatment for over 72 months, 55.5% patients had their viral load suppressed and 78.6% patients kept CD4 counts over 200 cells/ml. It seems that the first-line ART could still possibly be effective after long-term treatment.

Though the first-line ART is potent method to fight against HIV, but the development of drug resistance could make ART less effective [24-27]. NNRTI associated drug resistance mutations could compromise the success of NNRTI-containing ART [28-30]. Among these mutations, K103N Y181C and G190A are the most frequent NNRTI associated drug resistance mutations. In a research on nevirapine-experienced individuals, the frequencies of these mutations were 43%, 46% and 26% respectively [31]. Among the three NNRTI associated mutations, K103N is one of the most clinically important NNRTI resistance mutations; it causes 20- to 50-fold resistance to most available NNRTIs [32,33]. In phenotypic experiments, K103N, Y181C and G190A were defined as the mutations that have almost the same replication fitness with wild type. The rank of fitness among mutant viruses was as follows: wild type (WT) ≥ Y181C ≥ K103N ≥ G190A ≥ V106A ≥ P236L ≥ G190S [34,35]. Besides the replication fitness, K103N can persist for a long time in naive patients, over 2 years in a present case report

Table 5 Correlated mutations in Single Genome Amplification dataset

	Position1	Mutation type	Position2	Ckaks	Lod
ART for 12 months					
	K103N	NRTI	D67N	5	2.93
			T69D	8	Inf
			K70R	16	9.37
		NNRTI	Y181C	26	15.23
			H221Y	17	9.96
	Y181C	NRTI	D67N	5	2.93
			T69D	8	Inf
			K70R	1.12	5.27
		NNRTI	K103N	2	29.44
			H221Y	17	9.96
	G190A	NRTI	None		
		NNRTI	K101E	29	16.98
ART for over 60 months	K103N	NRTI	T69D	12	Inf
		NNRTI	K219R	88	6.75
	Y181C	NRTI	D67N	11.5	14.12
			T69D	2	Inf
		NNRTI	K103N	2.25	9.41
			H221Y	26	15.96
	G190A	NRTI	M41L	21.25	88.84
			D67N	7.33	13.51
			T69D	12	Inf
		NNRTI	K101E	13.8	42.37
			K103N	12	11.47
			Y181C	6.67	24.56
			H221Y	3.33	12.28

Note: **Ckaks** indicates the ka/ks ratio of two mutations. Here, it stands for the ka/ks ratio for M184V and the correlated mutations.
Lod is the confident score for positive selection, If LOD >2, the positive selection is significant.
Inf indicates the maximum infinity.

[36]. K103N also can be found in blood mononuclear cell (PBMC) DNA, with no K103N observed in plasma [37,38]. All the previous research indicated that K103N can steadily exist in plasma and PBMC, and quasispecies with K103N could be more possibly to survive in the surrounding with NVP.

In our research, the result was different with that in vitro study. We found that during the long-term ART treatment, the frequency of K103N, Y181C and G190A were not kept steady, the fact is the frequency of quasispecies with K103N decreased, and could even vanish in SGA sequences, while the proportion of Y181C and G190A could increase from 0% to nearly 100%. This result was also identified in a 204-patinets long-term cohort study.

Based on the results, we estimated that among the three strong NNRTI drug resistance mutations, K103N, Y181C and G190A, there may be some competition process in long-term ART. In the initial period of NVP-containing ART, K103N, Y181C and G190A emerged in different rate among quasispecies which K103N and G190A had a higher rate than Y181C [39]. Consider the fact that three mutations have similar replication fitness and the replication fitness which are associated with mutant prevalence in vivo [40-42]. Mutation emerged late would develop to the proper proportion associated with its replication fitness, while the proportion of mutation emerged earlier would reduced because the late emerged mutation took part of its dominant role. Then these three mutations would finally break the imbalanced and unequal proportion which was established in initial ART period.

The result of cKa/Ks ratio could provide another support for the competition hypothesis. Among the K103N, Y181C and G190A, they were not always positively correlated with each other, but may turn to negative correlation with the time of receiving ART. It indicated that although in vitro study, the three mutations all had high replication rate and less viral fitness reduction than other NNRTI mutations, variants with these mutations were not so strong in vivo when existed in plasma at same time, they were not always favored by variant under ART pressure. Some competition effect among them may change the frequency of these mutations.

Here is a question according to the research of Jiong Wang [42], the reduced fitness for G190A mutants may not explain the increased frequency of G190A variants over time. It is true that G190A alone can reduce viral fitness, but another research of Jiong Wang [23] found that the variant with K101E + G190S replicated better in the presence of NNRTIs than in the absence of drug, it indicate that mutation K101E may have some effect on the mutant of Codon 190 to enhance the viral fitness. In our study, the frequency of K101E had a similar trend with that of G190A in SGA result, and nearly 30% (3/9, 4/16, 7/23, 10/27) K101E emerged with G190A in standard genotyping result. This may partly explain the question that the increasing of G190A frequency in long-term ART.

The further mechanism and detail of the competition process were remaining unclear; we may need next-generation sequencing and other techniques to go deep in this question. At least we believe this changing of NNRTI mutations is crucial in long-term ART treatment, especially for the country with limited antiviral drugs.

Abbreviations

HIV: Human immunodeficiency virus; ART: Antiretroviral therapy; NRTI: Nucleoside reverse transcriptase inhibitors; NNRTI: Non-nucleoside reverse transcriptase inhibitors; PCR: Polymerase chain reaction; TAMs: Thymidine analogue mutations.

Competing interests

The authors declare that they have no competing interests.

Authors' contributions

Conceived and designed the experiments: YCW HX YMS. Performed the experiments: YCW. Analyzed the data: YCW YF. Contributed reagents/materials/analysis tools: PFM, JL, JJW, YHR, and QBZ. Wrote the manuscript: YCW HX. All authors read and approved the final manuscript.

Acknowledgments

We thank Prof. Chunfu Yang (International Laboratory Branch USA CDC) for suggestions and comments. We also thank Pengfei Ma, Peng Hong and Cui He who provided technical support for this work. Jenny Hsi provided outstanding administrative support.

Funding

This work was supported by grants from the Ministry of Science and Technology of China (2008ZX10001-004), Chinese State Key Laboratory for Infectious Disease Develop Grant (2011SKLID102) and Ministry of Science and Technology of China (2012ZX10001-002). This study was also supported by grants from the Guangxi Honor Scholar.

Author details

[1]Beijing Center for Diseases Prevention and Control, Beijing, China. [2]State Key Laboratory for Infectious Disease Prevention and Control, National Center for AIDS/STD Control and Prevention, Chinese Center for Disease Control and Prevention, Collaborative Innovation Center for Diagnosis and Treatment of Infectious Diseases, Beijing, China. [3]Henan Center for Disease Control and Prevention, Zhengzhou, China. [4]Anhui Center for Disease Control and Prevention, Hefei, China.

References

1. Zhang FJ, Pan J, Yu L, Wen Y, Zhao Y: **Current progress of China's free ART program.** *Cell Res* 2005, **15**(11–12):877–882.
2. National Center for AIDS/STD Control and Prevention, China CDC: **2011 Estimates for the HIV/AIDS Epidemic in China.** *Chin J AIDS STD* 2012, **18**(1):1–5.
3. Zhang FJ: **National Free HIV Antiretroviral Treatment Handbook.** *People's Medical Publishing House* 2008, 25–26.
4. World Health Organization: *Antiretroviral therapy for HIV infection in adults and adolescents: recommendations for a public health approach.* Geneva, Switzerland: WHO, HIV Department; 2006. Available at: http://www.who.int/hiv/pub/guidelines/artadultguidelines.pdf. Accessed 12 December 2007.
5. Taylor S, Boffito M, Khoo S, Smit E, Back D: **Stopping antiretroviral therapy.** *AIDS* 2007, **21**:1673–1682.
6. Panel on Antiretroviral Guidelines for Adults and Adolescents: *Guidelines for the use of antiretroviral agents in HIV-1-infected adults and adolescents.* Department of Health and Human Services; 2012. Available at http://www. Siripassorn. AIDS Research and Therapy 2013, 10:4 Page 8 of 9: Accessed [December 5, 2011].
7. van Griensven J, Zachariah R, Rasschaert F, Mugabo J, Atte EF, Reid T: **Stavudine- and nevirapine-related drug toxicity while on generic fixed-dose antiretroviral treatment: incidence, timing and risk factors in a three-year cohort in kigali, rwanda.** *Trans R Soc Trop Med Hyg* 2010, **104**:148–153.
8. Manosuthi W, Sungkanuparph S, Tansuphaswadikul S, Inthong Y, Prasithsirikul W, Chottanapund S, Mankatitham W, Chimsuntorn S, Sittibusaya C, Moolasart V, Chumpathat N, Termvises P, Chaovavanich A: **Incidence and risk factors of nevirapineassociated skin rashes among HIV-infected patients with CD4 cell counts <250 cells/microL.** *Int J STD AIDS* 2007, **18**:782–786.
9. Antinori A, Baldini F, Girardi E, Cingolani A, Zaccarelli M, Di Giambenedetto S, Barracchini A, De Longis P, Murri R, Tozzi V, Ammassari A, Rizzo MG, Ippolito G, De Luca A: **Female sex and the use of anti-allergic agents increase the risk of developing cutaneous rash associated with nevirapine therapy.** *AIDS* 2001, **15**:1579–1581.
10. Johnson VA, Brun-Vezinet F, Clotet B, Gunthard HF, Kuritzkes DR, Pillay D, Schapiro JM, Richman DD: **Update of the drug resistance mutations in HIV-1: December 2009.** *Top HIV Med* 2009, **17**:138–145.
11. Antinori A, Zaccarelli M, Cingolani A, Forbici F, Rizzo MG, Trotta MP, Di Giambenedetto S, Narciso P, Ammassari A, Girardi E, De Luca A, Perno CF: **Cross-resistance among nonnucleoside reverse transcriptase inhibitors limits recycling efavirenz after nevirapine failure.** *AIDS Res Hum Retroviruses* 2002, **18**:835–838.
12. Sinha S, Shekhar RC, Ahmad H: **Prevalence of HIV drug resistance mutation in the northern Indian population after failure of the first line antiretroviral therapy.** *Curr HIV Res* 2012, **10**(6):532–538.
13. Manasa J, Katzenstein D, Cassol S, Newell ML, de Oliveira T: **Primary drug resistance in South Africa: data from 10 years of surveys.** *AIDS Res Hum Retroviruses* 2012, **28**(6):558–565. doi:10.1089/AID.2011.0284. Epub 2012 Mar 12.
14. Lehman DA, Wamalwa DC, McCoy CO, Matsen FA, Langat A, Chohan BH, Benki-Nugent S, Custers-Allen R, Bushman FD, John-Stewart GC, Overbaugh J: **Low-frequency nevirapine resistance at multiple sites may predict treatment failure in infants on nevirapine-based treatment.** *J Acquir Immune Defic Syndr* 2012, **60**(3):225–233. doi 10.1097/QAI.0b013e3182515730.
15. Jiong W, Bambara RA, Demeter LM, Dykes C: **Reduced Fitness in Cell Culture of HIV-1 with Nonnucleoside ReverseTranscriptase Inhibitor-Resistant Mutations Correlates with RelativeLevels of ReverseTranscriptase Content andRNase H Activity in Virions.** *J Virol* 2010, **84**(18):9377–9389.
16. Xu HT, Oliveira M, Quan Y, Bar-Magen T, Wainberg MA: **Differential impact of the HIV-1 non-nucleoside reverse transcriptase inhibitor mutations K103Nand M230L on viral replication and enzyme function.** *J Antimicrob Chemother* 2010, **65**(11):2291–2299. Epub 2010 Sep 18.
17. Bannister WP, Ruiz L, Cozzi-Lepri A, Mocroft A, Kirk O, Staszewski S, Loveday C, Karlsson A, Monforte A, Clotet B, Lundgren JD, EuroSIDA study group: **Comparison of genotypic resistance profiles and virological response between patients starting nevirapine and efavirenz in EuroSIDA.** *AIDS* 2008, **22**(3):367–376.
18. Ceccherini-Silberstein F, Svicher V, Sing T, Artese A, Santoro MM, Forbici F, Bertoli A, Alcaro S, Palamara G, d'Arminio Monforte A, Balzarini J, Antinori A, Lengauer T, Perno CF: **Characterization and structural analysis of novel mutations in human immunodeficiency virus type 1 reverse transcriptase involved in the regulation of resistance to nonnucleoside inhibitors.** *J Virol* 2007, **81**(20):11507–11519.
19. Salazar-Gonzalez JF, Bailes E, Pham KT, Salazar MG, Guffey MB, Keele BF, Derdeyn CA, Farmer P, Hunter E, Allen S, Manigart O, Mulenga J, Anderson JA, Swanstrom R, Haynes BF, Athreya GS, Korber BT, Sharp PM, Shaw GM, Hahn BH: **Deciphering Human Immunodeficiency Virus Type 1 Transmission andEarly Envelope Diversification by Single-Genome Amplificationand Sequencing.** *J Virol* 2008, **82**(8):3952–3970.
20. Butler DM, Pacold ME, Jordan PS, Richman DD, Smith DM: **The efficiency of single genome amplification and sequencing is improved by quantitation and use of a bioinformatics tool.** *J Virol Methods* 2009, **162**(1–2):280–283.
21. Hurst LD: **The Ka/Ks ratio: diagnosing the form of sequence evolution.** *Trends Genet* 2002, **18**:486.
22. Chen L, Perlina A, Lee CJ: **Positive selection detection in 40,000 Human Immunodeficiency Virus (HIV) type 1 sequences automatically identifies drug resistance and positive fitness mutations in HIV protease and reverse transcriptase.** *J Virol* 2004, **2004**:3722–3732.
23. Wang J, Li D, Bambara RA, Dykes C: **Reverse transcriptase backbone can alter the polymerization and RNase activities of non-nucleoside reverse transcriptase mutants K101E + G190S.** *J Gen Virol* 2013, **94**(Pt 10):2297–2308.
24. Zhang F, Haberer JE, Wang Y, Zhao Y, Ma Y, Zhao D, Yu L, Goosby EP: **The Chinese free antiretroviral treatment program: challenges and responses.** *AIDS* 2007, **21**(Suppl 8):S143–S148.
25. DeGruttola V, Dix L, D'Aquila R, Holder D, Phillips A, Ait-Khaled M, Baxter J, Clevenbergh P, Hammer S, Harrigan R, Katzenstein D, Lanier R, Miller M, Para M, Yerly S, Zolopa A, Murray J, Patick A, Miller V, Castillo S, Pedneault L, Mellors J: **The relation between baseline HIV drug resistance and response to antiretroviral therapy: re-analysis of retrospective and prospective studies using a standardized data analysis plan.** *Antivir Ther* 2000, **5**:41–48.
26. D'Aquila RT, Johnson VA, Welles SL, Japour AJ, Kuritzkes DR, DeGruttola V, Reichelderfer PS, Coombs RW, Crumpacker CS, Kahn JO, Richman DD: **Zidovudine resistance and HIV-1 disease progression during antiretroviral therapy. AIDS Clinical Trials Group Protocol 116B/117 Team and the Virology Committee Resistance Working Group.** *Ann Intern Med* 1995, **122**:401–408.

27. Zolopa AR, Shafer RW, Warford A, Montoya JG, Hsu P, Katzenstein D, Merigan TC, Efron B: **HIV-1genotypic resistance patterns predict response to saquinavir-ritonavir therapy in patients in whom previous protease inhibitor therapy had failed.** *Ann Intern Med* 1999, **131**:813–821.
28. Jourdain G, Ngo-Giang-Huong N, Le Coeur S, Bowonwatanuwong C, Kantipong P, Leechanachai P, Ariyadej S, Leenasirimakul P, Hammer S, Lallemant M, Perinatal HIV Prevention Trial Group: **Intrapartum exposure to nevirapine and subsequent maternal responses to nevirapine-based antiretroviral therapy.** *N Engl J Med* 2004, **351**:229–240.
29. Lockman S, Shapiro RL, Smeaton LM, Wester C, Thior I, Stevens L, Chand F, Makhema J, Moffat C, Asmelash A, Ndase P, Arimi P, van Widenfelt E, Mazhani L, Novitsky V, Lagakos S, Essex M: **Response to antiretroviral therapy after a single, peripartum dose of nevirapine.** *N Engl J Med* 2007, **356**:135–147.
30. Stringer JSA, McConnell MS, Kiarie J, Bolu O, Anekthananon T, Jariyasethpong T, Potter D, Mutsotso W, Borkowf CB, Mbori-Ngacha D, Muiruri P, Ong'ech JO, Zulu I, Njobvu L, Jetsawang B, Pathak S, Bulterys M, Shaffer N, Weidle PJ: **Effectiveness of non-nucleoside reverse-transcriptase inhibitor-based antiretroviral therapy in women previously exposed to a single intrapartum dose ofnevirapine: a multi-countrym, Prospective Cohort Study.** *PLoS Med* 2010, **7**:e1000233.
31. Reuman EC, Rhee SY, Holmes SP, Shafer RW: **Constrained patterns of covariation and clustering of HIV-1 non-nucleoside reverse transcriptase inhibitor resistance mutations.** *J Antimicrob Chemother* 2010, **65**(7):1477–1485.
32. Casado JL, Hertogs K, Ruiz L, Dronda F, Van Cauwenberge A, Arnó A, Garcia-Arata I, Bloor S, Bonjoch A, Blazquez J, Clotet B, Larder B: **Non-nucleoside reverse transcriptase inhibitor resistance among patients failing a nevirapine plus protease inhibitor-containing regimen.** *AIDS* 2000, **14**:F1–F7.
33. Joly V, Moroni M, Concia E, Lazzarin A, Hirschel B, Jost J, Chiodo F, Bentwich Z, Love WC, Hawkins DA, Wilkins EG, Gatell AJ, Vetter N, Greenwald C, Freimuth WW, de Cian W: **Delavirdine in combination with zidovudine in treatment of human immunodeficiency virus type 1-infected patients: evaluation of efficacy and emergence of viral resistance in a randomized, comparative phase III trial.** *Antimicrob Agents Chemother* 2000, **44**:3155–3157.
34. Wang J, Bambara RA, Demeter LM, Dykes C: **Reduced fitness in cell culture of HIV-1 with nonnucleoside reverse transcriptase inhibitor-resistant mutations correlates with relative levels of reverse transcriptase content and RNase H activity in Virions[J].** *J Virol* 2010, **9**:9377–9389.
35. Xu HT, Oliveira M, Quan YJ, Bar-Magen T, Wainberg MA: **Differential impact of the HIV-1 non-nucleoside reverse transcriptase inhibitor mutations K103Nand M230L on viral replication and enzyme function[J].** *Antimicrob Chemother* 2010, **65**(11):2291–2299.
36. Zaccarelli M, Marconi P, Visco-Comandini U, Liuzzi G, Sette P, Acinapura R, Mosti S, Ammassari A, Perno CF, Antinori A: **Evidence of dual sexual transmission of multi-resistant HIV with two years persistence of resistance to NRTI and NNRTI: a case report.** *Infection* 2008, **36**(2):178–180.
37. Saladini F, Vicenti I, Razzolini F, Zazzi M: **Detection of residual human immunodeficiency virus type 1 reverse transcriptase K103N minority species in plasma RNA and peripheral blood mononuclear cell DNA following discontinuation of non-nucleoside therapy.** *Clin Microbiol Infect* 2010, **16**(7):848–851.
38. Loubser S, Balfe P, Sherman G, Hammer S, Kuhn L, Morris L: **Decay of K103N mutants in cellular DNA and plasma RNA after single-dose nevirapine to reduce mother-to-child HIV transmission.** *AIDS* 2006, **20**(7):995–1002.
39. Boltz VF, Zheng Y, Lockmanc S, Hong F, Halvas EK, McIntyre J, Currier JS, Chibowa MC, Kanyama C, Nair A, Owino-Ong'or W, Hughes M, Coffin JM, Mellors JW: **Role of low-frequency HIV-1 variants in failure of nevirapine-containing antiviral therapy in women previously exposed to single-dose nevirapine.** *Proc Natl Acad Sci U S A* 2011, **108**(22):9202–9207.
40. Archer RH, Dykes C, Gerondelis P, Lloyd A, Fay P, Reichman RC, Bambara RA, Demeter LM: **Mutants of human immunodeficiency virus type 1 (HIV-1) reverse transcriptase resistant to nonnucleoside reverse transcriptase inhibitors demonstrate altered rates of RNase H cleavage that correlate with HIV-1 replication fitness in cell culture.** *J Virol* 2000, **74**:8390–8401.
41. Gerondelis P, Archer RH, Palaniappan C, Reichman RC, Fay PJ, Bambara RA, Demeter LM: **The P236L delavirdine-resistant human immunodeficiency virus type 1 mutant is replication defective and demonstrates alterations in both RNA 5'-end- and DNA 3'-end-directed RNase H activities.** *J Virol* 1999, **73**:5803–5813.
42. Wang J, Dykes C, Domaoal RA, Koval CE, Bambara RA, Demeter LM: **The HIV-1 reverse transcriptase mutants G190S and G190A, which confer resistance to non-nucleoside reverse transcriptase inhibitors, demonstrate reductions in RNase H activity and DNA synthesis from tRNA(Lys, 3) that correlate with reductions in replication efficiency.** *Virology* 2006, **348**:462–474.

23

Defining the fitness of HIV-1 isolates with dual/mixed co-receptor usage

Immaculate L Nankya[1,2,3], Denis M Tebit[1,4], Awet Abraha[1], Fred Kyeyune[1,2,3], Richard Gibson[1], Oyebisi Jegede[1,5], Gabrielle Nickel[1] and Eric J Arts[1,2*]

Abstract

Background: CCR5-using (r5) HIV-1 predominates during asymptomatic disease followed by occasional emergence of CXCR4-using (x4) or dual tropic (r5x4) virus. We examined the contribution of the x4 and r5 components to replicative fitness of HIV-1 isolates.

Methods: Dual tropic r5x4 viruses were predicted from average HIV-1 env sequences of two primary subtype C HIV-1 isolates (C19 and C27) and from two patient plasma samples (B12 and B19). Chimeric Env viruses with an NL4-3 backbone were constructed from the B12 and B19 env sequences. To determine replicative fitness, these primary and chimeric dual tropic HIV-1 were then competed against HIV-1 reference isolates in U87.CD4 cells expressing CXCR4 or CCR5 or in PBMCs ± entry inhibitors. Contribution of the x4 and r5 clones within the quasispecies of these chimeric or primary HIV-1 isolates were then compared to the frequency of x4, r5, and dual tropic clones within the quasispecies as predicted by phenotypic assays, clonal sequencing, and 454 deep sequencing.

Results: In the primary HIV-1 isolates (C19 and C27), subtype C dual tropic clones dominated over x4 clones while pure r5 clones were absent. In two subtype B chimeric viruses (B12 and B19), r5 clones were >100-fold more abundant than x4 or r5/x4 clones. The dual tropic C19 and C27 HIV-1 isolates outcompeted r5 primary HIV-1 isolates, B2 and C3 in PBMCs. When AMD3100 was added or when only U87.CD4.CCR5 cells were used, the B2 and C3 reference viruses now out-competed the r5 component of the dual tropic C19 and C27. In contrast, the same replicative fitness was observed with dualtropic B12 and B19 HIV-1 isolates relative to x4 HIV-1 A8 and E6 or the r5 B2 and C3 viruses, even when the r5 or x4 component was inhibited by maraviroc (or AMD3100) or in U87.CD4.CXCR4 (or CCR5) cells.

Conclusions: In the dual tropic HIV-1 isolates, the x4 replicative fitness is higher than r5 clones but the x4 or x4/r5 clones are typically at low frequency in the intrapatient virus population. Ex vivo HIV propagation promotes outgrowth of the x4 clones and provides an over-estimate of x4 dominance in replicative fitness within dual tropic viruses.

Keywords: HIV-1 fitness, Co-receptor usage, Entry inhibitors

Background

Human immunodeficiency virus entry into host cells involves binding to CD4 and one of two coreceptors, namely CCR5 and CXCR4, hence the two viral phenotypes, the r5- and x4-using viruses. CCR5 is expressed in conjunction with surface CD4 on activated lymphocytes, macrophages, dendritic cells, and brain cells, while CXCR4 with CD4 are found on the surface of resting T cells and monocytes [1–3]. Although other chemokine receptors can mediate low level HIV-1 entry [4, 5], CCR5 and CXCR4 remain the primary co-receptors for all diverse HIV-1 subtypes as well as other primary lentiviruses, e.g. HIV-2, simian immunodeficiency virus from chimpanzees, sooty mangabeys, and African green monkeys [6–9]. The r5 HIV-1 variants are preferentially transmitted and predominate during the asymptomatic period of infection whereas x4 HIV-1 emerges late in disease and in less than 50 % of patients [10–13].

*Correspondence: eja3@case.edu
[1] Division of Infectious Diseases, Department of Medicine, Case Western Reserve University, 10900 Euclid Ave., Cleveland, OH 44106, USA
Full list of author information is available at the end of the article

HIV-1 entry into host cells is almost exclusively triggered by Env glycoproteins. In fact, expression of only HIV-1 Env in an effector cell can mediate fusion with a target cell expressing CD4 and a co-receptor (reviewed in [14]). During virus assembly, the Env gp160 precursor is cleaved by cellular proteases into the membrane spanning gp41 and the soluble gp120 subunits, which remain covalently linked through a disulfide bridge [15]. On the virus particle, Env gp120/gp41 form trimer spikes that mediate virus attachment to the receptor complex on the cell surface (reviewed in [14]). First, a conserved C4 region in gp120 interacts with the amino-terminal extracellular immunoglobulin-like domain of the CD4 receptor. Upon interaction with CD4, the V3 loop of gp120 can engage the second extracellular loop of CCR5 (or CXCR4) while a gp120 conformational change exposes a second Env site (comprised in part by the C2 region) to bind with the N terminus of the co-receptor.

Although the V3 loop appears to define selective binding of either CCR5 or CXCR4, specificity for a particular co-receptor also appears to extend to other regions throughout gp120 [16–18]. Specifically, the V1/V2 loops on HIV-1 gp120 can influence co-receptor usage but not as efficiently as the V3 domain [19–21]. Differential interaction with the co-receptors may be related to the higher negative charge of the second extracellular loop of CXCR4 compared to that of CCR5, which may in turn favor binding to a more positively charged gp120 V3 loop [22, 23]. Several algorithms/models have been developed to predict HIV-1 co-receptor usage from the amino sequence in Env. Geno2Pheno and PSSM are algorithms based solely on the V3 loop sequence and are generally greater than 85 % accurate in predicting co-receptor usage by HIV-1 subtype B strains [24–27]. Both of these models are heavily weighted by positive charges at amino acid positions 11 and/or 25 in the V3 loop, which are nearly absolute in predicting CXCR4 usage. In addition, Phenoseq a new program has the ability to predict coreceptor usage for all the major subtypes.

The switch from r5 to x4 virus has been associated with rapid depletion of CD4+ T cells [28, 29]. Patients harboring x4 viruses progress to AIDS more rapidly than those harboring exclusively r5 viruses implying that CXCR4 utilization is linked to a stronger pathogenic phenotype and a switch to CXCR4 utilization is a causative factor in disease progression, this has been mainly studied in subtype B [28, 30, 31]. However, this hypothesis is quite controversial considering that CD4 cell decline is observed in nearly all HIV-infected patients despite the fact that only 50 % switch from r5 to x4 viruses and only late in disease among subtype B individuals. A switch in coreceptor usage rarely occurs in subtype C. Three main hypotheses for the switch in coreceptor usage have been proposed. The transmission-mutation hypothesis proposes that predominance of r5 viruses during transmission and early infection is due to active selection of r5 and that the coreceptor switch is a result of virus evolution during the course of disease [29]. The target cell-based hypothesis is based on the inability of quiescent, naïve CXCR4+/CD4+ T cells to support HIV-1 replication whereas the memory CCR5+/CD4+ T cells are activated at a higher frequency and as such, support greater HIV-1 replication [32, 33]. With the depletion of the memory T cell population, there would be a shift in cells that support x4 versus r5 replication. Finally, the immune-control hypothesis assumes that x4 viruses are recognized better by the immune system than r5 viruses [34, 35]. Thus, x4 viruses would only emerge later in infection due in part to poor virologic control by a dysfunctional immune response. This hypothesis also suggests that emergence of x4 over r5 variants relates to higher replicative fitness [36]. However, increased sensitivity of CXCR4-using virus compared to CCR5-using virus to autologous neutralizing antibodies is not supported by other studies [37].

These hypotheses generally focus on the displacement of r5 HIV-1 by x4 HIV-1 late in disease progression but do not necessarily account for dual tropic HIV-1 variants. An HIV-1 isolate that utilizes both CCR5 and CXCR4 for entry is commonly referred to as dual tropic (r5x4). However, the intrapatient dual/mixed (dm) may be any combination of HIV-1 clones using just CCR5 or CXCR4 for entry (x4 or r5 HIV-1) in addition to clones capable of infecting both CD4+/CCR5+ and CD4+/CXCR4+ cells (r5x4 HIV-1). The contribution of the r5, x4, and r5x4 to the replicative fitness of an HIV-1 isolate is poorly understood but could be consequential to disease progression. Dominance of pure x4 variants within the intrapatient HIV-1 population at any time, even in late disease is relatively rare. Instead, most HIV-1 isolates that appear to prefer CXCR4 for host cell entry still retain the ability to infect CD4+/CCR5+ cells.

In previous studies, we performed hundreds of competitions between HIV-1 isolates of all group M subtypes with a focus of subtype C strains [38–40]. Subtype C isolates were substantially less fit than all other group M isolates when competed in head-to-head pair-wise competitions in PBMC cultures using a set of r5 and x4 HIV-1 isolates [40]. Two subtype C HIV-1 isolates (C19 and C27) capable of infecting CD4+/CXCR4+ cells were dual tropic (i.e. also capable of infecting CD4+/CCR5+ cells). Thus, the reduced fitness of at least two of these "x4" subtype C isolates may be related to the r5x4 phenotype, especially if there was a high proportion of pure r5 HIV-1 isolates in the C19 and C27 HIV-1 isolates. In almost all cases, x4 HIV-1 have faster replication kinetics than r5 HIV-1 isolates when performing dual infections of PBMCs [40, 41]. This dual infection is not a "true" competition considering that the r5 and x4 viruses likely replicate in different susceptible cells within the PBMC population. In this study, we examined the impact of both the "CXCR4"-using and "CCR5"-using clones to the replicative fitness of r5x4 HIV-1 isolates in CD4+/CCR5+ cells, CD4+/CXCR4+ cells, and in the mixed cell population found in PBMCs. We also competed the r5x4 HIV-1 isolates against r5 or x4 primary HIV-1 isolates in the presence of AMD3100 (CXCR4 antagonist) or MVC (CCR5 antagonist) to further confirm relative fitness of each phenotype in the dual tropic HIV-1 isolates. Finally, the contribution of the r5 and x4 component to replicative fitness of the primary HIV-1 isolates was compared to the sum of its parts by characterizing or predicting the co-receptor usage of the representative clones in these dual tropic virus populations.

Dual tropic and dm viruses are commonly observed in HIV infected patients and are frequently responsible for failure of maraviroc treatment. Treatment failure of maraviroc can result from the emergence of resistant CCR5 (r5)- using viruses with reduced susceptibility to MVC [42–45]. The contribution of the CCR5(r5)- and CXCR4(x4)-using component of the intrapatient HIV-1 population to overall virus replication in susceptible cells is poorly understood. Each component of the dual tropic and dm virus can replicate in different T cell and macrophage subsets. In this study, we have determined the contribution of the r5-using and x4-using components of dm and dual tropic HIV on replicative fitness and determine if a specific phenotype may be dominant in disease.

Results

Identification of dual tropic HIV-1 isolates from patient samples

Two methods were employed to isolate HIV-1 from patient samples and then screen for viral tropism. The first method involved initial co-cultivation of PBMCs from an HIV-infected patient with PBMCs from an HIV-negative donor (Fig. 1a). These standard co-cultivations were performed on a set of patient samples from Zimbabwe as previously described [40]. This initial analysis screened over 28 HIV-1 isolates and found 10 that were syncytium inducing (SI) and capable of replicating on MT2 cells [46]. These primary SI HIV-1 were then equalized for RT activity (see "Methods") and added to U87.CD4 cells expressing either CCR5 or CXCR4 [40] (Fig. 1b). Two (C19 and C27) of 10 primary HIV-1 isolates were dual tropic, i.e. capable of infecting and replicating in U87.CD4 cells expressing either CXCR4 or CCR5 as a co-receptor. HIV-1 C23 showed CCR5 (r5) just above the limit of detection whereas the remaining strains in this cohort were CXCR4 (x4) as previously described.

As part of another study that screened for co-receptor usage, HIV-1 env chimeric viruses were produced by homologous recombination in yeast rather than propagating HIV-1 from patient samples (Fig. 1c). The yeast-based recombination/gap repair cloning method can efficiently replace the yeast URA3 gene with the gp120 coding region of the env gene in our pREC_nfl_HIV-$1_{NL4\text{-}3}\Delta$gp120/URA3 vector (see "Methods") [44, 47]. The efficiency of this cloning method limits the genetic bottleneck introduced by prolonged PBMC co-cultivation and subsequent virus propagations. Following env cloning, the pREC_nfl_env_{Ptx} vectors from each patient sample (Ptx—patient x) were purified from pooled yeast colonies (>1,000) and transfected into 293T cells. We have recently described an efficient cell-to-cell fusion assay to screen for co-receptor usage using the U87.CD4.CXCR4 or U87.CD4.CCR5 as target cells [48]. In our preliminary screen of 11 patient-derived env chimeric viruses, we identified three dual tropic HIV Envs (B9, B12, and B19), five r5s, and two x4s (Fig. 1d). The pREC_nfl_env vectors of B9, B12, and B19 were co-transfected with the complementing vector (pCMV_cplt) to produce replication-competent chimeric HIV as described [47]. This virus was then used to infect U87.CD4.CXCR4 and U87.CD4.CCR5 cells to confirm co-receptor usage. HIV-1 env_B9 did not replicate in either cell line.

The x4 and r5 titers of each dual tropic primary and dual tropic env chimeric HIV-1 isolate along with a set of reference HIV-1 isolates were measured by standard $TCID_{50}$ assays on U87.CD4.CXCR4 and U87.CD4.CCR5 cells, respectively (Fig. 1e). The dual tropic C19 and C27 viruses had equal infectious r5 and x4 titers whereas the dual tropic env_B12 and env_B19 viruses had higher r5 than x4 titers. Interestingly, the infectious titers derived from $TCID_{50}$ assays using HIV-negative PBMCs was the same as the highest infectious titers from either U87.CD4.CXCR4 or U87.CD4.CCR5 cells. For at least the C19 and C27 viruses, the IU/ml on PBMCs did not reflect the simple addition of r5 and x4 infectious units suggesting that the clones within these dual tropic HIV-1 isolates may be primarily dual tropic rather than a mix of r5- and x4-only HIV-1 clones (Additional file 1: Table S1).

Phylogenetic analyses of the dm HIV-1 isolates and env chimeric viruses

Alignment of the env sequences confirmed that the bulk populations of the dual tropic C19 and C27 were subtype C whereas dual tropic env_B12 and env_B19 aligned with other subtype B HIV-1 sequences (Fig. 2a). In addition, the B12, B19, C19, and C27 viruses were not clonal but rather a population of related env sequences, based on approximately 10–15 sequenced clones from each (Fig. 2b–e).

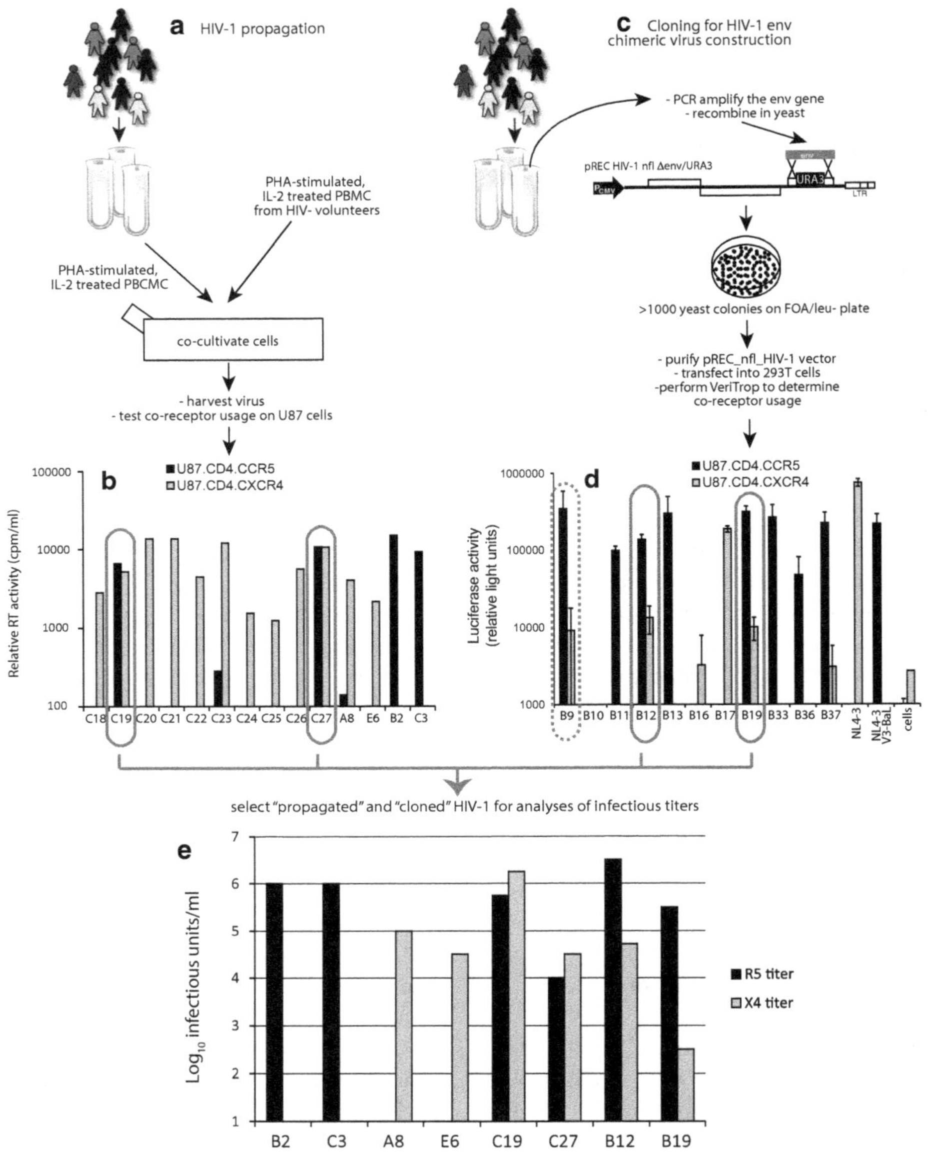

Fig. 1 Identification of dual/mixed isolates following HIV-1 propagation or construction of env chimeric viruses. **a** HIV-1 subtype C isolates from Zimbabwe were propagated by PBMC co-cultivation as described [46] and in the "Methods". **c** The HIV-1 env coding region of HIV-1 subtype B infected patients was PCR amplified and then cloned into pREC_nfl_HIV-$1_{nl4\text{-}3}\Delta$gp120/URA3 via yeast recombination/gap repair [47]. The propagated HIV-1 isolates (**a**) and cloned env genes expressed following 293T transfection (**c**) were screened for co-receptor usage by infection(1) (**b**) or cell-to-cell fusion (**d**) (Veritrop; [48]) on U87.CD4 cells expressing either CXCR4 or CCR5(2). In the virus infection system (**b**), virus production was monitored by RT activity in supernatant [87]. In the cell-to-cell fusion assay (**d**), the ability of pREC_nfl_env_{ptX} to modulate receptor binding and cell fusion was monitored by firefly luciferase activity, i.e. Rev/Tat in the effector cell controlling Luc expression under the control of the HIV-1 LTR and rescued via the RRE housed in an intron with Luc [80]. Two primary HIV-1 isolates and two env chimeric viruses were propagated to measure infectious titers on PBMCs (Additional file 1: Table S1), U87.CD4.CCR5 and U87.CD4.CXCR4 cells (**e**) using the classical Reed–Munch approach [79].

Contribution of x4 and r5 variants to replicative fitness in dual tropic and mixed r5x4 primary HIV-1 isolate

In a previous study, we performed two pairwise competition experiments in PBMC cultures with 14 primary r5 and 15 x4 HIV-1 isolates [40]. The phylogenetic relationships of these are shown in Fig. 2. To summarize, both the r5 and x4 HIV-1 subtype C isolates were less fit than the r5 and x4 HIV-1 isolates (respectively) of different group M subtypes. The poor replicative fitness of subtype C isolates has now been observed in over 2,000

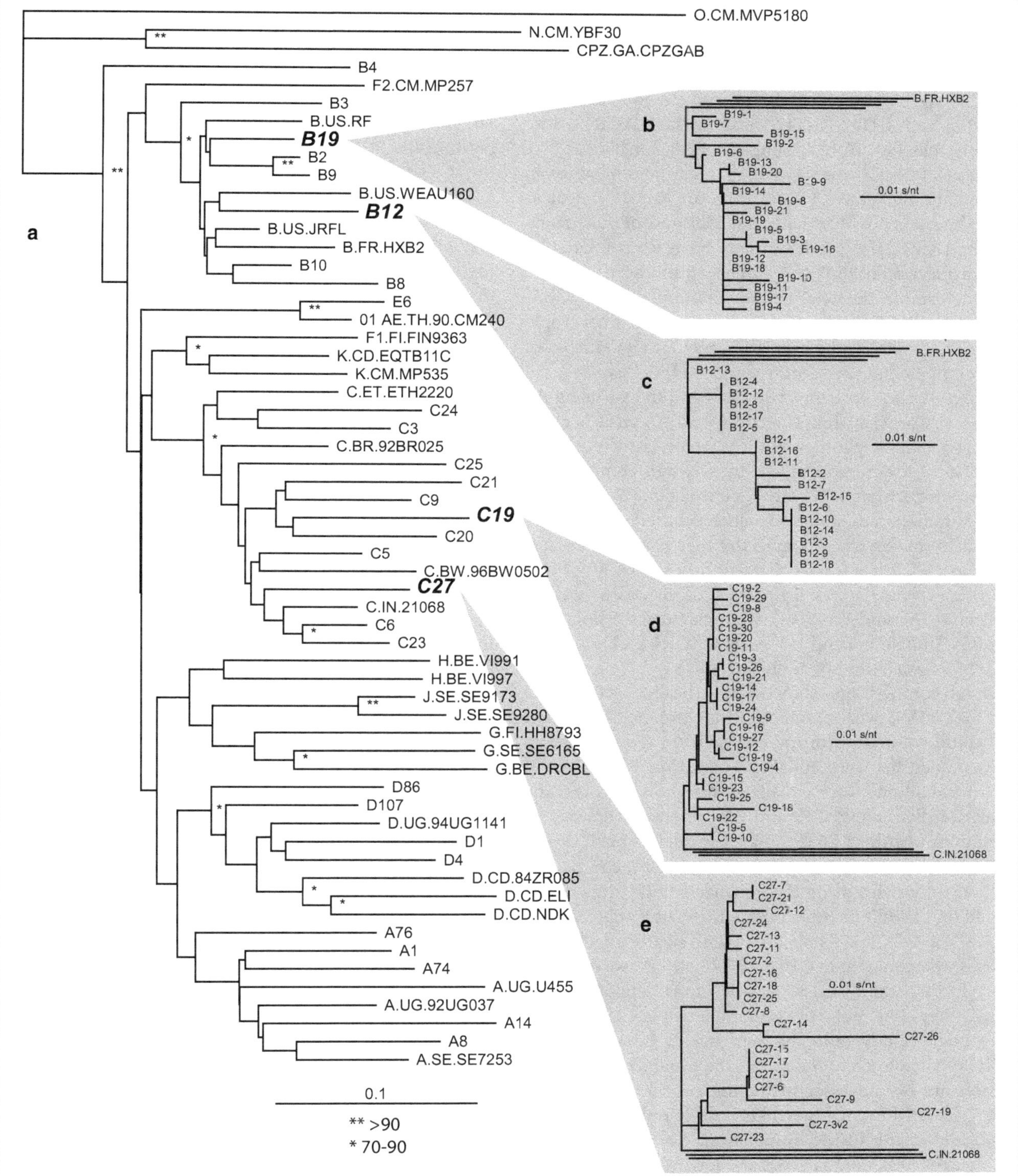

Fig. 2 Neighbor joining phylogenic trees of two dual tropic HIV-1 isolates, two HIV-1 env chimeric viruses, and of the sampled clones in their virus population. Alignments and phylogenetic trees were constructed for the C2-V3 region (350 nt) of the four reference strains, r5 B2, r5 C3, x4 A8, and x4 E6, the two dual tropic HIV-1 isolates (C19 and C27), the two HIV-1 env chimeric viruses (B12 and B19) and set of reference strains (**a**). As described in the "Methods", the Env coding region of two dual/mixed (dm) HIV-1 isolates were PCR amplified and cloned into pREC env via yeast-based recombination. The C2-V3 sequences from 21 B19 (**b**), 18 B19 (**c**), 26 C19 (**d**), 21 © clones (**e**) were aligned using MUSCLE and then schematic represented in phylogenetic trees.

head-to-head competitions with over 40 primary subtype C HIV-1 isolates [38–40, 49]. Although ten x4 HIV-1 subtype C isolates were dramatically less fit than any other x4 HIV-1 isolate, we also noted that two isolates, C19 and C27 were of a dual tropic phenotype and capable of infecting both CD4+/CCR5+ and CD4+/CXCR4+ susceptible cells [40]. When competing r5 against x4 HIV-1 isolates in PBMCs, the x4 viruses, regardless of subtype, had higher replicative fitness than an r5 HIV-1 isolate [40]. Thus, it is possible that reduced fitness of dual tropic C19 and C27 HIV-1 isolates may have been related to high proportion of r5 HIV-1 clones within these viruses.

To determine the relative contribution of the CCR5-using and CXCR4-using phenotypes in these dual tropic r5x4 HIV-1 isolates, the r5x4 C19 and C27 HIV-1 isolates were competed against four reference HIV-1 isolates, the r5-using B2 and C3 primary isolates and the x4-using A8 and E6 viruses (Fig. 1e). The control x4 A8 virus is characterized as having a high replicative fitness whereas the x4 E6 is of lower replicative fitness when compared in direct competition with other x4 isolates [39, 40]. Our control r5 B2 virus was also selected based on a higher replicative fitness as compared to other r5 HIV-1 isolates whereas r5 C3 has low replicative fitness [39, 40]. First, the titers of dual tropic C19 and C27 viruses as well as control x4 A8 and E6 HIV-1 were calculated using both PBMCs ("full" titer) and U87.CD4.CXCR4 ("x4" titer) for $TCID_{50}$ assays (Additional file 1: Table S1).

Direct competitions showed that the dual tropic C19 and C27 HIV-1 were completely outcompeted by A8 but still could compete with the x4 E6 HIV-1 (Fig. 3a), when virus inoculums were equalized based on PBMC titers. When inoculums were equalized based on x4 titers, the fitness of dual tropic C19 and C27 further decreased in competition with x4 E6 (Fig. 3a). The dual tropic C19 and C27 were then competed in PBMCs against the r5 B2 and C3 control viruses using the equalized "full" titers determined on PBMCs or the equalized "r5" titers determined on U87.CD4.CCR5. As observed with nearly all x4-using viruses, the dual tropic C19 and C27 HIV-1 isolates were more fit than the r5 C3 virus when inoculating with the PBMC titers (Fig. 3b). However, dual tropic C19 and C27 were only slightly more fit than the r5 B2 HIV-1. The "CXCR4"-using component of the dual tropic HIV-1 isolates are not necessarily in competition with these r5 HIV-1 in PBMC since they likely infect different susceptible cells in the PBMC population. Competitions with the control r5 B2 HIV-1 suggest a low frequency of an r5 phenotype in the dual tropic C19 and C27 viruses. When using U87.CD4.CCR5-derived titers, it was not surprising that C19 and C27 could further out replicate the r5 B2 and C3 viruses (Fig. 3b) in competition considering the fivefold increase in C19 and C27 inocula to equalize their "r5" titer with the titer of pure r5 B2 and C3 viruses.

In the competitions performed in PBMC cultures with PBMC-derived titers, C19 and C27 could replicate and compete with either the r5 (B2 and C3) or the x4 (A8 and E6) viruses (Fig. 3). In Fig. 4, we performed the same competitions as in Fig. 3 but prevented replication of either the "CXCR4"-using component (panel A) or the "CCR5"-using component (panel C) of the dual tropic C19 and C27 viruses. First, the C19+A8, C19+E6, C27+A8, and C27+E6 dual infections were added in equal "x4" titers (determined on U87.CD4.CXCR4 cells) to PBMC cultures in the presence of high maraviroc (MVC) concentrations. As described in Fig. 4b, the IC_{99} concentration of MVC, a CCR5 antagonist [50, 51], resulted in complete inhibition of the r5 B2 and C3 viruses but no apparent inhibition of C19 and C27 in PBMCs. Lack of C19 and C27 inhibition by MVC suggests that the majority of the HIV-1 clones in these quasispecies may be dual tropic (r5/x4) and fully capable of infecting CXCR4+ cells in the PBMC cultures such that MVC does not inhibit any virus replication. The composition of the quaispecies in terms of co-receptor usage is described below (Fig. 1). Interestingly, there was no significant difference in the replicative fitness of C19 or C27 (versus control x4 A8 or E6 HIV-1) when comparing results of competitions performed in PBMCs, PBMCs + MVC, or in U87.CD4.CXCR4 cells (Fig. 4a). The latter condition would only support replication of the control x4 viruses and the "CXCR4"-using component of the dual tropic viruses. The reference viruses A8 and E6 were significantly more fit than the "CXCR4"-using component of the dual tropic C19 and C27 viruses regardless of the above conditions (Fig. 3a).

To limit replication to only the "CCR5"-using component of the dual tropic viruses, we performed competitions in PBMCs + AMD3100 or in U87.CD4.CCR5 cell cultures with the "r5" titers of these viruses. AMD3100, a CXCR4 antagonist [52, 53], showed strong inhibition of x4 A8 and E6 viruses as well as the dual tropic C19 and C27 viruses whereas the r5 B2 and C3 viruses were largely unaffected (Fig. 4d). Reduction in B2 and C3 replication, as compared to no-drug controls, relates to the cellular toxicity from high AMD3100 concentrations, i.e. required for complete inhibition of x4 virus replication but this did not have an effect on the competition experiments as later shown with the B12 and B19 viruses. Whereas the dual tropic C19 and C27 could easily out replicate the r5 B2 and C3 viruses in PBMC cultures, the "CCR5"-using component of these viruses were significantly less fit than B2 and C3 (Fig. 4c). This data is consistent with the relatively weak fitness of r5 subtype C HIV-1 isolates [38–40, 49]. Again these were based only

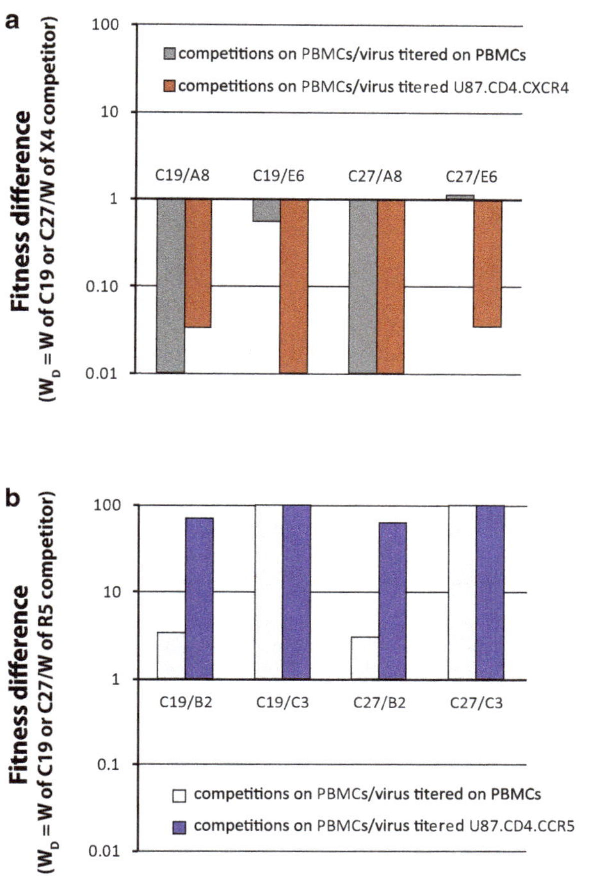

Fig. 3 Relative replicative fitness of the dual tropic C19 and C27 HIV-1 when competed against reference strains on PBMCs. **a** The dual tropic HIV-1 isolates, C19 and C27 were competed against the x4 reference strains, A8 and E6 on PBMC using equal MOIs (0.004) of each virus tittered on U87.CD4.CXCR4 cells or PBMCs (same donor and blood draw as those used in competition). **b** A similar set of competitions on PBMCs involved the same dm viruses competed against the r5 reference strains, B2 and C3 using equal MOIs tittered on U87.CD4.CCR5 cells or PBMCs. Fitness difference (or ratio) is shown with all competitions where the relative fitness of the dual tropic HIV-1 isolate is plotted as a ratio to the relative fitness of the reference virus in the competition. The titers of all dual tropic and reference HIV-1 isolates are shown in Additional file 1: Table S1.

on the r5 phenotype present as r5 or r5/x4 clones in the quasispecies in C19 and C27. Thus, use of AMD3100 with PBMCs or U87.CD4.CCR5 cells would limit replication to only the CCR5-using and r5/x4 components on CCR5+ cells. In PBMCs (without drug) where the "CXCR4" component was not inhibited, the C19 and C27 were 50- to 100-fold more fit than the r5 B2 and C3 controls. After eliminating replication of the pure CXCR4-component with AMD3100, the r5 competitors, B2 and C3 were now significantly more fit than the "CCR5"-using phenotype of the dual tropic C19 and C27 viruses (Fig. 4c). The 10,000-fold shift in fitness when inhibiting the "CXCR4"-using component of the primary C19 and C27 isolates (Fig. 4c) would suggest that the majority of these dual mixed virus populations were comprised of dual tropic clones (e.g. clones that use either CXCR4 or CCR5 for entry, thus r5x4) and that the "CXCR4"-using phenotype (in absence of inhibition) was dominant in determining fitness.

Co-receptor usage of the C19 and C27 quasispecies

The predicted amino acid sequences of the V3 loop of each C19 and C27 clone (Fig. 2) were aligned and then used in various algorithms to predict co-receptor usage. Based on the C27 consensus sequence, five "groups" of C19 clones were identified based on a unique V3 loop amino acid profile (Additional file 1: Fig. S1). There were three "groups" of clones in the C27 isolate. The five C19 groups all had Ser and Lys at position 11 and 25 and were predicted x4 by the 11/25 rule (positive charge at either or both sites) whereas two neutral amino acids, G11 and A25 predicted a pure r5 phenotype in all of the C27 clones (Additional file 1: Fig. S1). Using the PSSM [54], Geno2Pheno algorithms [25], and PhenoSeq [55], all C19 and C27 clones were predicted to use at least CXCR4 for entry and that CXCR4-using clones may dominate the virus population (PSSM predicted a possible dual tropism) (Additional file 1: Fig. S1).

The predicted co-receptor usage was then compared to actual co-receptor usage of the HIV-1 clones from C19 and C27. The HIV-1 Env genes sequenced in Fig. 2a and used for co-receptor prediction in Additional file 1: Fig. S1, were introduced into pREC_nfl_HIV-$1_{nl4\text{-}3}\Delta$env/URA3 via yeast-based recombination and described above [42]. This Env expression vector was then used to pseudotype virus produced from 293T cells co-transfected with the pNL luc-AM vector [56]. Equal virus titers (based on RT activity) were used to infect U87.CD4 cells expressing either CCR5 or CXCR4. Three (C19-14, C19-30, and C19-29) of 26 C19 clones and 2 of 20 C27 env clones were non-functional. Of the functional clones, none of the C19 or C27 clones were purely CCR5 tropic whereas several clones were "pure" CXCR4-using, i.e. C19-17, -28, -10, -25 (Fig. 5c) and C27-7, -21, -8, -26 (Fig. 5d).

For these analyses, we sequenced approximately 500 nt for each clone and identified 15 unique C19 Env sequence patterns, five of these were described as "groups" I–V (Fig. 5a). Eleven unique sequences and four "groups" (I–IV) were identified in the C27 HIV-1 isolates (Fig. 5b). In general, the clones within the same group (sharing the same C2-V3 nt sequence) showed similar co-receptor usage profiles (compare Fig. 5a with c; b with d). However, this was not always the case. For example in group

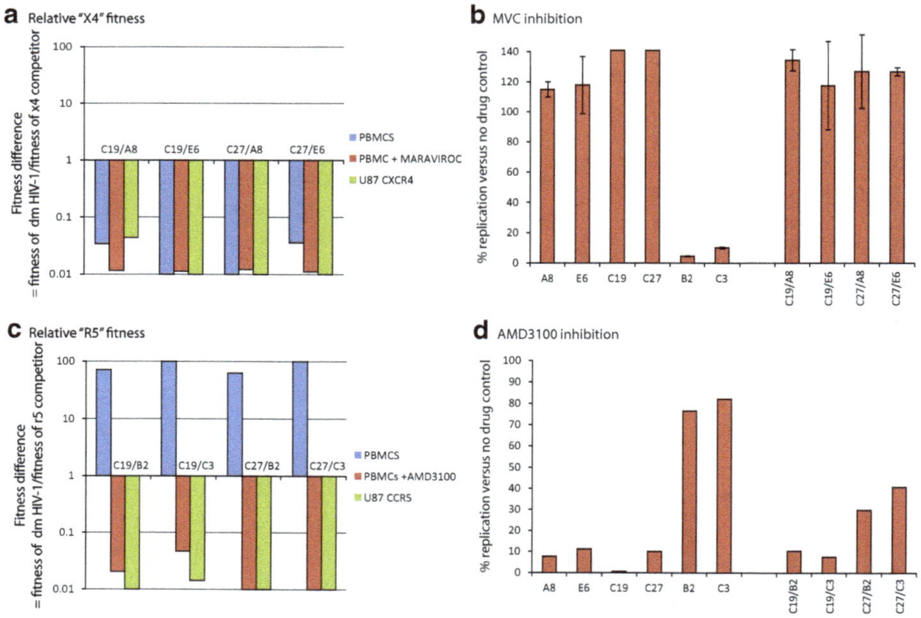

Fig. 4 Fitness of the dual tropic HIV-1 isolate when blocking the virus component using CCR5 or CXCR4. **a** The primary dual tropic HIV-1 isolates were competed against the x4 [50] titereds (all titered on U87.CD4.CXCR4 cells) in U87.CD4.CXCR4 cultures or in PHA-stimulated, IL-2 treated PBMC cultures with or without maraviroc. The fitness differences are plotted as described in Fig. 2 and in the "Methods". **b** The level of maraviroc inhibition of the monoinfections or dual infections was measured by relative RT activity in the cell free supernatant and plotted as a percentage of the no drug control. **c** The primary dual tropic HIV-1 isolates and r5 reference strains were also titered on U87.CD4.CCR5 cells and then competed together in PHA-stimulated, IL-2 treated PBMC cultures with or without AMD3100. The same dual infection with the same MOI (0.004) was repeated in U87.CD4.CCR5 cultures. The fitness differences are plotted as described in Fig. 2 and "Methods". **d** The level of AMD3100 inhibition of the monoinfections or dual infections was measured by relative RT activity in the cell free supernatant and plotted as a percentage of the no drug control. All experiments were performed in triplicate with the exception of **c**, **d** (performed in duplicate) due to limited supply of AMD3100.

I, C19-17 and C19-28 appeared to be pure x4 tropic whereas clones C19-11, -20, and -24 could infect both CCR5 and CXCR4 expressing cells (r5x4). It is important to note that clones that share sequence identity in the C2-V3 region may still differ in the remaining ~2,200 nt of Env (not sequenced), specifically in the V1V2 region which has been shown to influence co-receptor usage. Nonetheless, similar co-receptor usage was observed for most clones that share at least the C2-V3 sequences.

Finally, we compared five assays to determine co-receptor usage of these primary isolates: (1) the relative infection by primary C19 and C27 HIV-1 isolate on U87.CD4.CCR5 cells and U87.CD4.CXCR4 cells (Fig. 1c, d), (2) the $TCID_{50}$ values derived on CCR5+ and CXCR4+ cells, (3) the relative inhibition by AMD3100 and MVC on PBMCs (Fig. 4b, d), (4) predicted co-receptor usage from the clones (Additional file 1: Fig. S1), and (5) the actual co-receptor usage of Env clones in the quasispecies (Fig. 5c, d). For these two dual tropic HIV-1 isolates, the vast majority of clones in the quasispecies were used both R5 and X4 co-receptors. As discussed below, the use of co-receptor antagonist coupled with the $TCID_{50}$ measurements on U87.CD4.CCR5 cells and U87.CD4.CXCR4 cells provides the best prediction of the co-receptor usage within the HIV-1 quasispecies. The C19 and C27 primary HIV-1 isolates achieved a dual/mixed phenotype through similar quasispecies compositions. Both had more clones using both co-receptors, very few using only CXCR4, and no pure r5 clones (Fig. 5c, d). As described in our fitness analyses, the CXCR4 usage phenotype of a dual tropic virus is largely dominant in replicative fitness such that when it is inhibited, there is a total loss in fitness of these isolates.

Contribution of the CXCR4 and CCR5 using variants to replicative fitness in env chimeric viruses

Predominance of the x4 and r5x4 clones in the C19 and C27 primary HIV-1 isolates may be related to inability of r5 clones to compete during propagation of these primary HIV-1 isolates (as previously described; [57]). As described above, we also identified two patients infected with dual tropic HIV-1 through env chimeric virus construction [42]. By this method, there is no propagation to result in selection. Bias in the HIV-1 env quasispecies composition could be introduced during PCR and cloning. However, the targets for primer annealing and yeast

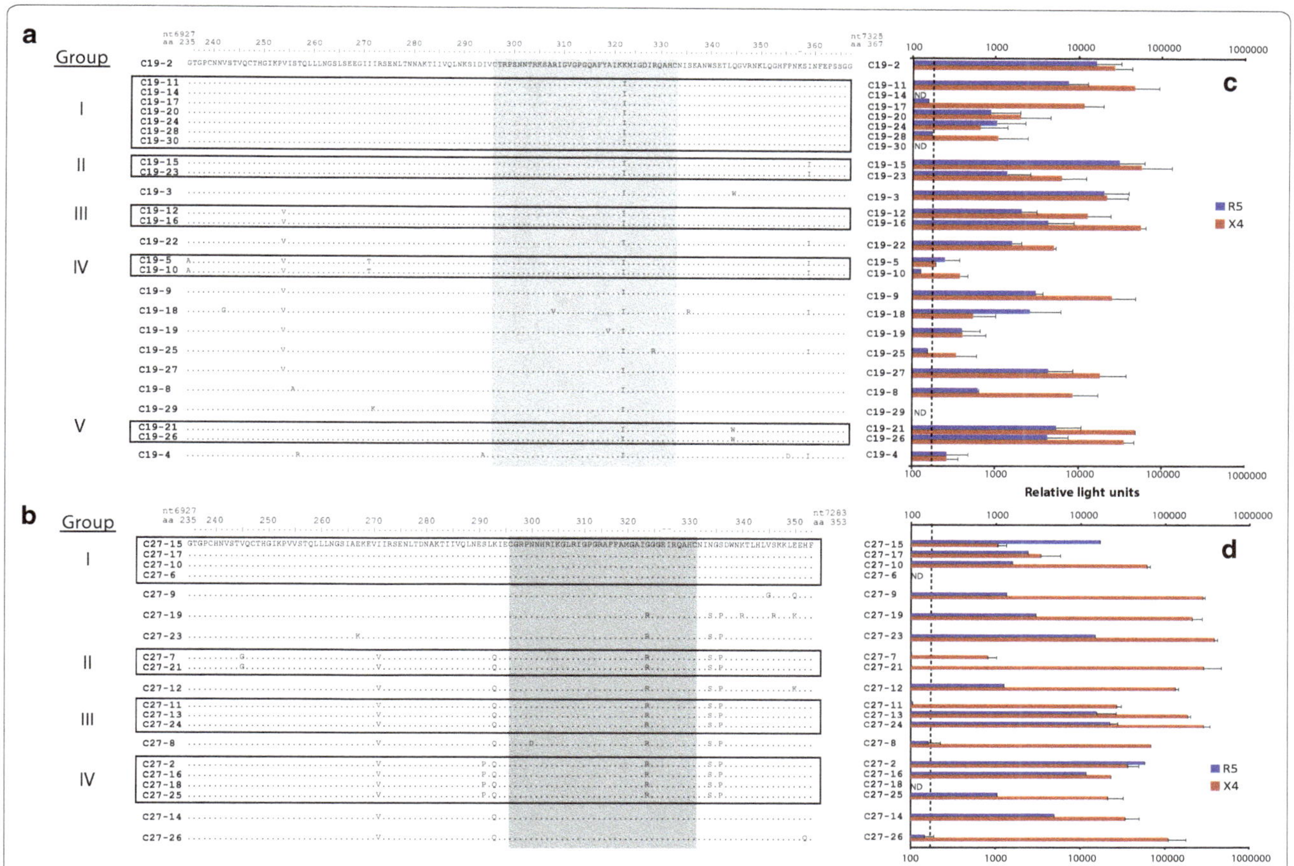

Fig. 5 Determining the co-receptor usage of C19 and C27 Env clones introduced into HIV-1 NL4-3 backbone via yeast-based recombination. The 26 C19 and 21 C27 env regions (same as those sequenced for Fig. 1) were cloned into pREC_env/URA3 via yeast-based recombination/gap repair [81, 82]. A 132 and 118 amino acid sequence of the C2-V3 region was used to group the C19 (**a**) and C27 (**b**) based on sequence identity/difference. The pREC_env expression vector was then used to pseudotype virus produced from 293T cells co-transfected with the pNL luc-AM vector [56]. Equal virus titers (based on RT activity) were used to infect U87.CD4 cells expressing either CCR5 or CXCR4. The infecting virus is reverse transcribed and integrated to express luciferase but is incapable of subsequent rounds of infection [56]. Luciferase activity (relative light units) was measured from lysed cells collected 72 h post infection with both the C19 (**c**) and C27 (**d**) Env pseudotyped virus infections. All assays were performed in triplicate. Background was subtracted from results and *dotted lines* on **c**, **d** represent the value three times the standard deviation of the background.

recombination on the HIV-1 genome were conserved for all HIV-1 strains [47]. In contrast to the C19 and C27 primary isolates, the B12 and B29 env chimeric viruses had higher r5 than x4 titers (Fig. 1e). Thus, there were minimal adjustments for equal "r5" titers and relative fitness of B12 and B19 env chimeric viruses were similar to B2 and C3. AMD3100 had minimal inhibition of B12 and B19 (adjusted for equal r5 titers) (Fig. 6d), which was expected based on the low x4-using component in the viral populations. The inhibition of "CXCR4"-using component (with AMD3100) (Fig. 6c) resulted in only a slight reduction in replicative fitness of the dual tropic B12 and B19 env chimeric viruses. This 2- to 10-fold decreased fitness in B12 and B19 with AMD3100 treatment was minimal compared to 10,000-fold loss in C19 and C27 fitness under the same conditions.

Due to the low "CXCR4"-using component levels in the B19 virus, equalizing x4 titers required the addition of >1,000-fold more volume of B19 (compared to B12) in competition with x4 control strains A8 and E6. Even with this high concentration of B19 virus over the A8 and E6 viruses, the B19 had only slightly greater fitness than A8 and equal fitness to E6 viruses whereas the B12 virus was slightly more fit than both A8 (by tenfold) and E6 (by threefold) in PBMCs (Fig. 6a). Inhibition by MVC appeared to be masked by very high levels of virus needed to reach equalized titers of the "CXCR4"-using component (Fig. 6b). This r5 HIV-1 concentration likely saturated the susceptible CCR5+/CD4+ cells in the PBMC culture. Nonetheless, some inhibition of the more abundant "CCR5"-using component in the B12 and B19 viruses did reduce the overall fitness of B12 and

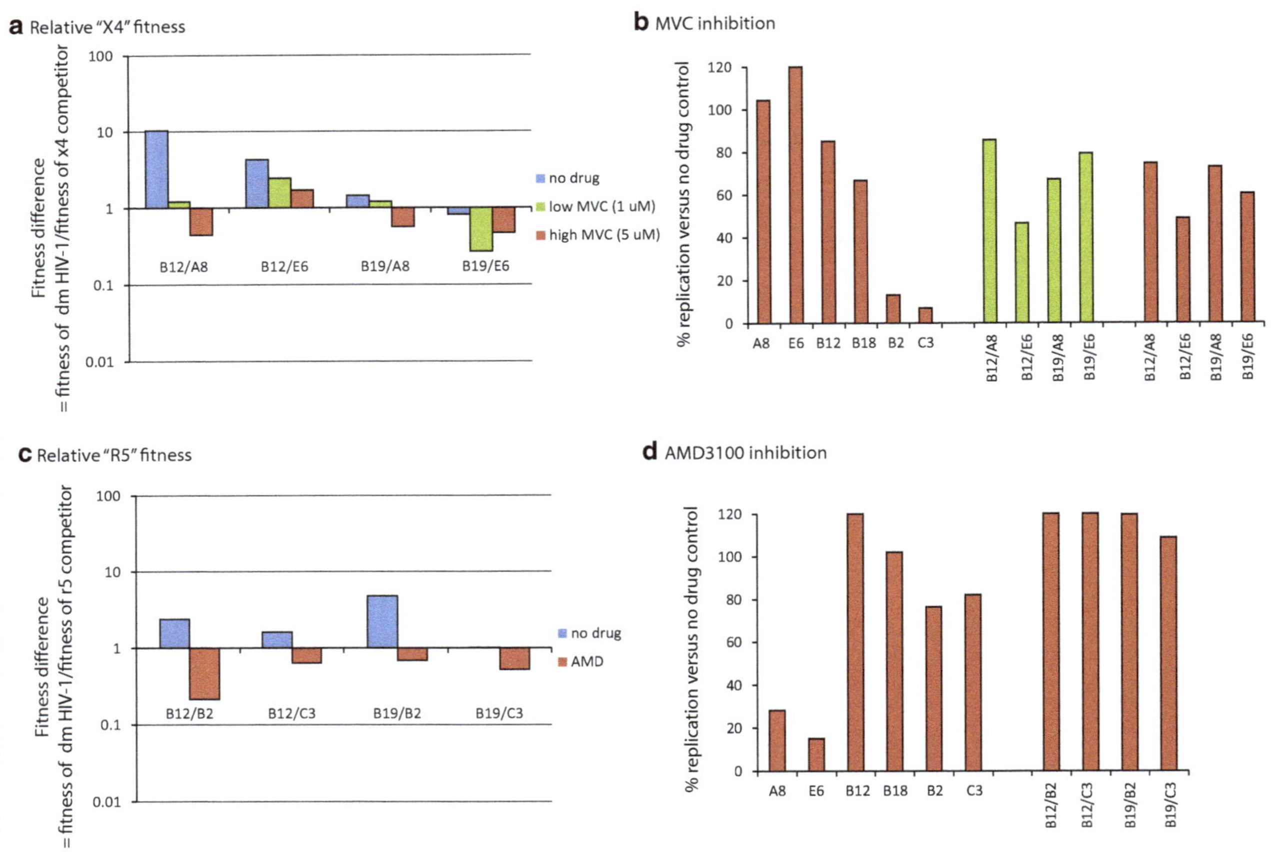

Fig. 6 Fitness of the dual tropic env chimeric virus when blocking the virus component using CCR5 or CXCR4. **a** The dm env **c**himeric viruses (B12 and B19) were competed against the x4 reference viruses (all titered on U87.CD4.CXCR4 cells) in U87.CD4.CXCR4 cultures or in PHA-stimulated, IL-2 treated PBMC cultures with or without maraviroc. The fitness differences are plotted as described in Fig. 2 and "Methods". **b** The level of maraviroc inhibition of the monoinfections or dual infections was measured by relative RT activity in the cell free supernatant and plotted as a percentage of the no drug control. **c** The env chimeric HIV-1 and r5 reference strains (B2 and C3) were titered on U87.CD4.CCR5 cells and then competed together in PHA-stimulated, IL-2 treated PBMC cultures with or without AMD3100. The same dual infection with the same MOI (0.004) was repeated in U87. CD4.CCR5 cultures. The fitness differences are plotted as described in Fig. 2 and "Methods". **d** The level of AMD3100 inhibition of the monoinfections or dual infections was measured by relative RT activity in the cell free supernatant and plotted as a percentage of the no drug control. All experiments were performed in triplicate with the exception of **c**, **d** (performed in duplicate) due to limited supply Of AMD3100.

B19 viruses compared to the A8 and E6 viruses (Fig. 6a). By reducing the MVC concentration, the B12 and B19 viruses regained fitness which again suggests that the "CCR5"-using component is contributing to the relative production of B12 and B19 in these competitions.

Prediction of low level x4 usage

With the B12 and B19 primary HIV-1 isolates, use of the co-receptor antagonists coupled with the $TCID_{50}$ measurements on U87.CD4.CCR5 cells and U87.CD4.CXCR4 cells provided the best prediction of co-receptor usage within the HIV-1 quasispecies. Thus, the x4-using or r5x4 component of the B12 and B19 chimeric env viruses was less than 1 and 0.1 % of the r5-using component, respectively. Based on the estimated low frequency of x4 or r5x4 clones, phenotypic analyses of co-receptor usage would require the cloning and analysis of >100 clones for B12 and >1,000 B19 clones (Table 1a, b) to identify r5 clones. Instead, we compared the predicted co-receptor usage for the B19 HIV-1 population found in: (1) env RT-PCR product from the original patient plasma sample, (2) in the pREC_nfl_envB12 plasmid population following yeast-based cloning of the B19 env PCR product, and (3) in the HIV-1 envB12 chimeric virus populations produced from 293T cells co-transfected with the pREC_nfl_envB12 + pCMV_cplt (see [42] for methods). The viral load in the B12 and B19 plasma samples was >50,000 copies/ml. Over 5,000 copies of RNA (from plasma and env chimeric virus) was reverse transcribed and then PCR amplified for subsequent 454 pyrosequencing of the

Table 1 Determination of predicted co-receptor usage in the HIV-1 isolate by 454 deep sequencing analyses

Culture	N	Plasmid	N	Plasma	N	Genotype		PSSM results			Geno2Pheno (5 %)	
						11/25	Prediction	% X4	% R5	Prediction	FPR (%)	Prediction
Predicted co-receptor usage for B19 clones[a]												
B19 C1	4,070	B19 P1	4,102	B19 R1	2,237	S/E	CCR5	0.11	0.62	CCR5 only	33.90	CCR5
B19 C2	25					S/E	CCR5	0.11	0.59	CCR5 only	10.90	CCR5
B19 C3	5					S/E	CCR5	0	0.1	CCR5 only	55	CCR5
B19 C4	3					S/E	CCR5	0.22	0.82	CCR5 only	41.20	CCR5
		B19 P2	3			S/E	CCR5	0.22	0.89	CCR5 only	50.50	CCR5
				B19 R2	*51*	*S/K*	*CXCR4*	0.24	0.92	CCR5 only	7.80	CCR5
				B19 R3	13	S/E	CCR5	0.22	0.86	CCR5 only	26.90	CCR5
				B19 R4	11	S/E	CCR5	0.11	0.42	CCR5 only	72	CCR5
				B19 R5	7	S/E	CCR5	0.11	0.46	CCR5 only	47.70	CCR5
				B19 R6	7	S/E	CCR5	0.11	0.46	CCR5 only	47.70	CCR5
				B19 R7	6	S/E	CCR5	0.11	0.46	CCR5 only	47.70	CCR5
				B19 R8	6	S/E	CCR5	0.11	0.46	CCR5 only	47.70	CCR5
				B19 R9	6	S/E	CCR5	0.11	0.46	CCR5 only	47.70	CCR5
				B19 R10	5	S/E	CCR5	0.11	0.6	CCR5 only	42.30	CCR5
				B19 R11	4	S/E	CCR5	0.11	0.47	CCR5 only	18.20	CCR5
				B19 R12	4	S/E	CCR5	0.09	0.39	CCR5 only	59.80	CCR5
				B19 R13	3	S/E	CCR5	0.11	0.46	CCR5 only	47.70	CCR5
				B19 R14	*3*	*S/K*	*CXCR4*	*0.29*	*0.95*	*CXCR4 capable*	*3.20*	*CXCR4*

Plasmid	N	Culture	N	Genotype		PSSM Results			Geno2Pheno (5 %)	
				11/25	Prediction	% X4	% R5	Prediction	FPR (%)	Prediction
Predicted co-receptor usage for B12 clones[a]										
B12_P1	3,611	B12_C1	1,405	S/Q	CCR5	0.31	0.96	CCR5 only	20.40	CCR5
B12_P2	55	B12_C2	19	S/Q	CCR5	0.31	0.96	CCR5 only	20.40	CCR5
B12_P3	24	B12_C3	10	S/Q	CCR5	0.31	0.96	CCR5 only	20.4	CCR5
B12_P4	21	B12_C4	6	S/Q	CCR5	0.27	0.95	CCR5 only	18.80	CCR5
		B12_C5	6	S/Q	CCR5	0.33	0.96	CCR5 only	22.60	CCR5
		B12_C6	6	S/Q	CCR5	0.31	0.96	CCR5 only	20.40	CCR5
		B12_C7	5	S/Q	CCR5	0.36	0.98	CCR5 only	10.50	CCR5
		B12_C8	5	S/Q	CCR5	0.36	0.98	CCR5 only	17.10	CCR5
B12_P10	3	B12_C9	5	S/Q	CCR5	0.33	0.96	CCR5 only	20.20	CCR5
B12_P17	3	B12_C10	4	S/Q	CCR5	0.31	0.96	CCR5 only	20.40	CCR5
		B12_C11	4	S/Q	CCR5	0.47	0.98	CCR5 only	36.90	CCR5
B12_P15	3	B12_C12	3	S/Q	CCR5	0.31	0.96	CCR5 only	20.40	CCR5
		B12_C13	3	S/Q	CCR5	0.51	0.98	CCR5 only	35.60	CCR5
B12_P8	4	B12_C14	3	S/Q	CCR5	0.33	0.96	CCR5 only	49.70	CCR5
		B12_C5	3	S/Q	CCR5	0.33	0.98	CCR5 only	14.40	CCR5
B12_P5	7	B12_C1	1,405	S/Q	CCR5	0.31	0.96	CCR5 only	20.40	CCR5
B12_P6	*6*	B12_C2	19	*S/K*	*CXCR4*	*0.53*	*0.99*	*CXCR4 capable*	*4.80*	*CXCR4*
B12_P7	4	B12_C3	10	S/E	CCR5	0.36	0.98	CCR5 only	*1.70*	*CXCR4*
B12_P9	3	B12_C4	6	S/Q	CCR5	0.29	0.95	CCR5 only	13.10	CCR5
B12_P11	3	B12_C5	6	S/Q	CCR5	0.31	0.96	CCR5 only	20.40	CCR5
B12_P12	3	B12_C6	6	S/Q	CCR5	0.42	0.98	CCR5 only	6.80	CCR5
B12_P13	3	B12_C7	5	S/Q	CCR5	0.31	0.96	CCR5 only	17.80	CCR5
B12_P14	3	B12_C8	5	S/Q	CCR5	0.33	0.96	CCR5 only	7.90	CCR5
B12_P16	3	B12_C9	5	S/Q	CCR5	0.29	0.95	CCR5 only	8.20	CCR5
B12_P18	3	B12_C10	4	S/Q	CCR5	0.51	0.98	CCR5 only	6.80	CCR5

Italics values indicate clones with different amino acids at the 11/25 positions

[a] The C2-V3 coding regions was RT-PCR amplified with barcoded 454 primers from the plasma RNA (only for B12), from the plasmid population following yeast recombination (no RT step), and from RNA of culture supernatant. Amino acid alignments grouped identical clones. Predictive co-receptor algorithms, 11/25, PSSM, and Geno2Pheno were run on the V3 loop amino acid sequences. *FPR* false positive rate for Geno2Pheno at 5 %.

V3 loop as described in the "Methods". Over 100,000 copies of DNA plasmid was sampled for 454. Unfortunately, the RT-PCR products of the B19 plasma sample (58,000 copies/ml) were unavailable for these analyses. An average depth of ~1,500–4,000 reads were obtained per sample. Only 105 nt of the V3 loop were analyzed and used to predict co-receptor usage based on 11/25 rule, subtype specific PSSM, Geno2Pheno (G2P, with a 5 % FPR), and PhenoSeq (Table 1a, b). For B19 plasma sample, 95 % of the 2,363 V3 reads were identical and predicted to be r5 by all three algorithms. Approximately 2 % of the reads (N = 51) had Lys at amino acid position 25 in the V3 loop and were predicted by PSSM and G2P to be x4 (Table 1a). Consistent with the low titers of x4 versus r5 in this B19 env chimeric virus (<0.1 %), we could not detect an x4 clone in ~4,100 V3 reads from the plasmid or the resulting virus. For B12 env chimeric virus, 10 clones (0.3 %) were predicted as x4 using by G2P but only 6 of these carried Lys at position 25 and were x4 using based on PSSM (Table 1b). Again, the percentage of predicted x4 or dual tropic clones in the B12 chimeric virus population was consistent with the relative x4 and r5 titers (Fig. 1e).

Discussion

HIV-1 disease progression is associated with the appearance of viral variants that are able to use an expanded repertoire of co-receptors for cell entry. Three phenotypes of HIV-1 isolates have been described: the r5 isolates that are more frequently transmitted and also predominate during the asymptomatic period of infection, the x4 variants that predominate in about 50 % of the infected individuals in the late phase of infection, dm and dual tropic isolates that could represent a transitional phenotype from r5 to x4. The x4, dual tropic and dm viruses have been associated with rapid CD4 declines and progression to AIDS and death but the prevalence/appearance of x4, dm and dual tropic HIV-1 was originally described for subtype B infections [28–31, 36]. A switch to an x4 or dual tropic phenotype in HIV-1 subtype C infections is quite infrequent [58] whereas subtype D HIV-1 infections have much higher prevalence of x4/dual tropic viruses, which also appear earlier in disease [59, 60]. However, Johnston et al. [61] screened 28 subtype C patients and 20 of these were found to be x4 or dual tropic. The high x4/dual tropism in this cohort was attributed to the fact that all these patients had been on antiretroviral therapy and for most of them, there was evidence of resistance. It is also important to note that the propagation of primary HIV-1 isolates on PHA-activated PBMCs commonly enriches for CXCR4-using virus even in HIV-1 populations with a low frequency x4 compared to r5 variants [57]. Early studies on HIV-1 tropism which defined the syncytia inducing (SI) and non-SI phenotypes relied on propagation which may have favored replication of the SI, T cell tropic HIV-1 clones (now defined as x4).

The rate of x4, dm or dual tropic HIV-1 outgrowth during propagations from patient samples typically depends on both the replicative fitness of x4 and r5 HIV-1 clones. This replicative fitness may also be one of many variables contributing to the appearance of x4 viruses during disease progression. As described earlier, other factors may include availability of target cells, co-receptor expression on susceptible cell subsets, differential immune response to x4 and r5 viruses, and preferential transmission of r5 variants followed by a slow evolution to x4 virus. Increased "in vivo" fitness of r5 HIV-1 variants over low frequency x4 variants in the intrapatient HIV-1 population is quite apparent based on various MVC treatment studies [62, 63]. Treatment failure of maraviroc can result from the emergence of resistant CCR5 (r5)-using viruses with reduced susceptibility to MVC [42–45]. However, the most common escape pathway for MVC resistance relates to the outgrowth of the intrinsically resistant x4 variants in a treated individual. In almost all cases, the x4 virus was found within the quasispecies prior to the treatment and often at a frequency requiring sensitive phenotypic or genotypic assays for detection [62, 63]. In the environment of MVC treatment, x4 emerged due to increased fitness over r5 and possibly dual tropic viruses in the intrapatient HIV-1 population. Based on these findings, the relative contribution of r5 and x4 virus components to the overall fitness of a primary isolate as well as the emergence of dual tropic HIV-1 isolate may have important implications on subsequent disease progression or response to MVC treatment.

In this study, we have measured the ex vivo replicative fitness of two dual tropic subtype C HIV-1 isolates and two dual tropic env chimeric viruses under different conditions. In our previous studies on replicative fitness involving pairwise competitions in PBMCs, it was important to standardize the initial virus inoculums via infectious titers, commonly calculated as $TCID_{50}$ values determined with PBMCs from the same donor and blood draw as those used in the competitions [57, 64]. Subsequent dual infections with two equal inocula of viruses of the same phenotype (i.e. r5 vs. r5 viruses or x4 vs. x4 viruses) will then compete for the same susceptible cell population within PBMCs. When dual infections are performed with an r5 and x4 virus, the viruses do not necessarily compete since they replicate in different cell populations within PBMCs and yet, the x4 viruses almost always replicate with faster kinetics to dominate the cultures simply because they have a stronger pathogenic phenotype [41, 57]. Thus, we wanted to assess the relative contribution of the CXCR4 and CCR5 components to the replicative fitness of dual tropic HIV-1 strains. We first screened for dual tropism in a collection of primary HIV-1 isolates and in env chimeric HIV-1 isolates constructed from patient plasma samples. We obtained two dual tropic primary HIV-1 isolates (C19 and C27) and two dual tropic env chimeric virus constructs (B12 and B19).

Co-cultivation of HIV + PBMCs with PBMCs derived from HIV-negative donors is a common method to obtain primary HIV-1 isolates. Several studies have indicated that x4 or dual tropic clones can expand more rapidly than r5 clones [57, 65]. As a consequence, x4 clones may predominate the primary HIV-1 isolates even if the original HIV-1 quasispecies in the patient PBMCs had very low frequency of x4 versus r5 clones. When we have examined the x4 frequency in several primary dual tropic HIV-1 isolates, the x4 or r5x4 clones typically predominate the quasispecies (as with C19 and C27) [57]. Because of this selection bias during virus propagation, we now clone the env gene from patient samples into a plasmid with the HIV-1 NL4-3 backbone and then produce virus by direct DNA transfection. Typical bacterial cloning of ~3 kbp fragment into a ~8 kbp DNA vector is quite inefficient, produces few bacterial colonies containing the plasmid with insert, and results in an undesired, severe genetic bottleneck on the HIV-1 env quasispecies. As previously described, cloning of this env product into the pREC_nfl_HIV-$1_{NL4\text{-}3}\Delta$gp120/URA3 construct via yeast homologous recombination/gap repair results in thousands of yeast colonies and a minimal genetic bottleneck in the env quasispecies [47]. Nonetheless, complementation with the patient-derived gp120 coding region (or entire env gene) and the NL4-3 backbone can occasionally result in a "dead" virus [66].

Using the primary HIV-1 isolates and the env chimeric viruses for fitness studies, we observed significant differences that reflected the r5, x4, and r5x4 composition in the quasispecies. Both x4r5 and x4 clones were observed in C19 and C27 primary HIV-1 isolates (1) as predicted by co-receptor usage algorithms applied to clonal sequencing analyses and (2) as determined by a phenotypic co-receptor usage assay applied to HIV-1 clones in the quasispecies. Interestingly, the "CXCR4"-using component was dominant over the "CCR5"-using component in determining replicative fitness of the r5x4 population in the C19 and C27 primary isolates (pure x4 clones were rare and r5 clones were absent). When the "CXCR4"-using component was completely inhibited in these primary HIV-1 isolates, the "CCR5"-using component of the r5x4 population could not compete with control r5 HIV-1 isolates. Interestingly, when competitions were limited to the "CCR5"- or "CXCR4"-using component in the primary r5x4 HIV-1 isolate, the replicative fitness was quite similar to related primary r5 and x4 HIV-1 isolates. The r5- and x4-using components of the C19 and C27 viruses were significantly less fit than the r5 B2 and C3 HIV-1 isolates or the x4 A8 and E6 HIV-1 isolates, respectively. We have published several studies showing that primary subtype C HIV-1 isolates are less fit than any other group M HIV-1 isolate (determined in head-to-head competitions in PBMCs from multiple donors) [38–40, 49]. It is interesting to note that from our unpublished and published data, subtype C competes well with other subtypes in ex vivo competition in langerhans cells implying that the transmission fitness of this subtype is comparable to that of other subtypes. However, after entry into cells, the pathogenic fitness of subtype C is lower than other subtypes, a possible explanation of the dominance of r5 tropism in subtype C which leads to a slower disease progression. In general, the less virulent r5 variants are more common during late subtype C infection.

Based on previous studies [67, 68] it appears that dual tropic isolates may be evolutionary intermediates. The early phase of intrapatient HIV-1 evolution consists predominantly of r5 variants possibly with a few r5x4 but likely minimal or no x4 variants [57, 69]. During the time of infection and possibly the absence of treatment, the r5x4 variants may increase in frequency and possibly mutate to a pure x4 variant [65, 70, 71]. However, previous studies also suggest that these r5x4 and x4 variants often represent separate lineages from CCR5 variants with deep roots within the intrapatient phylogenetic tree [72]. The actual mutational pathways from a single HIV-1 clone that leads to a phenotypic switch from r5 to x4 may arise with significant cost to replicative fitness [73]. These findings imply that this shift in tropism may be under selective pressure, i.e. increased availability of CXCR4+ versus CCR5+ susceptible cells. In our studies it appears that the "CXCR4"-using component of the r5x4 clones in the C19 and C27 were dominant over the "CCR5"-using component in determining replicative fitness. The "CXCR4"-using component of the dual tropic C19 and C27 HIV-1 isolates were generally less fit than the control x4 A8 and E6 HIV-1 isolates. However, we cannot assume that this reduced fitness was due to the initial mutation pattern leading to a switch in r5 to x4 since subtype C HIV are generally less fit than any other group M HIV-1 isolate.

The findings with C19 and C27 primary HIV-1 isolates might suggest that the "CXCR4"-using component of a dual tropic HIV-1 would dominate over the "CCR5"-using component in replicative fitness. However, this finding is misleading for patients harboring mixed X4 and R5 HIV viruses. As noted earlier, the primary HIV-1 isolates such as C19 and C27 primarily contain x4 or r5x4 clones and only low levels of r5 clones due to selection during PBMC co-cultivation/propagation. Within patients, x4 or r5x4 HIV-1 are often found at low frequency in the quasispecies. Thus, we constructed the B12 and B19 env chimeric viruses from patients with mixed X4 and R5 HIV-1. In these viruses, the r5 clones were 100- and 1,000-fold more abundant than the x4 or r5x4 clones. These findings were confirmed by (1) measuring infectious titers in both U87.CD4.CCR5 cells and U87.CD4.CXCR4 cells and by (2) predicting co-receptor usage from approximately 1,000–4,000 V3 loop sequence reads (derived by 454 pyrosequencing of ~10,000 patient-derived DNA templates). In the B12 and B19 env chimeric viruses, the CCR5 component derived from the pure r5 clones did contribute to overall replicative fitness. The more dominant "CXCR4" component in the C19 and C27 resulted in the ability to compete with the control x4 A8 and E6 HIV-1. In contrast, high levels of "CCR5" versus the "CXCR4" component in the B12 and B19 env chimeric virus resulted in low replicative fitness when competed against x4 A8 and E6 HIV-1. In general, x4 HIV-1 out replicates r5 HIV-1 in PBMC cultures. When adjusting for the r5 or x4 titers, the "r5" or "x4" components of B12 and B19 HIV-1 had similar fitness and were able to compete with the r5 (B2 and C3) and x4 (A8 and E6) control strains. These findings are consistent with our previous studies in that subtype B x4 or r5 HIV-1 isolates have, on average, higher replicative fitness than HIV-1 isolates from other group M subtypes [38–40].

Previous studies suggest a dominance of the "CXCR4"-using over the "CCR5"-using phenotype in HIV-1 defined as dual tropic/mixed tropic. As a consequence, a proposed x4 dominance in mixed X4 and R5 HIV-1 has been implicated in MVC treatment outcome and disease progression. Again, our findings with the C19 and C27 viruses suggest that use of primary HIV-1 isolates may over-emphasize this x4 dominance. The x4 or x4r5 HIV clones are typically dominant within the intrapatient quasispecies of some patients during late infection [65, 74]. Otherwise, x4 or x4r5 HIV clones are found at low frequencies compared to the pure r5 clones in the intrapatient quasispecies during asymptomatic disease. Furthermore, "CXCR4"- using HIV isolates are rare in subtype A and C [27, 58, 75] but more frequent in subtype B and D infected patients [59]. The x4 HIV strains typically have faster replication kinetics than r5 HIV but due to limited CCR5+/CXCR4+/CD4+ cells in PBMC cultures, these two HIV-1 phenotypes are not in direct competition in our studies. When we equalize for r5 or x4 titers in the dual tropic HIV-1 and limited replication to the "CCR5"-using and "CXCR4"-using components, we found that fitness of C19 and C27 virus reflected that of other subtype C HIV-1 isolates, i.e. less fit than most group M HIV-1 isolates. In contrast, even the low level of x4 or x4/r5 B12 and B19 HIV-1 had replicative fitness comparable to the control x4 viruses. However, without adjusting virus titers for the "CXCR4-using" component, this low level of x4 HIV-1 had minimal impact on replicative fitness of this env chimeric virus which was dominated by r5 clones. These findings suggest that detection of low frequency x4 clones in the HIV-1 quasipecies is not necessarily synonymous with rapid HIV replication kinetics and faster disease progressions. However, the overall replicative fitness in PBMCs regardless of the x4 and r5 composition remains a strong correlation of disease progression [41, 57, 76–78].

Conclusions

In this study, we show that x4 component is dominant in replicative fitness but is typically of low frequency compared to r5 HIV-1 in most dual tropic HIV-1 quasispecies. Based on findings in this study, the emergence of dual/mixed tropic viruses may have important implications on response to maraviroc containing regimens. Furthermore, although the "CXCR4"-using phenotype is of low frequency in the dual/mixed population, it may have a selective advantage in patients failing maraviroc. Based on our findings that the "CXCR4"-using phenotype is the major determinant of replicative fitness, this may have important implications on disease progression.

Methods

Cells

293T cells (human embryonic kidney cells) were grown on Dulbeco's Modified Eagle's medium (DMEM) supplemented with 10 % fetal bovine serum (FBS) (Cellgro), 100 U/ml of penicillin and 100 μg/ml of streptomycin (Cellgro). U87.CD4 (human glioma cells) expressing either CCR5 or CXCR4, obtained from the NIH AIDS Research and Reference Reagent Program (distributed by Dr. D Littman) were maintained in complete DMEM medium supplemented with 1 mg/ml of geneticin G418 (Life Technologies, Inc.) and 5 μg/ml puromycin to maintain receptor and coreceptor expression [5]. Peripheral blood mononuclear cells (PBMCs) from HIV-negative blood donors were obtained by Ficoll-Hypague density centrifugation of heparin treated venous blood. These were stimulated with 2 μg/ml of phytohemagglutinin (PHA; Gibco BRL) and 1 μg/ml of interleukin-2 (IL-2; Gibco BRL) in complete RPMI 1640 containing 2 mM L-glutamine for 3–4 days.

Virus propagation, chimeric virus production, and titers

Subtype C syncytium inducing (SI) HIV-1 isolates obtained from patients who had been on reverse transcriptase inhibitors for an average of 14.4 months [46] as well as the non-SI and SI-using reference viruses [38, 40] (Table 1) were grown in PHA-activated PBMCs over a period of 2 weeks. RT assays were performed at different time points to measure virus production. As determined by Abraha et al. [40], co-receptor usage was then estimated by exposing U87.CD4.CCR5 and CXCR4 cells to each virus.

In a subtype B cohort analyses, RNA was extracted from plasma samples from 11 untreated, HIV-infected patients (investigators were blinded to all patient demographics). The HIV-1 env gene was then reverse transcribed-PCR amplified from the plasma RNA with the Env-End primer as described [44]. The gp120 regions were then PCR amplified using primers F_gp120 (5′-GACAGGTTAATTGATAGACTA-3′) and B_gp120 (5′-CTTCCTGCTGCTCCCAAGAAC-3′). Briefly, these gp120 PCR products were cotransformed with SacII-linearized pREC_NFL_Δgp120/URA3 into Saccharomyces cerevisiae MYA-906 cells (ATCC). Following homologous recombination, plasmids were extracted from the yeast cells and transformed into electro-competent Escherichia coli Stbl4 cells (Invitrogen). Individual bacterial colonies were grown, and plasmids were extracted using Qiagen miniprep kits. The cloning procedures have been extensively described [44, 47]. Of the 11 plasma samples from HIV-infected patients, we obtained 3 pREC_nfl_gp120 vectors harboring a functional HIV-1 env gene from the patient. The pREC_nfl_gp120 vectors were then co-transfected into 293T cells along with the complementing vector, pCMV_cplt to produce infectious virus as described [47]. To avoid confusion, we will refer to the viruses with an NL4-3 backbone and containing the patient's gp120 coding region as env chimeric viruses.

$TCID_{50}$ determination for all the viruses was performed on PHA/IL-2 stimulated HIV negative donor PBMCs as well as on U87.CD4.CCR5 and CXCR4 cells. For PBMCs, 100,000 cells were added to each of the wells in a 96 well plate. Ten-fold serial dilutions of each virus were made and 100 μl were added to each well containing the cells with each dilution performed in triplicates [64]. The viruses were grown in RPMI-1640 complete media. Similar dilutions were made for the U87 cells, 10,000 cells per well were plated in 96 well plates in DMEM complete media containing G418 and puromycin 24 h prior to infection. At the time of infection, media containing selection antibiotics was removed and replaced with DMEM with no selection. Supernatants were harvested at different time points to measure RT activity. $TCID_{50}$ for each virus was calculated using the Reed and Muech method [79].

Veritrop cell-to-cell fusion assay

A new cell fusion assay to measure co-receptor usage to a 2 % level has been recently described [48]. Briefly, 2 ug of pREC_nfl_env_{ptX} is transfected into 293T cells using Fugene as described [48]. After 24 h, the transfection reagent is removed by cell washing and the 293T cells are layered over U87.CD4.CCR5 and CXCR4 cells transfected with pDM1.1 [80]. Luciferase is only produced from pDM1.1 in the presence of Tat and Rev derived from the 293T cells fused with U87 cells transfected with the pREC_nfl vector, i.e. expressing the entire HIV-1 proteome.

Determination of fitness of the dual tropic isolates

Fitness of the dual tropic isolates was determined on both PBMCs and U87.CD4.CCR5 and CXCR4 cells using dual competition assays described previously [38–41, 57]. Briefly, for PBMCs, to determine the effect of the "CCR5"-using phenotype on fitness, the dual-tropic isolates were competed against r5-using isolates (C3 and B2) at a multiplicity of infection (MOI) of 0.004 in the presence or absence of AMD3100, a CXCR4 coreceptor antagonist. AMD3100 was used at a concentration of 0.1 μM (>the inhibitory dose for 99 % inhibition or IC_{99}). To determine the role of the "CXCR4"-using phenotype in fitness of the dual tropic isolates, the dual-tropic isolates were competed against x4-using isolates (E6 and A8) in the presence or absence of maraviroc at an MOI of 0.004. Maraviroc was used at a concentration of 1 μM (IC_{99}).

On U87 cells, the role of the "CCR5" phenotype on fitness of the dual tropic isolates was determined by competing the dual tropic isolates against the r5 using competitor (B2 and C3) viruses on U87.CD4.CCR5 cells at an MOI of 0.004. The same isolates were competed against the x4-using competitor viruses (E6 and A8) on U87.CD4.CXCR4 cells at an MOI of 0.004. For all the competition experiments, mono-infections representing each of the viruses in the competition were included. Virus production was monitored over a period of time by measuring RT activity at different time points. At the time of peak virus production, the cells were harvested and DNA was extracted using the Qiagen DNA extraction kit.

Determination of viral fitness using heteroduplex tracking assay

To determine viral fitness, the env gene was PCR amplified in the C2-V3 region using a nested PCR. For the first round ENV B (5′-AGAAAGAGCAGAAGACAGTGGCAATGA) and antisense primer ED 14 (5′-TCTTGCCTGGAGCTGTTTGATGCCCCAGAC) were used to amplify a 1,400 bp of the *env* gene. The second round PCR was performed using a sense primer E80 (5′-CCAATTCCCATACATTATTGTG) and an antisense primer E125 (5′-CAATTTCTGGGTCCCCTCCTGAGG) amplifying a 480 bp fragment of the C2-V3 region. PCR conditions were as described. The PCR products were run on a 1 % agarose gel stained with 1 % ethidium bromide and viewed under UV illumination. C2-V3 fragment amplified from subtypes D and E with a ^{32}P labeled E80 and unlabeled E125 primer were used as probes. To determine the relative virus production for each virus in the competition, a heteroduplex tracking assay (HTA) was used as previously described [38–41]. Heretoduplexes were separated on a 6 % non-denaturing gel and quantified using a Molecular Imager FX (BioRad) phosphoimager. Virus production for each of the virus in the competition (f_o) was divided by the initial proportion in the inoculum (i_o) to get the relative fitness value ($w = f_o/i_o$) [38–41]. The relative fitness value of each isolate in the competition is a measure of the fitness difference W_D between the two HIV-1 variants ($W_D = W_M/W_L$), where W_M and W_L correspond to the relative fitness of the more and less fit virus.

Plasmid generation and env sequencing

The env gene (gp160) was PCR amplified from each of the dual-tropic isolates by nested PCR to obtain a 2,750 bp fragment. The first round PCR was amplified using Env A 5′-GGCTTAGGCATCTCCTATGGCAGGAAGAA (5,954–5,982 positions of the HXB2 genome) and Env M 5′-TAGCCCTTCCAGTCCCCCCTTTTCTTTTA (9,068–9,096). The second round PCR was carried out with Kpn-1Env TGTGGGTCACAGTCTATTATGG (6,325–6,346) and Env-End 5′-CTTTTTGACCACTTGCCACCCAT (8,797–8,819) primers. This PCR product was then cloned into a yeast vector by homologous recombination as described elsewhere. Briefly, the PCR amplified gp160 was cloned into a SacII linearized pREC_nfl_HIV-1_{nl4-3}env/URA3 vector by homologous recombination as already described [81, 82]. Thirty colonies were picked for each of the dual-tropic isolates. For each of these, the C2-V3 region was sequenced as described above and then analyzed to determine coreceptor usage via the 11/25 rule or with the webPSSM [54] and Geno2Pheno algorithms [25]. Sequences were aligned using ClustalX [83] and MUSCLE [84, 85] followed by phylogenetic tree constructions using TreeView [86].

Pyrosequencing of the B12 and B19 env chimeric viruses was performed on PCR amplicons of the C2-V3 region. Nested PCR products for sequencing were generated using the external products described above as templates with custom designed fusion oligos that contained the 454 adaptor sequences (Roche Lib-A Primer A and Primer B), followed by a 10 basepair Multiplex Identifier (MID) sequence to permit sample pooling, and lastly the HIV-1 template specific oligos E110 and E125 (5′-CTGTTAAATGGCAGTCTAGCAGAA-3′ and 5′-CAATTTCTGGGTCCCCTCCTGAGG-3′, respectively). Samples were quantified by fluorometry with the Quant-iT PicoGreen dsDNA Assay Kit (Life Technologies), pooled in equimolar concentrations, and sequenced on a 454 GS Junior System (Roche Diagnostics) using the GS Junior Titanium Sequencing chemistry. The resulting reads were trimmed to exclude the MIDs and primer sequence, and low-quality reads were filtered using the GS Run Processor according to length and quality scores. Multisequence alignments of reads were constructed using MUSCLE (PMID: 15034147), and all phylogenetic analysis was performed with MEGA5 (PMID: 21546353).

Pseudotyping single cycle assays

The pNL luc-AM vector described by Pugach et al. [56] was cotransfected along with one of each pREC env clonal plasmid (thirty for each dual tropic isolate) into 293T cells using effectene transfection kit (Qiagen, Valencia, CA, USA). Pseudovirus-containing supernatants were harvested from each well at 72 h post transfection and then used to infect both U87.CD4.CCR5 and U87.CD4.CXCR4 cells in triplicate. After 72 h at 37°C in 5 % CO_2, the supernatant was removed and cells were washed with 200 µl of phosphate buffered saline (PBS, Cellgro). 100 µl of cellgro lysis buffer was added to lyse the cells. 50 µl of the Luciferin Steady Glo substrate was added to 50 µl of lysate supernatant to measure luciferase activity.

Abbreviations

r5: CCR5-using; x4: CXCR4-using; dm: dual mixed; HIV: human immunodeficiency virus; Env: envelope glycoprotein; PBMC: peripheral blood mononuclear cells; MVC: maraviroc; $TCID_{50}$: infectious dose of 50 % infectivity in tissue culture.

Authors' contributions

All authors were involved in the preparation of this manuscript. ILN led the studies described herein and performed the majority of the experimentation. DMT and AA were involved in determining replicative fitness. FK propagated the viruses. RG and OJ performed the phenotypic co-receptor experiments. GN performed all of the sequence and phylogenetic analyses. EJA together with ILN conceived the project, supervised the research, and wrote the manuscript. All authors read and approved the final manuscript.

Author details

[1] Division of Infectious Diseases, Department of Medicine, Case Western Reserve University, 10900 Euclid Ave., Cleveland, OH 44106, USA. [2] Virology Program, Department of Molecular Biology and Microbiology, Case Western Reserve University, Cleveland, OH, USA. [3] Joint Clinical Research Centre, Kampala, Uganda. [4] Present Address: Myles Thaler Center for AIDS and Human Retrovirus Research, Department of Microbiology, Immunology and Cancer Biology, University of Virginia, Charlottesville, VA, USA. [5] Laboratory of Virology and Infectious Disease, Rockefeller University, New York, USA.

Acknowledgements
This work was supported by the Case/UHC CFAR Biosafety Core (AI36219) and by research Grants awarded to EJA (NIH/NIAID AI49170).

Competing interests
Dr. Eric J. Arts has filed a patent on the chimeric virus construction and phenotypic assay used to measure co-receptor assay. None of the other authors have competing financial interests.

References
1. Cilliers T, Morris L (2002) Coreceptor usage and biological phenotypes of HIV-1 isolates. Clin Chem Lab Med 40:911–917
2. Alkhatib G (2009) The biology of CCR5 and CXCR4. Curr Opin HIV AIDS 4:96–103
3. Lee B, Sharron M, Montaner LJ, Weissman D, Doms RW (1999) Quantification of CD4, CCR5, and CXCR4 levels on lymphocyte subsets, dendritic cells, and differentially conditioned monocyte-derived macrophages. Proc Natl Acad Sci USA 96:5215–5220
4. Doranz BJ, Rucker J, Yi Y, Smyth RJ, Samson M, Peiper SC et al (1996) A dual-tropic primary HIV-1 isolate that uses fusin and the beta-chemokine receptors CKR-5, CKR-3, and CKR-2b as fusion cofactors. Cell 85:1149–1158
5. Deng H, Liu R, Ellmeier W, Choe S, Unutmaz D, Burkhart M et al (1996) Identification of a major co-receptor for primary isolates of HIV-1. Nature (London) 381:661–666
6. Dragic T, Litwin V, Allaway GP, Martin SR, Huang Y, Nagashima KA et al (1996) HIV-1 entry into CD4+ cells is mediated by the chemokine receptor CC-CKR-5. Nature (London) 381:667–673
7. Marcon L, Choe H, Martin KA, Farzan M, Ponath PD, Wu L et al (1997) Utilization of C–C chemokine receptor 5 by the envelope glycoproteins of a pathogenic simian immunodeficiency virus, SIVmac239. J Virol 71:2522–2527
8. Kuhmann SE, Madani N, Diop OM, Platt EJ, Morvan J, Muller-Trutwin MC et al (2001) Frequent substitution polymorphisms in African green monkey CCR5 cluster at critical sites for infections by simian immunodeficiency virus SIVagm, implying ancient virus-host coevolution. J Virol 75:8449–8460
9. Deng HK, Unutmaz D, Kewalramani VN, Littman DR (1997) Expression cloning of new receptors used by simian and human immunodeficiency viruses. Nature (London) 388:296–300
10. Schuitemaker H, Koot M, Kootstra NA, Dercksen MW, de Goede RE, van Steenwijk RP et al (1992) Biological phenotype of human immunodeficiency virus type 1 clones at different stages of infection: progression of disease is associated with a shift from monocytotropic to T-cell-tropic virus population. J Virol 66:1354–1360
11. Fredriksson R, Stalhanske P, von Gegerfelt A, Lind B, Aman P, Rassart E et al (1991) Biological characterization of infectious molecular clones derived from a human immunodeficiency virus type-1 isolate with rapid/high replicative capacity. Virology 181:55–61
12. Karlsson A, Parsmyr K, Sandstrom E, Fenyo EM, Albert J (1994) MT-2 cell tropism as prognostic marker for disease progression in human immunodeficiency virus type 1 infection (see comments). J Clin Microbiol 32:364–370
13. Tersmette M, de Goede RE, Al BJ, Winkel IN, Gruters RA, Cuypers HT et al (1988) Differential syncytium-inducing capacity of human immunodeficiency virus isolates: frequent detection of syncytium-inducing isolates in patients with acquired immunodeficiency syndrome (AIDS) and AIDS-related complex. J Virol 62:2026–2032
14. Feng Y, Broder CC, Kennedy PE, Berger EA (1996) HIV-1 entry cofactor: functional cDNA cloning of a seven-transmembrane. G protein-coupled receptor. Science 272:872–877
15. Hallenberger S, Bosch V, Angliker H, Shaw E, Klenk HD, Garten W (1992) Inhibition of furin-mediated cleavage activation of HIV-1 glycoprotein gp160. Nature (London) 360:358–361
16. Fouchier RA, Groenink M, Kootstra NA, Tersmette M, Huisman HG, Miedema F et al (1992) Phenotype-associated sequence variation in the third variable domain of the human immunodeficiency virus type 1 gp120 molecule. J Virol 66:3183–3187
17. Huang CC, Tang M, Zhang MY, Majeed S, Montabana E, Stanfield RL et al (2005) Structure of a V3-containing HIV-1 gp120 core. Science 310:1025–1028
18. Lobritz MA, Ratcliff AN, Arts EJ (2010) HIV-1 entry, inhibitors, and resistance. Viruses 2:1069–1105
19. Cho MW, Lee MK, Carney MC, Berson JF, Doms RW, Martin MA (1998) Identification of determinants on a dualtropic human immunodeficiency virus type 1 envelope glycoprotein that confer usage of CXCR4. J Virol 72:2509–2515
20. Nabatov AA, Pollakis G, Linnemann T, Kliphius A, Chalaby MI, Paxton WA (2004) Intrapatient alterations in the human immunodeficiency virus type 1 gp120 V1V2 and V3 regions differentially modulate coreceptor usage, virus inhibition by CC/CXC chemokines, soluble CD4, and the b12 and 2G12 monoclonal antibodies. J Virol 78:524–530
21. Cornelissen M, Hogervorst E, Zorgdrager F, Hartman S, Goudsmit J (1995) Maintenance of syncytium-inducing phenotype of HIV type 1 is associated with positively charged residues in the HIV type 1 gp120 V2 domain without fixed positions, elongation, or relocated N-linked glycosylation sites. AIDS Res Hum Retroviruses 11:1169–1175
22. Moore JP, Stevenson M (2000) New targets for inhibitors of HIV-1 replication. Nat Rev Mol Cell Biol 1:40–49
23. Doms RW, Moore JP (2000) HIV-1 membrane fusion: targets of opportunity. J Cell Biol 151:F9–F14
24. Garrido C, Roulet V, Chueca N, Poveda E, Aguilera A, Skrabal K et al (2008) Evaluation of eight different bioinformatics tools to predict viral tropism in different human immunodeficiency virus type 1 subtypes. J Clin Microbiol 46:887–891
25. Lengauer T, Sander O, Sierra S, Thielen A, Kaiser R (2007) Bioinformatics prediction of HIV coreceptor usage. Nat Biotechnol 25:1407–1410
26. Bunnik EM, Swenson LC, Edo-Matas D, Huang W, Dong W, Frantzell A et al (2011) Detection of inferred. PLoS Pathog 7:e1002106
27. Lin NH, Becerril C, Giguel F, Novitsky V, Moyo S, Makhema J et al (2012) Env sequence determinants in CXCR4-using human immunodeficiency virus type-1 subtype C. Virology 433:296–307
28. Penn ML, Grivel JC, Schramm B, Goldsmith MA, Margolis L (1999) CXCR4 utilization is sufficient to trigger CD4+ T cell depletion in HIV-1-infected human lymphoid tissue. Proc Natl Acad Sci USA 96:663–668
29. Regoes RR, Bonhoeffer S (2005) The HIV coreceptor switch: a population dynamical perspective. Trends Microbiol 13:269–277
30. Scarlatti G, Tresoldi E, Bjorndal A, Fredriksson R, Colognesi C, Deng HK et al (1997) In vivo evolution of HIV-1 co-receptor usage and sensitivity to chemokine-mediated suppression. Nat Med 3:1259–1265
31. Connor RI, Sheridan KE, Ceradini D, Choe S, Landau NR (1997) Change in coreceptor use correlates with disease progression in HIV-1–infected individuals. J Exp Med 185:621–628
32. Cayota A, Vuillier F, Scott-Algara D, Dighiero G (1990) Preferential replication of HIV-1 in memory CD4+ subpopulation. Lancet 336:941
33. Riley JL, Levine BL, Craighead N, Francomano T, Kim D, Carroll RG et al (1998) Naive and memory CD4 T cells differ in their susceptibilities to human immunodeficiency virus type 1 infection following CD28 costimulation: implications for transmission and pathogenesis. J Virol 72:8273–8280
34. Cornelissen M, Mulder-Kampinga G, Veenstra J, Zorgdrager F, Kuiken C, Hartman S et al (1995) Syncytium-inducing (SI) phenotype suppression at seroconversion after intramuscular inoculation of a non-syncytium-inducing/SI phenotypically mixed human immunodeficiency virus population. J Virol 69:1810–1818
35. Groenink M, Moore JP, Broersen S, Schuitemaker H (1995) Equal levels of gp120 retention and neutralization resistance of phenotypically distinct primary human immunodeficiency virus type 1 variants upon soluble CD4 treatment. J Virol 69:523–527
36. Tersmette M, Miedema F (1990) Interactions between HIV and the host immune system in the pathogenesis of AIDS. AIDS 4(Suppl 1):S57–S66
37. Trkola A, Ketas T, Kewalramani VN, Endorf F, Binley JM, Katinger H et al (1998) Neutralization sensitivity of human immunodeficiency virus type 1 primary isolates to antibodies and CD4-based reagents is independent of coreceptor usage. J Virol 72:1876–1885
38. Ball SC, Abraha A, Collins KR, Marozsan AJ, Baird H, Quinones-Mateu ME et al (2003) Comparing the ex vivo fitness of CCR5-tropic human

immunodeficiency virus type 1 isolates of subtypes B and C 1. J Virol 77:1021–1038
39. Arien KK, Abraha A, Quinones-Mateu ME, Kestens L, Vanham G, Arts EJ (2005) The replicative fitness of primary human immunodeficiency virus type 1 (HIV-1) group M, HIV-1 group O, and HIV-2 isolates. J Virol 79:8979–8990
40. Abraha A, Nankya IL, Gibson R, Demers K, Tebit DM, Johnston E, Katzenstein D, Siddiqui A, Herrera C, Fischetti L, Shattock RJ, Arts EJ (2009) CCR5- and CXCR4-tropic subtype C human immunodeficiency virus type 1 isolates have a lower level of pathogenic fitness than other dominant group M subtypes: implications for the epidemic. J Virol 83(11):5592–5605. doi:10.1128/JVI.02051-08
41. Quinones-Mateu ME, Ball SC, Marozsan AJ, Torre VS, Albright JL, Vanham G et al (2000) A dual infection/competition assay shows a correlation between ex vivo human immunodeficiency virus type 1 fitness and disease progression. J Virol 74:9222–9233
42. Roche M, Jakobsen MR, Ellett A, Salimiseyedabad H, Jubb B, Westby M et al (2011) HIV-1 predisposed to acquiring resistance to maraviroc (MVC) and other CCR5 antagonists in vitro has an inherent, low-level ability to utilize MVC-bound CCR5 for entry. Retrovirology 8:89
43. Roche M, Salimi H, Duncan R, Wilkinson BL, Chikere K, Moore MS et al (2013) A common mechanism of clinical HIV-1 resistance to the CCR5 antagonist maraviroc despite divergent resistance levels and lack of common gp120 resistance mutations. Retrovirology 10:43
44. Ratcliff AN, Shi W, Arts EJ (2013) HIV-1 resistance to maraviroc conferred by a CD4 binding site mutation in the envelope glycoprotein gp120. J Virol 87:923–934
45. Westby M, Smith-Burchnell C, Mori J, Lewis M, Mosley M, Stockdale M et al (2007) Reduced maximal inhibition in phenotypic susceptibility assays indicates that viral strains resistant to the CCR5 antagonist maraviroc utilize inhibitor-bound receptor for entry. J Virol 81:2359–2371
46. Johnston ER, Zijenah LS, Mutetwa S, Kantor R, Kittinunvorakoon C, Katzenstein DA (2003) High frequency of syncytium-inducing and CXCR4-tropic viruses among human immunodeficiency virus type 1 subtype C-infected patients receiving antiretroviral treatment. J Virol 77:7682–7688
47. Dudley DM, Gao Y, Nelson KN, Henry KR, Nankya I, Gibson RM et al (2009) A novel yeast-based recombination method to clone and propagate diverse HIV-1 isolates. Biotechniques 46:458–467
48. Weber J, Vazquez AC, Winner D, Gibson RM, Rhea AM, Rose JD et al (2013) Sensitive cell-based assay for determination of human immunodeficiency virus type 1 coreceptor tropism. J Clin Microbiol 51:1517–1527
49. Marozsan AJ, Moore DM, Lobritz MA, Fraundorf E, Abraha A, Reeves JD et al (2005) Differences in the fitness of two diverse wild-type human immunodeficiency virus type 1 isolates are related to the efficiency of cell binding and entry. J Virol 79:7121–7134
50. Dorr P, Westby M, Dobbs S, Griffin P, Irvine B, Macartney M et al (2005) Maraviroc (UK-427,857), a potent, orally bioavailable, and selective small-molecule inhibitor of chemokine receptor CCR5 with broad-spectrum anti-human immunodeficiency virus type 1 activity. Antimicrob Agents Chemother 49:4721–4732
51. Fatkenheuer G, Pozniak AL, Johnson MA, Plettenberg A, Staszewski S, Hoepelman AI et al (2005) Efficacy of short-term monotherapy with maraviroc, a new CCR5 antagonist, in patients infected with HIV-1. Nat Med 11:1170–1172
52. Donzella GA, Schols D, Lin SW, Este JA, Nagashima KA, Maddon PJ et al (1998) AMD3100, a small molecule inhibitor of HIV-1 entry via the CXCR4 co- receptor. Nat Med 4:72–77
53. Blanco J, Barretina J, Henson G, Bridger G, De Clercq E, Clotet B et al (2000) The CXCR4 antagonist AMD3100 efficiently inhibits cell-surface-expressed human immunodeficiency virus type 1 envelope-induced apoptosis. Antimicrob Agents Chemother 44:51–56
54. Jensen MA, Li FS, 't Wout AB, Nickle DC, Shriner D, He HX et al (2003) Improved coreceptor usage prediction and genotypic monitoring of R5-to-X4 transition by motif analysis of human immunodeficiency virus type 1 env V3 loop sequences. J Virol 77:13376–13388
55. Cashin K, Gray LR, Jakobsen MR, Sterjovski J, Churchill MJ, Gorry PR (2013) CoRSeqV3-C: a novel HIV-1 subtype C specific V3 sequence based coreceptor usage prediction algorithm. Retrovirology 10:24
56. Pugach P, Marozsan AJ, Ketas TJ, Landes EL, Moore JP, Kuhmann SE (2007) HIV-1 clones resistant to a small molecule CCR5 inhibitor use the inhibitor-bound form of CCR5 for entry. Virology 361:212–228
57. Troyer RM, Collins KR, Abraha A, Fraundorf E, Moore DM, Krizan RW et al (2005) Changes in human immunodeficiency virus type 1 fitness and genetic diversity during disease progression. J Virol 79:9006–9018
58. Ping LH, Nelson JA, Hoffman IF, Schock J, Lamers SL, Goodman M et al (1999) Characterization of V3 sequence heterogeneity in subtype C human immunodeficiency virus type 1 isolates from Malawi: underrepresentation of X4 variants. J Virol 73:6271–6281
59. Kaleebu P, Nankya IL, Yirrell DL, Shafer LA, Kyosiimire-Lugemwa J, Lule DB et al (2007) Relation between chemokine receptor use, disease stage, and HIV-1 subtypes A and D: results from a rural Ugandan cohort. J Acquir Immune Defic Syndr 45:28–33
60. Huang W, Eshleman SH, Toma J, Fransen S, Stawiski E, Paxinos EE et al (2007) Coreceptor tropism in human immunodeficiency virus type 1 subtype D: high prevalence of CXCR4 tropism and heterogeneous composition of viral populations. J Virol 81:7885–7893
61. Johnston SH, Lobritz MA, Nguyen S, Lassen K, Delair S, Posta F et al (2009) A quantitative affinity-profiling system that reveals distinct CD4/CCR5 usage patterns among human immunodeficiency virus type 1 and simian immunodeficiency virus strains. J Virol 83:11016–11026
62. Westby M, Lewis M, Whitcomb J, Youle M, Pozniak AL, James IT et al (2006) Emergence of CXCR4-using human immunodeficiency virus type 1 (HIV-1) variants in a minority of HIV-1-infected patients following treatment with the CCR5 antagonist maraviroc is from a pretreatment CXCR4-using virus reservoir. J Virol 80:4909–4920
63. Vandekerckhove L, Verhofstede C, Demecheleer E, De WS, Florence E, Fransen K et al (2011) Comparison of phenotypic and genotypic tropism determination in triple-class-experienced HIV patients eligible for maraviroc treatment. J Antimicrob Chemother 66:265–272
64. Marozsan AJ, Fraundorf E, Abraha A, Baird H, Moore D, Troyer R et al (2004) Relationships between infectious titer, capsid protein levels, and reverse transcriptase activities of diverse human immunodeficiency virus type 1 isolates. J Virol 78:11130–11141
65. van't Wout AB, Blaak H, Ran LJ, Brouwer M, Kuiken C, Schuitemaker H (1998) Evolution of syncytium-inducing and non-syncytium-inducing biological virus clones in relation to replication kinetics during the course of human immunodeficiency virus type 1 infection. J Virol 72:5099–5107
66. Troyer RM, McNevin J, Liu Y, Zhang SC, Krizan RW, Abraha A et al (2009) Variable fitness impact of HIV-1 escape mutations to cytotoxic T lymphocyte (CTL) response. PLoS Pathog 5:e1000365
67. Singh A, Collman RG (2000) Heterogeneous spectrum of coreceptor usage among variants within a dualtropic human immunodeficiency virus type 1 primary-isolate quasispecies. J Virol 74:10229–10235
68. Yi Y, Shaheen F, Collman RG (2005) Preferential use of CXCR4 by R5X4 human immunodeficiency virus type 1 isolates for infection of primary lymphocytes. J Virol 79:1480–1486
69. Shankarappa R, Margolick JB, Gange SJ, Rodrigo AG, Upchurch D, Farzadegan H et al (1999) Consistent viral evolutionary changes associated with the progression of human immunodeficiency virus type 1 infection. J Virol 73:10489–10502
70. Shankarappa R, Gupta P, Learn GH Jr, Rodrigo AG, Rinaldo CR Jr, Gorry MC et al (1998) Evolution of human immunodeficiency virus type 1 envelope sequences in infected individuals with differing disease progression profiles. Virology 241:251–259
71. Stalmeijer EH, van Rij RP, Boeser-Nunnink B, Visser JA, Naarding MA, Schols D et al (2004) In vivo evolution of X4 human immunodeficiency virus type 1 variants in the natural course of infection coincides with decreasing sensitivity to CXCR4 antagonists. J Virol 78:2722–2728
72. Archer J, Rambaut A, Taillon BE, Harrigan PR, Lewis M, Robertson DL (2010) The evolutionary analysis of emerging low frequency HIV-1 CXCR4 using variants through time–an ultra-deep approach. PLoS Comput Biol 6:e1001022
73. Pastore C, Ramos A, Mosier DE (2004) Intrinsic obstacles to human immunodeficiency virus type 1 coreceptor switching. J Virol 78:7565–7574
74. Tersmette M, Gruters RA, de Wolf F, de Goede RE, Lange JM, Schellekens PT et al (1989) Evidence for a role of virulent human immunodeficiency virus (HIV) variants in the pathogenesis of acquired immunodeficiency syndrome: studies on sequential HIV isolates. J Virol 63:2118–2125
75. Peeters M, Vincent R, Perret JL, Lasky M, Patrel D, Liegeois F et al (1999) Evidence for differences in MT2 cell tropism according to genetic sub-

types of HIV-1: syncytium-inducing variants seem rare among subtype C HIV-1 viruses. J Acquir Immune Defic Syndr Hum Retrovirol 20:115–121
76. Lassen KG, Lobritz MA, Bailey JR, Johnston S, Nguyen S, Lee B et al (2009) Elite suppressor-derived HIV-1 envelope glycoproteins exhibit reduced entry efficiency and kinetics. PLoS Pathog 5:e1000377
77. Blaak H, Brouwer M, Ran LJ, de Wolf F, Schuitemaker H (1998) In vitro replication kinetics of human immunodeficiency virus type 1 (HIV-1) variants in relation to virus load in long-term survivors of HIV-1 infection. J Infect Dis 177:600–610
78. Blaak H, van't Wout AB, Brouwer M, Hooibrink B, Hovenkamp E, Schuitemaker H (2000) In vivo HIV-1 infection of CD45RA(+)CD4(+) T cells is established primarily by syncytium-inducing variants and correlates with the rate of CD4(+) T cell decline. Proc Natl Acad Sci USA 97:1269–1274
79. Reed LJ, Muench H (1938) A simple method of estimating fifty percent endpoints. Am J Hyg 27:493–497
80. Lalonde MS, Lobritz MA, Ratcliff A, Chamanian M, Athanassiou Z, Tyagi M et al (2011) Inhibition of both HIV-1 reverse transcription and gene expression by a cyclic peptide that binds the Tat-transactivating response element (TAR) RNA. PLoS Pathog 7:e10002038
81. Marozsan AJ, Arts EJ (2003) Development of a yeast-based recombination cloning/system for the analysis of gene products from diverse human immunodeficiency virus type 1 isolates. J Virol Methods 111:111–120
82. Moore DM, Arts EJ, Gao Y, Marozsan AJ (2005) A yeast recombination-based cloning system to produce chimeric HIV-1 viruses and express HIV-1 genes. In: Tuofu Z (ed) Human retrovirus protocols: virology and molecular biology. Humana Press, Totowa, pp 369–386
83. Thompson JD, Gibson TJ, Plewniak F, Jeanmougin F, Higgins DG (1997) The CLUSTAL_X windows interface: flexible strategies for multiple sequence alignment aided by quality analysis tools. Nucleic Acids Res 25:4876–4882
84. Edgar RC (2004) MUSCLE: a multiple sequence alignment method with reduced time and space complexity. BMC Bioinformatics 5:113
85. Edgar RC (2004) MUSCLE: multiple sequence alignment with high accuracy and high throughput. Nucleic Acids Res 32:1792–1797
86. Page RD (1996) TreeView: an application to display phylogenetic trees on personal computers. Comput Appl Biosci 12:357–358
87. Torre VS, Marozsan AJ, Albright JL, Collins KR, Hartley O, Offord RE, Quiñones-Mateu ME, Arts EJ (2000) Variable sensitivity of CCR5-tropic human immunodeficiency virus type 1 isolates to inhibition by RANTES analogs. J Virol 74(10):4868–4876

24

The impact of HIV/AIDS on compliance with antidepressant treatment in major depressive disorder

Francois N Slabbert[1], Brian H Harvey[2,3], Christiaan B Brink[2] and Martie S Lubbe[1*]

Abstract

Background: MDD and HIV/AIDS have a high prevalence worldwide with severe consequences for patients. In both conditions, compliance with treatment is key to successfully treat these disorders. In the current study, we examine the effect of MDD on the compliance with ADs in patients diagnosed with co-morbid HIV/AIDS and how different classes of ADs influence compliance in this group of patients.

Methods: A prospective, cohort study design was used to analyse nationally representative medicine claims data submitted to a privately-owned South African Pharmaceutical Benefit Management (PBM) company. Two groups were distinguished in the database, namely patients with only MDD and patients with both MDD and HIV/AIDS, over a six-year study period. The study population was determined by the following inclusion criteria: patients older than 18 years, MDD should be diagnosed by a psychiatrist supported by an appropriate ICD-10 code, and all patients have to be on combination antiretroviral treatment (cARV) treatment. The medicine possession ratio (MPR) was used as proxy to determine patient compliance with AD medication.

Results: 127 patients (i.e. 0.24%) met the criteria of co-morbid MDD and HIV/AIDS. Females have a significantly higher prevalence of MDD and HIV/AIDS when compared to males. Patients diagnosed with both HIV/AIDS and MDD (74.43. ± 32.03, 95% CI: 71.51-77.34) have a statistical significantly ($p < 0.0001$) lower compliance with AD treatment vs. MDD patients (80.94% ± 29.44, 95% CI: 80.56-81.33), but the practical significance thereof, is low (Cohen's d = 0.2255). In this group only 26.83% of TCA had acceptable compliance compared to the 58.57% of SNRIs. Noteworthy observations were that 75% ($p < 0.0217$; Cramer's V = 0.0388) of venlafaxine and 28.6% ($p < 0.0197$; Cramer's V = –0.0705) of the paroxetine items were compliant in patients diagnosed with both HIV/AIDS and MDD.

Conclusions: AD compliance is statistical significantly lower in depressed HIV/AIDS vs. depressed non-HIV/AIDS patients. However, these differences is of low practical or clinical significance, meaning that depressed HIV/AIDS patients would have missed approximately two AD doses (6.5% of a 30-day treatment period) more than the non-HIV/AIDS depressed patient over the same treatment period.

Keywords: Major depressive disorder, HIV/AIDS, Compliance, Antidepressants, Venlafaxine

* Correspondence: Martie.Lubbe@nwu.ac.za
[1]Medicines Usage Group (MUSA), North-West University, Potchefstroom 2520, South Africa
Full list of author information is available at the end of the article

Background

In 2012, the UNAIDS World AIDS Day Report estimated that approximately 34 million people worldwide are infected with human immunodeficiency virus (HIV), whereas 69% of these infected patients live in sub-Saharan Africa [1]. In the United States, more than one million individuals are infected with HIV and acquired immunodeficiency syndrome (AIDS, collectively HIV/AIDS), while nearly 50 000 more contract HIV each year [2]. In South Africa, the prevalence of HIV/AIDS is estimated to be 17.3% in the age group 15 to 49 years and approximately 5.6 million people in the country are living with HIV/AIDS [3]. South Africa is one of the countries with the highest HIV/AIDS-related mortality rates in the world, with approximately 270 000 deaths reported in 2011 [3].

Apart from the huge impact on the health system, HIV/AIDS also affects individual patients, causing a great deal of suffering in both their social lives as well as mental and physical health. It is therefore not surprising that HIV/AIDS is co-morbid with various psychosocial disorders, such as major depressive disorder (MDD) [4]. MDD is one of the main causes of psychiatric morbidity in HIV/AIDS patients [4]. In a six-month follow-up study in HIV/AIDS-infected patients in South Africa, Olley and co-workers described a 34.9% prevalence of MDD [5]. Elsewhere in the literature, however, there is some controversy over the prevalence of MDD in HIV/AIDS patients, with the prevalence rate varying between 3 and 54% [4,6,7]. Further studies in this regard are therefore urgently needed.

The co-morbidity between chronic illnesses and MDD is a well-recognised phenomenon. Chronically ill patients display two to three times higher rates of MDD when compared to healthy individuals of the same age and gender [8-10]. Diabetes, asthma, epilepsy, cancer, coronary heart disease, hypertension and HIV/AIDS are among the most common chronic illnesses that are associated with an increased prevalence of MDD [11,12]. Considering the symptomatology of depression, depressed patients tend to neglect themselves due to fatigue, low energy levels, impaired memory and the sense of helplessness [13]. Patients with a chronic illness and co-morbid MDD have a significantly decreased compliance with self-care treatment regimens [14], which negatively affects long-term treatment outcomes and is ultimately associated with impaired daily functioning and a decreased quality of life [15,16].

HIV-positive patients have twice the incidence of MDD compared to HIV-negative individuals [17-20]. In particular, late stage HIV (CD4 count of <200 cells/μL) is associated with a significantly higher incidence of MDD, with a number of studies showing as much as a two and a half-fold increase in the incidence of MDD [21-24]. A recent study by Lopes and co-workers found that HIV-positive men were more likely to have a major depressive disorder/dysthymia (OR = 3.77; 95% CI, 1.16-12.27) when compared to HIV-negative males [25]. The reason for this is likely to be multifactorial, although chronic-psychosocial stress (e.g. discrimination, isolation, violence, stigmatisation, hopelessness and drug abuse) [26] associated with HIV/AIDS can induce inflammation in the central nervous system (CNS), which is a major etiological factor [27]. Exposure to chronic psychosocial stress induces the continuous release of cortisol, and activates the hypothalamic-pituitary-adrenal (HPA) axis as well as the sympathetic autonomic nervous system, which in turn activates immune cells in both CNS and in the periphery [28,29]. Depressed patients express elevated levels and an imbalance of cytokines, especially interleukin-1 (IL-1) and tumour necrosis factor alpha (TNF α), which leads to cognitive and mood impairment [30-32]. Further evidence supporting inflammation as an etiological factor in depression, is that patients receiving interferon Alfa (IFN-α) therapy for various types of cancer develop severe depression, INF being an inflammatory mediator [33-35]. Cerebral HIV infection will induce chronic inflammation in the brain and this causes the release of IFN and other cytokines, with depression as a result [27]. Therefore, HIV/AIDS patients with chronic increased cytokine levels as a result of viral infection, can be expected to be particularly vulnerable to develop depression [36].

The introduction of combination antiretroviral therapy (cART) has been successful in improving morbidity and decreasing the mortality rate of HIV/AIDS, which provides a glimmer of hope [37-39]. Importantly, however, cART can suppress HIV-1 RNA levels and increase CD4 T cell lymphocytes only if the cART is associated with excellent compliance and persistence [40-43]. Patients who are HIV positive must maintain a compliance rate of at least 95% in order to prevent virologic failure, increase CD4 T cell lymphocyte count, and decrease viral load and opportunistic infections [44-47]. Another risk associated with non-compliance with ART is the increased risk of viral resistance that ultimately leads to treatment failure [48-51]. On the other hand, compliance with AD treatment is just as important. Patients who fail to comply with their AD treatment have a two-fold increased risk for relapse [52], are more likely to experience antidepressant withdrawal syndrome [53], and have a significantly increased mortality and morbidity rate associated with MDD [54]. Consequently, poor compliance with either ART or AD treatment will significantly compromise a successful treatment outcome.

The current literature regarding the prevalence of HIV/AIDS and MDD is quite limited. Therefore, this study will firstly strive to determine the prevalence of

HIV/AIDS-positive patients within the MDD-diagnosed population in the private health sector of South Africa. Secondly, the study will investigate how AD compliance is affected by MDD in HIV/AIDS-positive patients when compared to depressed non-HIV/AIDS patients and, lastly, whether AD compliance has any association with gender and antidepressant class in this population.

Results

The research cohort consisted of two groups, namely MDD patients with HIV/AIDS (n = 127) and patients with only MDD (n = 12 270) (Table 1). These patients received over the study period respectively 466 and 22 831 AD items (Table 2).

The mean MPR of antidepressants (ADs) was statistical significantly lower ($p < 0.0001$; $d = 0.2255$) in MDD patients with HIV/AIDS (74.43% ± 32.03, 95% Cl: 71.51-77.34) than in patients with only MDD (80.94% ± 29.44, 95% Cl: 80.56-81.33). These differences were of low practical significance. In MDD patients with HIV/AIDS, antidepressant compliance (MPR) was statistical significantly lower with medium practical significance in females (69.35% ± 29.69, 95% Cl: 66.03-72.67) than in males (84.51% ± 34.18, 95% Cl: 79.10-89.91) from the same cohort ($p < 0.0001$; $d = 0.4755$). Age was not a significant predictor of AD compliance in MDD patients with HIV/AIDS ($p < 0.9519$) and those with only MDD ($p = 0.1111$), as shown in Table 2.

In Table 3, a significant association was found between AD class and AD compliance in MDD patients with HIV/AIDS, with compliance figures as follows; tricyclic antidepressants (TCA) 26.83%; selective serotonin re-uptake inhibitors (SSRIs) 44.93%; diverse antidepressants 52.70%; and serotonin and noradrenalin re-uptake inhibitors (SNRIs) 58.57% ($p < 0.0001$; Cramer's $V = 0.3450$).

The following ADs, as depicted in Table 4, were associated with unacceptably low levels of compliance in MDD patients with HIV/AIDS vs. patients with only MDD, as observed from the compliance ratio: amitriptyline 23.53% vs. 39.34% ($p < 0.0618$; Cramer's $V = -0.0494$); trazodone 27.27% vs. 50.72% ($p < -0.0239$; Cramer's $V = -0.0630$); paroxetine 28.57% vs. 54.19% ($p < 0.0197$; Cramer's $V = -0.0705$); duloxetine 36.67% vs. 55.51% ($p < 0.0391$; Cramer's $V = -0.0426$); escitalopram 44.16% vs. 52.74% ($p < 0.0.0359$; Cramer's $V = -0.0254$); bupropion 78.26% vs. 50.46% ($p < 0.0082$; Cramer's $V = 0.0698$) and venlafaxine 75.00% vs. 56.93% ($p < 0.0217$; Cramer's $V = 0.0388$).

Table 1 Patient demographics

Total number of patients in the study population						
Illness	**n**	**%**				
MDD + HIV	127	0.24				
MDD	12270	22.94				
HIV	41086	76.82				
Gender classification of the study population						
	Male		**Female**			
Illness	**n**	**%**	**n**	**%**		
MDD + HIV	37	29.13	90	70.87		
MDD	3496	28.49	8774	71.51		
HIV	18268	44.46	22818	55.54		
Age classification of the study population						
	>18 ≤ 40 years		**>40 ≤ 60 years**		**>60 years**	
Illness	**n**	**%**	**n**	**%**	**n**	**%**
MDD + HIV	31	24.41	75	59.06	21	16.54
MDD	2662	21.7	21176	47.03	3837	31.27
HIV	16586	40.37	21176	5154	1652	4.02

Discussion

This study focused on the prevalence of HIV/AIDS-positive patients within the MDD-diagnosed population in this section of the private health sector of South Africa. Secondly, the study investigated how AD compliance is affected by MDD in HIV/AIDS-positive patients when compared to depressed non-HIV/AIDS patients, and whether AD compliance has any correlation with gender and antidepressant class in this population. These goals were attained in that we were able to confirm the co-morbidity between MDD and HIV/AIDS-positive patients; however, due to the strict inclusion criteria, the numbers of patients were small, which provided a limited picture of the overall prevalence between MDD and HIV/AIDS-positive patients.

This study found that patients diagnosed with both HIV/AIDS and MDD (74.43. ± 32.03, 95% Cl: 71.51-77.34) have a statistical significantly lower compliance with AD treatment when compared to patients diagnosed only with MDD (80.94% ± 29.44, 95% Cl: 80.56-81.33). However, these differences is of low practical or clinical significance, meaning that depressed HIV/AIDS patients would have missed approximately two AD doses (~6.5% of a 30-day treatment period) more than the non-HIV/AIDS depressed patient over the same treatment period. The current study confirms that patients suffering from both MDD and HIV/AIDS have a decreased compliance with MDD treatment. This trend is confirmed in the literature as several authors have found similar results, namely that patients suffering from both conditions are less compliant to AD treatment regimens [14,20,55,56]. Our data also seem to suggest, in Table 4, that patients with HIV/AIDS are less compliant with ADs that present with multi-receptor pharmacology, i.e. TCAs (26.83% compliance; Table 3) and paroxetine (compliance 28.57%, Table 4), while they are more compliant with pharmacologically 'clean' ADs, such as the venlafaxine (75% compliance, Table 4). The TCAs display a

Table 2 The effect of illness, gender and age on medicine possession ratio (MPR)

Mean MPR of ADs in MDD patients with/without HIV/AIDS (dispensed items)					
Illness	**n**	**Mean ± SD (%)**	**95% CI**	**p***	**Cohen's d-value**
HIV/AIDS + MDD	466	74.43 ± 32.03	71.51-77.34	0.0001	0.2255
MDD	22831	80.94 ± 29.44	80.56-81.33		
Mean MPR of ADs in MDD patients with HIV/AIDS vs. gender (dispensed items)					
Gender	**n**	**Mean ± SD (%)**	**95% CI**	**p***	**Cohen's d-value**
Female	310	69.35 ± 29.69	66.03-72.67	0.0001	0.4755
Male	156	84.51 ± 34.18	79.10-89.91		
Mean MPR of ADs in MDD patients without HIV/AIDS vs. gender (dispensed items)					
Gender	**n**	**Mean ± SD (%)**	**95% CI**	***p****	
Female	16600	80.97 ± 29.72	80.52-81.43	0.8067	
Male	6231	80.87 ± 28.65	80.16-81.58		
Mean MPR of ADs in MDD patients with HIV/AIDS vs. age group (dispensed items)					
Age (years)	**n**	**Mean ± SD (%)**	**95% CI**	***p*****	
> 18 ≤ 40	126	74.57 ± 32.39	68.86-80.29	0.9519	
>40 ≤ 60	284	74.61 ± 33.07	70.74-78.47		
>60	56	73.16 ± 25.74	66.27-80.06.		
Mean MPR of ADs in MDD patients without HIV/AIDS vs. age group (dispensed items)					
Age (years)	**n**	**Mean ± SD (%)**	**95% CI**	***p*****	
>18 ≤ 40	4320	81.39 ± 28.89	80.56-82.28	0.1111	
>40 ≤ 60	10929	80.52 ± 29.85	79.96-81.08		
>60	7582	81.30 ± 29.15	80.65-81.92		

*Two-sample *t*-test.
**One-way ANOVA.

high binding affinity for non-specific receptors such as muscarinic (mAch), histaminic (HA-1) and alpha-1 adrenoceptors, which are responsible for side effects such as dry mouth, constipation and sedation [57]. Similarly, paroxetine demonstrates an affinity for mAch receptors similar to that of imipramine and has marked anticholinergic adverse effects [57]. Our data infer that the reduced compliance with these antidepressants may have a biological basis, in particular an apparent increase in cholinergic sensitivity in the HIV/AIDS population. Indeed, cholinomimetic antibodies of the immunoglobulin (IgA) class are present in HIV/AIDS patients [58,59], suggesting that these patients may indeed be hypersensitive to drugs with activity on the cholinergic system [60]. Importantly,

Table 3 The influence of AD class on AD compliance in MDD patients with/without HIV/AIDS (dispensed items)

MDD patients with HIV/AIDS (dispensed items)					
Antidepressant class	**n**	**Acceptable (%)**	**Unacceptable (%)**	***p******	**Cramer's *V***
SSRIs	207	44.93	55.07	<0.0001	0.3450
Diverse antidepressants	148	52.70	37.30		
SNRIs	70	58.57	41.43		
TCA	41	26.83	73.17		
MDD patients without HIV/AIDS (dispensed items)					
Antidepressant class	**n**	**Acceptable (%)**	**Unacceptable (%)**	***p******	**Cramer's *V***
SSRIs	9435	51.64	48.36	0.0001	0.0942
SNRIs	5777	56.36	43.64		
Diverse antidepressants	5460	48.24	51.76		
TCA	2159	43.72	56.28		

***Chi-square.

Table 4 Percentage of the top 10 most frequently dispensed antidepressants with acceptable vs. non-acceptable compliance in MDD patients with/without HIV/AIDS (dispensed items)

	HIV + MDD				MDD					
	n	Acceptable	n	Unacceptable	n	Acceptable	n	Unacceptable	P***	Cramer's V
Mirtazapine	40	51.28	38	48.72	848	46.41	979	53.59	0.3987	0.0193
Escitalopram	34	44.16	43	55.84	1781	52.74	1596	47.26	0.1359	−0.0254
Venlafaxine	30	75.00	10	25.00	1972	56.93	1492	43.07	0.0217	0.0388
Citalopram	25	51.02	18	48.92	1002	51.46	945	48.54	0.9511	−0.0014
Fluoxetine	19	41.30	25	58.70	724	47.95	786	52.05	0.3743	−0.0225
Bupropion	18	78.26	5	21.74	714	50.46	701	49.54	0.0082	0.0698
Duloxetine	11	36.67	19	63.33	1284	55.51	1029	44.49	0.0391	−0.0426
Amitriptyline	8	23.53	26	76.47	548	39.34	845	60.66	0.0618	−0.0494
Trazodone	6	27.27	16	72.73	596	50.72	579	49.28	0.0293	−0.0630
Paroxetine	6	28.57	15	71.43	582	54.19	492	45.81	0.0197	−0.0705

***Chi-square.

TCA and paroxetine non-compliance with TCAs and paroxetine can evoke a cholinergic overdrive [57,61], which may augment the hyper-cholinergic state present in HIV/AIDS patients, leading to a greater adverse experience and subsequent non-compliance. Furthermore, since MDD is associated with increased cholinergic drive [62,63], it is clear that poor compliance in this population may worsen the mood disorder. For the successful treatment of both MDD and HIV/AIDS, compliance with treatment is therefore of utmost importance. Poor compliance with treatment can lead to a drastic decline in quality of life, increased social impairment, low occupational functioning and heightened social isolation, increased suicide ideation and ultimately to suicide [21,55,56,64-66].

Another interesting result is that the class of antidepressant plays a significant role in predicting compliance when treating patients with MDD and HIV/AIDS. The tricyclic antidepressant (TCA) class is associated with the weakest compliance ratio (26.83%), whereas the SNRIs present with the highest compliance ratio (58.57%). According to our results, SSRIs represent the class of ADs with the highest prescription frequency (44.42%, N = 466). Both escitalopram and citalopram are considered as first-line treatment for treating MDD in HIV/AIDS patients because of a limited effect on the cytochrome P450 system, thereby reducing drug-drug interactions with ARV treatment [67-69]. Moreover, a number of studies have proposed that MDD associated with HIV/AIDS should be treated with fluoxetine and paroxetine [70-72]. However, their use is limited by drug-drug interaction with protease inhibitors (PIs) due to their potent inhibition of CYP2D6, thereby increasing levels of PIs and associated toxicity [57,67,73]. However, in this study, the SSRIs as a group displayed a relatively weak compliance ratio (44.93%; $p < 0.0001$; Table 3) compared to the SNRIs, which displayed a significantly higher compliance ratio (58.57%; $p < 0.0001$; Table 3). These findings indicate that the SSRIs have more adverse effects in this population than originally predicted, possibly related to their anticholinergic (paroxetine), antihistaminic (citalopram) and general serotonergic properties [57]. In fact, considering the latter point, neuropsychiatric symptoms may be evident in HIV-treated patients, especially those on efavirenz, and respond to treatment with the antiserotonergic agent, cyproheptadine, suggesting increased serotonergic activity/sensitivity in these patients [74]. Furthermore, inappropriate AD discontinuation and non-compliance are also associated with increased serotonergic activity [75] that may amplify the adverse experience associated with HIV/AIDS-related neurotransmitter dysregulation. What is more important considering our data is that SNRIs are currently considered a second-line treatment for MDD in HIV/AIDS patients [68,69], while our data (preliminary as they may be) suggest a possible re-evaluation of these guidelines. Indeed, further studies in this regard are warranted.

Only 127 patients (i.e. 0.24% of the total population in the database) met the criteria of co-morbid MDD and HIV/AIDS. Currently, there exists great controversy in the literature regarding the co-morbidity between depression and HIV/AIDS, with a number of articles placing the co-morbidity rate between 0 and 54% [4,6,7,55]. This finding again highlights the complicated co-morbidity between MDD and HIV/AIDS, the different approaches, methodology and reporting of results used in several studies with regard to the selection of a study population, the demographics and the behaviour of the defined population. Furthermore, the low prevalence rate found in this study might suggest a severe under diagnoses of MDD in HIV/AIDS patients and that MDD symptoms might be mistaken rather as symptoms of HIV/AIDS [76,77].

We also observed that female patients (n = 90) were more than double that of male patients (n = 37). Female patients diagnosed with both MDD and HIV/AIDS displayed significantly lower compliance with AD treatment when compared to male patients of the same group, and displayed almost double the prevalence of both MDD and HIV/AIDS than male counterparts. Some of the reasons given for the poor compliance rate to AD treatment in women are the risk of adverse effects (e.g. weight gain and sexual dysfunction), low socio-economic status, younger age, drug abuse and divorce marital status [78]. Similar to our findings, two separate studies found that almost double the number of women with MDD and HIV/AIDS are likely to die from an HIV/AIDS-related cause when compared to HIV-positive women without depression [79], while females have a significantly higher frequency of MDD and HIV/AIDS vs. males with a combined diagnosis [80,81]. Some authors have suggested that lower levels of testosterone might play a role in the large prevalence of MDD in females when compared to men [82]. In support of this, males with hypogonadism have a significantly higher prevalence of MDD and anxiety disorders when compared to healthy males [83,84]. Moreover, testosterone-replacement therapy in hypogonadal men significantly improves these symptoms [83,85,86]. Importantly, studies have found benefits in administering testosterone to depressed women [87,88], thereby supporting the role of testosterone as a causal factor for MDD in women. However, a study in depressed HIV/AIDS patients has shown that testosterone displayed no significant effect on mood [56].

Examining individual ADs dispensed to patients who are suffering from both MDD and HIV/AIDS, mirtazapine was the most frequently dispensed AD (n = 78), followed closely by escitalopram (n = 77). Although mirtazapine is not a first-line AD for the treatment of MDD, its side effect profile seems to play a valuable role in late-stage HIV/AIDS patients with co-morbid MDD, with side effects such as constipation, weight gain and sedation helping to improve diarrhoea, diminished appetite and insomnia, respectively [67].

The strength of the current study is that only patients diagnosed with MDD by a psychiatrist were included in the study population. This article has shed light on the current practice of AD treatment in HIV/AIDS patients with medical aids. The most important findings include that HIV/AIDS with co-morbid MDD have reduced compliance with ADs, especially those exhibiting multi-receptor pharmacology, most notably TCAs and certain SSRIs such as paroxetine. Secondly, MDD patients with co-morbid HIV/AIDS display significantly higher compliance with venlafaxine, contrary to current clinical practice where guidelines suggest SSRIs and SNRIs as first and second line treatment options, respectively. Further clarification with respect to duloxetine is needed as it performed poorly in our analysis. Lastly, female patients are more prone to develop MDD and are notably less compliant with AD treatment.

The authors recognise a few limitations in the current study. Firstly, the numbers of patients with both MDD and HIV/AIDS were relatively small and not a full representation of the national population. Several factors contributed to the small sample size, such as the use of very strict inclusion criteria, only a portion of all the medical aids is listed with the PBM utilised in this study, depressed patients using psychological treatment for MDD were not taken into account, while the study population consisted of only patients contributing to a private medical aid/insurance. Secondly, the use of a database limits the further extraction of patient information regarding the stage of HIV/AIDS in which the patient is and whether there was an improvement or deterioration in the patient's mood.

Conclusion

This study confirms that AD compliance is lower in depressed HIV/AIDS vs. depressed non-HIV/AIDS patients, correlating with global trends regarding non-compliance of patients with a chronic disease and co-morbid disorders. However, this study indicated that the clinical and practical significance of the differences is low. Moreover, the fact that the prevalence of MDD patients with co-morbid HIV/AIDS was limited in this study again highlights the need for more research in various population groups with a focus on the socio-economic status of the patients. Although our data are preliminary and warrant further study, it does reveal evidence that venlafaxine may be a valid choice of antidepressant in HIV/AIDS patients suffering from MDD and should be considered as first-line antidepressant in such cases. Moreover, our data suggest that multi-target antidepressants such as TCAs and select SSRIs may increase the risk of non-compliance in this population. Lastly, when prescribing ADs to females, special consideration should be given to counselling them on both their illness and treatment so that they clearly understand the benefits of compliance to treatment.

Methods

We conducted a prospective, cohort study analysing nationally representative medicine claims data submitted to a privately-owned South African Pharmaceutical Benefit Management (PBM) company. The data represent a third of South African patients with private medical aids. No distinction was made between races. Two groups were distinguished in the database over a six-year study period (1 January 2006 to 31 December 2011), namely patients with only MDD (n = 12 270) and MDD patients with HIV/AIDS (n = 127).

We queried data for patient demographics (gender and date of birth) and pertinent prescription information (such as drug trade name, days supplied, dispensing date, quantity of medicine prescribed, and ICD-10 code per claim). The following automated validation processes were applied by the PBM that ascertained the quality of data: data integrity validation, eligibility management, medicine utilisation and clinical management, pricing and formulary management. There were no missing data fields in the datasets. The variables 'birth date' and 'dispensing date' were used to calculate the age of patients on the date of treatment and the number of days between refills.

A study population was selected according the following inclusion criteria: patients older than 18 years, MDD should be diagnosed by a psychiatrist supported by an appropriate ICD-10 code. The ICD-10 codes are based on the International Classification of Diseases, 10th edition published by the World Health Organization [89]. In this study, the ICD-10 codes F32 (Depressive episode) and F33 (Recurrent depressive disorder) were used to identify patients with MDD as diagnosed by a psychiatrist, as well as B20-B24 (Human immunodeficiency virus [HIV/AIDS] disease), and all patients on cARV treatment. Thereby it was ensured that data were excluded where ADs may have been used for other indications, such as amitriptyline for the treatment of chronic pain.

For the purpose of this study, the medicine possession ratio (MPR) was used to determine AD compliance of patients. The MPR is a well-established method to calculate drug compliance in pharmacoepidemiological studies, including chronic diseases such as MDD [90], hypertension [91], and schizophrenia [92]. However, it is important to note that the compliance value obtained from the MPR only gives an indication of the possession of medicine by the patient, and that appropriate consumption of medicine is assumed to ensue from possession. The usage of medicine claims data to determine MPR calculations is valuable in that it is acceptably accurate, convenient, objective, non-invasive and relatively inexpensive to obtain when a large study population is needed. It is therefore suitable for the calculation of MPR as an indication of patient compliance with medication therapy [93,94]. However, the MPR has a number of limitations. Firstly, MPR can only be calculated if a patient has filled more than two prescriptions. Secondly, MPR can only assess whether the medication was used consistently. Lastly, the MPR cannot measure whether a patient was compliant with the instructions given by the medical practitioner [95].

The MPR is defined as the number of days for which medication is supplied within the refill interval (medicine treatment period) divided by the number of days in the refill interval [96,97].

$$\text{MPR} = \frac{\text{Number of days in refill interval}}{\text{Sum the days of supplied medication}} \times 100$$

The MPR is considered acceptable if the calculated value is ≥ 80%, but ≤ 110%. An MPR of less than 80% indicates the presence of refill gaps so that possession is considered unacceptably low (undersupply), whereas an MPR greater than 110% is considered unacceptably high (oversupply). Conversely, a patient was considered compliant (acceptable group) with his/her AD treatment if the MPR was ≥ 80% and ≤ 110%, and AD treatment period was longer than 120 days. Therefore, distinguishing between compliant MPR group and patients out of this range will be considered as the non-compliant MPR group or unacceptable group.

Data management and analysis were performed in SAS Version 9.1.3 (SAS Institute, Cary, NC) [98]. All statistical significance was considered with a probability of $p < 0.05$. The practical significance of results was computed when the p-value was statistically significant ($p \leq 0.05$).

Variables (age groups, gender and active ingredients) were expressed using descriptive statistics such as frequencies (n), percentages (%), means, standard deviations and 95% confidence intervals (CI). The patient's age was determined at time of first dispensing and divided into three groups: > 18 to ≤ 40 years; > 40 to ≤ 60 years; > 60 years.

The dataset is very large, therefore all the statistical methods used in this study rely on the Central Limit Theorem, which states that the average of a large number of independent random variables is approximately normally distributed around the true population mean [99]. Therefore, the two-sample t-test allowed us to compare the mean MPR of male and female patients. The one-way ANOVA was used to test differences between the mean MPR of different age groups and AD classes. It was operationalised with the general linear model (GLM) procedure of the SAS Version 9.1.3. If a difference was indicated, a Tukey's multiple comparison test was performed to determine which groups differ significantly from each other. Cohen's d was used to evaluate effect size between means (with d ≥ 0.8 defined as a large effect with practical significance). The Chi-square test ($\chi 2$) was used to determine whether an association exists between proportions of two or more groups (compliance vs. active ingredients). The Cramer's V statistic was used to test the practical significance of this association (with Cramer's V ≥ 0.5 defined as practical significance).

This study was approved by the Research Ethics Committee of the North-West University (NWU-0046-08-550) and the Board of Directors of the South African Pharmaceutical Benefit Management (PBM). Data were analysed anonymously.

Competing interests
The authors declare that they have no competing interests.

Authors' contributions
FN Slabbert has been involved in the design of the study, drafted the manuscript, and carried out the analyses and interpretation of data. MS Lubbe made a substantial contribution in the design of the study and developed the methodology. BH Harvey and CB Brink revised the manuscript and have given extensive intellectual inputs. All authors read and approved the final manuscript.

Authors' information
FN Slabbert: BPharm, MSc (Pharmacology). PhD student and junior research scientist, School of Pharmacy, North-West University (Potchefstroom Campus).
MS Lubbe: BPharm, MPharm, PhD (Pharmacy Practice). Leader: Medicine Usage in South Africa, professor at the School of Pharmacy, North-West University (Potchefstroom Campus).
BH Harvey: BPharm, BSc (Hons), MSc (Pharmacology), PhD (Pharmacology). Center of Excellence for Pharmaceutical Sciences, Co-director – MRC unit on Anxiety and Stress Disorders. Professor of Pharmacology. School of Pharmacy, North-West University (Potchefstroom Campus).
CB Brink: BPharm, MSc (Pharmacology), PhD (Pharmacology). Secretary-general: WCP2014. President: SASBCP. Chair: IUPHAR-Ed. Professor of Pharmacology. School of Pharmacy, North-West University (Potchefstroom Campus).

Acknowledgements
We thank Dr Suria Ellis from Statistical Consultation Services and Mrs Marike Cockeran from Medicine Usage in South Africa, North-West University (Potchefstroom Campus) for statistical support, and Anne-Marie Bekker for administrative support regarding the database. The authors acknowledge the North-West University, National Research Foundation and the South African Medical Research Council for financial support.

Author details
[1]Medicines Usage Group (MUSA), North-West University, Potchefstroom 2520, South Africa. [2]Division of Pharmacology, North-West University, Potchefstroom 2520, South Africa. [3]Centre of Excellence for Pharmaceutical Sciences, School of Pharmacy, North-West University, Potchefstroom 2520, South Africa.

References

1. UNAIDS. UNAIDS World AIDS Day Report 2012; UNAIDS Fact Sheet 2012; Kaiser Family Foundation. . In Book UNAIDS World AIDS Day Report 2012; UNAIDS Fact Sheet 2012; Kaiser Family Foundation. (Editor ed.^eds.). City; 2012 [http://www.unaids.org/sites/default/files/en/media/unaids/contentassets/documents/epidemiology/2012/gr2012/20121120_FactSheet_Global_en.pdf]
2. Centers for Disease Control and Prevention. HIV surveillance report: Diagnoses of HIV infection and AIDS in the United States and dependent areas, 2009. [http://www.cdc.gov/hiv]
3. World Health Organistation. Data on the size of the HIV/AIDS epidemic: Number of people (all ages) living with HIV by country [http://apps.who.int/gho/data/view.main.22100]
4. Kinyanda E, Hoskins S, Nakku J, Nawaz S, Patel V. Prevalence and risk factors of major depressive disorder in HIV/AIDS as seen in semi-urban Entebbe district, Uganda. BMC Psychiatry. 2011, 11.
5. Olley BO, Seedat S, Stein DJ. Persistence of psychiatric disorders in a cohort of HIV/AIDS patients in South Africa: a 6-month follow-up study. J Psychosom Res. 2006;61:479–84.
6. Cysique LA, Deutsch R, Atkinson JH, Young C, Marcotte TD, Dawson L, et al. Incident major depression does not affect neuropsychological functioning in HIV-infected men. J Int Neuropsychol Soc. 2006;13:1–11.
7. Gibbie T, Hay M, Hutchison CW, Mijch A. Depression, social support and adherence to highly active antiretroviral therapy in people living with HIV/AIDS. Sex Health. 2007;4:227–32.
8. Ali S, Stone MA, Peters JL, Davies MJ, Khunti K. The prevalence of co-morbid depression in adults with Type 2 diabetes: a systematic review and meta-analysis. Diabet Med. 2006;23:1165–73.
9. Schleifer SJ, Macari-Hinson MM. The nature and course of depression following myocardial infarction. Arch Intern Med. 1989;149:1785–9.
10. Spijkerman T, de Jonge P, van den Brink RH, Jansen JH, May JF, Crijns HJ, et al. Depression following myocardial infarction: first-ever versus ongoing and recurrent episodes. Gen Hosp Psychiatry. 2005;27:411–7.
11. Von Korff M, Scott KM, Gureje O. Global perspectives on mental-physical comorbidity in the WHO world mental health surveys. Cambridge, UK: Cambridge University Press; 2009.
12. Springer SA, Dushaj A, Azar MM. The impact of DSM-IV mental disorders on adherence to combination antiretroviral therapy among adult persons living with HIV/AIDS: a systematic review. AIDS Behav. 2012;16:2119–43.
13. Katon WJ. Clinical and health services relationships between major depression, depressive symptoms, and general medical illness. Biol Psychiatry. 2003;54:216–26.
14. DiMatteo MR, Lepper HS, Croghan TW. Depression is a risk factor for noncompliance with medical treatment - Meta-analysis of the effects of anxiety and depression on patient adherence. Arch Intern Med. 2000;160:2101–7.
15. Plummer ML, Watson-Jones D, Lees S, Baisley K, Matari S, Changalucha J, et al. A qualitative study of participant adherence in a randomized controlled trial of herpes suppressive therapy for HIV prevention in Tanzania. AIDS care. 2010;22:499–508.
16. Singh N, Berman SM, Swindells S, Justis JC, Mohr JA, Squier C, et al. Adherence of human immunodeficiency virus-infected patients to antiretroviral therapy. Clin Infect Dis. 1999;29:824–30.
17. Ellis RJ, Rosario D, Clifford DB, McArthur JC Simpson D, Alexander T, et al. Continued high prevalence and adverse clinical impact of human immunodeficiency virus-associated sensory neuropathy in the era of combination antiretroviral therapy: the CHARTER Study. Arch Neurol. 2010;67:552–8.
18. Orlando M, Burnam MA, Beckman R, Morton SC, London AS, Bing EG, et al. Re-estimating the prevalence of psychiatric disorders in a nationally representative sample of persons receiving care for HIV: results from the HIV Cost and Services Utilization Study. Int J Methods Psychiatr Res. 2002;11:75–82.
19. Lima VD, Geller J, Rangsberg DR, Patterson TL, Daniel M, Kerr T, et al. The effect of adherence on the association between depressive symptoms and mortality among HIV-infected individuals first initiating HAART. AIDS. 2007;21:1175–83.
20. Sin NL, DiMatteo MR. Depression treatment enhances adherence to antiretroviral therapy: a meta-analysis. Ann Behav Med. 2014;47:259–69.
21. Alciati A, Starace F, Scaramelli B, Campaniello M, Adriani B, Mellado C, et al. Has there been a decrease in the prevalence of mood disorders in HIV-seropositive individuals since the introduction of combination therapy? Eur Psychiatry. 2001;16:491–6.
22. Ickovics JR, Hamburger ME, Vlahov D, Schoenbaum EE, Schuman P, Boland RJ, et al. Mortality, CD4 cell count decline, and depressive symptoms among HIV-seropositive women - Longitudinal analysis from the HIV epidemiology research study. JAMA. 2001;285:1466–74.
23. Lyketsos CG, Hoover DR, Guccione M, Dew MA, Wesch JE, Bing EG, et al. Changes in depressive symptoms as AIDS develops. The Multicenter AIDS Cohort Study. Am J Psychiatry. 1996;153(11):1430–7.
24. Lyketsos CG, Hoover DR, Guccione M. Depression and survival among HIV-infected persons. Jama-J Am Med Assoc. 1996;275:35–6.
25. Lopes M, Olfson M, Rabkin J, Hasin DS, Alegria AA, Lin KH, et al. Gender, HIV status, and psychiatric disorders: Results from the National Epidemiologic Survey on Alcohol and Related Conditions. J Clin Psychiatry. 2012;73:384–91.
26. Schuster R, Bornovalova M, Hunt E. The influence of depression on the progression of HIV: direct and indirect effects. Behav Modif. 2012;36:123–45.
27. Harvey BH, Meyer CL, Gallichio VS, Manji HK. Lithium salts in AIDS and AIDS-related dementia. Psychopharmacol Bull. 2002;36:5–26.
28. Leonard BE. The concept of depression as a dysfunction of the immune system. Curr Immunol Rev. 2010;6:205–12.
29. Weinstock M. Intrauterine factors as determinants of depressive disorder. Isr J Psychiatr Rel. 2010;47:36–45.
30. Loftis JM, Huckans M, Morasco BJ. Neuroimmune mechanisms of cytokine-induced depression: current theories and novel treatment strategies. Neurobiol Dis. 2010;37:519–33.
31. Khairova RA, Machado-Vieira R, Du J, Manji HK. A potential role for pro-inflammatory cytokines in regulating synaptic plasticity in major depressive disorder. Int J Neuropsychopharmacol. 2009;12:561–78.
32. Krishnadas R, Cavanagh J. Depression: an inflammatory illness? J Neurol Neurosurg Psychiatry. 2012;83:495–502.

33. Capuron L, Ravaud A, Dantzer R. Early Depressive Symptoms in Cancer Patients Receiving Interleukin 2 and/or Interferon Alfa-2b Therapy. J Clin Oncol. 2000;18:2143–51.
34. Capuron L, Ravaud A, Miller AH, Dantzer R. Baseline mood and psychosocial characteristics of patients developing depressive symptoms during interleukin-2 and/or interferon-alpha cancer therapy. Brain Behav Immun. 2004;18:205–13.
35. Sotelo JL, Musselman D, Nemeroff C. The biology of depression in cancer and the relationship between depression and cancer progression. Int Rev Psychiatry. 2014;26:16–30.
36. Del Guerra FB, Fonseca JL, Figueiredo VM, Ziff EB, Konkiewitz EC. Human immunodeficiency virus-associated depression: contributions of immuno-inflammatory, monoaminergic, neurodegenerative, and neurotrophic pathways. J Neurovirol. 2013;19:314–27.
37. Crum NF, Riffenburgh RH, Wegner S, Agan BK, Tasker SA, Spooner KM, et al. Comparisons of causes of death and mortality rates among HIV-infected persons: Analysis of the pre-, early, and late HAART (highly active antiretroviral therapy) eras. Jaids-J Acq Imm Def. 2006;41:194–200.
38. Lima VD, Harrigan R, Bangsberg DR, Hogg RS, Gross R, Yip B, et al. The combined effect of modern highly active antiretroviral therapy regimens and adherence on mortality over time. J Acquir Immune Defic Syndr. 2009;50:529–36.
39. Bhaskaran K, Hamouda O, Sannes M, Boufassa F, Johnson AM, Lambert PC, et al. Changes in the risk of death after HIV seroconversion compared with mortality in the general population. JAMA. 2008;300:51–9.
40. Bae JW, Guyer W, Grimm K, Altice FL. Medication persistence in the treatment of HIV infection: a review of the literature and implications for future clinical care and research. AIDS. 2011;25:279–90.
41. de Bruin M, Hospers HJ, van Breukelen GJ, Kok G, Koevoets WM, Prins JM. Electronic monitoring-based counseling to enhance adherence among HIV-infected patients: a randomized controlled trial. Health Psychol. 2010;29:421–8.
42. Angelino AF, Treisman GJ. Issues in co-morbid severe mental illnesses in HIV infected individuals. Int Rev Psychiatry. 2008;20:95–101.
43. Treisman GJ, Angelino AF, Hutton HE. Psychiatric issues in the management of patients with HIV infection. JAMA. 2001;286:2857–64.
44. Paterson DL, Swindells S, Mohr J, Brester M, Vergis EN, Squier C, et al. Adherence to protease inhibitor therapy and outcomes in patients with HIV infection. Ann Intern Med. 2000;133:21–30.
45. Nachega JB, Hislop M, Dowdy DW, Chaisson RE, Regensberg L, Maartens G. Adherence to nonnucleoside reverse transcriptase inhibitor-based HIV therapy and virologic outcomes. Ann Intern Med. 2007;146:564–73.
46. Mannheimer S, Friedland G, Matts J, Child C, Chesney M. The consistency of adherence to antiretroviral therapy predicts biologic outcomes for human immunodeficiency virus-infected persons in clinical trials. Clin Infect Dis. 2002;34:1115–21.
47. Nieuwkerk PT, Oort FJ. Self-reported adherence to antiretroviral therapy for HIV-1 infection and virologic treatment response: A meta-analysis. J Acquir Immune Defic Syndr. 2005;38:445–8.
48. Gonzalez JS, Batchelder AW, Psaros C, Safren SA. Depression and HIV/AIDS treatment nonadherence: a review and meta-analysis. J Acquir Immune Defic Syndr. 2011;58:181–7.
49. Marcus EN. The silent epidemic: The health effects of illiteracy. N Engl J Med. 2006;355:339–41.
50. Chesney MA. The elusive gold standard. Future perspectives for HIV adherence assessment and intervention. J Acquir Immune Defic Syndr. 2006;43 Suppl 1:S149–155.
51. Schneider J, Kaplan SH, Greenfield S, Li W, Wilson IB. Better physician-patient relationships are associated with higher reported adherence to antiretroviral therapy in patients with HIV infection. J Gen Intern Med. 2004;19:1096–103.
52. Nierenberg AA. Long-term management of chronic depression. J Clin Psychiatry. 2001;62 Suppl 6:17–21.
53. Warner CH, Bobo W, Warner C, Reid S, Rachal J. Antidepressant discontinuation syndrome. Am Fam Physician. 2006;74:449–56.
54. Akerblad AC, Bengtsson F, Holgersson M, von Knorring L, Ekselius L. Identification of primary care patients at risk of nonadherence to antidepressant treatment. Patient Prefer Adherence. 2008;2:379–86.
55. Chandler G, Himelhoch S, Moore RD. Substance abuse and psychiatric disorders in HIV-positive patients: Epidemiology and impact on antiretroviral therapy. Drugs. 2006;66(6):769–89.
56. Rabkin JG. HIV and depression: 2008 review and update. Curr HIV/AIDS Rep. 2008;5:163–71.
57. Harvey BH. The neurobiology and pharmacology of depression. A comparative overview of serotonin selective antidepressants. S Afr Med J. 1997;87:540–50. 552.
58. Borda E, Sterin-Borda L, Vernava D, Rodriquez M, Perez-Bianco R, De Bracco MME. Parasympathomimetic activity of sera from HIV-infected hemophilic patients with or without diarrhea. Immunol Infect Dis. 1993;3:321–6.
59. de Bracco MM, Borda E, Galassi N, Perez-Bianco R, Sterin-Borda L. Autoantibodies in HIV-infected patients that modulate the cholinergic activity of heart and gut tissue. Autoimmunity. 1993;14:307–14.
60. Sales ME, Sterin-Borda L, Bracco MME, Rodriguez M, Narbaitz M, Borda E. IgA from HIV+ haemophilic patients triggers intracellular signals coupled to the cholinergic system of the intestine. Clin Exp Immunol. 1997;110:189–95.
61. Harvey BH, McEwen BS, Stein DJ. Neurobiology of antidepressant withdrawal: implications for the longitudinal outcome of depression. Biol Psychiatry. 2003;54:1105–17.
62. Furey ML, Khanna A, Hoffman EM, Drevets WC. Scopolamine produces larger antidepressant and antianxiety effects in women than in men. Neuropsychopharmacology. 2010;35:2479–88.
63. Mineur YS, Obayemi A, Wigestrand MB, Fote GM, Calarco CA, Li AM, et al. Cholinergic signaling in the hippocampus regulates social stress resilience and anxiety- and depression-like behavior. Proc Natl Acad Sci U S A. 2013;110:3573–8.
64. Carrico AW, Antoni MH, Duran RE, Ironson G, Penedo F, Fletcher MA, et al. Reductions in depressed mood and denial coping during cognitive behavioral stress management with HIV-positive gay men treated with HAART. Ann Behav Med. 2006;31:155–64.
65. Cooperman NA, Simoni JM. Suicidal ideation and attempted suicide among women living with HIV/AIDS. J Behav Med. 2005;28:149–56.
66. Haller DL, Miles DR. Suicidal ideation among psychiatric patients with HIV: Psychiatric morbidity and quality of life. AIDS Behav. 2003;7:101–8.
67. Thompson A, Silverman B, Dzeng L, Treisman G. Psychotropic medications and HIV. Clin Infect Dis. 2006;42:1305–10.
68. Freudenreich O, Goforth HW, Cozza KL, Mimiaga MJ, Safren SA, Bachmann G, et al. Psychiatric treatment of persons with HIV/AIDS: An HIV-psychiatry consensus survey of current practices. Psychosomatics. 2010;51:480–8.
69. Relf MV, Eisbach S, Okine KN, Ward T. Evidence-based clinical practice guidelines for managing depression in persons living with HIV. J Assoc Nurses AIDS Care. 2013;24:S15–28.
70. Caballero J, Nahata MC. Use of selective serotonin-reuptake inhibitors in the treatment of depression in adults with HIV. Ann Pharmacother. 2005;39:141–5.
71. Elliott AJ, Uldall KK, Bergam K, Russo J, Claypoole K, Roy-Byrne PP. Randomized, placebo-controlled trial of paroxetine versus imipramine in depressed HIV-positive outpatients. Am J Psychiatry. 1998;155:367–72.
72. Treisman G, Fishman M, Lyketsos C, McHugh PR. Evaluation and treatment of psychiatric disorders associated with HIV infection. Res Publ Assoc Res Nerv Ment Dis. 1994;72:239–50.
73. Yanofski J, Croarkin P. Choosing antidepressants for HIV and AIDS patients: Insights on safety and side effects. Psychiatry (Edgmont). 2008;5:61–6.
74. Dabaghzadeh F, Ghaeli P, Khalili H, Alimadadi A, Jafari S, Akhondzadeh S, et al. Cyproheptadine for prevention of neuropsychiatric adverse effects of efavirenz: a randomized clinical trial. AIDS Patient Care STDS. 2013;27:146–54.
75. Harvey BH, Slabbert FN. New insights on the antidepressant discontinuation syndrome. Hum Psychopharmacol. 2014, in press.
76. Asch SM, Kilbourne AM, Gifford AL, Burnam MA, Turner B, Shapiro MF, et al. Underdiagnosis of depression in HIV: Who are we missing? J Gen Intern Med. 2003;18:450–60.
77. Pyne JM, Asch SM, Lincourt K, Kilbourne AM, Bowman C, Atkinson H, et al. Quality indicators for depression care in HIV patients. AIDS Care. 2008;20:1075–83.
78. Demyttenaere K. Compliance during treatment with antidepressants. J Affect Disord. 1997;43:27–39.
79. Cook JA, Grey D, Burke J, Cohen MH, Gurtman AC, Richardson JL, et al. Depressive symptoms and AIDS-related mortality among a multisite cohort of HIV-positive women. Am J Public Health. 2004;94:1133–40.
80. McKnight-Eily LR, Presley-Cantrell L, Elam-Evans LD, Chapman DP, Kaslow NJ, Perry GS. Prevalence and correlates of current depressive symptomatology and lifetime diagnosis of depression in black women. Womens Health Issues. 2009;19:243–52.

81. Weissman MM, Bland RC, Canino GJ, Faravelli C, Greenwald S, Hwu HG, et al. Cross-national epidemiology of major depression and bipolar disorder. JAMA. 1996;276:293–9.
82. McHenry J, Carrier N, Hull E, Kabbaj M. Sex differences in anxiety and depression: role of testosterone. Front Neuroendocrinol. 2014;35:42–57.
83. Zarrouf FA, Artz S, Griffith J, Sirbu C, Kommor M. Testosterone and depression: systematic review and meta-analysis. J Psychiatr Pract. 2009;15:289–305.
84. DiBlasio CJ, Hammett J, Malcolm JB, Judge BA, Womack JH, Kincade MC, et al. Prevalence and predictive factors for the development of de novo psychiatric illness in patients receiving androgen deprivation therapy for prostate cancer. Can J Urol. 2008;15:4249–56. discussion 4256.
85. Pope HG, Cohane GH, Kanayama G, Siegel AJ, Hudson JI. Testosterone gel supplementation for men with refractory depression: A randomized, placebo-controlled trial. Am J Psychiat. 2003;160:105–11.
86. Wang C, Alexander G, Berman N, Salehian B, Davidson T, McDonald V, et al. Testosterone replacement therapy improves mood in hypogonadal men: A clinical research center study. J Clin Endocrinol Metab. 1996;81:3578–83.
87. Miller KK, Perlis RH, Papakostas GI, Mischoulon D, Losifescu DV, Brick DJ, et al. Low-dose transdermal testosterone augmentation therapy improves depression severity in women. CNS Spectr. 2009;14:688–94.
88. Shifren JL, Braunstein GD, Simon JA, Casson PR, Buster JE, Redmond GP, et al. Transdermal testosterone treatment in women with impaired sexual function after oophorectomy. N Engl J Med. 2000;343:682–8.
89. World Health Organization: ICD-10 Version: 2010. [http://www.who.int/classifications/icd/icdonlineversions/en/]
90. Serna MC, Cruz I, Real J, Gasco E, Galvan L. Duration and adherence of antidepressant treatment (2003 to 2007) based on prescription database. Eur Psychiatry. 2010;25:206–13.
91. Cramer JA, Benedict A, Muszbek N, Keskinaslan A, Khan ZM. The significance of compliance and persistence in the treatment of diabetes, hypertension and dyslipidaemia: A review. Int J Clin Pract. 2008;62:76–87.
92. Weiden PJ, Kozma C, Grogg A, Locklear J. Partial compliance and risk of rehospitalization among California Medicaid patients with schizophrenia. Psychiatr Serv. 2004;55:886–91.
93. Medic G, Higashi K, Littlewood KJ, Diez T, Granstrom O, Kahn RS. Dosing frequency and adherence in chronic psychiatric disease: systematic review and meta-analysis. Neuropsychiatr Dis Treat. 2013;9:119–31.
94. Prukkanone B, Vos T, Burgess P, Chaiyakunapruk N, Bertram M. Adherence to antidepressant therapy for major depressive patients in a psychiatric hospital in Thailand. BMC Psychiatry. 2010;10:64.
95. Zhao B, Wong EC, Palaniappan L. Estimating patient adherence to medication with electronic health records data and pharmacy claims combined. SAS Global Forum 2013. [http://support.sas.com/resources/papers/proceedings13/167-2013.pdf]
96. Steiner JF, Prochazka AV. The assessment of refill compliance using pharmacy records: methods, validity, and applications. J Clin Epidemiol. 1997;50:105–16.
97. Steyn, HS. Manual for the determination of effect size indices and practical significance. Potchefstroom, North-West University. http://www.nwu.ac.za/content/statcs-effect-size. Date of access: 25 Sep. 2012.
98. SAS Institute Inc., 2002-2010. SAS for Windows 9.3 Cary, NC.
99. Lumley T, Diehr P, Emerson S, Chen L. The importance of the normality assumption in large public health data sets. Annu Rev Public Health. 2002;23:151–69.

Permissions

All chapters in this book were first published in AIDS R&T, by BioMed Central; hereby published with permission under the Creative Commons Attribution License or equivalent. Every chapter published in this book has been scrutinized by our experts. Their significance has been extensively debated. The topics covered herein carry significant findings which will fuel the growth of the discipline. They may even be implemented as practical applications or may be referred to as a beginning point for another development.

The contributors of this book come from diverse backgrounds, making this book a truly international effort. This book will bring forth new frontiers with its revolutionizing research information and detailed analysis of the nascent developments around the world.

We would like to thank all the contributing authors for lending their expertise to make the book truly unique. They have played a crucial role in the development of this book. Without their invaluable contributions this book wouldn't have been possible. They have made vital efforts to compile up to date information on the varied aspects of this subject to make this book a valuable addition to the collection of many professionals and students.

This book was conceptualized with the vision of imparting up-to-date information and advanced data in this field. To ensure the same, a matchless editorial board was set up. Every individual on the board went through rigorous rounds of assessment to prove their worth. After which they invested a large part of their time researching and compiling the most relevant data for our readers.

The editorial board has been involved in producing this book since its inception. They have spent rigorous hours researching and exploring the diverse topics which have resulted in the successful publishing of this book. They have passed on their knowledge of decades through this book. To expedite this challenging task, the publisher supported the team at every step. A small team of assistant editors was also appointed to further simplify the editing procedure and attain best results for the readers.

Apart from the editorial board, the designing team has also invested a significant amount of their time in understanding the subject and creating the most relevant covers. They scrutinized every image to scout for the most suitable representation of the subject and create an appropriate cover for the book.

The publishing team has been an ardent support to the editorial, designing and production team. Their endless efforts to recruit the best for this project, has resulted in the accomplishment of this book. They are a veteran in the field of academics and their pool of knowledge is as vast as their experience in printing. Their expertise and guidance has proved useful at every step. Their uncompromising quality standards have made this book an exceptional effort. Their encouragement from time to time has been an inspiration for everyone.

The publisher and the editorial board hope that this book will prove to be a valuable piece of knowledge for researchers, students, practitioners and scholars across the globe.

List of Contributors

Avina Sarna
Population Council, 142 Golf Links, New Delhi 110048, India

Stanley Luchters, Matthew Chersich and Marleen Temerman
International Centre for Reproductive Health, Department of Obstetrics and Gynaecology, Ghent University, Ghent, Belgium

Melissa Pickett
UCLA Center for Health Policy Research, Los Angeles, USA

Matthew Chersich
Centre for Health Policy, School of Public Health, Faculty of Health Sciences, University of the Witwatersrand, Johannesburg, South Africa

Jerry Okal and Scott Geibel
Population Council, Nairobi, Kenya

Nzioki Kingola
International Centre of Reproductive Health, Mombasa, Kenya

Amin S Hassan, Helen M Nabwera, Shalton M Mwaringa, Eduard J Sanders and James A Berkley
KEMRI/Wellcome Trust Research Programme, Kilifi, Kenya

Clare A Obonyo
Kilifi District Hospital, Kilifi, Kenya

Eduard J Sanders and James A Berkley
Centre for Clinical Vaccinology and Tropical Medicine, University of Oxford, Oxford, UK

Tobias F Rinke de Wit
PharmAccess Foundation, Amsterdam, Netherlands

Tobias F Rinke de Wit
Academic Medical Center, University of Amsterdam, Amsterdam, Netherlands

Patricia A Cane
Health Protection Agency, London, UK

José R Arribas
Consulta Medicina Interna 2, Hospital La Paz, IdiPAZ, Paseo de la Castellana 261, 28046, Madrid, Spain

Manuela Doroana
Serviço de Doenças Infecciosas, Hospital de Santa Maria, Av Prof Egas Moniz, 1649-035, Lisbon, Portugal

Dan Turner
Infectious Diseases Unit, Tel-Aviv Sourasky Medical Center, 6 Weizmann Street, Tel-Aviv 64239, Israels

Linos Vandekerckhove
AIDS Reference Centre, Ghent University Hospital, De Pintelaan 185, 9000, Ghent, Belgium

Adrian Streinu-Cercel
HIV/AIDS Academy, Str Dr Calistrat Grozovici, Nr 1, 021105, Bucharest, Romania

Edwin A Higuita, Maria T Rugeles and Carlos J Montoya
Immunovirology Group, School of Medicine, University of Antioquia, Medellin, Colombia

Fabián A Jaimes
Department of Internal Medicine and Academic Group of Clinical Epidemiology (GRAEPIC), School of Medicine, University of Antioquia, Medellín, Colombia

Fabián A Jaimes
Clinical Research Unit, Hospital Pablo Tobón Uribe, Medellin, Colombia

Odalis Asin-Milan, Annie Chamberland, Yi Wei, Alpha Haidara, Mohamed Sylla and Cécile L Tremblay
Centre de recherche, Centre hospitalier de l'Université de Montréal (CRCHUM), Montréal, QC, Canada

Odalis Asin-Milan, Annie Chamberland, Alpha Haidara, Mohamed Sylla and Cécile L Tremblay
Department of Microbiology and Immunology, Faculty of Medicine, Université de Montréal, Montréal, QC, Canada

Cécile L Tremblay
Laboratoire de santé publique du Québec/Institut national de santé publique du Québec (INSPQ), Québec, Canada
CRCHUM - Hôtel-Dieu, Pavillon Jeanne-Mance, bureau 7-355, 3840 rue St-Urbain, Montréal, QC H2W 1T8, Canada

Sibhatu Biadgilign
Department of Epidemiology and Biostatistics, College of Medical and Health Science, Jimma University, Jimma, Ethiopia

Ayalu A Reda
Department of Public Health, College of Health Sciences, Haramaya University, Harar, Ethiopia

Tesfaye Digaffe
Department of Medical Laboratory Science, College of Health Sciences, Harar, Ethiopia

Erica N Johnson, Mollie P Roediger, Michael L Landrum, Nancy F Crum-Cianflone, Amy C Weintrob, Anuradha Ganesan, Jason F Okulicz, Grace E Macalino and Brian K Agan
Department of Preventive Medicine and Biometrics, Infectious Disease Clinical Research Program, Uniformed Services University of the Health Sciences, Bethesda, MD, USA

Erica N Johnson, Michael L Landrum and Jason F Okulicz
Infectious Disease Service, San Antonio Military Medical Center, San Antonio, TX, USA

Mollie P Roediger
Biostatistics Division, University of Minnesota, Minnesota, MN, USA

Nancy F Crum-Cianflone
Naval Health Research Center, San Diego, CA, USA

Amy C Weintrob and Anuradha Ganesan
Infectious Disease Clinic, Walter Reed National Military Medical Center, Bethesda, MD, USA

Maurice Musheke and Virginia Bond
Zambia AIDS-related TB Research Project, University of Zambia, Lusaka, Zambia

Maurice Musheke and Sonja Merten
Swiss Tropical and Public Health Institute, Socinstrasse 57, Basel CH-4002, Switzerland

Maurice Musheke and Sonja Merten
University of Basel, Faculty of Science, Basel CH-4003, Switzerland

Virginia Bond
Department of Global Health and Development, London School of Hygiene and Tropical Medicine, Keppel Street, London WC1E 7HT, UK

Lillian Seu, Gabriel M Ortiz and Joseph M McCune
Division of Experimental Medicine, Department of Medicine, University of California, San Francisco, CA 94110, USA

Lillian Seu
Department of Bioengineering and Therapeutic Sciences, University of California, San Francisco, CA 94110, USA

Gabriel M Ortiz
Division of Hospital Medicine, Department of Medicine, University of California, San Francisco, CA 94110, USA

Trevor D Burt
Division of Neonatology, Department of Pediatrics, University of California, San Francisco, CA 94110, USA
Eli and Edythe Broad Center of Regeneration Medicine and Stem Cell Research, University of California, San Francisco, CA 94110, USA

Steven G Deeks and Jeffrey N Martin
Positive Health Program, Department of Medicine, University of California, San Francisco, CA 94110, USA

Jeffrey N Martin
Department of Epidemiology and Biostatistics, University of California, San Francisco, CA 94110, USA

Krittaecho Siripassorn, Weerawat Manosuthi, Aranya Pakdee, Sunanta Natprom, Anuttra Chaovavanich, Narongsak Hengphadpanadamrong, Khobchok Woratanarat and Aroon Lueangniyomkul
Department of Internal Medicine, Bamrasnaradura Infectious Diseases Institute, 126 Tiwanon Road, Nonthaburi 11000, Thailand

Kiat Ruxrungtham
Department of Medicine, Faculty of Medicine, Division of Allergy and Clinical Immunology, Chulalongkorn University, Bangkok, Thailand

Asres Berhan and Yifru Berhan
Hawassa University, Hawassa, Ethiopia

Yifru Berhan
Hawassa University College of Medicine and Health Sciences, Hawassa, Ethiopia

Claudia Beisel, Martin Heuer, Benjamin Otto, Johannes Jochum, Stefan Schmiedel, Sandra Hertling, Olaf Degen, Stefan Lüth, Jan van Lunzen and Julian Schulze zur Wiesch
Department of Medicine, Infectious Diseases Unit, University Medical Center Hamburg-Eppendorf, Martinistr. 52, 20246 Hamburg, Germany

Nilay Patel, Aadia Rana, Alyssa Thomas, John C Barnhart, Timothy P Flanigan, Jacob J van den Berg and Philip A Chan
Alpert Medical School of Brown University, Division of Infectious Diseases, The Miriam Hospital, 1125 North Main Street, Providence, RI 02904, USA

Davide Motta, Nigritella Brianese, Emanuele Focà and Carlo Torti
Institute of Infectious and Tropical Diseases, University of Brescia, Brescia, Italy

Franco Maggiolo and Giuliana Cologni
Department of Infectious Diseases, Ospedali Riuniti, Bergamo, Italy

Massimiliano Fabbiani and Simona Di Giambenedetto
Institute of Clinical Infectious Diseases, Catholic University of Sacred Heart, vRome, Italy

Massimo Di Pietro
Infectious Diseases Clinic, Santa Maria Annunziata Hospital, Florence, Italy

Nicoletta Ladisa
Clinic of Infectious Diseases, Policlinico di Bari, Bari, Italy

Laura Sighinolfi
Department of Infectious Diseases, S. Anna Hospital, Ferrara, Italy

Silvia Costarelli
Department of Infectious Diseases, Istituti Ospitalieri, Cremona, Italy

Paola Nasta and Filippo Castelnuovo
Spedali Civili di Brescia, Brescia, Italy

Carlo Torti
Unit of Infectious Diseases, University "Magna Graecia", Catanzaro, Italy

Rong Chu, Edward J Mills, Joseph Beyene, Eleanor Pullenayegum, P J Devereaux and Lehana Thabane
Department of Clinical Epidemiology and Biostatistics, McMaster University, Hamilton, Canada

Rong Chu, Eleanor Pullenayegum and Lehana Thabane
Biostatistics Unit, 3rd Floor Martha, Room H325, St Joseph's Healthcare Hamilton, 50 Charlton Avenue East, Hamilton, ON L8N 4A6, Canada

Edward J Mills
Faculty of Health Sciences, University of Ottawa, Ottawa, Canada

Celestin Bakanda
The AIDS Support Organization (TASO), Kampala, Uganda

Jean B Nachega
Department of Medicine and Centre for Infectious Diseases, Stellenbosch University, Cape Town, South Africa
Departments of Epidemiology and International Health, Johns Hopkins Bloomberg School of Public Health, Baltimore, MD, USA

P J Devereaux
Hamilton Health Sciences, Population Health Research Institute, Hamilton, Canada

Agete Tadewos
Referral hospital laboratory, Hawassa University College of Medicine and Health Science, Hawassa, Southern Ethiopia

Zelalem Addis
School of Biomedical and Laboratory Sciences, University of Gondar College of Medicine and Health Science, Gondar, Ethiopia

Henock Ambachew
Department of Medical laboratory Technology, Hawassa University College of Medicine and Health Science, Hawassa, Southern Ethiopia

Sandip Banerjee
Department of Animal and Range, Hawassa University College of Agriculture Sciences, Hawassa, Southern Ethiopia

Zvenyika AR Gomo
Department of Chemical Pathology, College of Health Sciences, University of Zimbabwe, Avondale, Harare, Zimbabwe

James G Hakim and Andrew Reid
Department of Medicine, College of Health Sciences, University of Zimbabwe, Avondale, Harare, Zimbabwe

Sarah A Walker and Diana M Gibb
MRC Clinical Trials Unit, London, UK

Willard Tinago and Gibson Mandozana
Department of Community Medicine, University of Zimbabwe, Harare, Zimbabwe

Cissy Kityo
Joint Clinical Research Centre, Kampala, Uganda

Paula Munderi
MRC Programme on AIDS/Uganda Virus Research Institute, Entebbe, Uganda

Elly Katabira
Infectious Disease Institute, Mulago Hospital, Kampala, Uganda

Charles F Gilks
Imperial College, London, UK

Amos K Laar
Department of Population, Family, and Reproductive Health, School of Public Health, University of Ghana, Accra, Ghana

Debra A DeBruin
Center for Bioethics, University of Minnesota, Minneapolis, USA

Susan Craddock
Department of Gender, Women, and Sexuality Studies, University of Minnesota, Minneapolis, USA

Kirsten A Donald
Division of Developmental Pediatrics, Department of Pediatrics and Child Health, University of Cape Town and Red Cross War Memorial Children's Hospital, Cape Town, South Africa

Kathleen G Walker and Jo M Wilmshurst
Division of Pediatric Neurology, Department of Pediatrics and Child Health, University of Cape Town and Red Cross War Memorial Children's Hospital, Cape Town, South Africa

Tracy Kilborn
Department of Pediatric Radiology, Red Cross War Memorial Children's Hospital, Cape Town, South Africa

Henri Carrara
Department of Public Health and Family Medicine, University of Cape Town, Cape Town, South Africa

Nelleke G Langerak
Department of Neurosurgery, University of Cape Town, Cape Town, South Africa

Brian Eley
Division of Pediatric Infectious Diseases, Department of Pediatrics and Child Health, University of Cape Town and Red Cross War Memorial Children's Hospital, Cape Town, South Africa

David Carballo and Pierre-Fréderic Keller
Department of Cardiology, University Hospital, Geneva, Switzerland

Cécile Delhumeau and Alexandra Calmy
HIV Metabolic Clinic, University Hospital, Geneva, Switzerland

Sebastian Carballo
General Internal Medicine, University Hospital, Geneva, Switzerland

Caroline Bähler and Dragona Radovanovic
AMIS Plus Data Center, Institute of Social and Preventive Medicine, University of Zurich, Zurich, Switzerland

Olivier Clerc
Infectious Diseases, University Hospital Center, Lausanne, Switzerland

Enos Bernasconi
Infectious Diseases, Regional Hospital, Lugano, Switzerland

Dominique Fasel
HIV Unit, Infectious diseases, University Hospital, Basel, Switzerland

Patrick Schmid
Infectious Diseases, University Hospital, Sankt Gallen, Switzerland

Alexia Cusini
Infectious Diseases, University Hospital, Bern, Switzerland

Jan Fehr and Bruno Ledergerber
Division of Infectious Diseases and Hospital Epidemiology, University Hospital, Zürich, University of Zurich, Zürich, Switzerland

Paul Erne
Cardiology Department, Peripherique Hospital, Lucern, Switzerland

Pierre-Fréderic Keller
Centre médical Ziggurat, Rue du Jura 11, 2900 Porrentruy, Switzerland

Margaret Ngwono Oluka, Faith Apolot Okalebo and Anastasia Nkatha Guantai
Department of Pharmacology and Pharmacognosy, University of Nairobi, Nairobi 00202, Kenya

R Scott McClelland and Susan M Graham
Departments of Medicine, Global Health, and Epidemiology, University of Washington, Seattle, USA and Institute of Tropical and Infectious Diseases, University of Nairobi, Nairobi, Kenya

Yuncong Wang
Beijing Center for Diseases Prevention and Control, Beijing, China

Yuncong Wang, Hui Xing, Lingjie Liao, Quanbi Zhao, Yi Feng, Pengfei Ma, Yuhua Ruan and Yiming Shao
State Key Laboratory for Infectious Disease Prevention and Control, National Center for AIDS/STD Control and Prevention, Chinese Center for Disease Control and Prevention, Collaborative Innovation Center for Diagnosis and Treatment of Infectious Diseases, Beijing, China

Zhe Wang and Jia Liu
Henan Center for Disease Control and Prevention, Zhengzhou, China

Bin Su and Jianjun Wu
Anhui Center for Disease Control and Prevention, Hefei, China

Immaculate L Nankya, Denis M Tebit, Awet Abraha, Fred Kyeyune, Richard Gibson, Oyebisi Jegede, Gabrielle Nickel and Eric J Arts
Division of Infectious Diseases, Department of Medicine, Case Western Reserve University, 10900 Euclid Ave., Cleveland, OH 44106, USA

Immaculate L Nankya, Fred Kyeyune and Eric J Arts
Virology Program, Department of Molecular Biology and Microbiology, Case Western Reserve University, Cleveland, OH, USA

Immaculate L Nankya and Fred Kyeyune
Joint Clinical Research Centre, Kampala, Uganda

Denis M Tebit
Myles Thaler Center for AIDS and Human Retrovirus Research, Department of Microbiology, Immunology and Cancer Biology, University of Virginia, Charlottesville, VA, USA

Oyebisi Jegede
Laboratory of Virology and Infectious Disease, Rockefeller University, New York, USA

Francois N Slabbert and Martie S Lubbe
Medicines Usage Group (MUSA), North-West University, Potchefstroom 2520, South Africa

Christiaan B Brink
Division of Pharmacology, North-West University, Potchefstroom 2520, South Africa

Brian H Harvey
Centre of Excellence for Pharmaceutical Sciences, School of Pharmacy, North-West University, Potchefstroom 2520, South Africa

Index

www.ingramcontent.com/pod-product-compliance
Lightning Source LLC
LaVergne TN
LVHW080919210926
848485LV00004B/687